Ocular Disease: Mechanisms and Management

Ocular Disease: Mechanisms and Management

Editor: Abigail Gipe

AMERICAN
MEDICAL PUBLISHERS
www.americanmedicalpublishers.com

AMERICAN
MEDICAL PUBLISHERS
www.americanmedicalpublishers.com

Cataloging-in-Publication Data

Ocular disease : mechanisms and management / edited by Abigail Gipe.
p. cm.
Includes bibliographical references and index.
ISBN 979-8-88740-348-9
1. Eye--Diseases. 2. Eye--Diseases--Treatment. 3. Vision disorders.
4. Therapeutics, Ophthalmological. 5. Ophthalmology. I. Gipe, Abigail.
RE46 .O28 2023
617.7--dc23

American Medical Publishers,
41 Flatbush Avenue,
1st Floor, New York,
NY 11217, USA

ISBN 979-8-88740-348-9 (Hardback)

Contents

Preface

The diseases or disorders that affect the human eye are called ocular diseases. The branch of medicine that specializes in the diagnosis and treatment of eye diseases is referred to as ophthalmology. The most common types of ocular diseases include cataract, glaucoma, uveitis, eye tumors, diabetic retinopathy, strabismus, etc. Infection, allergy, vitamin deficiency, chemical irritants, genetics, smoking etc. are some of the prominent causes of eye diseases. The examination and management of ocular diseases involve the use of diagnostic methods such as ocular tonometry to determine intraocular pressure, refraction assessment, visual acuity, etc. Optical coherence tomography (OCT) is a specialized test used to access ocular structures. OCT scans are used to examine the efficacy of managing diabetic retinopathy, age-related macular degeneration, and glaucoma. Some other tools to examine the eye and help in the diagnosis include retinal topography and fluorescein angiography. The topics covered in this extensive book deal with the mechanisms and management of ocular diseases and ophthalmology. It will prove to be immensely beneficial to students and researchers in the field of ophthalmology.

The information shared in this book is based on empirical researches made by veterans in this field of study. The elaborative information provided in this book will help the readers further their scope of knowledge leading to advancements in this field.

Finally, I would like to thank my fellow researchers who gave constructive feedback and my family members who supported me at every step of my research.

Editor

1

Genotype-Phenotype Analysis and Mutation Spectrum in a Cohort of Chinese Patients with Congenital Nystagmus

Xiao-Fang Wang [1†], Hui Chen [1†], Peng-Juan Huang [1], Zhuo-Kun Feng [1], Zi-Qi Hua [1], Xiang Feng [1], Fang Han [2], Xiao-Tao Xu [1], Ren-Juan Shen [2], Yang Li [2], Zi-Bing Jin [1,2] and Huan-Yun Yu [1*]*

[1] *School of Ophthalmology and Optometry, The Eye Hospital, Wenzhou Medical University, Wenzhou, China,* [2] *Beijing Ophthalmology and Visual Sciences Key Laboratory, Beijing Institute of Ophthalmology, Beijing Tongren Eye Center, Beijing Tongren Hospital, Capital Medical University, Beijing, China*

***Correspondence:**
Huan-Yun Yu
huanyunyu@126.com
Zi-Bing Jin
jinzibing@foxmail.com

† These authors have contributed equally to this work

Purpose: Congenital nystagmus (CN) is a genetically and clinically heterogeneous ocular disorder that manifests as involuntary, periodic oscillations of the eyes. To date, only *FRMD7* and *GPR143* have been reported to be responsible for causing CN. Here, we aimed to identify the disease-causing mutations and describe the clinical features in the affected members in our study.

Methods: All the subjects underwent a detailed ophthalmic examination. Direct sequencing of all coding exons and splice site regions in *FRMD7* and *GPR143* and a mutation assessment were performed in each patient.

Results: We found 14 mutations in 14/37 (37.8%) probands, including nine mutations in the *FRMD7* gene and five mutations in the *GPR143* gene, seven of which are novel, including c.284G>A(R95K), c.964C>T(P322S), c.284+10T>G, c.901T>C (Y301H), and c.2014_2023delTCACCCATGG(S672Pfs*12) in *FRMD7*, and c.250+1G>C, and c.485G>A (W162*) in *GPR143*. The mutation detection rate was 87.5% (7/8) of familial vs. 24.1% (7/29) of sporadic cases. Ten mutations in 24 (41.7%) non-syndromic subjects and 4 mutations in 13(30.8%) syndromic subjects were detected. A total of 77.8% (7/9) of mutations in *FRMD7* were concentrated within the FERM and FA domains, while all mutations in *GPR143* were located in exons 1, 2, 4 and 6. We observed that visual acuity tended to be worse in the *GPR143* group than in the *FRMD7* group, and no obvious difference in other clinical manifestations was found through comparisons in different groups of patients.

Conclusions: This study identified 14 mutations (seven novel and seven known) in eight familial and 29 sporadic patients with congenital nystagmus, expanding the mutational spectrum and validating *FRMD7* and *GPR143* as mutation hotspots. These findings also revealed a significant difference in the screening rate between different groups of participants, providing new insights for the strategy of genetic screening and early clinical diagnosis of CN.

Keywords: congenital nystagmus, *FRMD7*, *GPR143*, mutation, genotype-phenotype

INTRODUCTION

Nystagmus is an involuntary, periodic oscillation of unilateral or bilateral eyes. It can be classified into congenital nystagmus (CN) and acquired nystagmus according to the age at onset. The prevalence of nystagmus in the general population has been estimated to be 24/10,000 of the population, and CN is the most common type of all forms of nystagmus (Sarvananthan et al., 2009; Watkins et al., 2012). CN usually appears at birth or in early childhood, and is predominantly characterized by horizontal pendular or jerk nystagmus with various degrees of visual impairment. Abnormal head position (AHP) that is often linked to an eccentric horizontal null position can be observed in patients with CN (Watkins et al., 2012; Brodsky and Dell'Osso, 2014; Papageorgiou et al., 2014; Richards and Wong, 2015). Previous studies have demonstrated that CN may occur as an isolated trait or may be accompanied by other ocular abnormalities such as ocular albinism, strabismus, aniridia, achromatopsia, congenital cataract, Leber congenital amaurosis, retinitis pigmentosa, cone-rod dystrophy and optic nerve hypoplasia (Sarvananthan et al., 2009; Brodsky and Dell'Osso, 2014; Richards and Wong, 2015). At present, although there have been a large number of studies focusing on CN over the past years, the mechanisms of pathogenesis remain unclear. A review in 2015 concluded two main hypotheses to explain this phenotype: dysfunction in the ocular motor control pathways and developmental abnormalities in the anterior visual pathway (Richards and Wong, 2015). Currently, no cure is available for CN, but many treatments, including non-surgical options (prisms, contact lenses, and afferent stimulation) and surgical extraocular muscle surgery, have been reported to improve visual acuity by directly or indirectly reducing but not eliminating nystagmus (Dell'Osso, 2002; Hertle et al., 2010).

Multiple modes of inheritance of CN have been reported in the literature, and X-linked CN is the most common form of hereditary nystagmus with significant clinical and genetic heterogeneity (Forssman, 1971). To date, only *FRMD7* and *GPR143* are considered the major disease-causing genes for CN. However, a recent study found that mutations within the C-terminal region of CASK disrupt the interaction, which is crucial for correct development of oculomotor control between *FRMD7* and CASK, leading to nystagmus (Schnur et al., 1998; Watkins et al., 2013). Mutations were first identified in the *FRMD7* (Xq26-27) gene in both X-linked and sporadic CN cases in 2006 (Tarpey et al., 2006). Since then, more than 90 mutations in the *FRMD7* gene have been reported to date. G-protein coupled receptor 143 (*GPR143*), also known as OA1, was primarily described to cause ocular albinism with nystagmus as a prominent concomitant symptom. Pigmentation loss in the iris and retina is usually not obvious in Asian individuals, therefore, nystagmus may be the main manifestation in patients with *GPR143* mutations (Zhou et al., 2008). Currently, over 100 mutations in *GPR143* have been collected in the HGMD (Human Gene Mutation Database) (http://www.hgmd.cf.ac.uk). The mutation detection rate was found to be 20–57% and 62.5–95% in *FRMD7* and *GPR143*, respectively, in X-linked cases, and much higher than the rates in sporadic cases. The genetic causes of sporadic cases are still poorly understood (Richards and Wong, 2015; Jia et al., 2017a).

In our study, *FRMD7* and *GPR143* mutation analysis and detailed clinical characteristics evaluation were performed in a group of Chinese patients with CN. A total of 9 mutations in the *FRMD7* gene and five mutations in the *GPR143* gene were identified in this study, including 7 novel and 7 previously reported mutations.

METHODS

Patient Enrolment and Clinical Evaluation

This study was in compliance with the Declaration of Helsinki and was approved by the Institutional Review Board. Informed written consent was obtained from all participants. All participants were enrolled from The Affiliated Eye Hospital of Wenzhou Medical University in this study. The average age was 12 ± 10 years, ranging between 1 year and 46 years old. After a detailed ophthalmic examination including visual acuity, intraocular pressure measurement, a slit-lamp examination, fundus photography, OCT and other specialist review. All the patients were diagnosed with congenital nystagmus by a specialist. Among these participants, 24 were non-syndromic CN cases, 13 were syndromic CN cases (11 cases with strabismus, four cases with ocular albinism, and two patients suffered from both strabismus and ocular albinism).

DNA Extraction

Dna was extracted from each participant's peripheral blood using a DNA extraction kit (TIANGEN, Beijing, China) following the manufacturer's instructions. Nanodrop 2000 (Thermal Fisher Scientific, Delaware, USA) was used to determine the concentration and purity of the extracted DNA.

Mutation Screening

The primers of all coding exons and splice site regions in *FRMD7* and *GPR143* were obtained from previous literature (Zhang Q. et al., 2007; Hu et al., 2011). After PCR amplification and direct sequencing of the coding regions and splice site junctions in *FRMD7* and *GPR143*, we analyzed the sequencing of results. The reference genomic sequence versions of *FRMD7* and *GPR143* used were NM_194277.3 and NM_000273.3 from the GenBank database. The potential pathogenicity of the detected mutations in this study was evaluated by the following bioinformatics tools: SIFT (http://sift.jcvi.org/), Polyphen-2 (http://genetics.bwh.harvard.edu/pph2/), Mutation Taster (http://mutationtaster.org/), and PROVEAN (http://provean.jcvi.org/index.php). Allele frequency was assessed by the ExAC database (http://exac.broadinstitute.org/), and 1,000 Genomes Project (ftp://1000genomes.ebi.ac.uk/vol1/ftp). Co-segregation analysis was performed for mutations detected in our study when members in families were available.

Multiple Sequence Alignment and Molecular Structural Modeling of Missense Mutations

Protein sequences were obtained from the NCBI database (https://www.ncbi.nlm.nih.gov/), and multiple sequence alignments were performed using Clustalx1.83 software. Sequence logos were made with WebLogo3 (http://weblogo.threeplusone.com/). Schematic of protein domain structures were created using DOG 2.0 (Ren et al., 2009). The crystal structures of several wild-type and mutant proteins were predicted by Swiss Model (https://swissmodel.expasy.org/), and the predicted PDB files were visualized by PyMol software (version 2.1.1).

Statistical Analysis

We used Mann–Whitney U-tests to compare the VA of the two groups. Onset age in two groups was analyzed using a *t*-test. Fisher's exact test was used to evaluate the significance of proportions (strabismus, stereopsis, and AHP) between groups. Non-parametric Kruskal-Wallis tests and Pearson chi-square tests were used to compare multiple groups.

RESULTS

Clinical Manifestation

A total of 37 patients with CN (29 male, eight female) were recruited for this study, and the mean age of the participants was 12 ± 10 years. Pedigrees of the 8 (21.6%) families followed an X-linked pattern of inheritance, and the remaining 29 (78.4%) sporadic patients had no positive family history. Different degrees of reduced visual acuity, stereopsis, and AHP were observed among the patients: eleven of them had associated strabismus (29.7%), four of them had associated ocular albinism (10.8%), and two patients had both conditions. A total of 93.8% (30/32) of these patients presented horizontal nystagmus, indicating that horizontal nystagmus was the most common form, which is consistent with previous reports (Zhao et al., 2016).

Mutation Identified in This Study

Sanger sequencing of *FRMD7* and *GPR143* in this Chinese cohort revealed 14 different mutations (nine in *GPR143*, five in *FRMD7*) in seven unrelated families and five sporadic cases. Seven mutations are novel: c.284G>A(R95K), c.964C>T(P322S), c.901T>C(Y301H), c.2014_2023delTCACCCATGG(S672Pfs*12), and c.284+10T>G in *FRMD7* and c.250+1G>C, and c.485G>A(W162*) in *GPR143*. The remaining seven mutations have been reported before. The molecular and clinical results of the 12 participants with identified mutation are shown in **Table 1**. Mutations identified in our study were assessed for pathogenicity with four different bioinformatics tools, as shown in **Table 2**. **Figure 1** illustrates the pedigrees and the sequencing data. **Figure 2** shows the sequence conservation of the *FRMD7* protein of three novel missense mutations and the structural modeling of the novel missense mutation c.284G>A.

FRMD7 Mutations

We detected a reported missense c.782G>A mutation in exon 9 in family 1 (III1) and family 2 (III1 and II2), which causes the substitution of arginine to glutamine at position 261 (p.R261Q). Li et al. (2008) already identified R261Q in two Chinese families with CN in 2008, and the pathogenicity of this mutation is well-established. In family 2, the unaffected mother of the proband carried c.782G>A, and the results demonstrated the co-segregation of the c.782G>A mutation with CN in family 2. The known missense mutation c.781C>G in exon 9 was found in family 3 (III1), which results in the substitution of an amino acid at a highly conserved position, p.R261G, and has been reported three times in the Chinese population, indicating the high possibility that it is a Chinese-specific variant (Zhang B. et al., 2007; Song et al., 2013; Zhao et al., 2016). The novel missense

TABLE 1 | Clinical features of subjects.

Subject	Sex	Age(years)	Onset age	BCVA	Nystagmus	AHP	Accompanying symptoms	Family history	Mutation gene
S1	Male	14	1	0.6/0.7	Horizontal jerk	Y	N	N	*FRMD7*
S2	Male	15	2	0.9/0.9	Horizontal jerk	Y	N	N	*FRMD7*
S3	Male	6	1	0.5/0.5	Horizontal jerk	Y	N	N	*FRMD7*
S4	Male	10	At birth	0.6/0.4	Horizontal jerk	Y	N	N	*FRMD7*
S5	Male	17	1	0.3/0.4	Horizontal jerk	Y	Strabismus	Y	*GPR143*
S6	Male	42	2	0.1/0.2	Horizontal jerk	Y	Albinism	N	*GPR143*
S7	Male	22	NA	0.2/0.2	NA	NA	N	N	*GPR143*
F1: III:1	Male	6	1 month	1.0/1.0	Horizontal jerk	Y	N	Y	*FRMD7*
F2: III:1	Male	6	3 months	NA	NA	Y	N	Y	*FRMD7*
F3: III:1	Male	10	1	0.5/0.4	Horizontal jerk	Y	N	Y	*FRMD7*
F4: II:3	Female	33	3	0.8/0.8	NA	N	N	Y	*FRMD7*
F5: III:1	Female	23	3	0.16/0.16	Horizontal jerk	N	Strabismus	Y	*FRMD7*
F6: III:1	Male	6	1	0.1/0.1	NA	N	Albinism	Y	*GPR143*
F7: III:2	Male	7	6 months	0.1/0.1	Horizontal pendular	Y	N	Y	*GPR143*

Y, present; N, absent; NA, not available.

TABLE 2 | Overview of the mutations found in *FRMD7* and *GPR143* and their assessment.

Gene	Exon/Intron	Domain	Mutation	Protein change	Type	State	Prediction				Allele frequency		References
							Mutation taster	PROVEAN	SIFT	PolyPhen-2	1000G	EXAC	
FRMD7	9	FERM-C	782G>A	R261Q	Missense	Hemizygous	Disease causing	Deleterious	Damaging	probably damaging	0	0	Li et al., 2008
FRMD7	9	FERM-C	781C>G	R261G	Missense	Hemizygous	Disease causing	Deleterious	Damaging	probably damaging	0	0	Zhang B. et al., 2007
FRMD7	9	FERM-C	811T>A	C271S	Missense	Hemizygous	Disease causing	Deleterious	Damaging	probably damaging	0	0	Jia et al., 2017b
FRMD7	9	FA	**901T>C**	Y301H	Missense	Hemizygous	Disease causing	Deleterious	Damaging	probably damaging	0	0	This study
FRMD7	4	FERM-M	**284G>A**	R95K	Missense	Heterozygous	Disease causing	Deleterious	Damaging	probably damaging	0	0	This study
FRMD7	Intron 4	FERM-M	**284+10T>G**	-	Splice	Heterozygous	Polymorphism	-	-	-	0	16	This study
FRMD7	10	FA	**c.964C>T**	P322S	Missense	Hemizygous	Disease causing	Deleterious	Damaging	probably damaging	0	0	This study
FRMD7	12	C-terminal	**2014_2023del TCACCCATGG**	S672Pfs*12	Frameshift	Hemizygous	Disease causing	-	-	-	0	0	This study
FRMD7	12	C-terminal	c.1403G>A	R468H	Missense	Heterozygous	Polymorphism	Neutral	Damaging	possibly damaging	6	2136	Zhao et al., 2016
GPR143	Intron 1	-	**c.250+1G>C**	-	Splice	Hemizygous	Disease causing	-	-	-	0	0	This study
GPR143	2	-	c.276G>A	W92*	Non-sense	Hemizygous	Disease causing	Deleterious	-	-	0	0	Zou et al., 2017
GPR143	4	-	**c.485G>A**	W162*	Non-sense	Hemizygous	Disease causing	Deleterious	-	-	0	0	This study
GPR143	6	-	c.703G>A	E235K	Missense	Hemizygous	Disease causing	Deleterious	Damaging	probably damaging	0	0	Schnur et al., 1998
GPR143	6	-	c.733C>T	R245*	Non-sense	Hemizygous	Disease causing	Deleterious	-	-	0	0	Kim et al., 2016

*Novel mutations are highlighted in bold. * = X.*

mutation c.284G>A, leading to a replacement of arginine by lysine at position 95, was detected in a female proband in family 4. A different substitution of amino acid arginine to methionine at 95 has ever been reported by Bai et al. (2017). The substitution occurred in the highly conserved domain FERM-M, and the predicted three-dimensional structure showed a change in the mutant protein. The Arg-95 residue was predicted to locate in the alpha helix of the FERM domain, and the side chain of Arg-95 projected outwards from the alpha helix forming hydrogen bonds with the side chains of Leu-89. In the mutant protein, two hydrogen bonds disappeared between Lys-95 and Leu-89, and Lys-95 side chains formed another one hydrogen bond with the amino acid residues Glu-92 and Gly-87, respectively (**Figure 2C**). Furthermore, all four software tools predicted the p.R95K mutation to be pathogenic (**Table 2**). In family 5, the heterozygous donor splice site mutation c.284+10T>G in intron4 was identified in the female proband (III1). This variant was considered to be possibly pathogenic in this family, because the frequency was <0.01. The other two family members (III2, III3) who were unable to give a peripheral blood sample in this study also showed similar clinical signs of CN and esotropia. In sporadic cases, four mutations, c.811T>A, c.901T>C, c.964C>T, and c.2014_2023delTCACCCATGG, were found in S1, S2, S3, and S4, respectively; the latter three are first reported here. The missense mutation c.811T>A in exon 9 which caused a protein change at p.C271S, has been described before in a previous Chinese study (Jia et al., 2017b). The two novel missense variants resulted in amino acid substitutions at p.Y301H and p.P322S, and both of them occurred in the highly conserved residue of the FERM-adjacent (FA) domain. Multiple sequence alignment suggested that these sites were evolutionarily conserved from Danio to humans (**Figures 2A,B**). The 10-bp deletion mutation (c.2014_2023delTCACCCATGG) in exon 12 caused a frameshift in the ORF, leading to pre-mature translation termination of the *FRMD7* protein at position 683 (p. S672Pfs*12) (**Figure 1A**). Apart from the mutations above, the c.1403G>A mutation that changed arginine to histidine at position 468 (p.R468H) was identified in three unrelated probands [III1 in family 1, III1 in family 4 and sporadic 2 (S2)] in our study, which was predicted to be non-pathogenic by PROVEAN and Mutation Taster and damaging by SIFT and PolyPhen-2. Based on the fact that its minor allele frequency (MAF)>0.01 and all three probands harbored another disease-causing mutation, in addition to published report (Zhao et al., 2016), the c.1403G>A mutation did not appear to be the main causative mutation in the three probands.

GPR143 Mutations

We detected the known non-sense mutation c.276G>A in exon 2 in the proband (III1) and his unaffected mother (II2) in family 6, which introduced a pre-mature stop codon into the ORF and generated a truncated protein. In family 7, III2 and his asymptomatic mother had the missense mutation c.703G>A (from glutamate to lysine), which was first described in a North American family (Schnur et al., 1998). All the pedigrees in which mothers' blood samples were available are consistent with X-linked transmission. In sporadic patients, two new mutations,

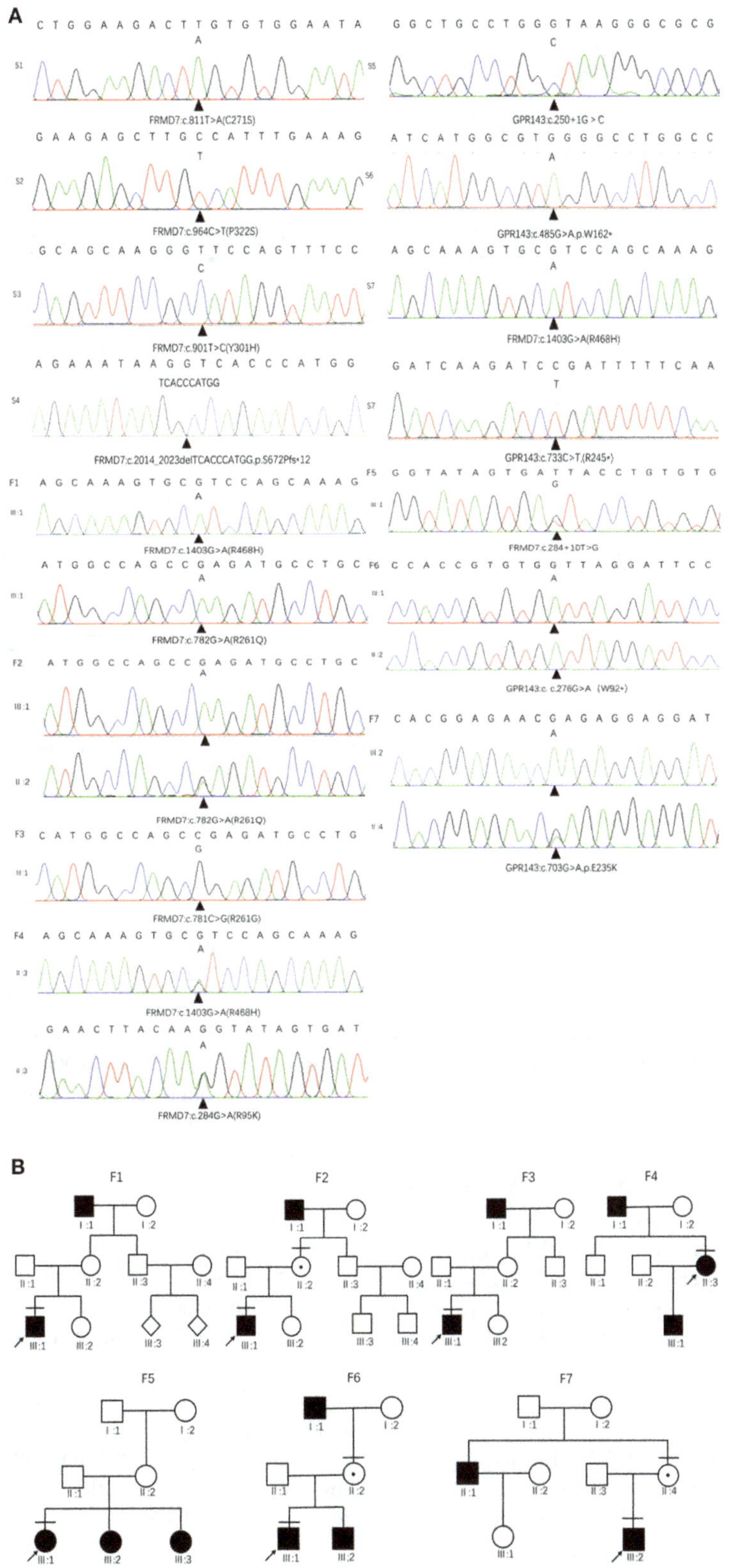

FIGURE 1 | Family pedigrees and Sanger sequencing results. **(A)** The chromatograms of sequencing results: F 1-F 7 represent family 1 to family 7, S 1-S 7 represent sporadic 1 to sporadic 7. **(B)** Pedigrees of *FRMD7* and *GPR143* mutation–positive families: F 1 Family 1; F 2, family 2; F 3, family 3; F 4, family 4; F5, family 5; F 6, family 6; F 7, family 7. Filled symbols indicate affected individuals, unfilled symbols indicate unaffected individuals, and a dotted circle indicates a heterozygous carrier. Bars over the symbols indicate subjects enrolled in this study. Arrows indicate the probands.

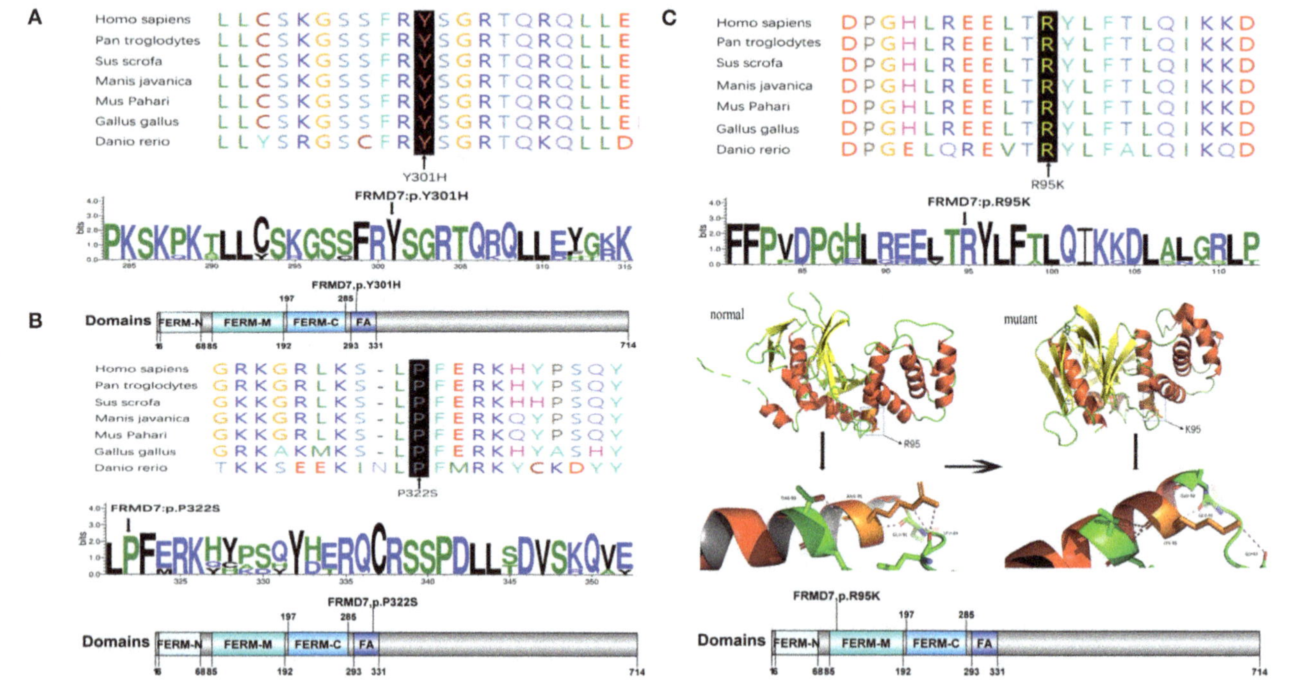

FIGURE 2 | Missense mutations identified in this study. One-dimensional and two-dimensional multiple sequence alignment of the *FRMD7* protein in different species and the predicted three-dimensional structure of the *FRMD7* protein show the high evolutionary conservation of amino acid residues. Black arrows show the location of the novel missense mutations identified in this study in the *FRMD7* protein. **(A)** The alignment of amino acids around residue p.301. **(B)** The alignment of amino acids around residue p.322. **(C)** The alignment of amino acids around residue p.95.The position of the missense mutation c.284G>A around residue p.R95K of *FRMD7* is highlighted in the 3D structure model. Hydrogen bonds between amino acids are shown as pink dashed lines. The normal protein is on the left, and the mutant protein is on the right.

a splice mutation c.250+1G>C on intron1 and a non-sense mutation c.485G>A truncating the translated protein at position 162, which were not present in the 1,000 Genomes Project or ExAC database and assessed to be pathogenic by prediction tools, were identified in S5 and S6. The known non-sense mutation c.733C>T created an early termination in the *GPR143* protein was present in S7.

Genotype-Phenotype Correlation Analysis

In our cohort of 37 participants with CN, 9 patients with *FRMD7* mutations and five patients with *GPR143* mutations were identified here. To further investigate the relationship of phenotype-to-genotype, we compared whether there was a statistical difference in terms of clinical characteristics between different groups of patients.

Onset Age

We found no significant difference ($p>0.05$) in onset age was observed between the *FRMD7* group and the *GPR143* group (*t*-test, $P = 0.2846$) or between the *FRMD7* group and the non-*FRMD7* group (*t*-test, $P = 0.4009 > 0.05$). The mean age of onset in our study was later than that in other studies.

Visual Acuity

We tested eight of nine patients (accurate visual acuity was not available for one child) in the *FRMD7* group and five patients in the *GPR143* group. The median logMAR visual acuity was −0.22 and −1.00 in these two groups of patients, respectively. The group with *GPR143* mutations had worse vision than in the group with *FRMD7* mutations (Mann–Whitney *U*-test, $P = 0.0062 < 0.05$). However, we did not see an obvious difference in patients' acuity between the *FRMD7* group and non-*FRMD7* group (Mann–Whitney *U*-test, $P = 0.5279 > 0.05$).

Strabismus

Only 1 case (11.11%) had esotropia in the *FRMD7* group. By comparison, in the *GPR143* group, one patient (20%) had exotropia, and two patients (40%) had ocular albinism (OA). No observable difference was found in the incidence of strabismus between the two groups (Fisher's exact test, $P > 0.99$). In the non-*FRMD7* group, strabismus was identified in nine of 23 (39.13%) patients (five with esotropia, four with exotropia), and no significant difference was observed between the *FRMD7* group and the non-*FRMD7* group (Fisher's exact test, $P = 0.21 > 0.05$).

Stereopsis

Seven of nine subjects were tested for stereopsis in the *FRMD7* group, and one subject (14.29%) with by esotropia demonstrated no stereopsis by the TNO and Titmus tests. In the *GPR143* group, two patients (100%) (test data were not available in the other three patients) with OA and exotropia were found to have no stereopsis in either TNO or Titmus test. In the non-*FRMD7* group, 59.09% (13/22) and 54.55% (12/22) did not have stereopsis by TNO test and Titmus test, respectively, and 61.54% (8/13) and 58.33% (7/12) of which had manifested strabismus in the TNO and Titmus tests, respectively. Fisher's exact test was performed between the *FRMD7* group and non-*FRMD7* group ($p = 0.08 > 0.05$), and statistical comparison between the *GPR143* group and *FRMD7* group was not considered due to the meager data.

Anomalous Head Posture

AHP was recorded in 7 (77.78%) patients in the *FRMD7* group compared with 3 (75%) patients in the *GPR143* group (Fisher's exact test, $P > 0.99$). Likewise, a similar proportion of AHP was achieved between the *FRMD7* group (7/9, 77.78%) and the non-*FRMD7* group (13/23, 56.52%) (Fisher's exact test, $p = 0.42 > 0.05$).

In addition to the subjects in our study, we also reviewed all samples as well as mutations in *FRMD7* reported in literature and conducted correlation analysis on patients with CN.

A total of 110 patients were recorded in the literature. We conducted two sets of analysis depending on the mutation locations and types in the patients in terms of VA, onset age, and the proportion of AHP. One-way analysis of variance (ANOVA) was performed and there were no significant differences among the FERM domain group, FA domain group, and other domain group (Kruskal-Wallis test, $p > 0.05$; Pearson chi-square test, $p > 0.05$). Similarly, we did not observe any differences among the missense group, non-sense group, deletion/insertion group, and splice group (Kruskal-Wallis test, $p > 0.05$; Pearson chi-square test, $p > 0.05$).

DISCUSSION

In this study, a total of fourteen mutations (nine mutations in the *FRMD7* gene and five mutations in the *GPR143* gene) in 37.8% (14/37) of the probands were identified. Seven of them were new mutations.

The mutation detection rate differs significantly between the familial cases (87.5%, 7/8) and the sporadic cases (24.1%, 7/29), and is higher than published studies. These data further support that *FRMD7* and *GPR143* are two major causative genes for CN. Tarpey et al. (2006) first detected mutations in 84.6% (22/26) of the familial cases and 7% (3/42) of the sporadic cases. Zhang Q. et al. (2007) detected mutations in 4 of 14 (28.5%) Chinese families with X-linked nystagmus. Self et al. (2007) identified mutations in 20% (2 of 10) of apparent X-linked families and 3.6% (1/28) singleton cases. A total of 33.3% (7/21) familial and 14.3% (4/28) of sporadic cases had mutations. In 2015, 40% (2/5) of X-linked IN families were found to have mutations, while no mutations were identified in 15 sporadic cases (AlMoallem et al., 2015). The screening rate was 38.89% (7/18) in another Chinese cohort published in 2017 (Jia et al., 2017b). Unexpectedly, 41.7% (10/24) of simple cases had mutations, comparable to 30.8% (4/13) of syndromic cases in this study. This illustrates that mutation screening is equally necessary in both X-linked cases and sporadic cases.

The *FRMD7* gene contains 12 exons and encodes a 714 amino acid protein that is composed of an N-terminal FERM domain, FERM-adjacent domain (FA), and C-terminal domain. The conserved FERM domain comprises three tightly folded clover-leaf structures (F1, F2, F3). Despite several studies, the specific functions of *FRMD7* protein are still uncertain. However, the two closest homologous proteins FARP1 and FARP2 have been found to be involved in the regulation of neural development, indicating that *FRMD7* may play a role in this process. A later study discovered that knockdown of *FRMD7* can cause abnormalities in neurite development, partially confirming the above conjecture, thus, mutations in *FRMD7* can influence neuronal functions, consequently leading to nystagmus (Betts-Henderson et al., 2010).

There are 98 mutations reported to date (Supplementary Excel 1 in **Supplementary Material**). Over half (51.02%) of the mutations are missense and are predicted to change the protein conformation, resulting in affecting the function of *FRMD7*. Non-sense, deletion/insertion, and splice mutations accounted for 6.12, 20.41, and 21.43%, respectively (**Figure 3B**). A significant number of mutations (80.6%) are primarily concentrated in the highly conserved FERM and FA domains (**Figure 3C**). In our study, 77.8% (7/9) were missense mutations, and all of them were located in the FERM and FA domains. Notably, the predicted molecular structural modeling of the c.284G>A mutation was similar with the normal protein. Lysine and arginine are both alkaline amino acids with similar molecular properties, but previous study has ever reported mutation of this locus causing nystagmus, and amino acids are well-conserved in the FERM domain, we therefore speculated that this variation of chemical bonds may affect the overall stability and functions of the protein (Bai et al., 2017). Of these 12 exons, exon 9 has been regarded as the mutational hot spot region, containing 21.4% of mutations (**Figure 3A**). Here, we found a higher proportion, with 4 (44.4%) mutations in exon 9. This indicates that alterations in this region severely affect the function of *FRMD7*. Remarkably, a new 10-bp deletion (c.2014_2023delTCACCCATGG) in exon 12 of C-terminal of *FRMD7* was detected in S4 in our study. As a whole, ten mutations have been identified in exon 12, all of which are predicted to result in severe loss of function of *FRMD7* due to the pre-mature termination of the protein. Only gross structural defects in this region may be responsible for the nystagmus phenotype. Therefore, we speculate that the specific biological function of this region may not be as important as the FERM and FA domains. In addition, we also noticed that c.781C>G and c.782G>A were most frequently reported in the Chinese population, and have not been found in other populations to date. c.782G>A were observed twice in 2 male probands of two unrelated families in our patients. The above findings to some extent suggest that these mutations are unique to Chinese people.

The *GPR143* gene consists of 9 exons and encodes the G protein-coupled receptor 143 that is present on the membrane of melanosomes in pigment cells. Recent research has proven that *GPR143* expression can be detected during the earliest stage of melanosome formation in the RPE. Mutations in *GPR143*

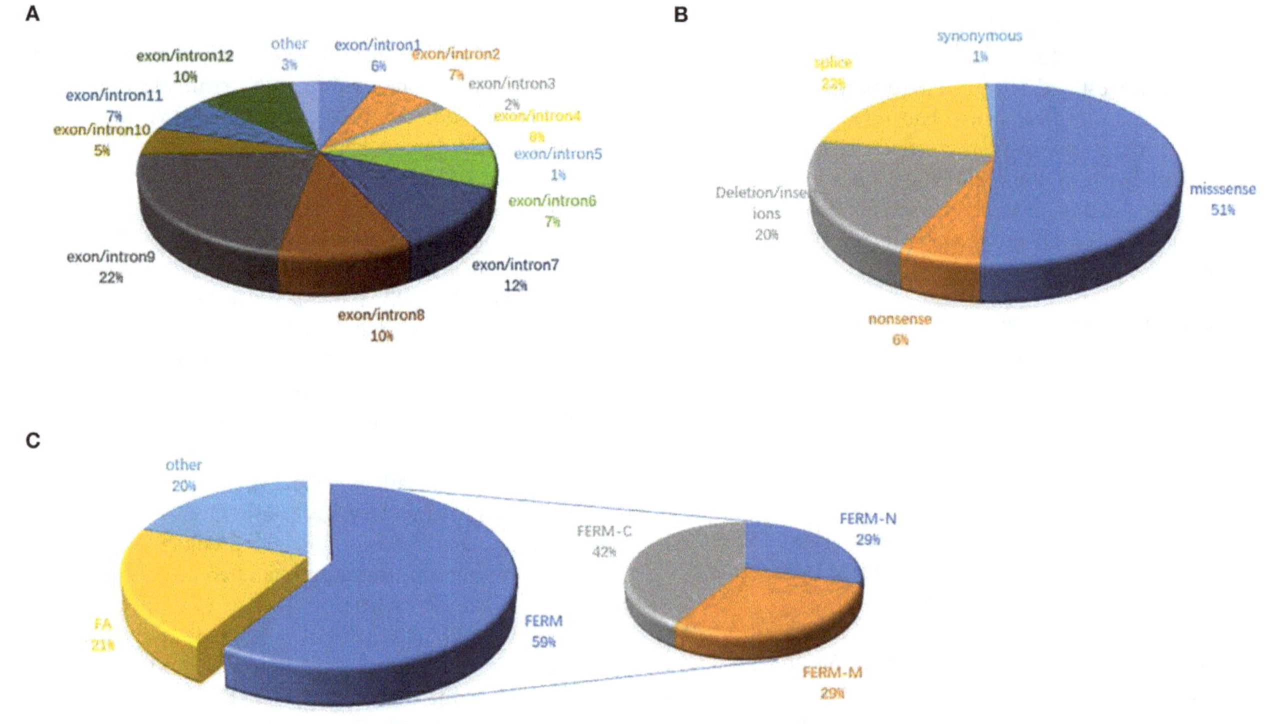

FIGURE 3 | *FRMD7* mutations published in the previous literature. **(A)** Distribution of *FRMD7* mutations identified before on exon/introns. **(B)** Proportions of different types of *FRMD7* mutations. **(C)** Distribution of *FRMD7* mutations identified before on domains in the *FRMD7* protein.

may cause isolated albinism in the eye or a series of other abnormalities, such as reduced visual acuity, nystagmus, and strabismus (Surace et al., 2000). The underlying pathogenic mechanisms of ocular abnormities caused by the GPR143 mutation have not been fully studied. It is well-known that melanin synthesis is disrupted in albinism, when this pathogenic condition occurs in the RPE, leading to severe defects in development and maintenance of vision eyes, including foveal hypoplasia, decreased numbers of photoreceptors and ganglion cells and misrouting of the optic tracts at the chiasm. However, mutations in GPR143, one of the genes associated with albinism, result in the impairment of visual pathway, but with intact melanin synthesis machinery (Schiaffino, 2010). This suggests that it is not the melanin synthesis and accumulation but the GPR143 signaling activity responsible for the developmental defects in retina. Researchers proposed that GPR143 signaling was the downstream of pigmentation, and all forms of albinism were dependent upon GPR143 signaling pathway to affect retinal development. Later studies found GPR143 signaling in RPE regulated the secretion of pigment epithelium-derived factor (PEDF) and vascular endothelial growth factor (VEGF) and exosome release. All of these signaling activities were involved in the protection from retinal diseases. However, it remains unclear that how the exosome release influences the retina (Locke et al., 2014; McKay, 2019; Figueroa and McKay, 2020). Mutations in GPR143 contributing to the aberrant protein function might disrupt the GPR143 signaling pathway leading to the developmental visual disorder. It was concluded that mutations in *GPR143* tend to cluster in exons 1-7; similarly, in this paper, all of these mutations in *GPR143* were found in exons 1, 2, 4, and 6. These results suggested that exons 1-7 are the most frequently mutated regions in the *GPR143* gene (Schnur et al., 1998; Fang et al., 2008).

However, several studies have reported that Chinese patients with *GPR143* mutations manifested CN as the most dominant, consistent phenotype. Researchers have proposed that the typical symptoms of OA caused by *GPR143* mutations are seldom observed in Asian populations, mainly because they have dark irises (**Table 3**) (Preising et al., 2001; Liu et al., 2007; Zhou et al., 2008; Peng et al., 2009; Xiao and Zhang, 2009; Hu et al., 2011; Gao et al., 2019). Three of five mutations (c.703G>A, c.733C>T, c.250+1G>C) in *GPR143* were detected in three cases without ocular albinism in our study. Unlike the study here, c.703G>A was reported to cause typical ocular albinism, while patients with the c.733C>T mutation exhibited foveal hypoplasia in previous studies (Schnur et al., 1998; Kim et al., 2016). In addition, Janecke et al. (2012) reported a patient misdiagnosed with CN first the time who was examined to have slight hypopigmentation in the fundus and was finally identified as ocular albinism through genetic screening. Herein, we summarized all the mutations in GPR143 identified in Chinses populations and phenotypes of the probands. It is believed that nystagmus, foveal hypoplasia, and hypopigmentation in the fundus are all associated with *GPR143* mutations (**Table 3**). We did not perform OCT to re-evaluate the three subjects more meticulously in our study due to the difficulty in children's examinations. Early and precise

TABLE 3 | Mutations identified in *GPR143* and the clinical characteristics of the probands in the Chinese population.

Mutation	Sex	Age(years)	BCVA	CN	Iris hypopigmentation	Fundus hypopigmentation	Macular hypoplasia	References
c.360+5G>T	Male	23	0.25/0.25	Y	Y	Y	Y	Gao et al., 2019
g.4572_5239del668bp	Male	5	0.2/0.2	Y	Y	Y	Y	Jiang et al., 2019
c.208_218del	Male	10	0.2/0.3	Y	Mild	N	Y	Jiang et al., 2019
g.4709_5711del1010bp	Male	52	0.1/0.1	Y	Mild	Y	Y	Jiang et al., 2019
c.659-2A>C	Male	10	0.1/0.1	Y	Mild	N	Y	Jiang et al., 2019
c.251G>A	Male	9	0.2/0.3	Y	Mild	N	Y	Jiang et al., 2019
c.733C>T	Male	7	0.1/0.1	Y	Mild	N	Y	Jiang et al., 2019
c.333G>A	Male	6 months	LP/LP	Y	Mild	Y	NA	Jia et al., 2017a
c.353G>A	Male	7	0.2/0.2	Y	N	Y	NA	Jia et al., 2017a
c.658+2T>G	Male	8 months	LP/LP	Y	Mild	Y	NA	Jia et al., 2017a
c.215_216 ins CGCTGC	Male	2 months	NA	Y	Mild	Y	NA	Jia et al., 2017a
c.17T>C	Male	10	0.3/0.3	Y	Mild	Y	NA	Jia et al., 2017a
c.333_360+14del42insCTT	Male	4	NA	Y	N	Y	Y	Zou et al., 2017
c.276G>A	Male	3	LP/LP	Y	N	Y	Y	Zou et al., 2017
c.793C>T	Male	24	0.15/0.15	Y	Y	Y	Y	Zou et al., 2017
exon 3_9del	Male	NA	NA	Y	N	N	N	Bu et al., 2016
c.494C>A	Male	4 months	NA	Y	N	Y	Y	Pan et al., 2016
c.333G>A	Female	36	0.1/0.1	Y	N	Y	Y	Han et al., 2015
c.360+1G>C	Male	7	0.1/0.1	Y	N	Y	Y	Han et al., 2015
c.659-1G>A	Male	10	0.3/0.2	Y	N	Y	Y	Han et al., 2015
c.43_50dupGACGCAGC	Male	8	0.3/0.3	Y	N	Y	Y	Han et al., 2015
c.703G> A	Male	29	0.3/0.4	Y	N	Y	Y	Han et al., 2015
g.24422G>C	Male	34	0.3/0.5	Y	Mild	Y	Y	Cai et al., 2013
c.943G>T	Male	6 months	NA	Y	Y	Y	Y	Wang et al., 2009
c.266C>T	Male	18	0.3/0.4	Y	N	N	N	Liu et al., 2007
c.807T>A	Male	42	0.2/0.2	Y	Mild	N	Y	Janecke et al., 2012
exon 1_2	Male	8	0.2/0.2	Y	N	Mild	Y	Xiao and Zhang, 2009
c.658+1G>T	Male	7	0.1/0.2	Y	Mild	Y	Y	Hu et al., 2011
c.849delT	Male	8	0.2/0.2	Y	N	N	N	Fang et al., 2008
c.238_240delCTC	Male	4	0.1/0.1	Y	NA	NA	NA	Fang et al., 2008
c.658+1G>A	Male	4	NA	Y	Mild	N	N	Fang et al., 2008
c.353G>A	Male	7	0.2/0.2	Y	Mild	N	Y	Fang et al., 2008
g.1103_7266del6164bp	Male	12	0.2/0.2	Y	N	N	N	Fang et al., 2008
g.25985_26546del562bp	Male	4	ND	Y	Mild	N	Y	Fang et al., 2008

Y, present; N, absent; NA, not available.

diagnosis is crucial to individual management and correct therapy. Several studies have shown that ultrahigh resolution OCT could detect minor differences in structural changes in the retina between albinism- and *FRMD7*- associated nystagmus (Thomas et al., 2014). Thus, comprehensive fundus examinations (OCT, fundus photograph) and molecular analysis are all required to distinguish between CN caused by *FRMD7* mutations and atypical OA caused by *GPR143* mutations more accurately. Targeted screening will be helpful to substantially increase the detection rate.

We did witness a considerable difference in visual acuity between the *FRMD7*-group and the *GPR143*-group. This result was in keeping with previous observational studies in which patients with *GPR143* mutations suffered more severe damage to vision, which may be explained by sensory defects in albinism-associated mechanisms, although this was not determined till now. GPR143 signaling might be essential for the process of RPE pigmentation protecting neurosensory retina. Although no typical albinism symptoms were observed, GPR143 mutation screening should be required for patients with poor visual function. In contrast to the earlier findings in 2011, comparisons of other clinical characteristics between the two groups are similar in our groups (Kumar et al., 2011).

Thomas et al. has described a lower proportion of AHP in the *FRMD7* group than the non-*FRMD7* group, which was not observed in our study. In addition, the remaining features of strabismus and stereopsis in the different groups here did not exhibit significant differences, which is compatible with previous studies (Thomas et al., 2008; Kumar et al., 2011). Noticeably, 100% of patients in *FRMD7* group and 61.54% (8/13) by TNO test and 58.33% (7/12) by Titmus test in the non-*FRMD7* group manifested strabismus in the group in which no stereopsis was recorded. This implies that strabismus has a strong adverse effect on binocular visual function. Excluding those with strabismus could be beneficial to improve the reliability of stereopsis phenotype analysis in different groups.

Unexpectedly, subjects with different mutation types exhibited no clear phenotypic-mutant link. In our study, we analyzed the clinical features of all the subjects reported before, but we did not conclude any differences among the non-sense, missense, deletion/insertion, and splice mutation groups. It seems that mutation types don not response to the severity of phenotype, and research by Thomas et al. (2008) also supported this finding. Other factors including the environment, modifier genes, and other unknown factors contributing to modulating the disease, may explain the phenotypic diversity.

In this research, we identified 14 mutations in two different genes, *FRMD7* and *GPR143*, and seven of them are novel. However, we cannot exclude the possibility that mutations are present in non-coding regions of *FRMD7* and *GPR143*. The combination of whole-genome and whole-exon sequencing is needed to identify novel candidate genes or variants in our unsolved cases.

However, several limitations in this study need to be acknowledged. First, it was difficult to obtain peripheral blood from some family members, and family segregation analysis was performed in only three families. Second, we did not re-evaluate patients without perfect clinical information, and the sample size may not be large enough, which might affect the credibility of the genotype–phenotype associations. Finally, the pathogenicity of new mutations was predicted by bioinformatic tools, and further experiments on cells and animals were not been performed in this study given the limited time and cost.

In conclusion, despite the limitations of this study, our research certainly provides another large-scale cohort with CN since the first four cohorts (Tarpey et al., 2006; Thomas et al., 2008; AlMoallem et al., 2015; Choi et al., 2018). For the first the time, we compared the phenotypes between groups with *FRMD7* and *GPR143* mutations and reviewed all the patients reported to explore the relationship of mutations and clinical characteristics. Here, 14 mutations were detected in 37.8% (14/37) of the probands (seven familiar cases, seven sporadic cases), seven of which are novel, demonstrating that mutations in *FRMD7* and *GPR143* appear to be two major causative factors in both X-linked and sporadic cases. Worse visual acuity was observed in patients with *GPR143* mutations than in patients with *FRMD7* mutations. These results broaden the mutation spectrum of *FRMD7* and *GPR143*, and add to our knowledge on Chinese patients with congenital nystagmus, providing new insights for the strategy of precise diagnosis and genetic counseling of CN.

ETHICS STATEMENT

The studies involving human participants were reviewed and approved by Ethics Committee of Eye Hospital of Wenzhou Medical University. Written informed consent to participate in this study was provided by the participants' legal guardian/next of kin.

AUTHOR CONTRIBUTIONS

Z-BJ conceived, supervised the study, and provided funding supports. H-YY and HC evaluated clinical characteristics for the enrolled patients. X-FW, P-JH, Z-KF, Z-QH, XF, X-TX, FH, and R-JS carried out the experiments. X-FW performed the data analysis and wrote the manuscript. Z-BJ and YL revised the manuscript. All authors contributed to the article and approved the submitted version.

ACKNOWLEDGMENTS

We thank all the subjects for their participation in this study.

REFERENCES

AlMoallem, B., Bauwens, M., Walraedt, S., Delbeke, P., De Zaeytijd, J., Kestelyn, P., et al. (2015). Novel FRMD7 mutations and genomic rearrangement expand the molecular pathogenesis of X-linked idiopathic infantile nystagmus. *Invest. Ophthalmol. Vis. Sci.* 56, 1701–1710. doi: 10.1167/iovs.14-15938

Bai, D., Shi, W., Qi, Z., Li, W., Wei, A., Cui, Y., et al. (2017). Clinical feature and waveform in infantile nystagmus syndrome in children with FRMD7 gene mutations. *Sci. China Life Sci.* 60, 707–713. doi: 10.1007/s11427-017-9089-5

Betts-Henderson, J., Bartesaghi, S., Crosier, M., Lindsay, S., Chen, H.-L., Salomoni, P., et al. (2010). The nystagmus-associated FRMD7 gene regulates neuronal outgrowth and development. *Hum. Mol. Genet.* 19, 342–351. doi: 10.1093/hmg/ddp500

Brodsky, M. C., and Dell'Osso, L. F. (2014). A unifying neurologic mechanism for infantile nystagmus. *JAMA Ophthalmol.* 132, 761–768. doi: 10.1001/jamaophthalmol.2013.5833

Bu, J., Liu, J., Jia, Y., and Wang, L. (2016). A previously unidentified deletion in G protein-coupled receptor 143 causing X-linked congenital nystagmus in a Chinese family. *Indian J. Ophthalmol.* 64, 813–817. doi: 10.4103/0301-4738.195593

Cai, C. Y., Zhu, H., Shi, W., Su, L., Shi, O., Cai, C. Q., et al. (2013). A novel splicing site mutation of the GPR143 gene in a Chinese X-linked ocular albinism pedigree. *Genet. Mol. Res.* 12, 5673–5679. doi: 10.4238/2013. November.18.16

Choi, J.-H., Jung, J.-H., Oh, E. H., Shin, J.-H., Kim, H.-S., Seo, J. H., et al. (2018). Genotype and phenotype spectrum ofFRMD7-associated infantile nystagmus syndrome. *Invest. Opthalmol. Vis. Sci.* 59, 3181–3188. doi: 10.1167/iovs.18-24207

Dell'Osso, L. F. (2002). Development of new treatments for congenital nystagmus. *Ann. N. Y. Acad. Sci.* 956, 361–379. doi: 10.1111/j.1749-6632.2002. tb02834.x

Fang, S., Guo, X., Jia, X., Xiao, X., Li, S., and Zhang, Q. (2008). Novel GPR143 mutations and clinical characteristics in six Chinese families with X-linked ocular albinism. *Mol. Vis.* 14, 1974–1982.

Figueroa, A. G., and McKay, B. S. (2020). A G-protein coupled receptor and macular degeneration. *Cells* 9:910. doi: 10.3390/cells9040910

Forssman, B. (1971). Hereditary studies of congenital nystagmus in a Swedish population. *Ann. Hum. Genet.* 35, 119–138. doi: 10.1111/j.1469-1809.1956.tb01385.x

Gao, X., Liu, T., Cheng, X., Dai, A., Liu, W., Li, R., et al. (2019). A novel GPR143 mutation in a Chinese family with X-linked ocular albinism type 1. *Mol. Med. Rep.* 21, 240–248. doi: 10.3892/mmr.2019.10813

Han, R., Wang, X., Wang, D., Wang, L., Yuan, Z., Ying, M., et al. (2015). GPR143 gene mutations in five Chinese families with X-linked congenital nystagmus. *Sci. Rep.* 5:12031. doi: 10.1038/srep12031

Hertle, R. W., Yang, D., Adams, K., and Caterino, R. (2010). Surgery for the treatment of vertical head posturing associated with infantile nystagmus syndrome: results in 24 patients. *Clin. Exp. Ophthalmol.* 39, 37–46. doi: 10.1111/j.1442-9071.2010.02380.x

Hu, J., Liang, D., Xue, J., Liu, J., and Wu, L. (2011). A novel GPR143 splicing mutation in a Chinese family with X-linked congenital nystagmus. *Mol. Vis.* 17, 715–722.

Janecke, A. R., Yan, N., Liao, X., Cai, S. P., Lan, C., Wang, Y., et al. (2012). A novel nonsense mutation of the GPR143 gene identified in a Chinese pedigree with ocular albinism. *PLoS ONE* 7:e43177. doi: 10.1371/journal.pone.0043177

Jia, X., Yuan, J., Jia, X., Ling, S., Li, S., and Guo, X. (2017a). GPR143 mutations in Chinese patients with ocular albinism type 1. *Mol. Med. Rep.* 15, 3069–3075. doi: 10.3892/mmr.2017.6366

Jia, X., Zhu, X., Li, Q., Jia, X., Li, S., and Guo, X. (2017b). Novel mutations of FRMD7 in Chinese patients with congenital motor nystagmus. *Mol. Med. Rep.* 16, 1753–1758. doi: 10.3892/mmr.2017.6824

Jiang, J., Yang, L., Li, H., Huang, L., and Li, N. (2019). Evaluation of the iris thickness changes for the Chinese families with GPR143 gene mutations. *Exp. Eye Res.* 189:107819. doi: 10.1016/j.exer.2019.107819

Kim, U. S., Cho, E., and Kim, H. J. (2016). A novel nonsense mutation of GPR143 gene in a Korean kindred with X-linked congenital nystagmus. *Int. J. Ophthalmol.* 9, 1367–1370. doi: 10.18240/ijo.2016.09.25

Kumar, A., Gottlob, I., McLean, R. J., Thomas, S., Thomas, M. G., and Proudlock, F. A. (2011). Clinical and oculomotor characteristics of albinism compared toFRMD7 associated infantile nystagmus. *Invest. Opthalmol. Vis. Sci.* 52, 2306–2313. doi: 10.1167/iovs.10-5685

Li, N., Wang, L., Cui, L., Zhang, L., Dai, S., Li, H., et al. (2008). Five novel mutations of the FRMD7 gene in Chinese families with X-linked infantile nystagmus. *Mol. Vis.* 14, 733–738.

Liu, J. Y., Ren, X., Yang, X., Guo, T., Yao, Q., Li, L., et al. (2007). Identification of a novel GPR143 mutation in a large Chinese family with congenital nystagmus as the most prominent and consistent manifestation. *J. Hum. Genet.* 52, 565–570. doi: 10.1007/s10038-007-0152-3

Locke, C. J., Congrove, N. R., Dismuke, W. M., Bowen, T. J., Stamer, W. D., and McKay, B. S. (2014). Controlled exosome release from the retinal pigment epithelium *in situ*. *Exp. Eye Res.* 129, 1–4. doi: 10.1016/j.exer.2014.10.010

McKay, B. S. (2019). Pigmentation and vision: is GPR143 in control? *J. Neurosci. Res.* 97, 77–87. doi: 10.1002/jnr.24246

Pan, Q., Yi, C., Xu, T., Liu, J., Jing, X., Hu, B., et al. (2016). A novel mutation, c.494C>A (p.Ala165Asp), in the GPR143 gene causes a mild phenotype in a Chinese X-linked ocular albinism patient. *Acta Ophthalmol.* 94, 417–418. doi: 10.1111/aos.12854

Papageorgiou, E., McLean, R. J., and Gottlob, I. (2014). Nystagmus in childhood. *Pediatr. Neonatol.* 55, 341–351. doi: 10.1016/j.pedneo. 2014.02.007

Peng, Y., Meng, Y., Wang, Z., Qin, M., Li, X., Dian, Y., et al. (2009). A novel GPR143 duplication mutation in a Chinese family with X-linked congenital nystagmus. *Mol. Vis.* 15, 810–814.

Preising, M., Op de Laak, J. P., and Lorenz, B. (2001). Deletion in the OA1 gene in a family with congenital X linked nystagmus. *Br. J. Ophthalmol.* 85, 1098–1103. doi: 10.1136/bjo.85.9.1098

Ren, J., Wen, L., Gao, X., Jin, C., Xue, Y., and Yao, X. (2009). DOG 1.0: illustrator of protein domain structures. *Cell Res.* 19, 271–273. doi: 10.1038/ cr.2009.6

Richards, M. D., and Wong, A. (2015). Infantile nystagmus syndrome: clinical characteristics, current theories of pathogenesis, diagnosis, and management. *Can. J. Ophthalmol.* 50, 400–408. doi: 10.1016/j.jcjo.2015.07.010

Sarvananthan, N., Surendran, M., Roberts, E. O., Jain, S., Thomas, S., Shah, N., et al. (2009). The prevalence of nystagmus: the leicestershire nystagmus survey. *Invest. Opthalmol. Vis. Sci.* 50, 5201–5206. doi: 10.1167/iovs.09-3486

Schiaffino, M. V. (2010). Signaling pathways in melanosome biogenesis and pathology. *Int. J. Biochem. Cell Biol.* 42, 1094–1104. doi: 10.1016/j.biocel.2010.03.023

Schnur, R. E., Gao, M., Wick, P. A., Keller, M., Benke, P. J., Edwards, M. J., et al. (1998). OA1 mutations and deletions in X-linked ocular albinism. *Am. J. Hum. Genet.* 62, 800–809. doi: 10.1086/301776

Self, J., Shawkat, F., Malpas, C., Thomas, N., Harris, C., Hodgkins, P., et al. (2007). Allelic variation of the FRMD7 gene in congenital idiopathic nystagmus. *Arch. Ophthalmol.* 125, 1255–1263. doi: 10.1001/archopht.125.9.1255

Song, F. W., Chen, B. B., Sun, Z. H., Wu, L. P., Zhao, S. J., Miao, Q., et al. (2013). Novel mutation c.980_983delATTA compound with c.986C>A mutation of the FRMD7 gene in a Chinese family with X-linked idiopathic congenital nystagmus. *J. Zhejiang Univ. Sci. B* 14, 479–486. doi: 10.1631/jzus.B1200259

Surace, E. M., Angeletti, B., Ballabio, A., and Marigo, V. (2000). Expression pattern of the ocular albinism type 1 (Oa1) gene in the murine retinal pigment epithelium. *Invest. Ophthalmol. Vis. Sci.* 41, 4333–4337. doi: 10.1097/00004397-200040010-00021

Tarpey, P., Thomas, S., Sarvananthan, N., Mallya, U., Lisgo, S., Talbot, C. J., et al. (2006). Mutations in FRMD7, a newly identified member of the FERM family, cause X-linked idiopathic congenital nystagmus. *Nat. Genet.* 38, 1242–1244. doi: 10.1038/ng1893

Thomas, M. G., Crosier, M., Lindsay, S., Kumar, A., Araki, M., Leroy, B. P., et al. (2014). Abnormal retinal development associated with FRMD7 mutations. *Hum. Mol. Genet.* 23, 4086–4093. doi: 10.1093/hmg/ddu122

Thomas, S., Proudlock, F. A., Sarvananthan, N., Roberts, E. O., Awan, M., McLean, R., et al. (2008). Phenotypical characteristics of idiopathic infantile nystagmus with and without mutations in FRMD7. *Brain* 131, 1259–1267. doi: 10.1093/brain/awn046

Wang, Y., Guo, X., Wei, A., Zhu, W., Li, W., and Lian, S. (2009). Identification of a novel mutation in a Chinese family with X-linked ocular albinism. *Eur. J. Ophthalmol.* 19, 124–128. doi: 10.1177/112067210901900118

Watkins, R. J., Patil, R., Goult, B. T., Thomas, M. G., Gottlob, I., and Shackleton, S. (2013). A novel interaction between FRMD7 and CASK: evidence for a causal role in idiopathic infantile nystagmus. *Hum. Mol. Genet.* 22, 2105–2118. doi: 10.1093/hmg/ddt060

Watkins, R. J., Thomas, M. G., Talbot, C. J., Gottlob, I., and Shackleton, S. (2012). The role of FRMD7 in idiopathic infantile nystagmus. *J. Ophthalmol.* 2012, 1–7. doi: 10.1155/2012/460956

Xiao, X., and Zhang, Q. (2009). Iris hyperpigmentation in a Chinese family with ocular albinism and theGPR143mutation. *Am. J. Med. Genet., Part A* 149A, 1786–1788. doi: 10.1002/ajmg.a.32818

Zhang, B., Liu, Z., Zhao, G., Xie, X., Yin, X., Hu, Z., et al. (2007). Novel mutations of the FRMD7 gene in X-linked congenital motor nystagmus. *Mol. Vis.* 13, 1674–1679.

Zhang, Q., Xiao, X., Li, S., and Guo, X. (2007). FRMD7 mutations in Chinese families with X-linked congenital motor nystagmus. *Mol. Vis.* 13, 1375-1378.

Zhao, H., Huang, X.-F., Zheng, Z.-L., Deng, W.-L., Lei, X.-L., Xing, D.-J., et al. (2016). Molecular genetic analysis of patients with sporadic and X-linked infantile nystagmus. *BMJ Open* 6:e010649. doi: 10.1136/bmjopen-2015-010649

Zhou, P., Wang, Z., Zhang, J., Hu, L., and Kong, X. (2008). Identification of a novel GPR143 deletion in a Chinese family with X-linked congenital nystagmus. *Mol. Vis.* 14, 1015–1019.

Zou, X., Li, H., Yang, L., Sun, Z., Yuan, Z., Li, H., et al. (2017). Molecular genetic and clinical evaluation of three Chinese families with X-linked ocular albinism. *Sci. Rep.* 7:33713. doi: 10.1038/srep33713

2

Ocular Characteristics of Patients with Bardet–Biedl Syndrome Caused by Pathogenic BBS Gene Variation in a Chinese Cohort

Xiaohong Meng[1,2†], Yanling Long[1,2†], Jiayun Ren[1,2], Gang Wang[1,2], Xin Yin[1,2] and Shiying Li[1,2]*

[1] Department of Ophthalmology, Southwest Hospital, Army Medical University (Third Military Medical University), Chongqing, China, [2] Key Laboratory of Visual Damage and Regeneration and Restoration of Chongqing, Chongqing, China

***Correspondence:**
Shiying Li
shiying_li@126.com

† These authors share first authorship

Bardet–Biedl syndrome (BBS; OMIM 209900) is a rare genetic disease causing damage to multiple organs and affecting patients' quality of life in late adolescence or early adulthood. In this study, the ocular characteristics including morphology and function, were analyzed in 12 BBS patients from 10 Chinese families by molecular diagnostics. A total of five known and twelve novel variants in four *BBS* genes (*BBS2*, 58.33%; *BBS4*, 8.33%; *BBS7*, 16.67%; and *BBS9*, 16.67%) were identified in 10 Chinese families with BBS. All patients had typical phenotypes of retinitis pigmentosa with unrecordable or severely damaged cone and rod responses on full-field flash electroretinography (ffERG). Most of the patients showed unremarkable reactions in pattern visual evoked potential (PVEP) and multifocal electroretinography (mfERG), while their flash visual evoked potentials (FVEP) indicated display residual visual function. Changes in the fundus morphology, including color fundus photography and autofluorescence (AF) imaging, were heterogeneous and not consistent with the patients' functional tests. Overall, our study expands the variation spectrum of the *BBS* gene, showing that the ocular characteristics of BBS patients are clinically highly heterogeneous, and demonstrates the usefulness of a combination of the ffERG and FVEP assessments of visual function in the advanced stage of retinopathy in BBS.

Keywords: Bardet–Biedl syndrome, ocular characteristics, morphology, visual function, gene variation

INTRODUCTION

Bardet–Biedl syndrome (BBS; OMIM 209900) is a genetic disease causing damage to multiple organs, including early onset progressive retinitis pigmentosa (RP), obesity, hypogonadal hypoplasia, hand and/or foot polydactyly, intellectual disability, abnormal renal development (Bardet, 1995; Biedl, 1995). Therefore, BBS patients' lives can be seriously threatened. However, while the diagnosis of BBS is often missed, it is usually fully recognized when patients visit an ophthalmologic clinic due to impaired vision or night blindness.

The ocular symptoms of BBS mainly manifest as RP since childhood. Fundus manifestations include optic disk pallor, bone spicule pigment deposits, thinning of the blood vessels, and retinal osteocyte pigmentation (Riise et al., 1996; Moore et al., 2005). Moreover, scotopic rod and maximal responses as well as cone responses are non-detectable in most BBS patients (Berezovsky et al., 2012; Scheidecker et al., 2015). A total of 24 causative genes of BBS have thus far been discovered (Weihbrecht et al., 2017; Bölükbaşı et al., 2018; Mary et al., 2019; Wormser et al., 2019). Most of them encode proteins necessary for the formation of the BBSome multi-subunit complex which localized at the cilia and basal body, and their connecting the cilium in the outer segment of photoreceptor has been thought to play a role in protein trafficking (Wei et al., 2012; Xu et al., 2015). Defects in any one subunit will adversely affect the formation or function of the BBSome, causing the BBS phenotype (Khan et al., 2016; Priya et al., 2016; Weihbrecht et al., 2017). Moreover, rhodopsin in BBS gene mutant mice was incorrectly located in the cells of the inner segment (IS) and outer nuclear layer (ONL), and the OS, IS, and ONL exhibited progressive loss (Nishimura et al., 2004; Datta et al., 2015). Currently, BBS treatment focuses on managing diabetes, hypertension, and metabolic syndrome to minimize the secondary effects of the disease on vulnerable organs.

Most BBS cases reported worldwide are concentrated in Europe and the Middle East (Farag and Teebi, 1988, 1989), whereas the disorder is very rare among the Chinese population. In this study, we conducted clinical and genetic analyses of 10 Chinese families (12 patients) with BBS and comprehensively evaluated visual function and fundus changes in these patients. We also investigated BBS genotype-phenotype differences between Chinese reports and those from abroad.

MATERIALS AND METHODS

Patient Recruitment

A total of 12 patients from 10 unrelated families with BBS treated at the Ophthalmology Department, Southwest Hospital, Army Medical University, Chongqing, China from 2012 to 2018 were retrospectively included in this study. The clinical diagnosis of BBS was made based on the potential patients presenting with four primary features or three primary features plus two secondary features. The primary features included retinal dystrophy, obesity, postaxial polydactyly, intellectual disability, gonadal abnormalities, and renal abnormalities. The secondary features included speech disorder/delay, sbtrabismus/cataracts/astigmatism, brachydactyly/syndactyly, developmental delay, polyuria/polydipsia (nephrogenic diabetes insipidus), ataxia/poor coordination/imbalance, mild spasticity (especially in the lower limbs), diabetes mellitus, dental crowding/hypodontia/small roots/high arched palate, left ventricular hypertrophy/congenital heart disease, hepatic fibrosis, short stature and hearing loss (Beales et al., 1999). If a patient was highly suspected to have BBS but one or two cardinal symptoms were missing, genetic analyses were performed for comprehensive analysis. We could clinically exclude the other syndromes such as Usher syndrome, Alström syndrome, Mckusick–Kaufman syndrome, Prader–Willi syndrome, and Joubert syndrome. Available family members of the probands were invited for clinical examination and genetic analysis. The research protocol was approved by the Ethics Review Board of Southwest Hospital (Chongqing, China, KY2020096), and the study was conducted in accordance with the provisions of the Declaration of Helsinki. Written informed consent was obtained from all participants. Assessment of ocular characteristics.

All patients underwent comprehensive ophthalmologic examinations, including best-corrected visual acuity (BCVA) tests with a decimal chart, indirect ophthalmoscopy, and slit lamp biomicroscopy. Color fundus photography, fundus fluorescein angiography (FFA), fundus autofluorescence (FAF; excitation: 488 nm), and Spectralis HRA-optical coherent tomography (OCT, Heidelberg Engineering, Dossenheim, Germany) imaging were used. Full-field flash electroretinography (ffERG; Diagnosys LLC, Lowell, MA, United States) and multifocal electroretinography (mfERG; VERIS Science 6.3.2; Electro-Diagnostic Imaging, Inc., Milpitas, CA, United States) were performed according to the ISCEV standard protocol (Hood et al., 2012; McCulloch et al., 2015). Pattern visual evoked potentials (PVEP) and flash visual evoked potentials (FVEP) were also recorded.

Molecular Genetic Analysis

Genomic DNA was extracted from the patients' peripheral blood using the Tiangen blood kit (Tiangen Biltech, Beijing, China) following the manufacturer's standard sequencing protocols. Targeted next generation sequencing (NGS) was then performed using a capture panel including 131 known inherited retinal disease (IRD) genes (**Supplementary Table 1**). All coding exons of these genes were captured using the GenCap Liquid Phase Capture Kit (MyGenostics Inc.) and sequenced on the Illumina NextSeq 500. Then, the sequencing data processing, single nucleotide variants (SNVs) and insertions/deletions (InDels) calling and annotation were performed based on the hg19/GRCh37 human reference genome by using Haplotype Caller in GATK software (V.3.7), VariantFiltration in GATK software(V.3.7) and ANNOVAR software (V.3.4), respectively. Then, the online bioinformatics analysis software used to classify the pathogenicity of the candidate variants according to the American College of Medical Genetics and Genomics (ACMG) guidelines, including Exome Aggregation Consortium (ExAC), 1000Genomes database (1000G), and Genome Aggregation Database (gnomAD) to check the allele frequency; The rs number were found in Single Nucleotide Polymorphism Database (dbSNP); The pathogenicity of missense and synonymous variations were analyzed using ClinVar, HGMD Professional and four software prediction programs: Sorting Intolerant from Tolerance (SIFT), Protein Variation Effect Analyzer (PROVEAN) (Choi and Chan, 2015), Polymorphism Phenotyping v2 (PolyPhen2), and MutationTaster (Schwarz et al., 2014). The predicted effect on the splicing of all missense and synonymous variations was assessed with the Human Splicing finder program version 3.1 (Desmet et al., 2009). Finally, the disease-causing variants were identified while fully considering the clinical phenotypic findings and co-segregation analysis (by Sanger sequencing) of the affected subjects.

TABLE 1 | Systemic manifestations of patients with BBS.

Patient	Sex	Age at diagnostic exam	Initial eye symptom	Age of onset of NB	Ocular disease	BMI (Kg/m^2)	Polydactyly	Intellectual disability	Gonad	Renal	Abnormal						
											Hear	Tooth	Short stature	Heart	Blood sugar	Blood pressure	Lipids
F1-II:1	M	21 y	NB	Since birth	RP	33.2	Yes	Yes	No	No	Yes	Yes	Yes	No	No	No	No
F2-II:1#	M	13 y	NB	Since birth	RP	19.53	No	Yes	No	No	No	Yes	No	No	No	No	No
F2-II:2	F	19 y	NB	Childhood	RP	24.44	Yes	No	OD	No	No	No	Yes	No	No	No	No
F3-II:1#	M	30 y	NB	Since birth	RP	26.72	No	No	EGD	No	Yes	No	No	No	No	No	No
F3-II:2*	M	29 y	NB	Since birth	RP	29.05	No	No	EGD	No	Yes	No	No	HSHR	No	SH	No
F4-II:1	F	37 y	NB	Since birth	RP	28.76	No	No	No	No	No	Yes	No	No	No	SH	No
F5-II:1	M	26 y	NB	Since birth	RP	32.30	Yes	No	-	-	-	Yes	Yes	-	-	-	-
F6-II:1	F	13 y	NB	3 y	RP	30.00	Yes	Yes	OC	-	-	Yes	Yes	-	SH	-	SH
F7-II:1	M	8 y	NB	Since birth	RP	26.30	-	No	-	-	-	Yes	Yes	-	-	-	-
F8-II:1	F	8 y	NB	8 y	RP	41.42	Yes	Yes	No	No	No	Yes	Yes	No	No	No	No
F9-II:1	M	27 y	NB	6 y	RP	26.12	Yes	No	No	No	No	Yes	No	No	No	No	No
F11F10-II:1	M	18 y	NB	Since birth	RP	30.42	Yes	No	No	RC	No	No	No	No	No	No	SH

EGD, external genital dysplasia; HSHR, high sinus heart rate; NB, night blindness; OC, ovarian cyst; OD, ovarian dysplasia; RC, renal cyst; SH, slightly higher.
**Bones and joints change. #Epilepsy, dorsal hemangioma. Not available.*

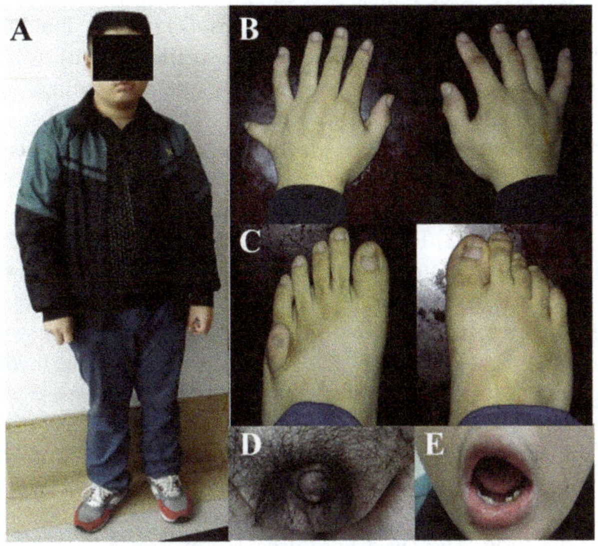

FIGURE 1 | Systemic manifestations of BBS patients. The Wechsler Intelligence Score showed that this patient (F1-II:1) only had an 6-year-old intellectual level, his physical signs are: **(A)** Obesity (BMI 33.2 Kg/m^2). **(B)** Polydactyly of the right hand and left foot. **(C)** Sexual organ dysplasia. **(D)** Dental dysplasia. **(E)** Abnormal tooth development.

RESULTS

Clinical Findings of BBS

We enrolled four women and eight men from 10 unrelated families. Their average age was 20.75 years (range: 8–37 years). The physical examination findings included obesity (12/12), hand and foot polydactyly (7/12), intellectual disability (4/12), abnormal tooth development (8/12), short stature (6/12), hearing loss (3/12), gonadal dysplasia (4/12), epilepsy (2/12), dorsal hemangioma (2/12), renal dysplasia (1/12), spinal dysplasia (1/12), gallstones (1/12), hyperlipidemia (1/12), hypertension (2/12), osteoarthritis-like changes (1/12), and heart abnormalities (1/12) (**Table 1** and **Figure 1**). Five patients had undergone surgical extra toe removal at an early age, and one side ovary was removed from F6-II:1 due to acute torsion of a unilateral polycystic ovary cyst. Three patients dropped out of school at an early age due to intellectual disability.

Ocular Characteristics

All BBS patients were misdiagnosed with amblyopia upon their first visit to our hospital, and their common initial eye symptom was night blindness, and most of they have vision decline and vision field defect. Three patients (F-II:1, F2-II:2, and F8-II:1) had strabismus, and four (F1-II:1, F4-II:1, F5-II:1, and F8-II:1) had concomitant cataracts. F1-II:1 had nystagmus and concomitant cataract, and F2-II:2 had nystagmus with strabismus. The BCVA ranged from light perception (LP) to 0.3, including low vision (10/24 eyes) and legal blindness (16/24 eyes). All patients presented with typical RP features, including pigmentary changes in their peripheral and midperipheral retina, attenuated arteriolar vessels, pallor of the optic disk, and macular lesions (**Figure 2**; Fundus). Solitary macular atrophy was found in F3-II:1 and F8-II:1, which was characterized by pigment disorder, retinal thinning, and local retinal pigment epithelial atrophy, with a normal pigment change in the posterior pole retina. The AF of all patients showed plaque hypoautofluorescence in the posterior pole. Plaque hypoautofluorescence in the macular area was enlarged in F1-II:1, F2-II:1, F2-II:2, F3-II:2, F4-II:1, F5-II:1, and F9-II:1 (**Figure 2**; FAF). Patients' fundus (F3-II:1 and F8-II:1) showed solitary enlarged macular lesions, while hypoautofluorescence of the macular area seemed to be normal in F10-II:1. OCT showed that the outer structure of the subfovea, including the myoid zone, ellipsoid zone, and external limiting membranes, was completely absent in F1-II:1; while most of the outer structure of the subfovea remained in F6-II:1; the rest of the patients showed different degrees of deletion of the outer structure of the subfovea (**Figure 2**; OCT). In the objective visual functional test, the ffERG displayed unrecordable waveforms in most of the patients (**Figure 3A**), and only F3-II:1 exhibited partial residual rod response. The mfERG waves were unrecordable in all patients assessed. The PVEP results showed a severely decreased amplitude and moderate delayed peak time in the P100 wave of F6-II:1, while the other patients had unrecordable PVEP due to nystagmus and fixation loss (**Supplementary Figure 2**). The FVEP showed mild delayed but visible P2 waves in patients assessed. Interestingly, all of the six patients who showed moderately reduced P2 wave amplitude, also had BCVA better than 0.01 (F2-II:1, F2-II:2, F3-II:1, F6-II:1, F7-II:1, and F8-II:1) (**Figure 3B** and **Table 2**).

Variant and Pedigree Analysis

Consanguineous marriage (F2) was noted in one of the 10 families in our cohort (**Figure 4**). After variant calling and data filtering, we identified 15 compound variants and two homozygous variants in the 12 patients with *BBS2* (F1–F5), *BBS4* (F6), *BBS7* (F7–F8), and *BBS9* (F9–F10) gene (**Table 3**), including five splice variations (c.263 + 2delT, c.534 + 1G > T, c.1198 + 1G > A, c.2059 + 1G > C, and c.2059 + 1G > T), three frameshift variations c.72delT(p.L25Cfs*16), c.563delT(p.I188Tfs*13), and c.1002delT(p.N335Ifs*47), four nonsense variations c.31C > T(p.Q11*), c.445C > T(p.R149*), c.1015C > T(p.R339*), and c.1395T > A(p.Y465*), four missense variations c.79A > C(p.T27P), c.728G > A(p.C243Y), c.932G > A(p.G311D), and c.944G > A(p.R315Q), one synonymous variation c.1278A > G(p.E426E). These variants were confirmed as perfectly co-segregated with the disease within the families in which they occurred (**Figure 4**) based on a recessive pattern of inheritance as ascertained by Sanger sequencing. Among the identified variants, c.563delT(p.I188Tfs*13), c.944G > A(p.R315Q), and c.1015C > T(p.R339*) in the *BBS2* gene (Katsanis et al., 2001; Xing et al., 2014; Shaheen et al., 2016), c.728G > A(p.C243Y) and c.1002delT(p.N335Ifs*47) in the *BBS7* gene (Chen et al., 2013; Wang et al., 2013) have been reported to be related to RP or BBS, while the rest of the 12 variants in the four genes were never been reported in ClinVar or HGMD Professional, so they were considered novel (*BBS2*, 41.67%; *BBS4*, 16.67%; *BBS7*, 8.33%; and *BBS9*, 33.33%). Moreover, according to the ACMG guidelines, except for c.79A > C(p.T27P) and c.1278A > G(p.E426E) which were

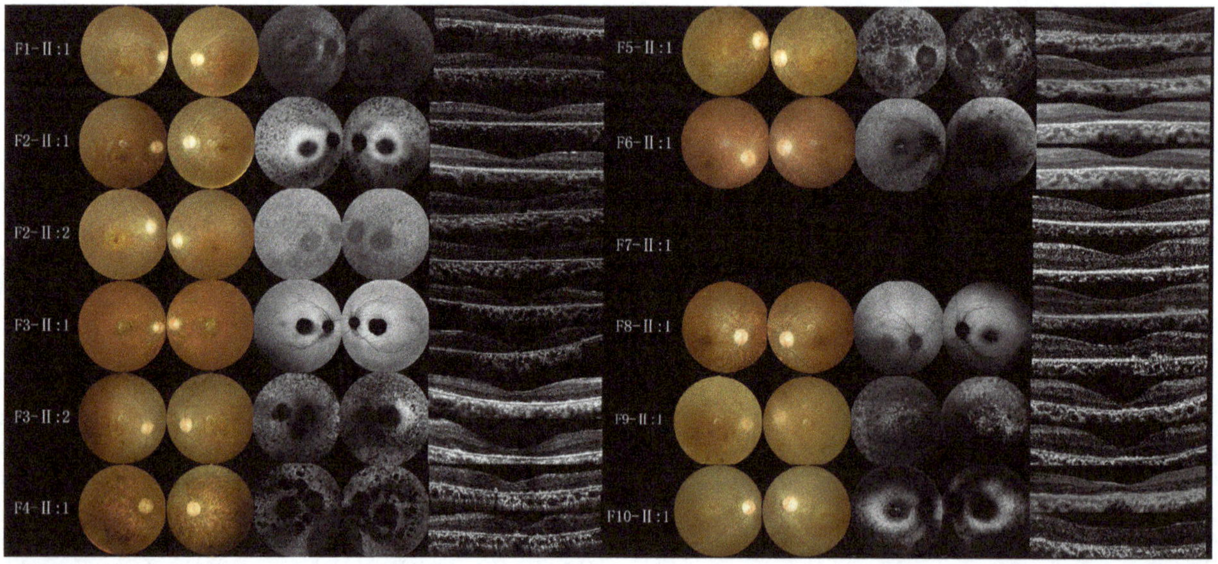

FIGURE 2 | Fundus photography, fundus autofluorescence imaging, and foveal optical coherence tomography scans of probands from the BBS families. All patients had macular lesions, with pigmentary changes in the peripheral and midperipheral retina, attenuated arteriolar vessels, and pallor of the optic disk (Fundus). Plaque hypoautofluorescence in the macular area was enlarged in F1-II:1, F2-II:1, F2-II:2, F3-II:2, F4-II:1, F5-II:1, F9-II:1 (FAF). OCT (OD and OS in the vertical order) showed the outer structure of the subfovea was completely absent in F1-II:1, most of the outer structure remained in F6-II:1, and different degrees of deletion of the outer structure of the subfovea were observed in the rest of the patients (OCT).

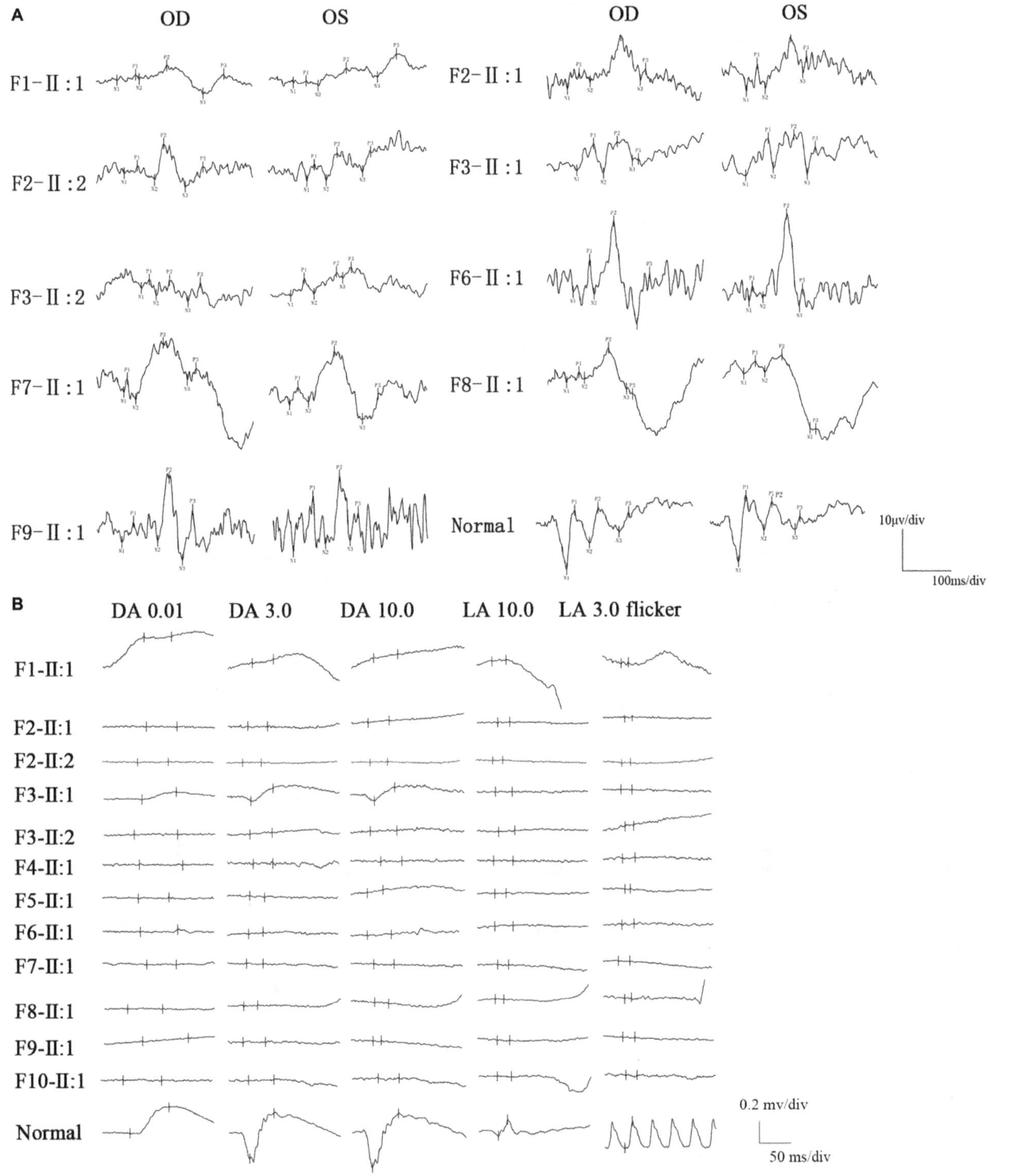

FIGURE 3 | FVEP and ffERG recordings in patients with BBS. **(A)** The FVEP showed mild delayed but visible P2 waves in patients who performed it. Interestingly, all of six patients who showed moderate reduced P2 wave amplitude, also had BCVA better than 0.01 (F2-II:1, F2-II:2, F3-II:1, F6-II:1, F7-II:1, F8-II:1). **(B)** The ffERG was unrecordable in most of the patients, only patient (F3-II:1) had partial residual rod response.

classified as uncertain significance, we classify the other 15 variants as pathogenic. Furthermore, in this study, the novel heterozygous variation c.534 + 1G > T in *BBS2* was detected in two families (F3 and F5), and, among the pathogenic *BBS* genes in the 10 probands, *BBS2* was the most common.

TABLE 2 | Fundus manifestation and evaluation of visual function in patients with BBS.

Patient	Ocular complications	BCVA RE/LE	Fundus	PVEP (P100 wave)	FVEP (P2 wave)	ffERG	mfERG
F1-II1	Nystagmus, cataract	CF/HM	MA, ODP, OCLPD	UR	Severe reduce amplitude, mild delay	UR	UR
F2-II:1	Strabism	0.05/0.2	MA, ODP, OCLPD	Severe decreased amplitude and moderate delay peak time	Moderate reduced amplitude, mild delay	UR	UR
F2-II:2	Pystagmus, strabism	0.05/0.1	MA, ODP, OCLPD	UR	Moderate reduced amplitude, mild delay	UR	UR
F3-II:1	–	0.02/0.01	MA, ODP, OCLPD	UR	Moderate reduced amplitude, mild delay	Partial residual rod response	UR
F3-II:2	–	LP/LP	MA, ODP, OCLPD	UR	Severe reduced amplitude, without delay	UR	UR
F4-II:1	Cataract	HM/HM	CS, RPE atrophy, ODP	–	–	UR	UR
F5-II:1	Cataract	0.05/0.05	MA, ODP, OCLPD	UR	–	UR	UR
F6-II:1	–	0.1/0.15	ODP, OCLPD	Moderately decreased amplitude and delayed peak time	Moderate reduce amplitude, mild delay	UR	–
F7-II:1	–	0.2/0.2	MA, ODP, OCLPD	–	Moderate reduceamplitude, mild delay	UR	–
F8-II:1	Exotropia	0.3/0.3	RPD	–	Moderate reduceamplitude, mild delay	UR	–
F9-II:1	Cataract	HM/HM	ODP, OCLPD,	–	Unstable and severe reduced amplitude, mild delay	UR	UR
F10-II	–	0.2/0.1	MA, ODP, OCLPD	–	–	UR	UR

BCVA, best-corrected visual acuity; CF, count finger; CS, choroid sclerosis; HM, hand move; LE, left eye; LP, light perception; MA, macular atrophy; RE, right eye; OCLPD, osteocyte cell-like pigment deposition; ODP, optic disk pallor; RPD, retinitis pigment disorder; UR, unrecorded; –, not available.

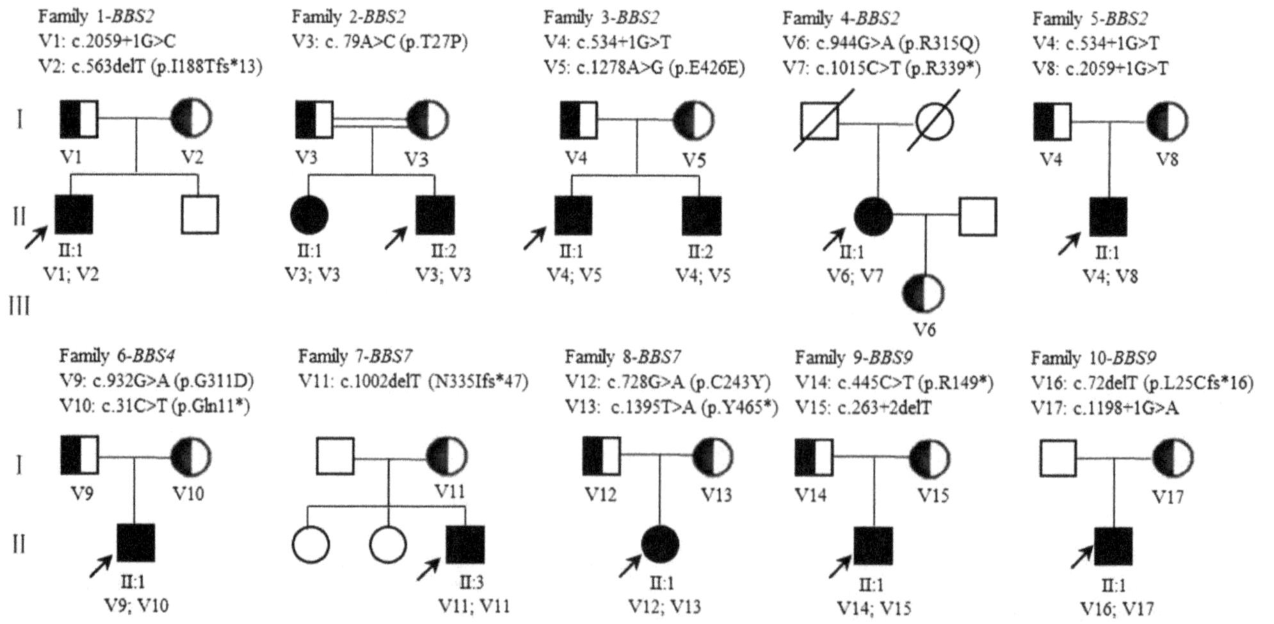

FIGURE 4 | Pedigrees of BBS families. The squares and circles indicate men and women, respectively. The black solid square or circle represent the affected individual. The half black solid circle or square represent variation carrier. The probands are indicated by arrows. V, variant. A double line indicates a consanguineous marriage (The parents of F2-II:1 and F2-II:2 are consanguineous). A diagonal indicates that the individual has died.

TABLE 3 | Identified variants in patients with BBS.

Patient	Gene*	Exon/ Intron	Nucleotide change	Protein change	Hom/ Het	PolyPhen-2	PROVEAN	SIFT	Mutation Taster	HSF	gnomAD	Rs	Report	ACMG
F1-II1	BBS2	Intron16	c.2059 + 1G > C		het	–	–	–	DC	MPADS	–	–	Novel	P (PVS1, PM2, PM3, PP1)
		Exon5	c.563delT	p.I188Tfs*13	het	–	–	–	DC	PADS	0.00001083	rs1367927635	Xing et al., 2014	P (PVS1, PS1, PM2, PM3)
F2-II:1, F2-II:2	BBS2	Exon1	c.79A > C	p.T27P	hom	benign	Neutral	Tolerated	Polymorphism	PADS	–	–	Novel	US (PM1, PM2, PP1, BP4)
F3-II:1, F3-II:2	BBS2	Intron4	c.534 + 1G > T		het	–	–	–	DC	MPADS	0.000101	rs773862084	Novel	P (PVS1, PM2, PP1)
		Exon11	c.1278A > G	p.E426E	het	–	Neutral	Tolerated	DC	PADS	–	–	Novel	US (PM2, PM3, PP1, BP4)
F4-II:1	BBS2	Exon9	c.944G > A	p.R315Q	het	PRD	Deleterious	Damaging	DC	PAAS	–	rs544773389	Katsanis et al., 2001	P (PS1, PM1, PM2, PM3, PP3)
		Exon9	c.1015C > T	p.R339*	het	–	–	–	DC	No impact	–	rs193922710	Shaheen et al., 2016	P (PVS1, PS1)
F5-II:1	BBS2	Intron16	c.2059 + 1G > T		het	–	–	–	DC	MPADS	–	–	Novel	P (PVS1, PM2, PM3, PP1)
		Intron4	c.534 + 1G > T		het	–	–	–	DC	MPADS	0.000101	rs773862084	Novel	P (PVS1, PM2, PP1)
F6-II:1	BBS4	Exon12	c.932G > A	p.G311D	het	PRD	Deleterious	Damaging	DC	No impact	–	–	Novel	P (PM1, PM2, PM3, PP1, PP3)
		Exon2	c.31C > T	p.Q11*	het	–	–	–	DC	PADS	–	–	Novel	P (PVS1, PM2, PP1)
F7-II:1	BBS7	Exon10	c.1002delT	p.N335Ifs*47	hom	–	–	–	DC	No impact	–	–	Chen et al., 2013	P (PVS1, PS1)
F8-II:1	BBS7	Exon8	c.728G > A	p.C243Y	het	PRD	Deleterios	Damaging	DC	No impact	0.00003974	rs727503821	Wang et al., 2013	P (PS1, PM2, PM3, PP1, PP3)
		Exon14	c.1395T > A	p.Y465*	het	–	–	–	DC	PADS	–	–	Novel	P (PVS1, PM2, PP1)
F9-II:1	BBS9	Exon6	c.445C > T	p.R149*	het	–	–	–	DC	PAAS	0.00001224	rs781174906	Novel	P (PVS1, PM2, PP1)
		Intron3	c.263 + 2delT		het	–	–	–	DC	MPADS	–	–	Novel	P (PVS1, PM2, PM3, PP1)
F10-II:1	BBS9	Exon2	c.72delT	p.L25Cfs*16	het	–	–	–	DC	No impact	–	–	Novel	P (PVS1, PM2, PM3, PP1)
		Intron10	c.1198 + 1G > A		het	–	–	–	DC	MPADS	–	–	Novel	P (PVS1, PM2, PM3)

*DC, disease causing; LP, likely pathogenic; MPADS, most probably affecting donor splicing; P, pathogenic; PAAS, potential alteration of acceptor splice site; PADS, potential alteration of donor splice site; POD, possibly damaging; PRD, probable damaging; –, not available; US, uncertain significance. *The transcripts of the four genes we used in this study for sequencing and refer were BBS2 (NM_031885.3), BBS4 (NM_033028.4), BBS7 (NM_176824.2), and BBS9 (NM_198428.2).*

Analysis of BBS Related Literatures

We performed a literature analysis of the BBS related literatures on both Chinese and foreigner patients (number of cases ≥ 7), focusing on the ocular characteristics shown in **Table 4**. The first report of a BBS case in the Chinese literature was in 1954. So far, more than 100 BBS patients distributed among 17 provinces in China have been reported (Wei et al., 1998), Among these cases, the initial eye symptoms were most of night blindness, vision decline, so as the foreign reports (Deveault et al., 2011; Berezovsky et al., 2012; Castro-Sánchez et al., 2015; Scheidecker et al., 2015; Esposito et al., 2017). The age at diagnostic exam ranged from 1 to 65 years, and most were later the actual age of onset. The consanguineous mating rate (10% in our study) ranged between 35 and 39% in these previous studies. Among these reports (**Table 4**), not all BBS cases met the criteria of four main characteristics or three main characteristics plus two secondary characteristics (Hulleman et al., 2016). However, the high penetrance of RP seemed to be universal among all the BBS patients. Moreover, compared with the other five main clinical manifestations, the proportion of renal abnormalities was found to be relatively low (Wei et al., 1998). Variations in *BBS1*, *BBS2*, and *BBS10* are the most common disease-causing genes among BBS patients in abroad (responsible for 50% of all cases). Thus far, our report, together with other local Chinese patient reports, suggests that the *BBS2* (20%) and *BBS7* (14.29%) genes are hot spot genes among Chinese BBS patients.

DISCUSSION

The detailed clinical and genetic characteristics of a cohort of 12 affected subjects from 10 Chinese families with BBS are illustrated in this study. To our knowledge, this is largest cohort of BBS patients by diagnosis using comprehensive clinical and genetic analysis to date in China. Although BBS has similar features and molecular overlap with Usher syndrome, Alström syndrome (OMIM 203800), McKusick-Kauffman (OMIM 604896) syndrome, Joubert syndrome (OMIM 213300, 608091, 608629, 609583, 610688, 611560, 61229, 612285, and 300804) or Meckel Gruber syndrome (OMIM 249000, 603294, 607361, and 611134), they are considered distinct clinical diseases, such as Alström syndrome (Pereiro et al., 2010) and Usher syndrome (Tsang et al., 2018) no polydactyly, or hypogonadism. Advanced gene sequencing technology has played an important role in helping distinguish between these similar genetic diseases. Although, *ALMS1* gene which belong to Alström syndrome was not tested genetically specially by the patients (F1-II:1, F3-II:1, and F3-II:2) which have hearing disturbances, the disease-causing gene of BBS we identified was co-segregated with the family members and phenotype. The BBS patients in our study did not all fully meet the clinical diagnosis criteria for BBS, especially with the low proportion of renal abnormalities. Wei et al. (1998) reviewed 65 Chinese cases published from 1956 to 1998, finding that renal abnormalities of patients accounted for only 10.6%, and only 44.6% of patients had five main features. Furthermore, the ratio of renal abnormalities in cases reported abroad has been very different (**Table 4**) (Imhoff et al., 2011), as the phenotypes of BBS cases in different regions have differed, including the unexpected high frequency of tooth anomalies in our cohort, which further confirmed the high heterogeneity phenotype of BBS patients.

In this study, we focus on the ocular characteristics of BBS patients and explore the similarities and differences between the cohort we reported and previous cases reported in China and abroad. It is always challenging for doctors to access the complete information regarding the development of the retina of BBS patients, since patients present with visual symptoms at a young age and their visit to an ocular department usually occurs later than their actual onset. Impaired vision and night blindness have been found to be the most common initial eye symptom in patients worldwide. In our study, 12 patients exhibited low vision and night blindness which was independent age and gender. Weihbrecht et al. (2017) reported more than 90% of individuals with BBS displayed rod-cone dystrophy with general early macular involvement. They also observed the retina morphology by fundus, FAF, and OCT, and accessed the retinal function via ffERG and mfERG. We found that the visual field could not be measured accurately in these BBS patients because the vision of these patients was considered too poor to perform the kinetic visual field testing. And in the objective vision function assessment via visual electrophysiology, the ffERG wave was mostly unrecordable. Scheidecker et al. (2015) reported macular atrophy in all BBS patients, and severely reduced and delayed ERG-light-adapted responses were found in most BBS patients. In general, FVEP testing can appraise the residual visual function of BBS patients, and FVEP changes seem to be consistent with BCVA impairment, suggesting the feasibility of using FVEP to assess residual visual function in patients with rod-cone dystrophy without detection of FERG response.

Researcher made effort to find the genotype-phenotype correlations in BBS families (**Table 4**) (Deveault et al., 2011; Daniels et al., 2012; Niederlova et al., 2019), but actually, it is high diversity among affected patients that existed the same genotype from one family (F2 and F3 in our study). In our study, we found that the clinical manifestations of the different genes did not differ significantly, and five patients with the same disease-causing gene in *BBS2* had completely different fundus morphological and functional changes. This indicated that the *BBS* genes and phenotypes are highly heterogeneous, which is consistent with previous findings (**Table 4**). In our study, we identified four pathogenic *BBS* genes (*BBS2, BBS4, BBS7*, and *BBS9*). Of those, *BBS2* was the most common in our cohort. We also identified a novel *BBS2* heterozygous variant c.534 + 1G > T in two families. Due to the small number of cases included in this study, it was not clear whether this is a hot spot variant of *BBS* in the Chinese population. However, the gene and its regional distributions, and even the distributions of hot spot variants have differed among studies (Mykytyn et al., 2002; Katsanis, 2004; Stoetzel et al., 2006; Ajmal et al., 2013). Yet variation in *BBS1*, *BBS2*, and *BBS10* are the most common

TABLE 4 | Clinical manifestations and disease-causing genes of patients with BBS from previous reports#.

Number (male/ female)	Age at diagnostic exam	Initial eye symptoms	RP	Polydactyly	Obesity	Intellectual disability	Abnormal Renal	Abnormal Gonad	Disease-causing gene (Top 3)	Report
Cases outside China										
83 (42/41)	mean age of 19 y, age range 50–64 y	Most are vision decline, nystagmus	100%	97%	92%	61%	53%	59%	BBS10 (*N* = 23), BBS1/BBS2 (*N* = 16), BBS12 (*N* = 12)	Deveault et al. (2011)
23 (15/8)	mean age of 15y, age range of 6~36 y	Most are night blindness, vision decline, vision field defect	100%	78%	91%	78%	30%	–	–	Berezovsky et al. (2012)
62 (30/32)	mean age of 21 y, age range 16–56 y	–	100%	–	–	–	–		BBS1 (*N* = 35), BBS2 (*N* = 6), BBS10 (*N* = 5)	Denniston et al. (2014)
52 (28/24)	mean age 6y	Most are night blindness, vision decline, vision field defect	100%	79%	88%	56%	23%	33%	BBS1(*N* = 33), BBS10 (*N* = 9), BBS12 (*N* = 8)	Castro-Sánchez et al. (2015)
7 (6/1)	mean age of 37 y, age range of 25~54 y	Most are vision decline	100%	100%	83%	42%	14%	42%	BBS10 (*N* = 3), BBS1/BBS5/ BBS6/BBS12 (*N* = 1)	Scheidecker et al. (2015)
12	mean age of 25y, age range of 9–65 y	vision decline	100%	–	–	–	75%	–	BBS1(*N* = 6), BBS1(*N* = 4), BBS2 (*N* = 2)	Esposito et al. (2017)
Domestic cases in China										
*65 (45/20)	1~37 y	–	72%	75%	89%	90%	10%	–	–	Wei et al. (1998)
2 (2/0)	32 y, 37 y	–	Yes	Yes	Yes	Yes	Yes	Yes	BBS7 (*N* = 2)	Yang et al. (2008)
6 (4/2)	–	–	Yes	Yes	Yes	Yes	–	16%	BBS2/BBS3 (*N* = 2), BBS6/BBS13 (*N* = 1)	Xing et al. (2014)
1 (0/1)	4 y	Night blindness, Vision decline	Yes	Yes	Yes	Yes	–	No	BBS4 (*N* = 1)	Li et al. (2014)
2 (1/1)	6 y	–	Yes	Yes	NO	Yes	Yes	Yes	BBS6 (*N* = 2)	Qi et al. (2017)
3 (1/2)	35 y, 37 y, 39 y	–	Yes	Yes	Yes	Yes	Yes	1M, the rest one are unknown	BBS7(*N* = 3)	Shen et al. (2019)
1 (1/0)	4 y	Night blindness, Vision decline, Vision field defect	Yes	Yes	Yes	NO	–	–	BBS2 (*N* = 1)	Dan et al. (2020)
5	–	–	20%	60%	80%	60%	–	–	BBS2 (*N* = 2), TM1M67/ BBS12 (*N* = 1)	Tang et al. (2020)
7 (6/1)	Mean age of 12 y, age range of 5~22 y	Night blindness, Vision field defect	Yes	Yes	Yes	Yes	1M, the rest are unknown	–	BBS2/BBS10 (*N* = 2)	Tao et al. (2020)

*N, number; –, not available. #Study aboard: number of patients ≥ 7, study in China: no limitation of number of patients. *This letter summarizes all cases of BBS reported in China since 1954.*

disease-causing genes among BBS patients abroad (responsible for 50% of all cases).

Overall, our study had some limitations. First, the number of enrolled patients was small. Second, we did not perform a longitudinal study regarding visual impairment. The changes in morphology and function of the retina should be followed up and correlated with different genes. Therefore, future studies with a larger sample size of BBS patients with BBS variants should be conducted using longitudinal clinical assessments and genotype-phenotype correlation analyses, not only in retina but also nephrology and endocrinology investigations and others to find some late syndromatic symptoms and signs (follow up by ophthalmologist, nephrologist and internist).

CONCLUSION

In our study, it demonstrated heterogeneous visual function and retinal morphology changes in these BBS patients. Our study expands the variation spectrum of *BBS*, and indicates that a combination of ffERG and FVEP may be helpful in evaluating the residual bioelectric activity of retina and visual pathway. To our knowledge, this is the largest cohort study with BBS patients in the Chinese population until now, we may conduct a large-scale screening BBS clinical cohort study among RP patients in China in the future.

ETHICS STATEMENT

The studies involving human participants were reviewed and approved by Ethics Review Board of Southwest Hospital, Army Medical University (Third Military Medical University) (Chongqing, China, KY2020096). Written informed consent was obtained from the individual(s), and minor(s)' legal guardian/next of kin, for the publication of any potentially identifiable images or data included in this article.

AUTHOR CONTRIBUTIONS

XM collected cases, evaluated clinical characteristics, molecular diagnosis, and wrote the manuscript. YL made the figures and tables, and management data. GW helped in data evaluating. JR and XY collected and organized the data. SL collected cases, and wrote and revised the manuscript.

ACKNOWLEDGMENTS

We acknowledge all the investigated family members for their cooperation, and very appreciate Minfang Zhang, Cheng Sun, Ziyang Li, and Min Wang for their help in this study.

REFERENCES

Ajmal, M., Khan, M. I., Neveling, K., Tayyab, A., Jaffar, S., Sadeque, A., et al. (2013). Exome sequencing identifies a novel and a recurrent *BBS1* mutation in Pakistani families with Bardet-Biedl syndrome. *Mol. Vis.* 19, 644–653.

Bardet, G. (1995). On congenital obesity syndrome with polydactyly and retinitis pigmentosa (a contribution to the study of clinical forms of hypophyseal obesity). *Obes. Res.* 3, 387–399. doi: 10.1002/j.1550-8528.1995.tb00165.x

Beales, P. L., Elcioglu, N., Woolf, A. S., Parker, D., and Flinter, F. A. (1999). New criteria for improved diagnosis of Bardet-Biedl syndrome: results of a population survey. *J. Med. Genet.* 36, 437–446.

Berezovsky, A., Rocha, D. M., Sacai, P. Y., Watanabe, S. S., Cavascan, N. N., and Salomão, S. R. (2012). Visual acuity and retinal function in patients with Bardet-Biedl syndrome. *Clinics* 67, 145–149. doi: 10.6061/clinics/2012(02)09

Biedl, A. (1995). A pair of siblings with adiposo-genital dystrophy. *Obes. Res.* 3:404. doi: 10.1136/bjo.81.5.378

Bölükbaşı, E. Y., Mumtaz, S., Afzal, M., Woehlbier, U., Malik, S., and Tolun, A. (2018). Homozygous mutation in CEP19, a gene mutated in morbid obesity, in Bardet-Biedl syndrome with predominant postaxial polydactyly. *J. Med. Genet.* 55, 189–197. doi: 10.1136/jmedgenet-2017-104758

Castro-Sánchez, S., Álvarez-Satta, M., Cortón, M., Guillén, E., Ayuso, C., and Valverde, D. (2015). Exploring genotype-phenotype relationships in Bardet-Biedl syndrome families. *J. Med. Genet.* 52:503. doi: 10.1136/jmedgenet-2015-103099

Chen, X., Zhao, K., Sheng, X., Li, Y., Gao, X., Zhang, X., et al. (2013). Targeted sequencing of 179 genes associated with hereditary retinal dystrophies and 10 candidate genes identifies novel and known mutations in patients with various retinal diseases. *Invest. Ophthalmol. Vis. Sci.* 54, 2186–2197. doi: 10.1167/iovs.12-10967

Choi, Y., and Chan, A. P. (2015). PROVEAN web server: a tool to predict the functional effect of amino acid substitutions and indels. *Bioinformatics* 31, 2745–2747. doi: 10.1093/bioinformatics/btv195

Dan, H., Huang, X., Xing, Y., and Shen, Y. (2020). Application of targeted panel sequencing and whole exome sequencing for 76 Chinese families with retinitis pigmentosa. *Mol. Genet. Genomic. Med.* 8:e1131. doi: 10.1002/mgg3.1131

Daniels, A. B., Sandberg, M. A., Chen, J., Weigel-DiFranco, C., Fielding, H. J., and Berson, E. L. (2012). Genotype-phenotype correlations in Bardet-Biedl syndrome. *Arch. Ophthalmol.* 130, 901–907. doi: 10.1001/archophthalmol.2012.89

Datta, P., Allamargot, C., Hudson, J. S., Andersen, E. K., Bhattarai, S., Drack, A. V., et al. (2015). Accumulation of non-outer segment proteins in the outer segment underlies photoreceptor degeneration in BardetBiedl syndrome. *Proc. Natl. Acad. Sci. U.S.A.* 112, E4400–E4409.

Denniston, A. K., Beales, P. L., Tomlins, P. J., Good, P., Langford, M., and Foggensteiner, L. (2014). Evaluation of visual function and needs in adult patients with bardet-biedl syndrome. *Retina* 34, 2282–2289. doi: 10.1097/IAE.0000000000000222

Desmet, F. O., Hamroun, D., Lalande, M., Collod-Béroud, G., Claustres, M., and Béroud, C. (2009). Human Splicing Finder: an online bioinformatics tool to predict splicing signals. *Nucleic. Acids. Res.* 37:e67. doi: 10.1093/nar/gkp215

Deveault, C., Billingsley, G., Duncan, J. L., Bin, J., Theal, R., Vincent, A., et al. (2011). BBS genotype-phenotype assessment of a multiethnic patient cohort calls for a revision of the disease definition. *Hum. Mutat.* 32, 610–619. doi: 10.1002/humu.21480

Esposito, G., Testa, F., Zacchia, M., Crispo, A. A., Di-Iorio, V., Capolongo, G., et al. (2017). Genetic characterization of Italian patients with Bardet-Biedl syndrome and correlation to ocular, renal and audio-vestibular phenotype: identification of eleven novel pathogenic sequence variants. *BMC. Med. Genet.* 17:10. doi: 10.1186/s12881-017-0372-0

Farag, T. I., and Teebi, A. S. (1988). Bardet-Biedl and laurence-moon syndromes in a mixed arab population. *Clin. Genet.* 33, 78–82. doi: 10.1111/j.1399-0004.1988.tb03414.x

Farag, T. I., and Teebi, A. S. (1989). High incidence of Bardet Biedl syndrome among the Bedouin. *Clin. Genet.* 36, 463–464. doi: 10.1111/j.1399-0004.1989.tb03378.x

Hood, D. C., Bach, M., Brigell, M., Keating, D., Kondo, M., Lyons, J. S., et al. (2012). ISCEV standard for clinical multifocal electroretinography (mfERG) (2011 edition). *Doc. Ophthalmol.* 124, 1–13. doi: 10.1007/s10633-011-9296-8

Hulleman, J. D., Nguyen, A., Ramprasad, V. L., Murugan, S., Gupta, R., Mahindrakar, A., et al. (2016). A novel H395R mutation in MKKS/BBS6 causes retinitis pigmentosa and polydactyly without other findings of Bardet-Biedl or McKusick-Kaufman syndrome. *Mol. Vis.* 22, 73–81.

Imhoff, O. V., Marion, C., Stoetzel, M., Durand, M., Holder, S., Sigaudy, P., et al. (2011). Bardet-Biedl syndrome: a study of the renal and cardiovascular phenotypes in a French cohort. *Clin. J. Am. Soc. Nephrol.* 6, 22–29. doi: 10.2215/CJN.03320410

Katsanis, N. (2004). The oligogenic properties of Bardet–Biedl syndrome. *Hum. Mol. Genet.* 13, 65–71. doi: 10.1093/hmg/ddh092

Katsanis, N., Ansley, S. J., Badano, J. L., Eichers, E. R., Lewis, R. A., Hoskins, B. E., et al. (2001). Triallelic inheritance in Bardet-Biedl syndrome, a Mendelian recessive disorder. *Science* 293, 2256–2259. doi: 10.1126/science.1063525

Khan, S. A., Muhammad, N., Khan, M. A., Kamal, A., Rehman, Z. U., and Khan, S. (2016). Genetics of human Bardet-Biedl syndrome, an updates. *Clin. Genet.* 90, 3–15. doi: 10.1111/cge.12737

Li, Q., Zhang, Y., Jia, L., and Peng, X. (2014). A novel nonsense mutation in BBS4 gene identified in a Chinese family with Bardet-Biedl syndrome. *Chin. Med. J.* 127, 4190–4196.

Mary, L., Chennen, K., Stoetzel, C., Antin, M., Leuvrey, A., Nourisson, E., et al. (2019). Bardet-Biedl syndrome: antenatal presentation of forty-five fetuses with biallelic pathogenic variants in known Bardet-Biedl syndrome genes. *Clin. Genet.* 95, 384–397. doi: 10.1111/cge.13500

McCulloch, D. L., Marmor, M. F., Brigell, M. G., Hamilton, R., Holder, G. E., Tzekov, R., et al. (2015). ISCEV Standard for full-field clinical electroretinography (2015 update). *Doc. Ophthalmol.* 130, 1–12. doi: 10.1007/s10633-014-9473-7

Moore, S. J., Green, J. S., Fan, Y., Bhogal, A. K., Dicks, E., Fernandez, B. A., et al. (2005). Clinical and genetic epidemiology of Bardet–Biedl syndrome in newfoundland: a 22-year prospective, population-based, cohort study. *Am. J. Med. Genet. A* 132, 352–360. doi: 10.1002/ajmg.a.30406

Mykytyn, K., Nishimura, D. Y., Searby, C. C., Shastri, M., Yen, H. J., Beck, J. S., et al. (2002). Identification of the gene (BBS1) most commonly involved in Bardet-Biedl syndrome, a complex human obesity syndrome. *Nat. Genet.* 31, 435–438. doi: 10.1038/ng935

Niederlova, V., Modrak, M., Tsyklauri, O., Huranova, M., and Stepanek, O. (2019). Meta-analysis of genotype-phenotype associations in Bardet-Biedl syndrome uncovers differences among causative genes. *Hum. Mutat.* 40, 2068–2087. doi: 10.1002/humu.23862

Nishimura, D. Y., Fath, M., Mullins, R. F., Searby, C., Andrews, M., Davis, R., et al. (2004). Bbs2-null mice have neurosensory deficits, a defect in social dominance, and retinopathy associated with mislocalization of rhodopsin. *Proc. Natl. Acad. Sci. U.S.A.* 23, 16588–16593. doi: 10.1073/pnas.0405496101

Pereiro, I., Hoskins, B. E., Marshall, J. D., Collin, G. B., Naggert, J. K., Piñeiro-Gallego, T., et al. (2010). Arrayed primer extension technology simplifies mutation detection in Bardet-Biedl and Alström syndrome. *Eur. J. Hum. Genet.* 19, 485–488. doi: 10.1038/ejhg.2010.207

Priya, S., Nampoothiri, S., Sen, P., and Sripriya, S. (2016). Bardet–Biedl syndrome: Genetics, molecular pathophysiology, and disease management. *Indian. J. Ophthalmol.* 64, 620–627. doi: 10.4103/0301-4738

Qi, Z., Shen, Y., Fu, Q., Li, W., Yang, W., Xu, W., et al. (2017). Whole-exome sequencing identified compound heterozygous variants in MMKS in a Chinese pedigree with Bardet-Biedl syndrome. *Sci. China. Life. Sci.* 60, 739–745. doi: 10.1007/s11427-017-9085-7

Riise, R., Andréasson, S., and Tornqvist, K. (1996). Full-field electroretinograms in individuals with the laurence-moon-Bardet-Biedl syndrome. *Acta Ophthalmol. Scand.* 74, 618–620. doi: 10.1111/j.1600-0420.1996.tb00747.x

Scheidecker, S., Hull, S., Perdomo, Y., Studer, F., Pelletier, V., Muller, J., et al. (2015). Predominantly cone-system dysfunction as rare form of retinal degeneration in patients with molecularly confirmed Bardet-Biedl syndrome. *Am. J. Ophthalmol.* 160, 364–372. doi: 10.1016/j.ajo.2015.05.007

Schwarz, J. M., Cooper, D. N., Schuelke, M., and Seelow, D. (2014). MutationTaster2: mutation prediction for the deep-sequencing age. *Nat. Methods* 11, 361–362. doi: 10.1038/nmeth.2890

Shaheen, R., Szymanska, K., Basu, B., Patel, N., Ewida, N., Faqeih, E., et al. (2016). Characterizing the morbid genome of ciliopathies. *Genome. Biol.* 17:242. doi: 10.1186/s13059-016-1099-5

Shen, T., Gao, J. M., Shou, T., Li, L., Zhang, J. P., Zhao, Q., et al. (2019). Identification of a homozygous BBS7 frameshift mutation in two (related) Chinese miao families with Bardet-Biedl syndrome. *J. Chin. Med. Assoc.* 82, 110–114. doi: 10.1097/jcma.0000000000000011

Stoetzel, C., Laurier, V., Davis, E. E., Muller, J., Rix, S., Badano, J. L., et al. (2006). BBS10 encodes a vertebrate-specific chaperonin-like protein and is a major BBS locus. *Nat. Genet.* 38, 521–524. doi: 10.1038/ng1771

Tang, X., Liu, C., Liu, X., Chen, J., Fan, X., Liu, J., et al. (2020). Phenotype and genotype spectra of a Chinese cohort with nephronophthisis-related ciliopathy. *J. Med. Genet.* 1–8. doi: 10.1136/jmedgenet-2020-107184

Tao, T., Wang, L., Chong, W., Yang, L., and Li, G. (2020). Characteristics of genotype and phenotype in Chinese patients with Bardet-Biedl syndrome. *Int. Ophthalmol.* 40, 2325–2343. doi: 10.1007/s10792-020-01415-3

Tsang, S. H., Aycinena, A. R. P., and Sharma, T. (2018). Ciliopathy: usher syndrome. *Adv. Exp. Med. Biol.* 1085, 167–170. doi: 10.1007/978-3-319-95046-4_32

Wang, X., Wang, H., Sun, V., Tuan, H. F., Keser, V., and Wang, K. (2013). Comprehensive molecular diagnosis of 179 Leber congenital amaurosis and juvenile retinitis pigmentosa patients by targeted next generation sequencing. *J. Med. Genet.* 50, 674–688. doi: 10.1136/jmedgenet-2013-101558

Wei, L. J., Pang, X., Duan, C., and Pang, X. (1998). Bardet-Biedl syndrome: a review of Chinese literature and a report of two cases. *Ophthalmic. Genet.* 19, 107–109. doi: 10.1076/opge.19.2.107.2315

Wei, Q., Zhang, Y., Li, Y., Zhang, Q., Ling, K., and Hu, J. (2012). The BBSome controls IFT assembly and turnaround in cilia. *Nat. Cell. Biol.* 14, 950–957. doi: 10.1038/ncb2560

Weihbrecht, K., Goar, W. A., Pak, T., Garrison, J. E., DeLuca, A. P., Stone, E. M., et al. (2017). Keeping an eye on Bardet-Biedl syndrome: a comprehensive review of the role of Bardet-Biedl syndrome genes in the eye. *Med. Res. Arch.* 5:10.18103/mra.v5i9.1526. doi: 10.18103/mra.v5i9.1526

Wormser, O., Gradstein, L., Yogev, Y., Perez, Y., Kadir, R., Goliand, I., et al. (2019). SCAPER localizes to primary cilia and its mutation affects cilia length, causing Bardet-Biedl syndrome. *Eur. J. Hum. Genet.* 27, 928–940. doi: 10.1038/s41431-019-0347-z

Xing, D. J., Zhang, H. X., Huang, N., Wu, K. C., Huang, X. F., Huang, F., et al. (2014). Comprehensive molecular diagnosis of Bardet-Biedl Syndrome by high-throughput targeted exome sequencing. *PLos One* 9:e90599. doi: 10.1371/journal.pone.0090599

Xu, Q., Zhang, Y., Wei, Q., Huang, Y., Li, Y., Ling, K., et al. (2015). BBS4 and BBS5 show functional redundancy in the BBSome to regulate the degradative sorting of ciliary sensory receptors. *Sci. Rep.* 5:11855. doi: 10.1038/srep11855

Yang, Z., Yang, Y., Zhao, P., Chen, K., Chen, B., Lin, Y., et al. (2008). A novel mutation in BBS7 gene causes Bardet-Biedl syndrome in a Chinese family. *Mol. Vis.* 14, 2304–2308.

3

Identification of Four Novel Variants and Determination of Genotype–Phenotype Correlations for ABCA4 Variants Associated with Inherited Retinal Degenerations

Qing Zhu[1], Xue Rui[2], Ya Li[1,3], Ya You[1,3], Xun-Lun Sheng[2] and Bo Lei[1,3]**

[1] Zhengzhou University People's Hospital, Henan Provincial People's Hospital, Zhengzhou, China, [2] Ningxia Clinical Research Center of Blinding Eye Disease, Ningxia Eye Hospital, People's Hospital of Ningxia Hui Autonomous Region, First Affiliated Hospital of Northwest University for Nationalities, Yinchuan, China, [3] Henan Branch of National Clinical Research Center for Ocular Diseases, Henan Eye Institute and Henan Eye Hospital, Henan Provincial People's Hospital, Zhengzhou, China

***Correspondence:**
Xun-Lun Sheng
shengxunlun@163.com
Bo Lei
bolei99@126.com

Purpose: The purpose of the study is to describe the genetic and clinical features of 17 patients with ABCA4-related inherited retinal degenerations (IRDs) and define the phenotype–genotype correlations.

Methods: In this multicenter retrospective study, 17 patients from 16 families were enrolled, and ABCA4 gene variants were detected using targeted next-generation sequencing using a custom designed panel for IRDs. Sanger sequencing and co-segregation analysis of the suspected pathogenic variants were performed with the family members. The pathogenicities of variants were evaluated according to the American College of Medical Genetics and Genomics guidelines (ACMG). Protein structure modifications mediated by the variants were studied using bioinformatic analyses.

Results: The probands were diagnosed with Stargardt disease 1 (7), cone-rod dystrophy type 3 (8), cone dystrophy (1), and retinitis pigmentosa 19 (1). Onset of symptoms occurred between 5 and 27 years of age (median age = 12.4 years). A total of 30 unique ABCA4 suspicious pathogenic variations were observed, including 18 missense mutations, seven frameshift mutations, two nonsense mutations, one canonical splice site mutation, one small in-frame deletion, and one insertion. Four novel ABCA4 variants were identified. Two novel frameshift variants, c.1290dupC (p.W431fs), and c.2967dupT (G990fs), were determined to be pathogenic. A novel missense variant c.G5761T (p.V1921L) was likely pathogenic, and another novel missense c.C170G (p.P57R) variant was of undetermined significance. All ABCA4 variants tested in this study inordinately changed the physico-chemical parameters and structure of protein based on *in silico* analysis.

Conclusion: ABCA4-related IRD is genetically and clinically highly heterogeneous. Four novel ABCA4 variants were identified. This study will expand the spectrum of disease-causing variants in ABCA4, which will further facilitate genetic counseling.

Keywords: ABCA4, inherited retinal degeneration, Stargardt diseases, cone-rod dystrophy, photoreceptor degeneration

INTRODUCTION

Inherited retinal degenerations (IRDs) are a group of blinding diseases that cause severe impairments of visual functions such as visual acuity and visual field. More than 270 disease-causing genes are associated with IRD (RetNet)[1]. Among them, ABCA4 is the most frequently identified gene (Kim et al., 2019; Pontikos et al., 2020). Mutations in the ABCA4 gene can cause various retinal diseases such as autosomal recessive (ar)-Stargardt disease (STGD1, OMIM # 248200), ar-cone-rod dystrophy (CORD3, OMIM # 604116), ar-cone dystrophy (COD), ar-retinitis pigmentosa (RP19, OMIM # 601718), and age-related macular degeneration-2 (ARMD2, OMIM # 153800) (van Driel et al., 1998; Baum et al., 2003; Burke and Tsang, 2011; Xin et al., 2015; Wang et al., 2018; Koyanagi et al., 2019).

ATP-binding cassette subfamily A member 4, denoted as ABCA4 (OMIM #601691), was first cloned by Allikmets et al. (Allikmets et al., 1997). The gene contains 50 exons, and it maps to position 22.1 (1p22.1) of the short (p) arm of chromosome 1 (Nasonkin et al., 1998). ABCA4 gene encodes a transmembrane protein that is exclusively expressed in photoreceptors and retina pigment epithelial cells (Lenis et al., 2018). The protein is composed of two non-equivalent tandem halves, and each half contains six transmembrane helices, a glycosylated extracytoplasmic domain (ECD) in the endolysosomes or disks, and a nucleotide binding domain in the cytoplasm. ATP-binding cassette transporter unidirectionally flips various compounds obtained from enzyme-catalyzed reactions of the visual cycle to the cytoplasm using the energy released from ATP hydrolysis (Kos and Ford, 2009; Quazi et al., 2012; Lenis et al., 2018). The misfolding and loss of functional activity of the transporter, caused by gene mutations, lead to accumulation of toxic substances such as all-trans-retinal and 11-cis-retinal in the outer segment of photoreceptor cells. Following diurnal phagocytosis of the distal outer segment of photoreceptors, excessive deposition of secondary toxic products, such as bisretinoid, eventually leads to the death of retinal pigment epithelium (Young and Bok, 1969; Weng et al., 1999; Quazi and Molday, 2014; Lenis et al., 2018). Different ABCA4 mutations lead to a broad range of IRD phenotypes (Rozet et al., 1998; van Driel et al., 1998; Xu et al., 2014; Garces et al., 2018). Phenotype severity mainly depends on the degree of influence of variations on protein functions (Fujinami et al., 2015).

Rapid advances in high-throughput next-generation sequencing technology have enabled an efficient and credible detection of gene mutations (Glöckle et al., 2014; Rong et al., 2018). Currently, 1,467 ABCA4 gene variants, containing a broad spectrum of IRD phenotypes, are present in the Human Gene Mutation Database[2] (updated on April, 2019). However, the pathogenicities of numerous reported variants have not been elucidated yet, making their accurate clinical diagnoses difficult, let alone those of novel variants. Additionally, the analyses of genotype–phenotype correlations for the highly heterogeneous variants and clinical features are a challenge.

Therefore, we conducted this retrospective study to determine the pathogenicities of ABCA4 gene variants and novel genotype–phenotype correlations.

MATERIALS AND METHODS

Ethical Approval

This multicenter retrospective study was conducted at the Henan Eye Hospital and the Ningxia Eye Hospital. The study was approved by the Medical Ethics Committees of both institutions, and it was conducted in accordance with the 1975 Declaration of Helsinki guidelines. Written informed consent was obtained from all included subjects or their guardians.

Subjects

Seventeen patients with retinal degeneration, carrying the ABCA4 gene variants and belonging to 16 unrelated Chinese families, were recruited in the study from ophthalmic clinics. Of these, 11 patients were enrolled from Henan Eye Hospital (B1–11) and six patients from Ningxia Eye Hospital (A1–6). Family history, if available, was obtained from the patients and unaffected family members. Detailed clinical data, including age of onset, disease duration, best-corrected visual acuity (BCVA), and result of color vision testing, fundus photography, fundus autofluorescence imaging, fundus fluorescein angiography, optical coherence tomography, and full-field electroretinogram, were collected. Diagnostic criteria were adapted from previous studies (Fishman, 1976; Hamel, 2007; Sahel et al., 2014; Aboshiha et al., 2016; Verbakel et al., 2018). Retina specialists performed phenotype subgroup classification on all 17 included subjects.

Mutation Screening

Whole genomic DNA was extracted from the peripheral blood of the subjects using the TIANamp Blood DNA kit DP318 (TIANGEN, Beijing, China) according to the manufacturer's protocol. A custom-designed posterior segment gene detection kit (PS400), containing 376 known causative IRD genes, their coding exons, flanking intronic sequences (50 bp), and all known intron mutations, was used for mutation screening. Sequence reads were aligned to the reference human genome (GRCh37/hg19) from the UCSC Genome Browser (Kent et al., 2002)[3] using the XYGeneRanger2.0 software. Suspicious disease-relevant gene variants were routinely confirmed using Sanger sequencing, and co-segregation analyses were conducted for all affected families.

In silico Analysis

All variants were classified according to the American College of Medical Genetics and Genomics (ACMG) standards and guidelines (Richards et al., 2015). To exclude the possibility of non-pathogenic polymorphism, the frequency of variations

[1] https://sph.uth.edu/retnet/

[2] http://www.hgmd.cf.ac.uk/ac/index.php

Abbreviations: IRDs, inherited retinal degenerations; ar, autosomal recessive; ACMG, American College of Medical Genetics and Genomics; ECD, extracytoplasmic domain; BCVA, best-corrected visual acuity.

[3] http://genome.ucsc.edu/

in the healthy control population was determined using the 1,000 Genomes Project (1,000 Genomes)[4] and the Genome Aggregation Database[5]. A variant was classified as benign if its minor allele frequency was ≥ 0.005. Prediction algorithms of the programs Polyphen-2[6], SIFT[7], PROVEAN[8], CADD[9], FATHMM (Shihab et al., 2013)[10], and MutationTaster[11] were used to test variants for disease relevance. Clustal Omega[12] was used to analyze the conservative loci. For the variants of uncertain significance. Human Splicing Finder (Desmet et al., 2009)[13] and Project HOPE (Venselaar et al., 2010)[14] were used to predict the splicing defects and structural effects of variants.

RESULTS

Clinical characteristics of patients are summarized in **Table 1**. Seven subjects were diagnosed with STGD1 (7/17, 41.2%), eight with CORD3 (8/17, 47%), one with RP19 (1/17, 5.9%), and one with COD (1/17, 5.9%). Hypopsia was the chief complaint in all 17 patients. The age of onset of diseases in patients ranged from 5 to 27 years with a median age of 12.4 years. The BCVA of the most recent evaluation ranged from 0.3 to 0.02 across the group. One RP19 patient (A1) and three patients with cone/cone-rod dystrophy had color vision disorders (A2, A4, and A5), all others possessed normal color vision.

Genotypic and phenotypic variations were observed in three patients, and others possessed a typical ABCA4-associated disease phenotype. Patient A1 was asymptomatic until 27 years of age. The patient was diagnosed with retinitis pigmentosa along with BCVA of 0.3 bilaterally. The patient carried heterozygous mutations for both ABCA4 (NM_000350: c.G2473A, p.G825R and c.G673A, p.V225M) and AHI1 (NM_001134830: c.G3267A, p.W1089X and c.T1979G, p.L660R), and color-vision testing revealed errors in the red-green axis. The cone-rod dystrophy patient (B1), who carried compound heterozygous variants (NM_000350: c.A2894G, p.N965S and c.2063dupA, p.N688fs) in the ABCA4 gene, complained of visual defects with strabismus for 25 years. Her latest BCVA was 0.05 bilaterally. Retinal degenerative features were observed in the fundus, and exposure of the underlying sclera was observed in the fovea of both eyes. Spectral domain optical coherence tomography scans through the fovea revealed retinal rupture with a subretinal cavitation in the fovea of the left eye (**Figure 1**). Patient B4, with two heterozygous missense mutations in ABCA4, had blurred vision in both eyes for 10 years, and fundus autofluorescence exhibited diffuse patches of macular atrophy with nascent fleck development in the mid-periphery (**Figure 1**), which is similar

[4]http://browser.1000genomes.org
[5]http://gnomad.broadinstitute.org/
[6]http://genetics.bwh.harvard.edu/pph2
[7]http://sift.jcvi.org
[8]http://provean.jcvi.org/index.php
[9]https://cadd.gs.washington.edu/
[10]http://fathmm.biocompute.org.uk/
[11]http://www.mutationtaster.org
[12]https://www.ebi.ac.uk/Tools/msa/clustalo/
[13]http://www.umd.be/HSF/
[14]https://www3.cmbi.umcn.nl/hope

TABLE 1 | Clinical characteristics, including ABCA4 variations, of the 17 patients in the study.

Patient	Diagnosis	Onset (y)	DD (y)	BCVA	ffERG[b]		ABCA4 Variation(s)
				OD/OS	Rods	Cones	
A1	RP19	27	7	0.3/0.3 +	NA	NA	c.G2473A; c.G673A
B1	CORD3	13	25	0.05/0.05	↓↓↓	↓↓↓	c.A2894G; c.2063dupA
B2	CORD3	20	13	0.04/0.05	↓↓	↓↓↓	c.A2894G; c.1290dupC
B3	CORD3	5	2	0.05/0.05	↓↓↓↓	↓↓↓↓	c.2967dupT; c.T4748C
B4	CORD3	17	10	0.06/0.05	↓	↓↓	c.C3322T; c.G1648A
B5	CORD3	12	6	0.05/0.02	↓	↓↓	c.A2894G; c.G3106A; c.A983T
A2	CORD3	9	1	0.15/0.15	↓↓	↓↓	1761-2A > G; c.C5512T
A3	CORD3	5	17	0.06/0.02	↓↓↓↓	↓↓↓↓	c.170_171insAA; c.C170G
A4	CORD3	10	10	0.05/0.15	NA	NA	c.1006delT; c.618_619insAAGGACATCGCCTGCAGC
A5	COD	13	4	0.15/0.12	↓	↓	c.A2894G; c.A1034G
B6[a]	STGD1	12	5	0.05/0.05	↓↓	↓↓↓	c.T1035G; c.A1034C
B7[a]	STGD1	12	0	0.05/0.05	↓	↓↓	c.T1035G; c.A1034C
B8	STGD1	11	1	0.05/0.07	NA	NA	c.C6118T; c.101_106del
B9	STGD1	6	10	0.04/0.05	NA	NA	c.4203delC; c.C203T
B10	STGD1	10	2	0.08/0.1	Normal	↓↓↓↓	c.1561delG; c.1760G > A
B11	STGD1	12	10	0.08/0.06	NA	NA	c.C5593T; c.G5761T; c.G3106A; c.C5318T
A6	STGD1	17	4	0.12/0.12	Normal	↓	c.C4070T; c.C4070T

y, years; DD, disease duration; OD, right eye; OS, left eye; ffERG, full-field electroretinogram; RP19, retinitis pigmentosa19; CORD3, cone-rod dystrophy 3; COD, cone dystrophy; STGD1, Stargardt disease 1; NA, not available; ↓↓↓↓, severely attenuated; ↓↓↓, moderate-severely attenuated; ↓↓, moderately/mild-moderately attenuated; ↓,mildly attenuated.
[a]Patients B4 and B5 are siblings.
[b]The right eye.

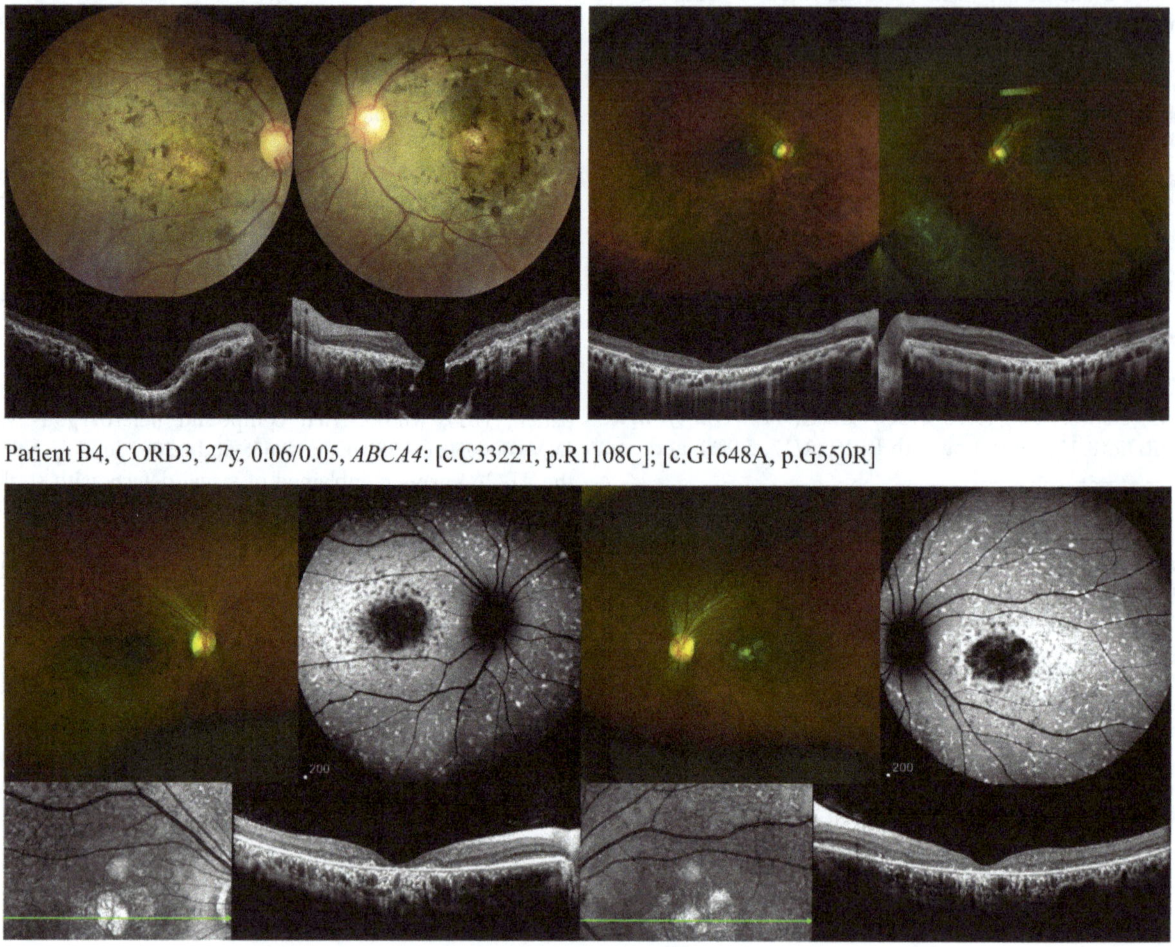

FIGURE 1 | Different ABCA4 mutations lead to a broad range of phenotypes of cone-rod dystrophy. Fundus of patient B1 exhibited a relatively pale and blonde appearance due to exposure of the underlying sclera and nummular pigmentary deposition in the fovea of both eyes. The fundus retinal pigmentation in patient B2 was mainly distributed in the mid-periphery. Wide-field color fundus photograph of patient B4 demonstrated diffuse pisciform flecks throughout the posterior pole, macular atrophy, and no obvious retinal pigmentation.

to the ABCA4 phenotype in the early stage of rapid-onset chorioretinopathy (Tanaka et al., 2018). Additionally, the STGD1 patients demonstrated typical fundus manifestations of macular atrophy with miscellaneous sizes (**Figure 2**).

We detected a total of 30 unique ABCA4 variants, including missense mutations (18), frameshift mutations (7), non-sense mutations (2), a splice site mutation (1), a small deletion (1), and an insertion (1). The 17 individuals, including one sibling pair, with at least two variants in the ABCA4 gene belonged to 16 families. Of the 30 rare ABCA4 variants, 24 were classified as pathogenic or likely pathogenic, and six were of uncertain significance. The pathogenicity of other mutated genes, except for the AHI1 in patient A1, was ruled out by phenotypic analysis. Frameshift mutations [c.1290dupC (p.W431fs) and c.2967dupT (G990fs)] and missense mutations [c.C170G (p.P57R) and c.G5761T (p.V1921L)] were novel unpublished variants (**Table 2**). The missense mutation c.A2894G (p.N965S) was detected four times without any exception in patients with cone/cone-rod dystrophy. The amino acid changes were primarily concentrated in ECD1 (47%, 14/30), and the amino acid variants were randomly distributed (**Figure 3**). Moreover, the HOPE online software revealed that all missense variants in this study inordinately changed the physico-chemical parameters or structure of ABCA4 (Appendix 1).

DISCUSSION

We identified four novel variants of the ABCA4 gene (**Figure 4**). According to ACMG standards and guidelines, two novel ABCA4 frameshift variants were pathogenic, one missense variant c.G5761T (p.V1921L) was likely pathogenic, and another missense variant c.C170G (p.P57R) was a variant of uncertain significance (**Appendix 2**).

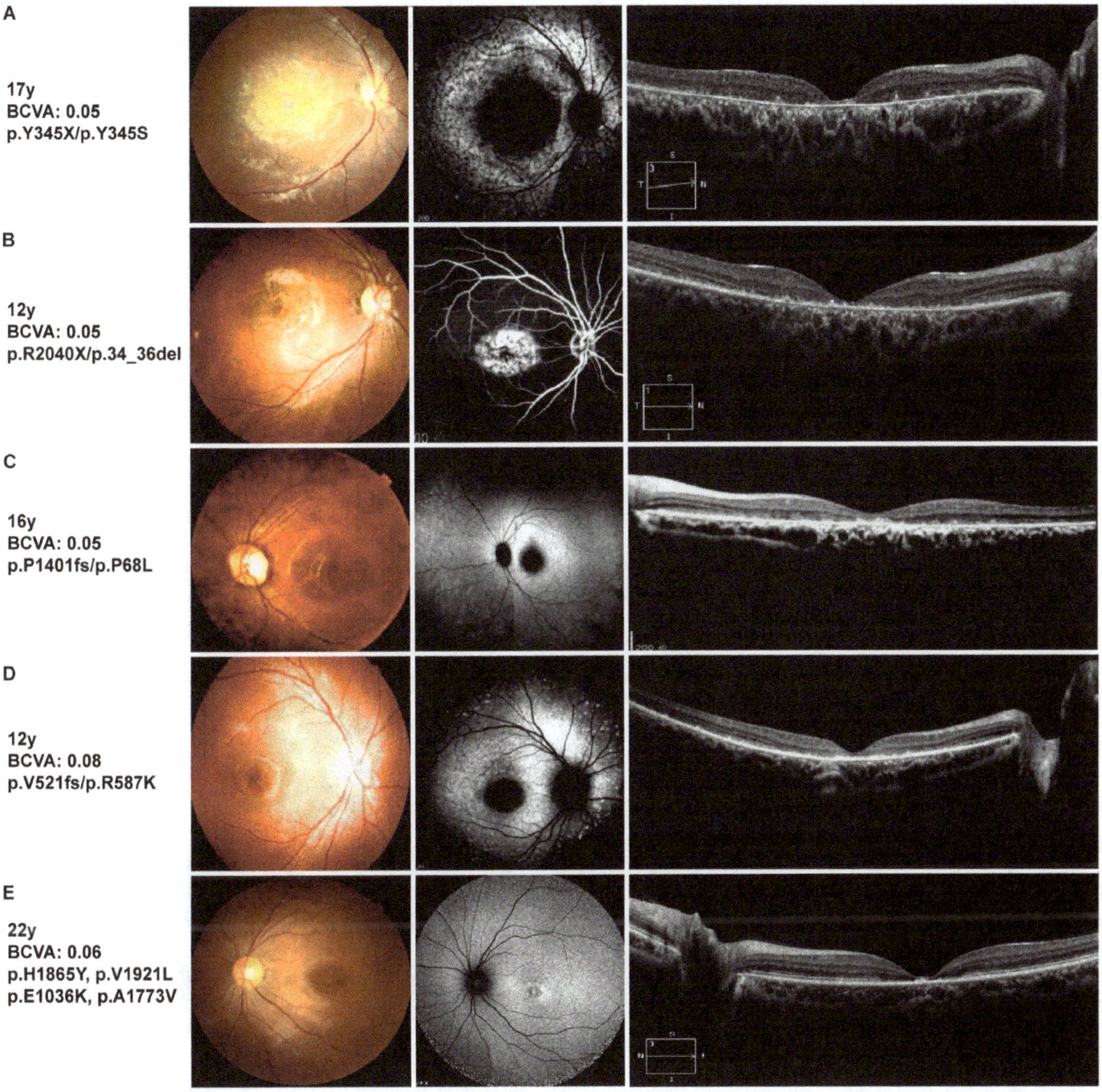

FIGURE 2 | Representative clinical features of STGD1 patients. Left: color fundus images, center: retinal autofluorescence imaging or fundus photography, right: optical coherence tomography images. **(A)** Patient B6, **(C)** Patient B9, and **(D)** Patient B10 harboring a compound heterozygous truncating mutation and missense mutation. Fundus autofluorescence shows hypo-autofluorescence at the fovea with different sizes of macula atrophy. Optical coherence tomography shows atrophy around the fovea of STGD1 with the most severe degeneration for patient B6. **(B)** Center-fluoresce in angiography of the right eye (AV-transit phase) of patient B8 showing a window defect in the area of bull's eye atrophy. The retinal deposits exhibit hyperfluorescence. **(E)** Fundus autofluorescence of patient B11, an individual with four ABCA4 missense mutations, showing a parafoveal hyperfluorescent ring.

The well-conserved VFVNFA motif (amino acids 2244–2249) present within the C-terminal of ABCA4 enables folding of the polypeptide into a functionally active protein (Zhong et al., 2009). Deletion of the C-terminal domain, including the VFVNFA motif, leads to a loss of ABCA4 functions, such as N-retinylidene-phosphatidylethanolamine substrate binding, ATP photoaffinity labeling, retinal-stimulated ATPase activity, and nucleotide binding domain interactions (Zhong et al., 2009; Patel et al., 2019). All frameshift and nonsense mutations of ABCA4 caused a removal of the C-terminal conserved sequence VFVNFA in the polypeptide. The downstream sequence of the VFVNFA motif also plays a role in regulating the functions of ABCA4 (Zhong et al., 2009). Protein-truncating mutations in ABCA4 leads to truncated protein products or protein loss due to nonsense-mediated RNA decay (Khajavi et al., 2006; Makelainen et al., 2019). Hence, the frameshift and nonsense ABCA4 mutations, which are defined as pathogenic according to ACMG guidelines, may have a great impact on gene expression

TABLE 2 | Pathogenicity analyses of ABCA4 (NM_000350) variants in the 17 Chinese patients.

Proband	Exon/ Intron	Nucleotide change	Protein Variant	Online Prediction: Polyphen[c] (Score)	SIFT (Score)	PROVEAN (Score)	CADD_Phred (Score)[d]	FATHMM (Score)	Mutation Taster	MAF in gnomAD[e] (%)	MAF in 1000G	Source[f]	Category
A1	16	c.G2473A	p.G825R	B (0.022)	T(0.411)	Neutral (−1.139)	12.55	Damaging (−2.4)	DC	0.0208	NA	rs368367104	VUS
	6	c.G673A	p.V225M	PrD (0.965)	D(0.006)	Neutral (−1.336)	17.34	Damaging (−2.9)	DC	0.2807	–	Koyanagi et al., 2019	VUS
B1	19	c.A2894G	p.N965S	PrD (0.961)	D(0.012)	Deleterious (−4.624)	25.9	Damaging (−3.59)	DC	0.04009	NA	Rosenberg et al., 2007	P
	14	c.2063dupA	p.N688fs	–	–	–	–		DC(NMD)	NA	NA	Xu et al., 2014	P
B2	19	c.A2894G	p.N965S	PrD (0.961)	D(0.012)	Deleterious (−4.624)	25.9	Damaging (−3.59)	DC	0.04009	NA	Rosenberg et al., 2007	P
	10	c.1290dupC	p.W431fs	–	–	–	–		DC(NMD)	NA	NA	Novel	P
B3	20	c.2967dupT	p.G990fs	–	–	–	–		DC(NMD)	NA	NA	Novel	P
	33	c.T4748C	p.L1583P	PoD (0.878)	D(0.002)	Deleterious (−4.466)	17.4	Damaging (−2.89)	DC	0.01087	NA	Kim et al., 2019	VUS
B4	22	c.C3322T	p.R1108C	PrD (0.937)	D(0.000)	Deleterious (−7.002)	25.8	Damaging (−3.73)	DC	0.005013	0.0599	Rozet et al., 1998	LP
	12	c.G1648A	p.G550R	PoD (0.523)	D(0.003)	Deleterious (−5.955)	18.07	Damaging (−5.12)	DC	0.000	NA	Shroyer et al., 2001	LP
B5	19	c.A2894G	p.N965S	PrD (0.961)	D(0.012)	Deleterious (−4.624)	25.9	Damaging (−3.59)	DC	0.04009	NA	Rosenberg et al., 2007	P
	21	c.G3106A	p.E1036K	B (0.010)	T(0.681)	Neutral (−0.820)	7.787	Damaging (−3.16)	DC	0.01631	NA	Nasonkin et al., 1998	LP
	8	c.A983T	p.E328V	B (0.236)	D(0.014)	Deleterious (−4.199)	15.46	Damaging (−2.83)	DC	0.005437	NA	Rivera et al., 2000	VUS
A2	IVS12	1761−2A > G	–	–	–	–	21.9	–	Acceptor splice sites abolished	0.005472	NA	Jiang et al., 2016	P
	39	c.C5512T	p.H1838Y	PrD (0.989)	D(0.001)	Deleterious (−4.625)	27.3	Damaging (−2.2)	DC	NA	NA	Lewis et al., 1999	LP
A3	3	c.170_171insAA	p.P57fs	–	–	–	–		DC(NMD)	NA	NA	Rong et al., 2018	P
	3	c.C170G	p.P57R	PoD(0.602)	D(0.006)	Deleterious (−5.667)	23	Damaging (−5.02)	DC	NA	NA	Novel	VUS
A4	8	c.1006delT	p.S336fs	–	–	–	–	–	DC(NMD)	NA	NA	Hu et al., 2019	P
	6	c.618_619ins AAGGACAT CGCCTGCAGC	p.E207delins KDIACSE	–	–	Deleterious (−7.314)	–	–	p	NA	NA	Tian et al., 2016	LP

(Continued)

TABLE 2 | Continued

				Online Prediction									
Proband	**Exon/ Intron**	**Nucleotide change**	**Protein Variant**	**Polyphen[c] (Score)**	**SIFT (Score)**	**PROVEAN (Score)**	**CADD_Phred (Score)[d]**	**FATHMM (Score)**	**Mutation Taster**	**MAF in gnomAD[e](%)**	**MAF in 1000G**	**Source[f]**	**Category**
A5	19	c.A2894G	p.N965S	PrD (0.961)	D(0.012)	Deleterious (−4.624)	25.9	Damaging (−3.59)	DC	0.04009	NA	Rosenberg et al., 2007	P
	8	c.A1034G	p.Y345C	PoD(0.808)	D(0.002)	Deleterious (−4.541)	21.6	Damaging (−2.77)	DC	NA	NA	rs1417184535	LP
B6a	8	c.T1035G	p.Y345X	–	–	–	36	–	DC(NMD)	NA	NA	Wang et al., 2018	P
	8	c.A1034C	p.Y345S	B (0.035)	D(0.003)	Deleterious (−4.529)	16.5	Damaging (−2.7)	DC	NA	NA	Jiang et al., 2016	LP
B7a	8	c.T1035G	p.Y345X	–	–	–	36	–	DC(NMD)	NA	NA	Wang et al., 2018	P
	8	c.A1034C	p.Y345S	B (0.035)	D(0.003)	Deleterious (−4.529)	16.5	Damaging (−2.7)	DC	NA	NA	Jiang et al., 2016	LP
B8	44	c.C6118T	p.R2040X	–	–	–	36	–	DC(NMD)	0.01504	NA	Baum et al., 2003	P
	2	c.101_106del	p.34_36del	–	–	Deleterious (−16.717)	–	–	DC	0.02719	NA	Huang et al., 2018	P
B9	28	c.4203delC	p.P1401fs	–	–	–	–	–	DC(NMD)	NA	NA	Jiang et al., 2016	P
	3	c.C203T	p.P68L	PoD(0.826)	D(0.003)	Deleterious (−6.677)	31	Damaging (−7.45)	DC	0.000	NA	Rivera et al., 2000	LP
B10	12	c.1561delG	p.V521fs	–	–	–	–	–	DC(NMD)	0.005437	NA	Xin et al., 2015	P
	12	c.1760G > A	p.R587K	B (0.270)	T(0.510)	Neutral (−1.224)	10.66	Damaging (−4.03)	DC	NA	NA	Fujinami et al., 2015	LP
B11	40	c.C5593T	p.H1865Y	B (0.006)	T(0.903)	Neutral (−0.888)	0.006	Damaging (−2.63)	p	0.1631	–	rs201707267	VUS
	41	c.G5761T	p.V1921L	PoD(0.625)	D(0.003)	Deleterious (−2.696)	27.9	Damaging (−3.66)	DC	NA	NA	Novel	LP
	21	c.G3106A	p.E1036K	B (0.01)	T(0.681)	Neutral (−0.820)	7.787	Damaging (−3.16)	DC	0.01631	NA	Nasonkin et al., 1998	LP
	38	c.C5318T	p.A1773V	PoD(0.892)	D(0.044)	Deleterious (−3.030)	21.3	Damaging (−1.73)	DC	0.005437	NA	Chacon-Camacho et al., 2013	P
A6	27	c.C4070T	p.A1357V	PoD(0.889)	D(0.001)	Deleterious (−3.710)	29.4	Damaging (−3.36)	DC	NA	NA	Noupuu et al., 2016	LP
	27	c.C4070T	p.A1357V	PoD(0.889)	D(0.001)	Deleterious (−3.711)	29.4	Damaging (−3.36)	DC	NA	NA	Noupuu et al., 2016	LP

MAF, minor allele frequency; B, benign; PrD, probably damaging; PoD, possibly damaging; T, tolerated; D, deleterious (<0.05); DC, disease causing; NMD, nonsense-mediated decay; p, polymorphism; NA, not appliable; –, not done; VUS, uncertain significance; LP, likely pathogenic; P, pathogenic. aSiblings. cHumVar. dThe threshold level was set to 10. eRefer to the frequency in East Asian population. fPublication or in dbSNP.

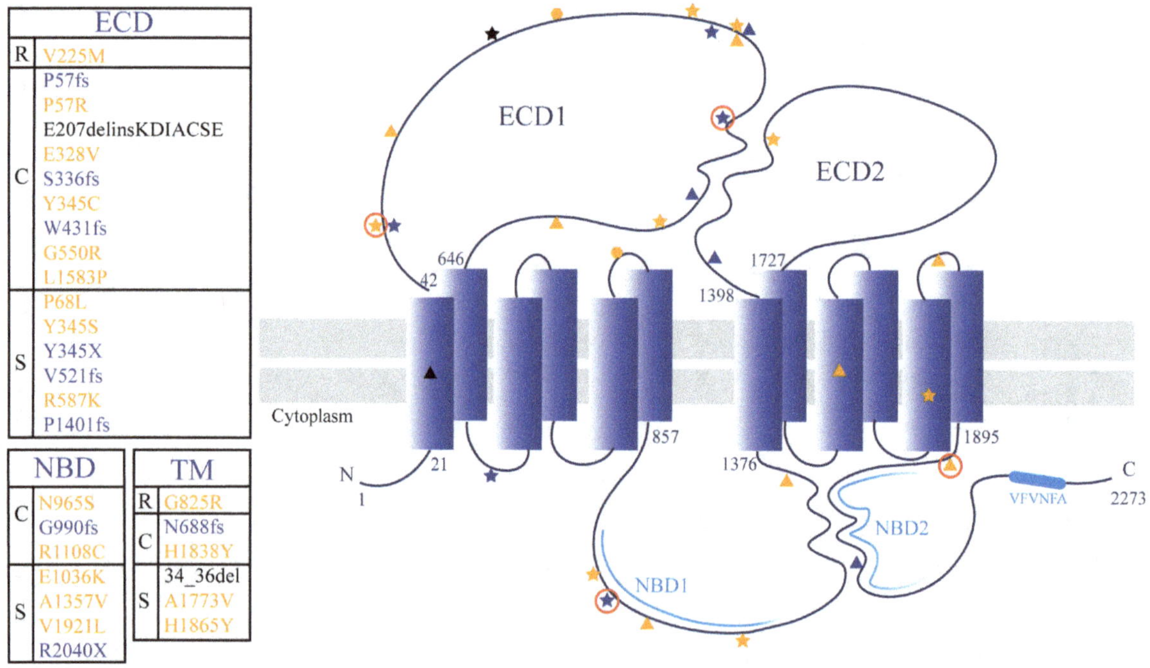

FIGURE 3 | Topological model of ABCA4 protein showing the distribution of detected mutations. The textbox on the left of the model shows correspondence between the locus and phenotype (R: RP19; C: CORD3/COD; S: STGD1). The sites associated with RP19, CORD3/COD, and STGD1 phenotypes are denoted with hexagon, pentagram, and triangle, respectively. Missense mutation, protein truncating mutation, and non-frame-shift deletion are colored yellow, blue, and black, respectively. The novel variants are circled in red.

and protein functions (**Table 2**). The allele frequencies of the small deletion mutation c.101_106del (p.34_36del) in two Chinese patient cohorts were 3.1% (Jiang et al., 2016) and 10.5% (Hu et al., 2019). This mutation, located in the transmembrane domain, is predicted to break the transmembrane helical structure, leading to ABCA4 transport dysfunction. The variant c.618_619insAAGGACATCGCCTGCAGC (p.E207delinsKDIACSE) inserted six amino acids in ECD1 of ABCA4, which was predicted to make ECD1 more hydrophobic and alter the protein structure. The mutation is associated with STGD1 disease (Tian et al., 2016).

The majority of identified ABCA4 sequence variants are missense mutations. Therefore, analysis of ABCA4-associated retinal degeneration is difficult. Additionally, determination of the pathogenicity of a particular variant is difficult. Testing the phenotypic associations of all amino acid substitutions along with experimental characterizations of their effects on protein functions would be extremely expensive and time consuming. Therefore, an online study of their putative effects would be conducive to prioritize the most probable disease-causing variations associated with these diseases. To further study the pathogenesis and possibility of amino acid substitutions that damage the protein, we analyzed the effects of variants on the protein using an online software (**Appendix 1**). Biochemical studies on ABCA4 missense mutations have reported that insertion of charged amino acids in transmembrane domains leads to a decrease in protein expression (Sun et al., 2000). Apart from the variations located in nucleotide-binding domains (Sun et al., 2000; Ahn et al., 2003), the missense mutations of ABCA4 gene, in or close to the transmembrane region, causing protein conformational changes can impair azido-ATP labeling to the nucleotide binding domains (Sun et al., 2000; Garces et al., 2018). Three cone–rod dystrophy patients (B1, B2, and B5) and one cone dystrophy patient (A5) harbored the missense mutation c.A2894G (p.N965S). The prevalence of the c.A2894G (p.N965S) mutation was higher in STGD1-affected individuals than in controls (Rosenberg et al., 2007; Jiang et al., 2016; Hu et al., 2019). Therefore, we hypothesized that patients carrying c.A2894G (p.N965S) might more likely manifest cone–rod dystrophy as the disease progresses, although the early stage may be an STGD1-like phenotype. The mutation, which is a replacement of asparagine with serine, resides in the conserved WalkerA sequence of nucleotide binding domain 1, which participates in nucleotide binding (Tsybovsky et al., 2013). An *in vivo* experiment concluded that p.N965S mutation causes a loss of substrate-dependent ATPase activity of ABCA4 and protein misfolding (Molday et al., 2018).

Patient B11 harbored four unique ABCA4 gene missense variants. The variant c.C5593T (p.H1865Y) and a novel variant c.G5761T (p.V1921L) were inherited from his healthy father. The missense variant c.G5761T (p.V1921L), adjacent to the transmembrane region, was likely pathogenic according to ACMG standards (**Table 2**). The variant c.C5593T (p.H1865Y), which has not been reported to date, was predicted as "tolerated" using a five-function prediction software. The other two missense mutations c.G3106A (p.E1036K) and c.C5318T (p.A1773V)

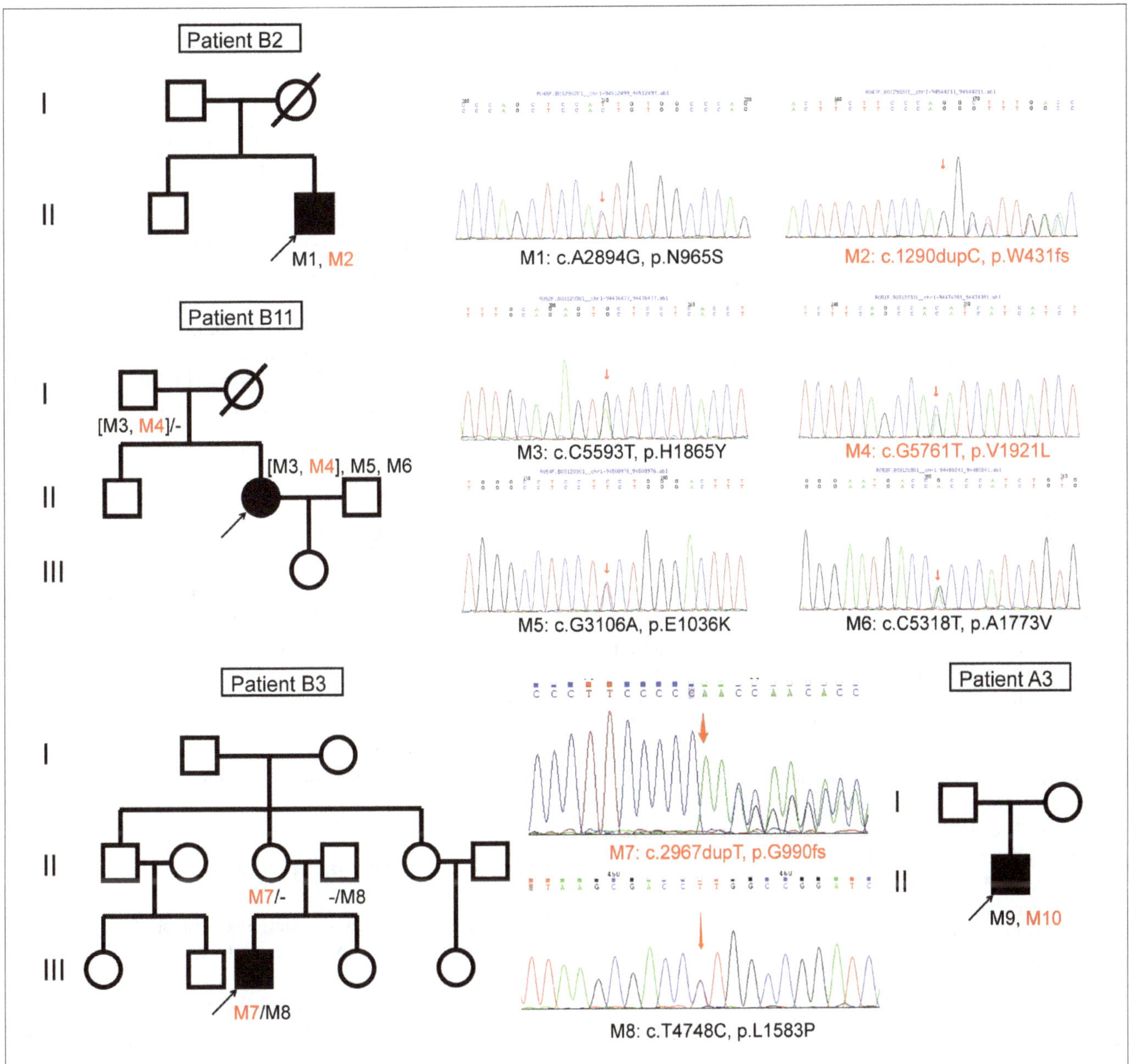

FIGURE 4 | Pedigrees of four Chinese families with inherited retinal disorders harboring the ABCA4 novel variants (red font).

were classified as STGD1 disease-related variants (Rivera et al., 2000; Chacon-Camacho et al., 2013). The variant c.C5318T (p.A1773V) was conserved and located in the transmembrane domain of the ABCA4 protein. The allele frequency of this mutation in an STGD1 patient cohort is significantly higher than that in the control group (Chacon-Camacho et al., 2013). According to bioinformatic analysis, it was disease causing. Homozygous p.Ala1773Val mutation leads to a severe phenotype, which is similar to that of patients harboring null ABCA4 variants (Lopez-Rubio et al., 2018). However, the fundus autofluorescence of patient B11 did not reveal extensive retinal atrophy (**Figure 2**), which may be related to the heterozygous state of the c.C5318T (p.A1773V) mutation. The trans variant may be a "milder" mutation. Patient A6 harbored a highly conserved ABCA4 homozygous mutation c.C4070T (p.A1357V), which was revealed to be consistently pathogenic using the six-function software. A patient harboring compound heterozygous variants of p.A1357V and p.G1961E has been reported to possess a foveal sparing (Noupuu et al., 2016). The p.G1961E mutation is usually associated with a late onset and mild phenotype (Lewis et al., 1999; Burke et al., 2012). Patient A6 was asymptomatic until 17 years of age, and the phenotype was milder compared with that of other patients. Considering this, we hypothesized that p.A1357V is not a severe mutation.

Genetic studies revealed that the patient A1 harbored variations in both ABCA4 and AHI1 genes. The two missense mutations c.G2473A (p.G825R) and c.G673A (p.V225M), located in ABCA4, were two variants of uncertain significance according to ACMG standards. Based on the analyses of the ABCA4 protein structure, p.G825R was located in the torsion angles of the transmembrane domain, which will force the local backbone into an incorrect conformation to disturb the local structure. p.V225M was located in ECD1, which will slightly destabilize the local conformation. The c.G3267A (p.W1089X) and c.T1979G (p.L660R) variants were identified in the AHI1 gene. The nonsense mutation was located in the SH3 domain of AHI1, and the missense mutation was located in the WD40 domain. Missense mutations in the WD40 domain of the AHI1 gene can underlie non-syndromic retinitis pigmentosa (Nguyen et al., 2017). ABCA4-related retinitis pigmentosa in patients is frequently caused by combinations of ABCA4 null mutations such as frameshift and splicing site mutations (van Driel et al., 1998; Shroyer et al., 2001; Huang et al., 2018). Thus, we suspect that the phenotype of patient A1 with retinitis pigmentosa may be a result of variations in both ABCA4 and AHI1 genes, which highlights the genotypic variability associated with ABCA4-related retinitis pigmentosa.

The missense mutations c.C203T (p.P68L), c.A1034G (p.Y345C), c.A1034C (p.Y345S), c.C5512T (p.H1838Y), c.G1648A (p.G550R), c.C4070T(p.A1357V), and c.C3322T (p.R1108C) have been conserved during evolution. The minor allele frequencies of these mutations in 1,000 Genomes and gnomAD database were less than 0.005. They were predicted as "deleterious" using SIFT, PROVEAN, CADD, FATHMM, and MutationTaster. Considering the lack of functional experiments to verify the effect of mutant residues and based on the results of HOPE, we classified them as "likely pathogenic" in accordance with the ACMG guidelines (**Table 2**). The missense mutations c.A983T (p.E328V) and c.T4748C (p.L1583P), and novel mutation c.C170G (p.P57R) were all located in ECD1 of ABCA4. The biological functions of the ECDs of ABCA4 were unknown, and the results of computer prediction were contradictory. The clinical significance of the three missense mutations was unclear.

According to the genotype–phenotype correlation model proposed by van Driel et al., the severity of the phenotype of ABCA4-related diseases is inversely proportional to the residual function of the mutant protein (van Driel et al., 1998). Hence, we could evaluate the severity and prognosis of ABCA4-related diseases using the genotype. Because the protein-truncating mutations cause nearly a complete loss of protein function, the residual function of protein caused by trans mutations primarily determines the severity of the phenotype. In this study, all 11 patients (B1, B2, B3, A3, A4, B6, B7, B8, B9, and B10) carried a severe ABCA4 gene variant, including frameshift mutations, nonsense mutations, and the missense mutation c. C5318T (p. A1773V). Additionally, the severity of the phenotype was related to the course of the disease; therefore, follow-up was highly recommended.

ABCA4-related retinal degeneration is genetically and clinically heterogeneous. The high allelic heterogeneity makes molecular genetic analysis of ABCA4-associated retinal disease challenging. We described the findings of mutational profiling of the ABCA4 gene and related clinical phenotypes, and we predicted the pathogenicities of newly discovered variants, which will expand the spectrum of disease-causing variants in ABCA4, and further facilitate genetic counseling. For the variants of unknown significance due to limited data, further experimental verification is needed to provide new insights into the molecular mechanisms of the disease, which may help in the development of precision medicine.

ETHICS STATEMENT

The studies involving human participants were reviewed and approved by The Medical Ethics Committee of People's Hospital of Ningxia Hui Autonomous Region and Henan Provincial Eye Hospital. Written informed consent to participate in this study was provided by the participants' legal guardian/next of kin. Written informed consent was obtained from the individual (s), and minor (s)' legal guardian/next of kin, for the publication of any potentially identifiable images or data included in this article.

AUTHOR CONTRIBUTIONS

BL and X-LS conceived and designed this study, directed the work, and finalized the manuscript. QZ and XR collected the clinical samples and clinical data. YL, YY, and QZ analyzed the sequencing data. QZ collected the information and drafted and revised the manuscript. All authors contributed to the article and approved the submitted version.

ACKNOWLEDGMENTS

We would like to thank all patients and their families for participating in this study. We would like to thank Editage (www.editage.com) for English language editing.

REFERENCES

Aboshiha, J., Dubis, A. M., Carroll, J., Hardcastle, A. J., and Michaelides, M. (2016). The cone dysfunction syndromes. *Br. J. Ophthalmol.* 100, 115–121. doi: 10.1136/bjophthalmol-2014-306505

Ahn, J., Beharry, S., Molday, L. L., and Molday, R. S. (2003). Functional interaction between the two halves of the photoreceptor-specific ATP binding cassette protein ABCR (ABCA4). Evidence for a non-exchangeable ADP in the first nucleotide binding domain. *J. Biol. Chem.* 278, 39600–39608. doi: 10.1074/jbc.M304236200

Allikmets, R., Singh, N., Sun, H., Shroyer, N. F., Hutchinson, A., Chidambaram, A., et al. (1997). A photoreceptor cell-specific ATP-binding transporter gene (*ABCR*) is mutated in recessive stargardt macular dystrophy. *Nat. Genet.* 15, 236–246. doi: 10.1038/ng0397-236

Baum, L., Chan, W. M., Li, W. Y., Lam, D. S. C., Wang, P. B., and Pang, C. P. (2003). *ABCA4* sequence variants in chinese patients with age-related macular degeneration or stargardt's disease. *Ophthalmologica.* 217, 111–114. doi: 10.1159/000068553

Burke, T. R., Fishman, G. A., Zernant, J., Schubert, C., Tsang, S. H., Smith, R. T., et al. (2012). Retinal phenotypes in patients homozygous for the G1961E mutation in the ABCA4 gene. *Invest. Ophthalmol. Vis. Sci.* 53, 4458–4467. doi: 10.1167/iovs.11-9166

Burke, T. R., and Tsang, S. H. (2011). Allelic and phenotypic heterogeneity in ABCA4 mutations. *Ophthalmic Genet.* 32, 165–174. doi: 10.3109/13816810.2011.565397

Chacon-Camacho, O. F., Granillo-Alvarez, M., Ayala-Ramirez, R., and Zenteno, J. C. (2013). ABCA4 mutational spectrum in Mexican patients with Stargardt disease: identification of 12 novel mutations and evidence of a founder effect for the common p.A1773V mutation. *Exp. Eye Res.* 109, 77–82. doi: 10.1016/j.exer.2013.02.006

Desmet, F. O., Hamroun, D., Lalande, M., Collod-Béroud, G., Claustres, M., and Béroud, C. (2009). Human splicing finder: an online bioinformatics tool to predict splicing signals. *Nucleic Acids Res.* 37:e67. doi: 10.1093/nar/gkp215

Fishman, G. A. (1976). Fundus flavimaculatus. a clinical classification. *Arch. Ophthalmol.* 94, 2061–2067. doi: 10.1001/archopht.1976.03910040721003

Fujinami, K., Zernant, J., Chana, R. K., Wright, G. A., Tsunoda, K., Ozawa, Y., et al. (2015). Clinical and molecular characteristics of childhood-onset stargardt disease. *Ophthalmology* 122, 326–334. doi: 10.1016/j.ophtha.2014.08.012

Garces, F., Jiang, K., Molday, L. L., Stohr, H., Weber, B. H., Lyons, C. J., et al. (2018). Correlating the expression and functional activity of ABCA4 disease variants with the phenotype of patients with stargardt disease. *Invest. Ophthalmol. Vis. Sci.* 59, 2305–2315. doi: 10.1167/iovs.17-23364

Glöckle, N., Kohl, S., Mohr, J., Scheurenbrand, T., Sprecher, A., Weisschuh, N., et al. (2014). Panel-based next generation sequencing as a reliable and efficient technique to detect mutations in unselected patients with retinal dystrophies. *Eur. J. Hum. Genet.* 22, 99–104. doi: 10.1038/ejhg.2013.72

Hamel, C. P. (2007). Cone rod dystrophies. *Orphanet J. Rare Dis.* 2:7. doi: 10.1186/1750-1172-2-7

Hu, F. Y., Li, J. K., Gao, F. J., Qi, Y. H., Xu, P., Zhang, Y. J., et al. (2019). ABCA4 Gene screening in a chinese cohort with stargardt disease: identification of 37 novel variants. *Front. Genet.* 10:773. doi: 10.3389/fgene.2019.00773

Huang, X., Yuan, L., Xu, H., Zheng, W., Cao, Y., Yi, J., et al. (2018). Identification of a novel mutation in the *ABCA4* gene in a chinese family with retinitis pigmentosa using exome sequencing. *Biosci. Rep.* 38. doi: 10.1042/BSR20171300

Jiang, F., Pan, Z., Xu, K., Tian, L., Xie, Y., Zhang, X., et al. (2016). Screening of ABCA4 gene in a chinese cohort with stargardt disease or cone-rod dystrophy with a report on 85 novel mutations. *Invest. Ophthalmol. Vis. Sci.* 57, 145–152. doi: 10.1167/iovs.15-18190

Kent, W. J., Sugnet, C. W., Furey, T. S., Roskin, K. M., Pringle, T. H., Zahler, A. M., et al. (2002). The human genome browser at UCSC. *Genome Res.* 12, 996–1006. doi: 10.1101/gr.229102

Khajavi, M., Inoue, K., and Lupski, J. R. (2006). Nonsense-mediated mRNA decay modulates clinical outcome of genetic disease. *Eur. J. Hum. Genet.* 14, 1074–1081. doi: 10.1038/sj.ejhg.5201649

Kim, M. S., Joo, K., Seong, M. W., Kim, M. J., Park, K. H., Park, S. S., et al. (2019). Genetic mutation profiles in korean patients with inherited retinal diseases. *J. Korean Med. Sci.* 34:e161. doi: 10.3346/jkms.2019.34.e161

Kos, V., and Ford, R. C. (2009). The ATP-binding cassette family: a structural perspective. *Cell Mol. Life. Sci.* 66, 3111-3126. doi: 10.1007/s00018-009-0064-69

Koyanagi, Y., Akiyama, M., Nishiguchi, K. M., Momozawa, Y., Kamatani, Y., Takata, S., et al. (2019). Genetic characteristics of retinitis pigmentosa in 1204 japanese patients. *J. Med. Genet.* 56, 662–670. doi: 10.1136/jmedgenet-2018-105691

Lenis, T. L., Hu, J., Ng, S. Y., Jiang, Z., Sarfare, S., Lloyd, M. B., et al. (2018). Expression of ABCA4 in the retinal pigment epithelium and its implications for stargardt macular degeneration. *Proc. Natl. Acad. Sci. U.S.A.* 115, E11120–E11127. doi: 10.1073/pnas.1802519115

Lewis, R. A., Shroyer, N. F., Singh, N., Allikmets, R., Hutchinson, A., Li, Y., et al. (1999). Genotype/phenotype analysis of a photoreceptor-specific ATP-binding cassette transporter gene, *ABCR*, in Stargardt disease. *Am. J. Hum. Genet.* 64, 422–434. doi: 10.1086/302251

Lopez-Rubio, S., Chacon-Camacho, O. F., Matsui, R., Guadarrama-Vallejo, D., Astiazaran, M. C., and Zenteno, J. C. (2018). Retinal phenotypic characterization of patients with ABCA4 retinopathydue to the homozygous p.Ala1773Val mutation. *Mol. Vis.* 24, 105–114.

Makelainen, S., Godia, M., Hellsand, M., Viluma, A., Hahn, D., Makdoumi, K., et al. (2019). An ABCA4 loss-of-function mutation causes a canine form of Stargardt disease. *PLoS Genet.* 15:e1007873. doi: 10.1371/journal.pgen.1007873

Molday, L. L., Wahl, D., Sarunic, M. V., and Molday, R. S. (2018). Localization and functional characterization of the p.Asn965Ser (N965S) ABCA4 variant in mice reveal pathogenic mechanisms underlying Stargardt macular degeneration. *Hum. Mol. Genet.* 27, 295–306. doi: 10.1093/hmg/ddx400

Nasonkin, I., Illing, M., Koehler, M. R., Schmid, M., Molday, R. S., and Weber, B. H. (1998). Mapping of the rod photoreceptor ABC transporter (ABCR) to 1p21–p22.1 and identification of novel mutations in stargardt's disease. Hum. Genet. 102, 21–26. doi: 10.1007/s004390050649

Nguyen, T. T., Hull, S., Roepman, R., van den Born, L. I., Oud, M. M., de Vrieze, E., et al. (2017). Missense mutations in the WD40 domain of AHI1 cause non-syndromic retinitis pigmentosa. *J. Med. Genet.* 54, 624–632. doi: 10.1136/jmedgenet-2016-104200

Noupuu, K., Lee, W., Zernant, J., Greenstein, V. C., Tsang, S., and Allikmets, R. (2016). Recessive Stargardt disease phenocopying hydroxychloroquine retinopathy. *Graefes Arch. Clin. Exp. Ophthalmol.* 254, 865–872. doi: 10.1007/s00417-015-3142-3148

Patel, M. J., Biswas, S. B., and Biswas-Fiss, E. E. (2019). Functional significance of the conserved C-Terminal VFVNFA motif in the retina-specific ABC transporter, ABCA4, and its role in inherited visual disease. *Biochem. Biophys. Res. Commun.* 519, 46–52. doi: 10.1016/j.bbrc.2019.08.121

Pontikos, N., Arno, G., Jurkute, N., Schiff, E., Ba-Abbad, R., Malka, S., et al. (2020). Genetic basis of inherited retinal disease in a molecularly characterized cohort of more than 3000 families from the United Kingdom. *Ophthalmology* 127, 1384–1394. doi: 10.1016/j.ophtha.2020.04.008

Quazi, F., Lenevich, S., and Molday, R. S. (2012). ABCA4 is an N-retinylidene-phosphatidylethanolamine and phosphatidylethanolamine importer. *Nat. Commun.* 3:925. doi: 10.1038/ncomms1927

Quazi, F., and Molday, R. S. (2014). ATP-binding cassette transporter ABCA4 and chemical isomerization protect photoreceptor cells from the toxic accumulation of excess 11-cis-retinal. *Proc. Natl. Acad. Sci. U S A.* 111, 5024–5029. doi: 10.1073/pnas.1400780111

Richards, S., Aziz, N., Bale, S., Bick, D., Das, S., Gastier-Foster, J., et al. (2015). Standards and guidelines for the interpretation of sequence variants: a joint consensus recommendation of the American College of Medical Genetics and Genomics and the Association for Molecular Pathology. *Genet. Med.* 17, 405–424. doi: 10.1038/gim.2015.30

Rivera, A., White, K., Stohr, H., Steiner, K., Hemmrich, N., Grimm, T., et al. (2000). A comprehensive survey of sequence variation in the ABCA4 (ABCR) gene in Stargardt disease and age-related macular degeneration. *Am. J. Hum. Genet.* 67, 800–813. doi: 10.1086/303090

Rong, W. N., Wang, X. G., and Sheng, X. L. (2018). ABCA4 mutations and phenotype of different hereditary retinopathies in 3 pedigrees. *Chin. J. Ophthalmol.* 54, 775–781. doi: 10.3760/cma.j.issn.0412-4081.2018.10.011

Rosenberg, T., Klie, F., Garred, P., and Schwartz, M. (2007). N965S is a common ABCA4 variant in stargardt-related retinopathies in the danish population. *Mol. Vis.* 13, 1962–1969.

Rozet, J. M., Gerber, S., Souied, E., Perrault, I., Châtelin, S., Ghazi, I., et al. (1998). Spectrum of ABCR gene mutations in autosomal recessive macular dystrophies. *Eur. J Hum. Geneti.* 6, 291–295. doi: 10.1038/sj.ejhg.5200221

Sahel, J.-A., Marazova, K., and Audo, I. (2014). Clinical characteristics and current therapies for inherited retinal degenerations. *Cold Spring Harb. Perspect. Med.* 5:a017111. doi: 10.1101/cshperspect.a017111

Shihab, H. A., Gough, J., Cooper, D. N., Stenson, P. D., Barker, G. L. A., Edwards, K. J., et al. (2013). Predicting the functional, molecular, and phenotypic consequences of amino acid substitutions using hidden Markov models. *Hum. Mutat.* 34, 57–65. doi: 10.1002/humu.22225

Shroyer, N. F., Lewis, R. A., Yatsenko, A. N., and Lupski, J. R. (2001). Null missense ABCR (ABCA4) mutations in a family with stargardt disease and retinitis pigmentosa. *Invest. Ophthalmol. Vis. Sci.* 42, 2757–2761.

Sun, H., Smallwood, P. M., and Nathans, J. (2000). Biochemical defects in ABCR protein variants associated with human retinopathies. *Nat. Genet.* 26, 242–246. doi: 10.1038/79994

Tanaka, K., Lee, W., Zernant, J., Schuerch, K., Ciccone, L., Tsang, S. H., et al. (2018). The rapid-onset chorioretinopathy phenotype of ABCA4 disease. *Ophthalmology* 125, 89–99. doi: 10.1016/j.ophtha.2017.07.019

Tian, L., Jiang, F., Xu, K., Zhang, X. H., Sun, T. Y., Lu, N., et al. (2016). Characteristics of ABCA4 genotype in Chinese patients with Stargardt disease. *Ophthalmol CHN* 25, 219–224.

Tsybovsky, Y., Orban, T., Molday, R. S., Taylor, D., and Palczewski, K. (2013). Molecular organization and ATP-induced conformational changes of ABCA4, the photoreceptor-specific ABC transporter. *Structure* 21, 854–860. doi: 10.1016/j.str.2013.03.001

van Driel, M. A., Maugeri, A., Klevering, B. J., Hoyng, C. B., and Cremers, F. P. (1998). ABCR unites what ophthalmologists divide(s). *Ophthalmic Genet.* 19, 117–122. doi: 10.1076/opge.19.3.117.2187

Venselaar, H., Te Beek, T. A., Kuipers, R. K., Hekkelman, M. L., and Vriend, G. (2010). Protein structure analysis of mutations causing inheritable diseases. an e-science approach with life scientist friendly interfaces. *BMC Bioinformatics* 11:548. doi: 10.1186/1471-2105-11-548

Verbakel, S. K., van Huet, R. A. C., Boon, C. J. F., den Hollander, A. I., Collin, R. W. J., Klaver, C. C. W., et al. (2018). Non-syndromic retinitis pigmentosa. *Prog. Retin. Eye Res.* 66, 157–186. doi: 10.1016/j.preteyeres.2018.03.005

Wang, X. G., Liu, H. J., Zhang, S. C., Qi, X. L., Pan, B., Zhuang, W. J., et al.(2018). Genotype and clinical phenotype analysis in patients with retinitis pigmentosa and cone rod dystrophy. *Chin. J. Ocul. Fundus. Dis.* 34, 526–535. doi: 10.3760/cma.j.issn.1005-1015.2018.06.002

Weng, J., Mata, N. L., Azarian, S. M., Tzekov, R. T., Birch, D. G., and Travis, G. H. (1999). Insights into the function of Rim protein in photoreceptors and etiology of Stargardt's disease from the phenotype in abcr knockout mice. *Cell* 98, 13–23. doi: 10.1016/s0092-8674(00)80602-80609

Xin, W., Xiao, X., Li, S., Jia, X., Guo, X., and Zhang, Q. (2015). Identification of genetic defects in 33 probands with stargardt disease by WES-based bioinformatics gene panel analysis. *PloS One* 10:e0132635. doi: 10.1371/journal.pone.0132635

Xu, Y., Guan, L., Shen, T., Zhang, J., Xiao, X., Jiang, H., et al. (2014). Mutations of 60 known causative genes in 157 families with retinitis pigmentosa based on exome sequencing. *Hum. Genet.* 133, 1255–1271. doi: 10.1007/s00439-014-1460-2

Young, R. W., and Bok, D. (1969). Participation of the retinal pigment epithelium in the rod outer segment renewal process. *J. Cell Biol.* 42, 392–403. doi: 10.1083/jcb.42.2.392

Zhong, M., Molday, L. L., and Molday, R. S. (2009). Role of the C terminus of the photoreceptor ABCA4 transporter in protein folding, function, and retinal degenerative diseases. *J. Biol. Chem.* 284, 3640–3649. doi: 10.1074/jbc.M806580200

4

Genotype Profile of Global EYS-Associated Inherited Retinal Dystrophy and Clinical Findings in a Large Chinese Cohort

Ke Xu[1], De-Fu Chen[2], Haoyu Chang[1], Ren-Juan Shen[1], Hua Gao[2], Xiao-Fang Wang[2], Zhuo-Kun Feng[2], Xiaohui Zhang[1], Yue Xie[1], Yang Li[1]* and Zi-Bing Jin[1]**

[1] *Beijing Ophthalmology and Visual Science Key Laboratory, Beijing Tongren Eye Center, Beijing Tongren Hospital, Beijing Institute of Ophthalmology, Capital Medical University, Beijing, China,* [2] *School of Ophthalmology and Optometry, The Eye Hospital, Wenzhou Medical University, Wenzhou, China*

***Correspondence:**
De-Fu Chen
ysgcdf@foxmail.com
Yang Li
yanglibio@aliyun.com
Zi-Bing Jin
jinzb502@ccmu.edu.cn

Purpose: The aim of this study was to probe the global profile of the EYS-associated genotype-phenotype trait in the worldwide reported IRD cases and to build a model for predicting disease progression as a reference for clinical consultation.

Methods: This retrospective study of 420 well-documented IRD cases with mutations in the *EYS* gene included 39 patients from a genotype-phenotype study of inherited retinal dystrophy (IRD) conducted at the Beijing Institute of Ophthalmology and 381 cases retrieved from global reports. All patients underwent ophthalmic evaluation. Mutations were revealed using next-generation sequencing, followed by Sanger DNA sequencing and real-time quantitative PCR analysis. Multiple regression models and statistical analysis were used to assess the genotype and phenotype characteristics and traits in this large cohort.

Results: A total of 420 well-defined patients with 841 identified mutations in the *EYS* gene were successfully obtained. The most common pathogenic variant was a frameshift c.4957dupA (p.S1653Kfs*2) in exon 26, with an allele frequency of 12.7% (107/841), followed by c.8805C > A (p.Y2935X) in exon 43, with an allele frequency of 5.9% (50/841). Two new hot spots were identified in the Chinese cohort, c.1750G > T (p.E584X) and c.7492G > C (p.A2498P). Several EYS mutation types were identified, with CNV being relatively common. The mean age of onset was 20.54 ± 11.33 (4–46) years. Clinical examinations revealed a typical progression of RPE atrophy from the peripheral area to the macula.

Conclusion: This large global cohort of 420 IRD cases, with 262 distinct variants, identified genotype-phenotype correlations and mutation spectra with hotspots in the *EYS* gene.

Keywords: inherited retinal dystrophy, copy number variations, mutation spectrum, hot spot mutation, genotype-phenotype trait, EYS mutation

INTRODUCTION

Inherited Retinal Dystrophy (IRD) includes a variety of genetic retinal disorders linked with disease-causing mutations. It is characterized by progressive retinal degeneration and photoreceptor loss (Bernardis et al., 2016; Broadgate et al., 2017), and has a global prevalence rate of 1 in 2000–3000 (Hartong et al., 2006). The primary form of progressive IRD is retinitis pigmentosa (RP) (OMIM #268000), with a global incidence of ~1 in 4,000 births and 2.5 million affected patients (Hartong et al., 2006; Dias et al., 2018). RP is a highly heterogeneous genetic disorder in humans (Bandah-Rozenfeld et al., 2010), with more than 100 causative genes identified (a detailed list is available at the RetNet database[1] and the RetinoGenetics database[2]) (Ran et al., 2014). RP shows a significant genetic heterogeneity, with multiple inherited patterns including autosomal recessive (AR), autosomal dominant (AD), and X-linked (XL) forms (Bunker et al., 1984; Grøndahl, 1987).

Mutations in the eyes shut homolog (*EYS*) gene, one of the most prevalent causes of RP, account for about 5-10% of ARRP (Audo et al., 2010; Barragán et al., 2010; Littink et al., 2010; Hosono et al., 2012). The *EYS* mutations were first reported as a genetic cause of ARRP in 2008 (Abd El-Aziz et al., 2008; Collin et al., 2008). The *EYS* gene has 43 exons and is located on chromosome 6q12. Spanning approximately 2 MB, this gene is one of the largest genes identified in the human genome (Abd El-Aziz et al., 2008; Barragán et al., 2010; Littink et al., 2010). The gene encodes a protein located in the outer segment of the photoreceptor cells (Abd El-Aziz et al., 2008) and is an ortholog of the Drosophila spacemaker (spam) protein. The protein is encoded by the longest isoform of the gene, containing 3165 amino acids, and is subdivided into 28 epidermal growth factor-like (EGF) domains and 5 Laminin A G-like domains at the C-terminus (Abd El-Aziz et al., 2008; Bandah-Rozenfeld et al., 2010; Barragán et al., 2010). Functionally, the EYS protein is indispensable for sustaining the morphological stability of the photoreceptor (Abd El-Aziz et al., 2008). However, the exact pathogenic role of the protein requires further elucidation.

The large number of EYS mutations reported to date in many independent studies prompted the present study aimed at assessing the effects of each mutation. The correlations between genotype and phenotype have not yet been well defined in patients with EYS mutations. We included 420 participants with *EYS* mutations in the present study to explore the possible correlations between genotypes and clinical phenotypes. Our findings provide a global profile of *EYS*-associated genotype-phenotype traits in patients with IRD and a model for predicting the progression of the disease as a reference for clinical consultation.

[1] https://sph.uth.edu/retnet/

[2] http://www.retinogenetics.org/

SUBJECTS AND METHODS

Study Subjects

The study was conducted in compliance with the protocols of the Medical Ethics Committee of Beijing Tongren Hospital and with the tenets of the Declaration of Helsinki. We classified 39 unrelated patients with *EYS* gene variants who had a diagnosis of *EYS*-IRD as group one (G1). This group included nine probands with family histories and 30 sporadic cases, making it the largest cohort of *EYS* patients with genetic and clinical information in Asia to date. Every study participant provided informed consent for the clinical and genetic studies. All patients' medical and family histories were taken carefully; these histories mainly covered the chief complaints of the initial ocular symptoms (such as low vision or night blindness), onset age of the disease, and clinical information about their available relatives. Ophthalmic examinations, including best-corrected visual acuity, slit-lamp biomicroscopy, subjective and objective optometry, and fundus photography, were performed for each participant. Some patients also underwent optical coherence tomography (OCT), full-field electroretinography (ERG), and autofluorescence imaging (AF).

We also retrospectively investigated 381 previously reported index probands from various populations who carried *EYS* mutations and included their available clinical information published until June 2020; these patients were classified as group two (G2). Detailed literature sources for the G2 group variants are provided in **Supplementary Table 1**. In brief, our study included 420 patients divided into two cohorts.

Targeted Exome Sequencing and Bioinformatics Analysis

Peripheral venous blood samples of each participant and their available family members were collected. Genomic DNA was extracted from the peripheral leukocytes according to standard extraction protocols using the Whole Blood Genomic DNA Extraction Kit (Vigorous, Beijing, China). The DNA concentration was quantified with a NanoDrop 2000 device (Thermal Fisher Scientific, DE) (Chen et al., 2020).

The participants' genetic information was analyzed with subsequent targeted exon sequencing (TES) to develop a sequencing panel including 188 known inherited retinal degeneration (IRD) genes (Sun et al., 2018). The Illumina library preparation, capture experiments, sequencing raw data analysis, and subsequent bioinformatics evaluation have been described previously (Sun et al., 2018). Multiple databases were used for annotation and evaluation of the variants, and the pathogenicity of missense variants was predicted *in silico* by Mutation Taster, PolyPhen-2, and SIFT. Variants with a potential splicing effect were predicted based on their ada-boost and random forest scores. We appraised the sequence variant classifications based on the American College of Medical Genetics and Genomics (ACMG) policies and guidelines (Richards et al., 2015). The HGMD database was used to query reported pathogenic mutations. Real-time quantitative PCR was performed for three probands to confirm the presumed copy number variations (CNV) of *EYS*. All the putative pathogenic EYS variants

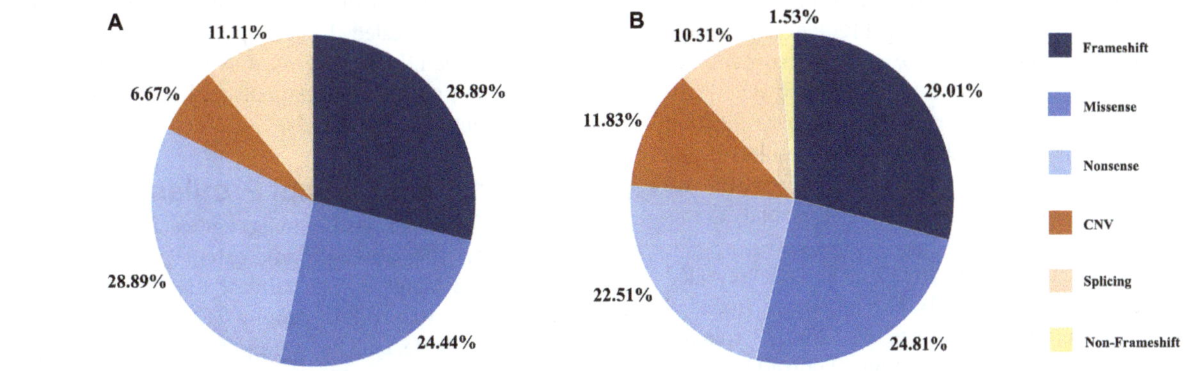

FIGURE 1 | Distribution of the variant types in this study. **(A)** Proportion of variant types in G1 cohort. **(B)** Proportion of variant types in two cohort, G1 and G2.

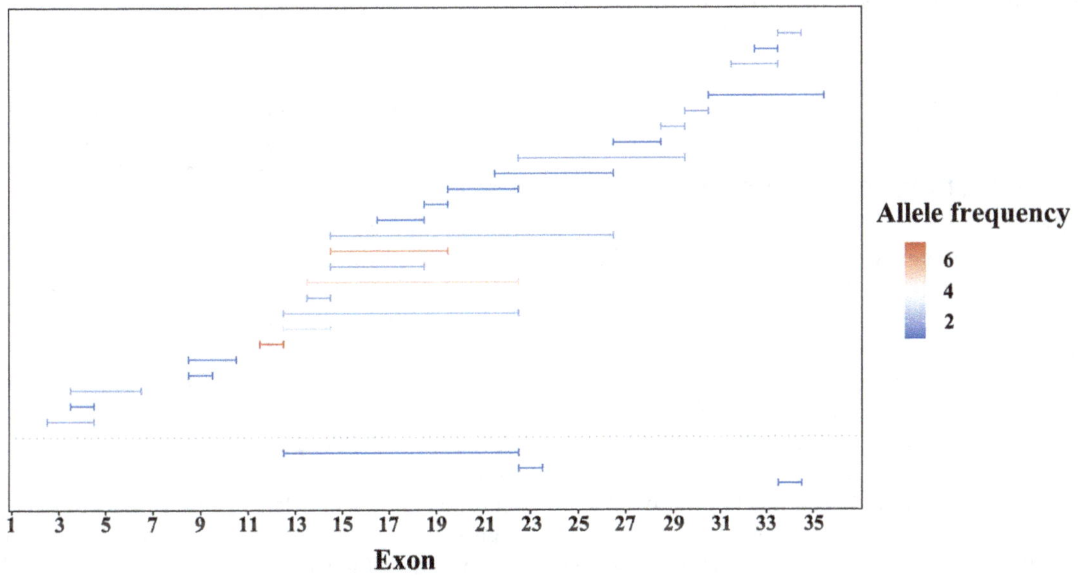

FIGURE 2 | Copy number variations (CNV) of *EYS* gene in this study. CNV in G1 cohort under the dotted line and G2 cohort above. Lengths of the horizontal line represents the CNV range. Color from blue to red indicate an increase in allele frequency.

(NM_001142800) were validated using Sanger sequencing. The available family members were evaluated for co-segregation.

Statistical Analysis

Statistical analyses were performed using SPSS version 22.0 software (IBM, Corp., Armonk, NY, United States). The best corrected visual acuity (BCVA) was converted to the logarithm of minimum angle of resolution (logMAR) unit for statistical analysis. Logistic regression analysis was performed to evaluate the visual progression by calculating the probability of low vision or blindness observed at different ages. The WHO criteria were used to set low vision and legal blindness as $0.05 \leq \text{BCVA} < 0.3$ and $\text{BCVA} < 0.05$, respectively. A p-value < 0.05 was considered statistically significant. The Kolmogorov-Smirnov test was performed to assess the normal distribution of visual acuity. The Wilcoxon Rank Sum Test was performed to evaluate the difference between genotypes.

RESULTS

Molecular Diagnosis in EYS Gene

In the G1 cohort, we identified 45 distinct causal or likely causal variants, including 11 missense, 13 nonsense, 13 frameshift, 5 splice-site, and 3 CNV mutations (**Figure 1A**). Of these 45 mutations, the most prevalent was c.6557G > A (p.G2186E), identified 7 times with an allele frequency 9% (7/78), followed by c.1750G > T (p.E584X) and c.7492G > C (p.A2498P) with allele frequencies of 6.4% (5/78), and variants c.7228 + 1G > A and c.8805C > A (p.Y2935X) with allele frequencies of 5.1% (4/78). This was the first report of 19 of these 45 variants and included 4 new missense, 7 new nonsense, 6 new frameshift, and 3 new CNV mutations. Two novel missense variants, c.359C > G (p.T120R) and c.9002C > T (p.A3001V), were identified in two unrelated probands. The *in silico* analysis programs of SIFT showed that these mutations could be damaging, while the

Mutation Taster and Polyphen2 programs indicated they were likely benign. The frequency of variant p.T120R was less than 0.005 in database ExAC and gnomAD, and the frequency of variant p.A3001V was not recorded in any public databases; therefore, according to the ACMG guidelines, the classification of these two mutations is uncertain. Detailed results of the frequency and pathogenicity analyses of G1 group variants are presented in **Supplementary Table 2**. Cosegregation analysis was performed in 39 families.

A summary of the genetic data from G1 and G2 revealed 262 variants among the 420 probands. The mutations included 76 frameshift, 65 missense, 59 nonsense, 31 CNV, 27 splicing change, and 4 non-frameshift indel mutations (**Figure 1B**). Most of these variants were clustered in exon 26 and exon 43. The most common pathogenic variant was a frameshift c.4957dupA (p.S1653Kfs*2) in exon 26, with an allele frequency of 12.7% (107/841), followed by a c.8805C > A (p.Y2935X) variant in exon 43, with an allele frequency was 5.9% (50/841). Mutations in exons 4, 16, and 32 were also common, whereas the remaining variants were distributed across the whole gene. CNV was more common in exons 12–22 (**Figure 2**).

Evaluation of Genotype–Phenotype Correlations

We stratified all patients into six groups to obtained a better assessment of the relationship between the genotypes of two mostly common pathogenic variants (M1: p.S1653Kfs*2 and M2: p.Y2935X) and the *EYS*-IRD phenotypes (e.g., BCVA, and onset age). Grouped as follows: group I, 40 patients, carried only one of the two mutation hot spots, M1; group II, 24 patients, carried M1 homozygous mutation; group III, 16 patients, carried only one of the two mutation hot spots, M2; group IV, 7 patients, carried M2 homozygous mutation; group V, 18 patients, carried M1 and M2 compound heterozygosity mutation; group VI, 315 patients, without carried the above two common mutation. Comparison of the differences in age of onset and the severity of the loss of visual acuity of six groups and sorting the age of onset from left to right (**Figure 3**) revealed that group I and group IV had an earlier onset age than the other groups. No significant difference was noted in the proportion of patients with specific degrees of visual impairment in each group.

Participants and Clinical Profiles in G1

In total, 39 affected *EYS*-IRD subjects were included in this study (G1 cohort); 30 were sporadic cases, 9 were ARRP, and all of them were Chinese. The clinical diagnosis was RP in 38 patients, and cone-rod dystrophy (CORD) in 1 patient (**Supplementary Table 1**). The average age of onset and age at first visit were 20.54 ± 11.33 (4–46) and 37.33 ± 11.36 (14–48) years, respectively. The average best corrected visual acuity (LogMAR) was 0.74 ± 1.06 (0–5) in this cohort. We identified the visual prognosis of *EYS*-IRD subjects by exploring the probability of low vision and blindness at different ages. The regression model was as follows: probability of low vision is $\mathrm{Ln}(P/1 - P) = 0.145 \times \text{age} - 7.163$ and probability of blindness is $\mathrm{Ln}\ (P/1 - P) = 0.098 \times \text{age} - 6.56$. When the cut-off probability was delimited as > 50%, the age of visual acuity when low vision and blindness were reached was 50 and 55 years.

All 38 probands with *EYS*-RP presented typical RP symptoms, with the most common initial symptom being nyctalopia. The visual field subsequently constricted and vision decreased. Lens opacities were present in 13 patients, with the youngest being 35 years old. No patients presented with nystagmus. Observation of the patients with different courses of disease by fundus photography revealed atrophy of the RPE in the peripheral retina and typical progression of RPE atrophy from the periphery to the macula, with disease aggravation and classic bone spicule pigmentation consistently appearing in the mid-peripheral retina; the macula was also sometimes affected in the later stages (**Figure 4**). The OCT images showed thinning of the outer retina, RPE atrophy with high reflection sediments, gradually reduction of the thickness of the ellipsoid and interdigitation zone until

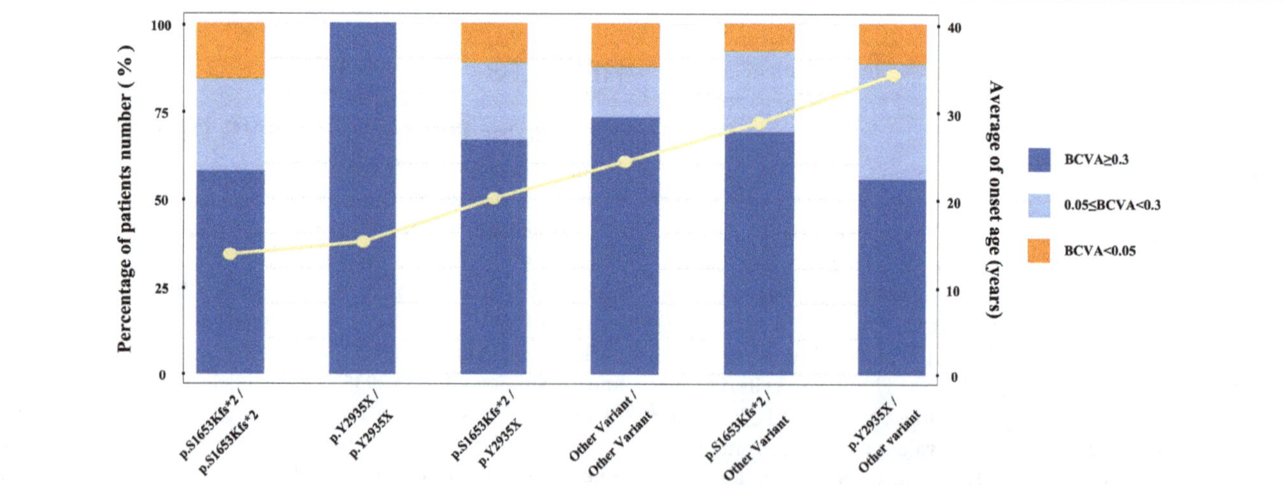

FIGURE 3 | Relationship between average age at onset and specific causative mutation. The histogram displays the proportion distribution of three visual impairment levels, represented in different colors. The yellow line represents the average age at onset.

it completely disappeared from the peripheral region to the macular fovea, and a relative preservation of the retinal layers in the central macula. In patient 191,025, we noticed some cysts in the left OCT, located in the inner nuclear layer. Four *EYS*-RP probands underwent AF examination. The course of their disease ranged from 5 to 31 years, and they showed progression of abnormal fundus autofluorescence consistent with the fundus appearance (**Figure 4**). ERGs were all extinguished except in patient 19,562, whose ERGs showed a severe decrease in rod and cone function.

Patient 10,364, carrying homozygous c.8805C > A (p.Y2935X), was the only EYS-CORD patient. This patient was 31 years old and had experienced vision impairment at 5 years old, without nyctalopia. Fundus photography showed a marked atrophy of the macula and pigment deposition in the peripheral retina. His OCT shown thinning of the full retinal layers, disappearance of the ellipsoid zone, atrophy of the RPE layer with high granular reflection, and enhancement of the reflection bands of the choroid tissue. AF showed a dark macular area and a hyperfluorescent ring within the vascular arcade. The ERG showed a severely decreased amplitude (**Figure 4**).

DISCUSSION

The eyes shut homolog (*EYS*; OMIM: 612424) is a major disease-causing gene for autosomal recessive retinitis pigmentosa, and is mainly found in Chinese and Japanese populations

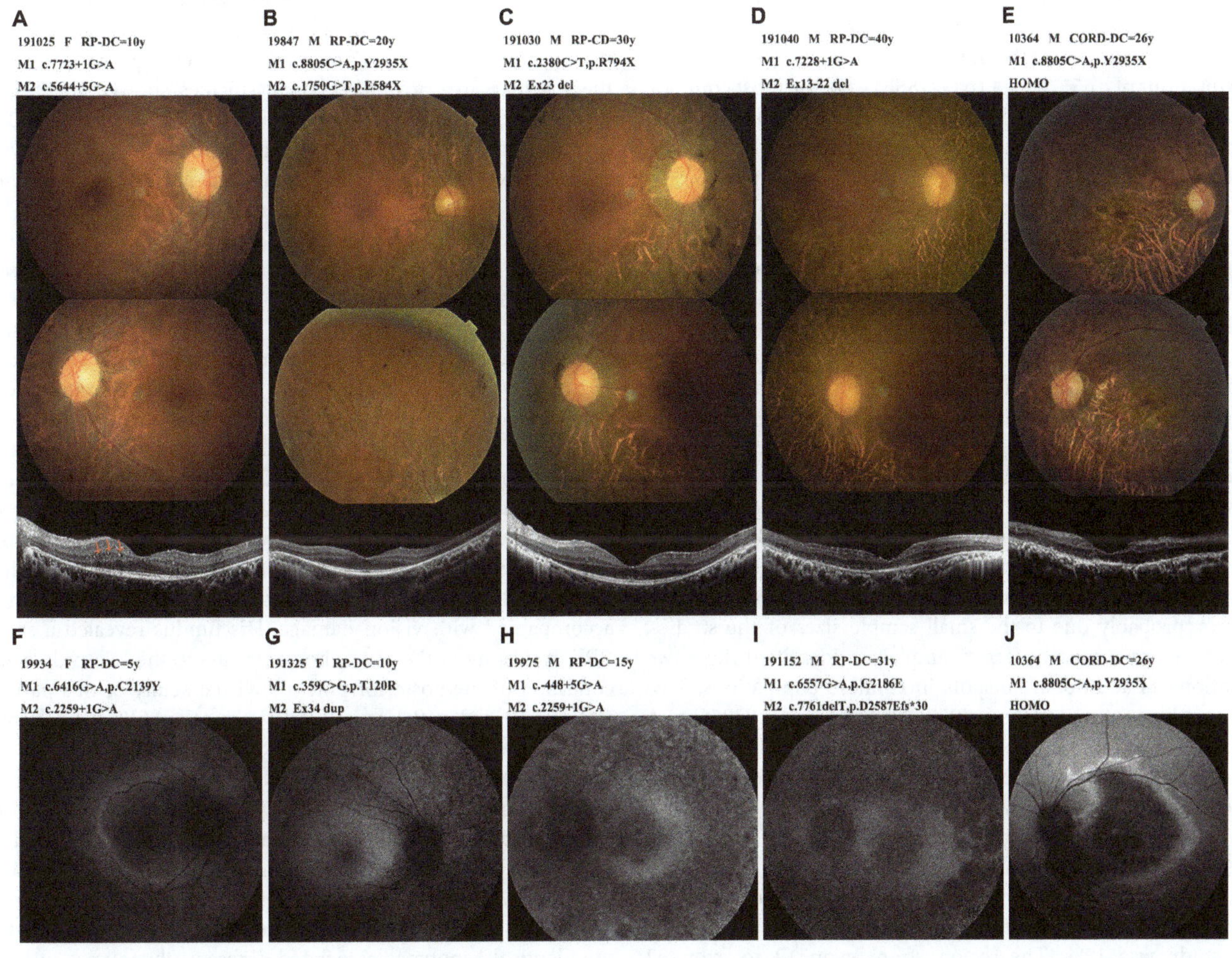

FIGURE 4 | The photographs characteristics of the patients with different courses. **(A)** A 22-year-old female (191025) diagnosed with RP, showed RPE atrophic changes outside the vessel arcade without pigmentation, OCT with some cysts in the inner nuclear layer (arrow-heads). **(B)** A 44-year-old male (19847) diagnosed with RP, pigmentations were scattered in the peripheral retina. OCT showed relatively preserved macular structure. **(C)** A 43-year-old male (191030) diagnosed with RP, extensive choroid atrophy with minimal residual RPE outside the macular region. OCT showed ellipsoid and interdigitation zone discontinuity. **(D)** A 47-year-old male (191040) diagnosed with RP, showed the fundus appearance of the end-stage of the disease, widespread RPE and choroidal atrophy, bone spicules and vascular thinning were evident, macular affected. OCT showed thinning of the outer retina, ellipsoid completely disappeared, RPE atrophied with high reflection sediments. **(E,J)** A 31-year-old male (10364) diagnosed with CORD, marked atrophy of macular, OCT showed full retinal layers thinned, severe atrophy of the outer retina. Dark macular area and a hyperfluorescent ring within the vascular arcade in AF. **(F,G,H,I)** Autofluorescence images from early to late-stage disease. Hyper auto-fluorescent ring at the posterior pole in the early stages, evolve into low fluorescence in the whole field of view. Abbreviations: DC, disease course. HOMO, homozygosis. M, mutation.

(Pontikos et al., 2020), where it has a prevalence ratio of about 11% (Abd El-Aziz et al., 2010; Xiao et al., 2019) and 32.8% (Hosono et al., 2012; Iwanami et al., 2012; Arai et al., 2015; Yang et al., 2020), respectively. In this study, we performed a comprehensive analysis of the phenotype characteristics in the largest cohort to date of 39 Chinese *EYS* gene mutant patients. We also combined data from 381 patients from all over the world to summarize the mutation spectrum and genotype–phenotype correlations of the *EYS* gene.

The *EYS* gene was first reported to cause retinitis pigmentosa and associated phenotypes in 2008 (Abd El-Aziz et al., 2008; Collin et al., 2008). At present, at least 390 disease-causing mutations of the *EYS* gene have been reported, according to the HGMD database. In the present study, 42% (19/45) of the mutations in G1 cohort were novel, suggesting that the *EYS* gene mutation spectrum remains to be explored. This extensive mutation spectrum may provide a basis for more effective targeting for future gene therapy.

Mutations of c.6557G > A (p.G2186E) were the most common in the G1 cohort, with a frequency of 9%. This mutation has been reported as a hotspot in Chinese patients with RP (Gu et al., 2016). Previous studies have also identified c.6557G > A (p.G2186E) mutations as a major cause of ARRP in Japanese and Korean populations (Suto et al., 2014; Yoon et al., 2015; Yang et al., 2020), this mutation has also been detected in Dutch patients (Littink et al., 2010; Pierrache et al., 2019). In the present study, we discovered that 6.4% of the Chinese patients in this group displayed a c.1750G > T (p.E584X) mutation, and this seems to be a frequent mutation in the Chinese population. By contrast, the prevalence of this variant was lower in the other Asian ethnic groups, including Japanese and Korean patients (Yoon et al., 2015; Hirashima et al., 2017). Another reported causal mutation, c.7492G > C (p.A2498P), shared the same allele frequency of 6.4%, but has been identified only in Chinese populations. These two mutations, c.1750G > T (p.E584X) and c.7492G > C (p.A2498P), were only rarely mentioned in previous reports, probably due to the small sample sizes of the studies. In the present study, the larger sample size identified these two mutations as additional hotspots in Chinese populations. Two Japanese hotspot mutations, c.4957_4958insA and c.8805C > A (Numa et al., 2020), were detected less frequently in the G1 cohort, indicating differences between the hotspots among patients in the Asian population.

We detected *EYS* gene mutations of various types, including missense, nonsense, splicing, frameshift, CNV, and non-frameshift mutations, but the proportions of different mutation types were similar (**Figure 1**). The ratio of CNV identified in this study was 12%. The regions from exon 12 to exon 22 and the C-terminal part of the amino acid chain are prone to produce large deletion or duplication variants; however, CNV analysis and validation is a challenging task, as traditional sequencing technologies, such as PCR-based or target enrichment sequencing, have limitations in detecting CNV (Huang et al., 2017; Jin et al., 2018). Therefore, the proportion of CNV in the EYS gene may be underestimated. Compared with the other pathogenic genes of autosomal recessive IRD, CNV is a relatively common event in *EYS* gene (Pieras et al., 2011).

In this study, we have identified novel genotype–phenotype correlations among globally distributed patients with EYS-IRD. Although the analysis is limited by the case numbers and the amount of clinical information, these results demonstrated that the onset age of patients with *EYS* gene mutation might be affected by the specific mutation, but the overall average onset age of patients with *EYS* mutations is 21 years old. Compared with *USH2A*, the most common pathogenic gene of IRD, the onset of *EYS* patients occurs at a later age, and the visual acuity is preserved until the fifth decade in most patients (Huang et al., 2015).

Overall, the fundus of all the patients showed a relatively consistent phenotype. Our comparison of the fundus features of patients in different periods. In the early stage of the disease, the peripheral retinal pigment epithelium underwent extensive atrophy, the posterior pole was relatively preserved, the macular area of the fundus was generally normal, and the fovea reflection disappeared before 50 years of age. In the later stage of the disease, the macular area atrophied. Bone spicules showed increasing density with disease progression. The OCT of patient 191,025 showed some small cysts in the inner nuclear layer; these cysts were caused by Muller cell atrophy and necrosis in the inner core layer, as previously described (Makiyama et al., 2014; Mucciolo et al., 2018), but most patients do not show these cysts; they are not typical OCT characteristics of patients with *EYS* gene mutations.

The *EYS* gene mutations are mainly related to RP, but some subjects show autosomal recessive CORD (Pierrache et al., 2019; Tian et al., 2020). In our study, only one patient in the G1 cohort had a CORD diagnosis (an incidence of 2.6%). Our CORD patient carried a homozygous c.8805C > A (p.Y2935X) mutant, the same mutation identified in a Japanese CORD patient reported previously, who carried compound heterozygous variants c.8805C > A (p.Y2935X) and c.4957dupA (p.S1653Kfs*2) (Katagiri et al., 2014). When compared with other *EYS*-RP patients, our CORD patient developed symptoms earlier, accompanied with vision damage. His fundus revealed a serve RPE dystrophy in the fovea; however, due to the relatively good condition of the posterior pole, the visual acuity of this patient was maintained at the same level as the other *EYS*-RP patients. Yang.et reported on 7 cases of CORD who carried c.8805C > A (p.Y2935X) heterozygous variant, the median onset age of these subjects was 40.0 (range 29.0–43.0), with a later age of onset compare with our CORD patient and other EYS-RP cohort. The fundus of all EYS-CORD patients showed earlier progressive and more severe RPE dystrophy in the fovea than peripheral retina, unanimously (Yang et al., 2020). Unfortunately, the reasons for the identical genotypes associated different phenotypes in both RP and CRD remain unclear.

CONCLUSION

In conclusion, our analysis of the extensive global data from 420 IRD patients and 262 distinct variants demonstrated the characteristic genotypes and phenotypes and mutation spectra with hotspots in the *EYS* gene. Our findings provide critical information for clinical genetic diagnosis, as well as for therapeutic management of EYS-associated retinal disease.

ETHICS STATEMENT

The studies involving human participants were reviewed and approved by Institutional Medical Ethics Committee. Written informed consent to participate in this study was provided by the participants' legal guardian/next of kin.

AUTHOR CONTRIBUTIONS

Z-BJ designed and supervised whole study. KX and D-FC collected the data and interpreted the results. HC, R-JS, HG, X-FW, Z-KF, XZ, and YX conducted the data analysis. KX wrote the manuscript. YL and Z-BJ revised the manuscript. All authors contributed to the article and approved the submitted version.

REFERENCES

Abd El-Aziz, M. M., Barragan, I., O'Driscoll, C. A., Goodstadt, L., Prigmore, E., Borrego, S., et al. (2008). EYS, encoding an ortholog of Drosophila spacemaker, is mutated in autosomal recessive retinitis pigmentosa. *Nat. Genet.* 40, 1285–1287. doi: 10.1038/ng.241

Abd El-Aziz, M. M., O'Driscoll, C. A., Kaye, R. S., Barragan, I., El-Ashry, M. F., Borrego, S., et al. (2010). Identification of novel mutations in the ortholog of Drosophila eyes shut gene (EYS) causing autosomal recessive retinitis pigmentosa. *Invest. Ophthalmol. Vis. Sci.* 51, 4266–4272. doi: 10.1167/iovs.09-5109

Arai, Y., Maeda, A., Hirami, Y., Ishigami, C., Kosugi, S., Mandai, M., et al. (2015). Retinitis pigmentosa with EYS mutations is the most prevalent inherited retinal dystrophy in japanese populations. *J. Ophthalmol.* 2015:819760.

Audo, I., Sahel, J. A., Mohand-Saïd, S., Lancelot, M. E., Antonio, A., Moskova-Doumanova, V., et al. (2010). EYS is a major gene for rod-cone dystrophies in France. *Hum. Mutat.* 31, E1406–E1435.

Bandah-Rozenfeld, D., Littink, K. W., Ben-Yosef, T., Strom, T. M., Chowers, I., Collin, R. W., et al. (2010). Novel null mutations in the EYS gene are a frequent cause of autosomal recessive retinitis pigmentosa in the Israeli population. *Invest. Ophthalmol. Vis. Sci.* 51, 4387–4394. doi: 10.1167/iovs.09-4732

Barragán, I., Borrego, S., Pieras, J. I., González-del Pozo, M., Santoyo, J., Ayuso, C., et al. (2010). Mutation spectrum of EYS in Spanish patients with autosomal recessive retinitis pigmentosa. *Hum. Mutat.* 31, E1772–E1800.

Bernardis, I., Chiesi, L., Tenedini, E., Artuso, L., Percesepe, A., Artusi, V., et al. (2016). Unravelling the complexity of inherited retinal dystrophies molecular testing: added value of targeted next-generation sequencing. *Biomed. Res. Int.* 2016:6341870.

Broadgate, S., Yu, J., Downes, S. M., and Halford, S. (2017). Unravelling the genetics of inherited retinal dystrophies: past, present and future. *Prog. Retin. Eye Res.* 59, 53–96. doi: 10.1016/j.preteyeres.2017.03.003

Bunker, C. H., Berson, E. L., Bromley, W. C., Hayes, R. P., and Roderick, T. H. (1984). Prevalence of retinitis pigmentosa in Maine. *Am. J. Ophthalmol.* 97, 357–365. doi: 10.1016/0002-9394(84)90636-6

Chen, Z. J., Lin, K. H., Lee, S. H., Shen, R. J., Feng, Z. K., Wang, X. F., et al. (2020). Mutation spectrum and genotype-phenotype correlation of inherited retinal dystrophy in Taiwan. *Clin. Exp. Ophthalmol.* 48, 486–499. doi: 10.1111/ceo.13708

Collin, R. W., Littink, K. W., Klevering, B. J., van den Born, L. I., Koenekoop, R. K., Zonneveld, M. N., et al. (2008). Identification of a 2 Mb human ortholog of Drosophila eyes shut/spacemaker that is mutated in patients with retinitis pigmentosa. *Am. J. Hum. Genet.* 83, 594–603. doi: 10.1016/j.ajhg.2008.10.014

Dias, M. F., Joo, K., Kemp, J. A., Fialho, S. L., da Silva, Cunha, A., et al. (2018). Molecular genetics and emerging therapies for retinitis pigmentosa: basic research and clinical perspectives. *Prog. Retin. Eye Res.* 63, 107–131. doi: 10.1016/j.preteyeres.2017.10.004

Grøndahl, J. (1987). Estimation of prognosis and prevalence of retinitis pigmentosa and Usher syndrome in Norway. *Clin. Genet.* 31, 255–264. doi: 10.1111/j.1399-0004.1987.tb02804.x

Gu, S., Tian, Y., Chen, X., and Zhao, C. (2016). Targeted next-generation sequencing extends the phenotypic and mutational spectrums for EYS mutations. *Mol. Vis.* 22, 646–657.

Hartong, D. T., Berson, E. L., and Dryja, T. P. (2006). Retinitis pigmentosa. *Lancet* 368, 1795–1809.

Hirashima, T., Miyata, M., Ishihara, K., Hasegawa, T., Sugahara, M., Ogino, K., et al. (2017). Choroidal vasculature in bietti crystalline dystrophy with CYP4V2 mutations and in retinitis pigmentosa With EYS mutations. *Invest. Ophthalmol. Vis. Sci.* 58, 3871–3878. doi: 10.1167/iovs.17-21515

Hosono, K., Ishigami, C., Takahashi, M., Park, D. H., Hirami, Y., Nakanishi, H., et al. (2012). Two novel mutations in the EYS gene are possible major causes of autosomal recessive retinitis pigmentosa in the Japanese population. *PLoS One* 7:e31036. doi: 10.1371/journal.pone.0031036

Huang, X. F., Huang, F., Wu, K. C., Wu, J., Chen, J., Pang, C. P., et al. (2015). Genotype-phenotype correlation and mutation spectrum in a large cohort of patients with inherited retinal dystrophy revealed by next-generation sequencing. *Genet. Med.* 17, 271–278. doi: 10.1038/gim.2014.138

Huang, X. F., Mao, J. Y., Huang, Z. Q., Rao, F. Q., Cheng, F. F., Li, F. F., et al. (2017). Genome-wide detection of copy number variations in unsolved inherited retinal disease. *Invest. Ophthalmol. Vis. Sci.* 58, 424–429. doi: 10.1167/iovs.16-20705

Iwanami, M., Oshikawa, M., Nishida, T., Nakadomari, S., and Kato, S. (2012). High prevalence of mutations in the EYS gene in Japanese patients with autosomal recessive retinitis pigmentosa. *Invest. Ophthalmol. Vis. Sci.* 53, 1033–1040. doi: 10.1167/iovs.11-9048

Jin, Z. B., Li, Z., Liu, Z., Jiang, Y., Cai, X. B., and Wu, J. (2018). Identification of de novo germline mutations and causal genes for sporadic diseases using trio-based whole-exome/genome sequencing. *Biol. Rev. Camb. Philos. Soc.* 93, 1014–1031. doi: 10.1111/brv.12383

Katagiri, S., Akahori, M., Hayashi, T., Yoshitake, K., Gekka, T., Ikeo, K., et al. (2014). Autosomal recessive cone-rod dystrophy associated with compound heterozygous mutations in the EYS gene. *Doc. Ophthalmol.* 128, 211–217. doi: 10.1007/s10633-014-9435-0

Littink, K. W., van den Born, L. I., Koenekoop, R. K., Collin, R. W., Zonneveld, M. N., Blokland, E. A., et al. (2010). Mutations in the EYS gene account for approximately 5% of autosomal recessive retinitis pigmentosa and cause a fairly homogeneous phenotype. *Ophthalmology* 117, 2026–2033, 2033.e1-7

Makiyama, Y., Oishi, A., Otani, A., Ogino, K., Nakagawa, S., Kurimoto, M., et al. (2014). Prevalence and spatial distribution of cystoid spaces in retinitis pigmentosa: investigation with spectral domain optical coherence tomography. *Retina* 34, 981–988. doi: 10.1097/iae.0000000000000010

Mucciolo, D. P., Sodi, A., Passerini, I., Murro, V., Cipollini, F., Borg, I., et al. (2018). Fundus phenotype in retinitis pigmentosa associated with EYS mutations. *Ophthalmic Genet.* 39, 589–602. doi: 10.1080/13816810.2018.1509351

Numa, S., Oishi, A., Higasa, K., Oishi, M., Miyata, M., Hasegawa, T., et al. (2020). EYS is a major gene involved in retinitis pigmentosa in Japan: genetic landscapes revealed by stepwise genetic screening. *Sci. Rep.* 10:20770.

Pieras, J. I., Barragán, I., Borrego, S., Audo, I., González-Del Pozo, M., Bernal, S., et al. (2011). Copy-number variations in EYS: a significant event in the appearance of arRP. *Invest. Ophthalmol. Vis. Sci.* 52, 5625–5631. doi: 10.1167/iovs.11-7292

Pierrache, L. H. M., Messchaert, M., Thiadens, A., Haer-Wigman, L., de Jong-Hesse, Y., van Zelst-Stams, W. A. G., et al. (2019). Extending the spectrum of EYS-associated retinal disease to macular dystrophy. *Invest. Ophthalmol. Vis. Sci.* 60, 2049–2063. doi: 10.1167/iovs.18-25531

Pontikos, N., Arno, G., Jurkute, N., Schiff, E., Ba-Abbad, R., Malka, S., et al. (2020). Genetic basis of inherited retinal disease in a molecularly characterized cohort of more than 3000 families from the United Kingdom. *Ophthalmology* 127, 1384–1394. doi: 10.1016/j.ophtha.2020.04.008

Ran, X., Cai, W. J., Huang, X. F., Liu, Q., Lu, F., Qu, J., et al. (2014). 'RetinoGenetics': a comprehensive mutation database for genes related to inherited retinal degeneration. *Database* 2014:bau047. doi: 10.1093/database/bau047

Richards, S., Aziz, N., Bale, S., Bick, D., Das, S., Gastier-Foster, J., et al. (2015). Standards and guidelines for the interpretation of sequence variants: a joint consensus recommendation of the American college of medical genetics and genomics and the association for molecular pathology. *Genet. Med.* 17, 405–424. doi: 10.1038/gim.2015.30

Sun, T., Xu, K., Ren, Y., Xie, Y., Zhang, X., Tian, L., et al. (2018). Comprehensive molecular screening in Chinese Usher syndrome patients. *Invest. Ophthalmol. Vis. Sci.* 59, 1229–1237. doi: 10.1167/iovs.17-23312

Suto, K., Hosono, K., Takahashi, M., Hirami, Y., Arai, Y., Nagase, Y., et al. (2014). Clinical phenotype in ten unrelated Japanese patients with mutations in the EYS gene. *Ophthalmic Genet.* 35, 25–34. doi: 10.3109/13816810.2013.768673

Tian, W., Li, X., Li, Y., Wang, L., Yang, Y., Sun, K., et al. (2020). Identification of novel mutations by targeted sequencing analysis. *Genet. Test. Mol. Biomarkers* 24, 745–753. doi: 10.1089/gtmb.2020.0186

Xiao, X., Cao, Y., Chen, S., Chen, M., Mai, X., Zheng, Y., et al. (2019). Whole exome sequencing reveals novel EYS mutations in Chinese patients with autosomal recessive retinitis pigmentosa. *Mol. Vis.* 25, 35–46.

Yang, L., Fujinami, K., Ueno, S., Kuniyoshi, K., Hayashi, T., Kondo, M., et al. (2020). Genetic spectrum of EYS-associated retinal disease in a large japanese cohort: identification of disease-associated variants with relatively high allele frequency. *Sci. Rep.* 10:5497.

Yoon, C. K., Kim, N. K., Joung, J. G., Shin, J. Y., Park, J. H., and Eum, H. H. (2015). The diagnostic application of targeted re-sequencing in Korean patients with retinitis pigmentosa. *BMC Genom.* 16:515.

5

Updating the Genetic Landscape of Inherited Retinal Dystrophies

Belén García Bohórquez[1,2], Elena Aller[1,2,3], Ana Rodríguez Muñoz[1,2], Teresa Jaijo[1,2,3], Gema García García[1,2] and José M. Millán[1,2]*

[1] Molecular, Cellular and Genomics Biomedicine, Health Research Institute La Fe, Valencia, Spain, [2] CIBER of Rare Diseases, Madrid, Spain, [3] Unit of Genetics, University Hospital La Fe, Valencia, Spain

***Correspondence:**
Gema García García
gegarcia@ciberer.es

Inherited retinal dystrophies (IRD) are a group of diseases characterized by the loss or dysfunction of photoreceptors and a high genetic and clinical heterogeneity. Currently, over 270 genes have been associated with IRD which makes genetic diagnosis very difficult. The recent advent of next generation sequencing has greatly facilitated the diagnostic process, enabling to provide the patients with accurate genetic counseling in some cases. We studied 92 patients who were clinically diagnosed with IRD with two different custom panels. In total, we resolved 53 patients (57.6%); in 12 patients (13%), we found only one mutation in a gene with a known autosomal recessive pattern of inheritance; and 27 patients (29.3%) remained unsolved. We identified 120 pathogenic or likely pathogenic variants; 30 of them were novel. Among the cone-rod dystrophy patients, *ABCA4* was the most common mutated gene, meanwhile, *USH2A* was the most prevalent among the retinitis pigmentosa patients. Interestingly, 10 families carried pathogenic variants in more than one IRD gene, and we identified two deep-intronic variants previously described as pathogenic in *ABCA4* and *CEP290*. In conclusion, the IRD study through custom panel sequencing demonstrates its efficacy for genetic diagnosis, as well as the importance of including deep-intronic regions in their design. This genetic diagnosis will allow patients to make accurate reproductive decisions, enroll in gene-based clinical trials, and benefit from future gene-based treatments.

Keywords: inherited retinal dystrophies, diagnosis, custom-panels, gene, pathogenic, deep-intronic

INTRODUCTION

Inherited retinal dystrophies (IRD) are a group of diseases characterized by the progressive death or dysfunction of photoreceptors that leads to vision loss and, in some cases, legal blindness. IRDs have a prevalence of one case in 3,000 individuals (Sahel et al., 2015). Depending on the photoreceptor initially affected, IRD can be classified into cone, rod-cone, or cone-rod dystrophies in those cases in which both are affected at one time. Moreover, they can manifest as either isolated (70–80% of the total) or part of one of the 80 syndromes that have been estimated to be associated with IRD (Ayuso and Millan, 2010; Tatour and Ben-Yosef, 2020).

This group of diseases has a wide clinical spectrum and number of involved genes, currently reaching 271 for syndromic and non-syndromic forms (Retnet[1], December 2020); explaining why IRDs have such a high clinical and genetic heterogeneity. Furthermore, there is a high inter and intrafamily variability, variable expression, and incomplete penetrance (Farrar et al., 2017). IRDs can follow different patterns of inheritance, including autosomal recessive, autosomal dominant,

[1]https://sph.uth.edu/retnet/sum-dis.htm#A-genes

X-linked, mitochondrial mode, and some other less common, such as uniparental isodisomy or digenic inheritance (Kajiwara et al., 1994; Dryja et al., 1997; Rivolta et al., 2002; Ayuso and Millan, 2010; Parmeggiani et al., 2011; Neveling et al., 2012). These issues, together with the fact that 50% are sporadic cases, make it even more complicated to determine the mode of inheritance, genetic diagnosis, and genetic counseling (Perea-Romero et al., 2021).

With the advent of next generation sequencing (NGS), the ratio of diagnosis has risen to 50–70%, which was difficult to achieve a few years ago (Carss et al., 2017; Sanchis-Juan et al., 2018; Rodríguez-Muñoz et al., 2020). Some different approaches, such as custom panel designs, whole exome sequencing (WES), and whole genome sequencing (WGS), have been implemented to study the molecular mechanisms of IRD. Currently, these new sequencing techniques are essential to obtain an early and accurate genetic diagnosis, which is necessary to offer a correct genetic counseling to patients and their families (Salmaninejad et al., 2019).

In this study, we analyzed 92 patients, who were previously clinically diagnosed with IRD, with two custom panels for the main aim of achieving genetic diagnoses.

MATERIALS AND METHODS

Cohort Selection

We selected 92 patients, belonging to 90 different Spanish families, with a clinical diagnosis of non-syndromic IRD, except for one who had a clinical suspicion of a syndromic IRD. Patient DNA was isolated from peripheral blood with the automatic extractor QIAsymphony (QIAGEN).

Patients underwent complete ophthalmologic examinations, including OCT (Heidelberg Spectralis OCT Bluepeak, Heidelberg, Germany; Topcon 3D OCT 2000, Tokyo, Japan; CIRRUS OCT Zeiss, Oberkochen, Germany), ERG (Roland RETI-port/scan21, Brandenburg, Germany), eye fundus (Visucam NM/FA Zeiss, Oberkochen, Germany), visual acuity measure (BCVA), and evoked potentials and visual fields (Carl Zeiss Humphrey Field Analyzer, Oberkochen, Germany). A clinical questionnaire, which collected the main IRD characteristics, and an informed consent were completed by each patient. This study was approved by the Hospital La Fe Ethics Committee, in agreement with the Declaration of Helsinki.

Panel Design and Sequencing

Sixty-three patients were sequenced with a gene panel version (PV1) that included 117 genes involved in a non-syndromic IRD, and their flanking intronic regions (±25 base pairs) (Rodríguez-Muñoz et al., 2020). Moreover, the panel of genes contained five intronic regions of *ABCA4*, *OFD1*, *USH2A*, *CEP290*, and *PRPF31*, in which pathogenic variants had been previously identified (Den Hollander et al., 2006; Littink et al., 2010; Vaché et al., 2012; Webb et al., 2012; Braun et al., 2013; **Supplementary Table 1**).

The remaining 29 cases were analyzed with an updated version of the custom panel (PV2) that had 114 genes and all the deep-intronic variants described in the last few years in *ABCA4* and *USH2A* (Vaché et al., 2012; Braun et al., 2013; Zernant et al., 2014; Bauwens et al., 2015, 2019; Liquori et al., 2016; Baux et al., 2017; Fadaie et al., 2019; Khan et al., 2019; Sangermano et al., 2019; **Supplementary Table 2**).

The patients' libraries were prepared in accordance with the SureSelect QXT protocol (Agilent Technologies) and sequenced on a MiSeq platform (Illumina, San Diego, CA) in 300 cycles with 2 × 150 base pairs reads.

Data Analysis

The reads alignment against the reference hg19 genome, variant calling, and annotation of all the identified variants were carried out with the *Alissa* resource (Agilent Technologies). The obtained variants were filtered based on a MAF (minor allele frequency) $\leq$ 0.01 according to the ExAC[2] and gnomAD[3] databases. In order to evaluate the pathogenicity of the detected variants, we also evaluated specific databases such as ClinVar[4], Locus Specific Data Base[5], and HGMD professional[6]. To evaluate the potential effect of novel missense variants, we used the *in silico* predictors included in Varsome[7]. The putative effect on the splicing process was performed with HSF (Human SplicingFinder[8]), NNSplice[9], and SpliceAI[10]. Finally, the IGV view finder[11] allowed the examination of all detected variants in every read.

The novel variants identified in this study were classified according to the standards of the American College of Medical Genetics and Genomics (ACMG) (Richards et al., 2015).

Copy Number Variation Analysis

A copy number variations (CNV) analysis was performed using the DECoN bioinformatic tool version 1.0.2 (Fowler et al., 2016).

We also studied large rearrangements by Multiplex Ligation-dependent Probe Amplification (MLPA; MRC Holland) in patients harboring one pathogenic variant in *USH2A* (probemixes P361 and P362), *EYS* (probemix P328-A3), and*ABCA4* (probemixes P151 and P152). The multiplex ligation-dependent probe amplification results were analyzed by the Coffalyser. Net software version 140721.1958 (MRC-Holland).

Sanger Sequencing and Segregation Analysis

The candidate variants identified in each patient were validated by Sanger sequencing (Big Dye Terminator v1.1 or v3.1, Applied

[2]http://exac.broadinstitute.org/
[3]https://gnomad.broadinstitute.org/
[4]https://www.ncbi.nlm.nih.gov/clinvar/
[5]https://grenada.lumc.nl/LSDB_list/lsdbs
[6]https://portal.biobase-international.com/cgi-bin/portal/login.cgi
[7]https://varsome.com/
[8]http://www.umd.be/HSF
[9]https://www.fruitfly.org/seq_tools/splice.html
[10]https://mobidetails.iurc.montp.inserm.fr/MD/
[11]http://software.broadinstitute.org/software/igv/

Biosystems by Life Technologies). Moreover, the deep-intronic variants, already described as pathogenic in *USH2A* and *ABCA4* (**Supplementary Table 3**; Vaché et al., 2012; Braun et al., 2013; Zernant et al., 2014; Bauwens et al., 2015, 2019; Liquori et al., 2016; Baux et al., 2017; Fadaie et al., 2019; Khan et al., 2019; Sangermano et al., 2019), were studied by Sanger sequencing in patients analyzed with PV1 who carried only one pathogenic variant in either or both genes.

Segregation analysis was performed when relatives' DNA was available.

RESULTS

We obtained a mean depth of 190× per patient. In 98.6% of the patients, at least 88% of the bases were covered with a sequencing depth of coverage ≥50× and 95% of the bases were covered with at least 20×. Moreover, we obtained a 70% of on-target reads.

We solved 53 patients belonging to 52 families (53/92, ratio of 57.6%): 17 (of 17 families) which had disease-causing variants in autosomal dominant genes, 33 (of 32 families) with autosomal recessive genes, two patients (of two families) who carried a pathogenic variant in an X-linked gene and one patient who carried two different pathogenic variants in two different autosomal dominant genes and two additional variants in an autosomal recessive gene (RPN-670). We reported five cases with more than two pathogenic variants in the same autosomal recessive gene, and we also described six patients who carry pathogenic variants in more than one IRD gene (**Table 1**). Among the unresolved patients, 13% carried one pathogenic variant in an autosomal recessive IRD gene, with a higher prevalence of cases with a heterozygous variant in *ABCA4,* followed by *USH2A* and *RPGRIP1* (**Table 2**). In the remaining 29.3% cases, no pathogenic variant was identified.

We identified a total of 120 pathogenic or likely pathogenic variants (of which, 85 were unique), including: 65 missense, 15 nonsense, 17 frameshift, 16 splice-site variants, two pathogenic deep-intronic variants, one in-frame deletion, one synonymous, and three CNV (**Figure 1**). Twenty-nine variants were first described in this study (**Tables 1–3**). In line with this, we identified a high number of mutated-genes, nine autosomal dominant genes (highest prevalence of *PRPH2*); 19 autosomal recessive genes, among which, *ABCA4* and *USH2A* stand out; and finally, one X-linked gene, *RPGR* (**Figure 2**). All identified novel variants were classified as pathogenic or likely pathogenic according to the ACMG criteria except for variant c.2470_2478del (p.Lys824_Glu826del) in *PDE6B*, which remained as a variant of uncertain significance. This patient harbored another heterozygous pathogenic variant in the same gene; however, we could not carry out the segregation analysis to confirm it as likely pathogenic.

Copy number variants analysis with the bioinformatic tool allowed us to detect two putative deletions: a deletion in *PRPF31*, which was properly validated with MLPA (patient RPN-717), and a homozygous deletion of exon 11 of *PROM1* in patient RPN-709. In this last patient, the exon 11 did not have reads in the alignment and was not amplified by PCR; however, there was PCR amplification for the flanking exons, thus, reinforcing the hypothesis of a homozygous deletion of the exon.

The individual RPN-728 presented nephropathy and alterations in the brain MRI (mild hypoplasia of the cerebellar vermis and slightly elongated superior cerebellar peduncles) in addition to retinal degeneration, suggesting a Joubert syndrome. The panel sequencing allowed us to identify two pathogenic variants in *CEP290*, c.4966_4967delGA (p.Glu1656Asnfs*3) and c.2817G > T (p.Lys939Asn). On the other hand, the panel analysis in the RPN-708 revealed a pathogenic variant in the *OTX2* gene (**Table 1**). Although this gene has been implicated in other diseases such as microphthalmia and retinal degeneration with pituitary dysfunction (OMIM: 610125; 610125), our patient only referred a macular dystrophy (MD) phenotype.

Because of the inclusion of the deep-intronic regions, we solved two cases who carried deep-intronic pathogenic variants in *ABCA4* and *CEP290* (RPN-750, RPN-734) (**Table 1**).

DISCUSSION

A total of 92 patients, previously clinically diagnosed with IRD, were analyzed by two IRD-custom panels. These gene panels allowed us to find a genetic diagnosis in 53 patients of 52 different families (**Table 1**), with a diagnostic ratio of 57.6%, which is within the average of other studies (50–70%) (Ellingford et al., 2016; Di Resta et al., 2018; Wang et al., 2018; Jespersgaard et al., 2019; Zenteno et al., 2020).

In recent years, several deep-intronic mutations have been described as pathogenic due to their effect in the splicing process by leading to the introduction of a pseudoexon (PE) in the coding sequence (Vaché et al., 2012; Braun et al., 2013; Zernant et al., 2014; Bauwens et al., 2015, 2019; Liquori et al., 2016; Baux et al., 2017; Fadaie et al., 2019; Khan et al., 2019; Sangermano et al., 2019). The inclusion of these regions in the present study allowed us to detect two deep intronic variants and, therefore, solve the molecular diagnosis in two more families. The variant *CEP290*: c.2991 + 1655A > G, detected in patient RPN-750, is one of the most prevalent in Leber congenital amaurosis (LCA) associated with *CEP290* (Den Hollander et al., 2006; Coppieters et al., 2010). Coppieters et al. reported this variant with a frequency of 49% in the *CEP290*-associated LCA cases. Also, we identified the deep-intronic variant c.4539 + 2064C > T in *ABCA4*. Deep-intronic variants in *ABCA4* were reported to be involved in 2.1–17.9% of the STGD cohorts (Braun et al., 2013; Zernant et al., 2014; Bauwens et al., 2015; Bax et al., 2015; Zaneveld et al., 2015; Schulz et al., 2017); our finding of 7.1% of cases within the STGD patients fits into the observed frequencies. Furthermore, the development of new therapeutical approaches, such as antisense oligonucleotides (AONs), entailed a new advantage for deep-intronic variants correction, which highlights the importance of detecting these changes for future treatments. In this sense, several studies have proven the therapeutic potential of AONs strategy and a phase I/II clinical trial for patients harboring the *CEP290* c.2991 + 1655A > G mutation using this type of therapy was conducted (Burke et al., 2012; Slijkerman et al., 2016;

TABLE 1 | Pathogenic variants identified in solved patients.

Family	Patient	Clinical diagnosis	Gene	Nucleotide change	Protein change	Zygosity	References
$FRPN-51[1]	RPN-129	STG	*ABCA4* (NM_000350.3)	c.1804C > T	p.(Arg602Trp)	Heterozygous	Lewis et al., 1999
				c.982G > T	p.(Glu328*)	Heterozygous	Fishman, 2003
	RPN-544	STG	*ABCA4* (NM_000350.3)	c.5882G > A	p.(Gly1961Glu)	Heterozygous	Allikmets et al., 1997
				c.982G > T	p.(Glu328*)	Heterozygous	Fishman, 2003
$FRPN-244[1]	RPN-646	RP	*RHO* (NM_000539.3)	c.328T > C	p.(Cys110Arg)	Heterozygous	To et al., 2004
FRPN-246[1]	RPN-649	MD/STG	*ABCA4* (NM_000350.3)	c.5917del	p.(Val1973*)	Homozygous	Rivolta et al., 2000
$FRPN-252[1]	RPN-657	STG	*ABCA4* (NM_000350.3)	**c.5714 + 1G > A**	**p.?**	**Heterozygous**	**This study**
				c.3386G > T	p.(Arg1129Leu)	Heterozygous	Allikmets et al., 1997
FRPN-254[1]	RPN-659	RP	*EYS* (NM_001142800.2)	**c.7736_7742del**	**p.(Thr2579Lysfs*36)**	**Homozygous**	**This study**
FRPN-255[1]	RPN-660	RP	*USH2A* (NM_206933.4)	c.4732C > T	p.(Arg1578Cys)	Heterozygous	Le Quesne Stabej et al., 2012
				c.1214del	p.(Asn405Ilefs*3)	Heterozygous	Schwartz et al., 2005
$FRPN-256[1]	RPN-661	RP/LCA	*CRB1* (NM_201253.3)	c.2416G > T	p.(Glu806*)	Homozygous	Corton et al., 2013
FRPN-258[1]	RPN-663	STG	*ABCA4* (NM_000350.3)	c.3386G > T	p.(Arg1129Leu)	Homozygous	Allikmets et al., 1997
				c.6718A > G	p.(Thr2240Ala)	Heterozygous	Zernant et al., 2011
FRPN-261[1]	RPN-666	Reverse BCAMD/ STG/RP	*ABCA4* (NM_000350.3)	c.5929G > A	p.(Gly1977Ser)	Heterozygous	Rozet et al., 1998
				c.5882G > A	p.(Gly1961Glu)	Heterozygous	Allikmets et al., 1997
FRPN-263[1]	RPN-668	CD	*CRB1* (NM_201253.3)	c.1604T > C	p.(Leu535Pro)	Heterozygous	Corton et al., 2013
				c.2843G > A	p.(Cys948Tyr)	Heterozygous	den Hollander et al., 1999
FRPN-265[1]	RPN-670	NA	*RP1* (NM_006269.2)	c.3157del	p.(Tyr1053Thrfs*4)	Heterozygous	Jacobson et al., 2000
			PRPH2 (NM_000322.5)	c.623G > A	p.(Gly208Asp)	Heterozygous	Kohl et al., 1997
			USH2A (NM_206933.4)	**c.6957 + 1G > C**	**p.?**	**Heterozygous**	**This study**
				c.4955C > T	**p.(Pro1652Leu)**	**Heterozygous**	**This study**
FRPN-266[1]	RPN-671	RP	*EYS* (NM_001142800.2)	c.5928-2A > G	p.?	Homozygous	González-del Pozo et al., 2011
FRPN-267[1]	RPN-672	RP	*CNGB1* (NM_001297.5)	**c.2492 + 2T > G**	**p.?**	**Homozygous**	**This study**
FRPN-268[1]	RPN-673	RP	*USH2A* (NM_206933.4)	c.2276G > T	p.(Cys759Phe)	Heterozygous	Rivolta et al., 2000
				c.13894C > T	**p.(Pro4632Ser)**	**Heterozygous**	**This study**
FRPN-269[1]	RPN-675	RP	*USH2A* (NM_206933.4)	c.4732C > T	p.(Arg1578Cys)	Heterozygous	Le Quesne Stabej et al., 2012
				c.12575G > A	p.(Arg4192His)	Heterozygous	Ávila-Fernández et al., 2010
FRPN-273[1]	RPN-679	STG	*ABCA4* (NM_000350.3)	**c.4880del**	**p.(Leu1627Argfs*35)**	**Heterozygous**	**This study**
				c.5714 + 5G > A	p.?	Heterozygous	Cremers, 1998
				c.2953G > A	**p.(Gly985Arg)**	**Heterozygous**	**This study**
FRPN-276[1]	RPN-682	MD	*BEST1* (NM_004183.4)	c.247G > T	p.(Val83Phe)	Heterozygous	Kinnick et al., 2011
FRPN-277[1]	RPN-683	RP	*RPGR* (NM_001034853.2)	**c.1366del**	**p.(Gln456Lysfs*20)**	**Hemizygous**	**This study**
FRPN-278[1]	RPN-684	RP	*EYS* (NM_001142800.2)	c.9468T > A	p.(Tyr3156*)	Homozygous	Collin et al., 2008
FRPN-279[1]	RPN-685	NA	*PRPH2* (NM_000322.5)	c.658C > T	p.(Arg220Trp)	Heterozygous	Payne et al., 1998
FRPN-280[1]	RPN-686	RP	*USH2A* (NM_206933.4)	c.12575G > A	p.(Arg4192His)	Homozygous	Ávila-Fernández et al., 2010
FRPN-281[1]	RPN-687	CRD/STG	*CRB1* (NM_201253.3)	**c.481G > A**	**p.(Ala161Thr)**	**Homozygous**	**This study**
FRPN-284[1]	RPN-692	RP Punctata albensces	*ABCA4* (NM_000350.3)	c.3386G > T	p.(Arg1129Leu)	Heterozygous	Allikmets et al., 1997
				c.6148G > C	p.(Val2050Leu)	Heterozygous	Lewis et al., 1999
$FRPN-286[1]	RPN-694	NA	*PRPH2* (NM_000322.5)	**c.440dup**	**p.(Gly148Trpfs*29)**	**Heterozygous**	**This study**
$FRPN-289[1]	RPN-697	STG	*ABCA4* (NM_000350.3)	c.3386G > T	p.(Arg1129Leu)	Heterozygous	Allikmets et al., 1997
				c.634C > T	p.(Arg212Cys)	Heterozygous	Gerber et al., 1998
FRPN-293[1]	RPN-701	RP	*PRPH2* (NM_000322.5)	**c.647C > A**	**p.(Pro216His)**	**Heterozygous**	**This study**
FRPN-294[1]	RPN-702	MD	*ELOVL4* (NM_022726.4)	c.59A > G	p.(Asn20Ser)	Heterozygous	Hu et al., 2020
FRPN-296[1]	RPN-704	CD	*GUCA1A* (NM_000409.5)	**c.66C > A**	**p.(Tyr22*)**	**Heterozygous**	**This study**
FRPN-298[1]	RPN-706	CRD	*CRB1* (NM_201253.3)	c.613_619del	p.(Ile205Aspfs*13)	Homozygous	Lotery, 2001
				c.2291G > A	p.(Arg764His)	Heterozygous	Corton et al., 2013

(Continued)

TABLE 1 | Continued

Family	Patient	Clinical diagnosis	Gene	Nucleotide change	Protein change	Zygosity	References
FRPN-299[1]	RPN-707	RP	*USH2A* (NM_206933.4)	c.13811 + 2T > G	p.?	Heterozygous	Besnard et al., 2014
				c.2276G > T	p.(Cys759Phe)	Heterozygous	Rivolta et al., 2000
FRPN-300[1]	RPN-708	NA	*OTX2* (NM_001270525.2)	**c.638T > A**	**p.(Leu213*)**	**Heterozygous**	**This study**
FRPN-301[1]	RPN-709	RP	*PROM1* (NM_006017.2)	**deletion exon 11**	**p.?**	**Homozygous**	**This study**
FRPN-302[1]	RPN-710	MD/BVMD	*PRPH2* (NM_000322.5)	c.641G > A	p.(Cys214Tyr)	Heterozygous	Trujillo et al., 2001
FRPN-303[1]	RPN-711	RP	*USH2A* (NM_206933.4)	c.14803C > T	p.(Arg4935*)	Heterozygous	Baux et al., 2007
				c.2332G > T	p.(Asp778Tyr)	Heterozygous	Lenassi et al., 2015
FRPN-307[1]	RPN-715	RP	*RHO* (NM_000539.3)	c.512C > A	p.(Pro171Gln)	Heterozygous	Antiñolo et al., 1994
$FRPN-308[2]	RPN-717	RP	*ABCA4* (NM_000350.3)	c.6148G > C	p.(Val2050Leu)	Heterozygous	Allikmets et al., 1997
			PRPF31 (NM_015629.3)	**Gene deletion**	**p.?**	**Heterozygous**	**This study**
FRPN-309[2]	RPN-718	RP	*USH2A* (NM_206933.4)	c.2276G > T	p.(Cys759Phe)	Homozygous	Rivolta et al., 2000
FRPN-312[2]	RPN-721	RP	*RHO* (NM_000539.3)	c.512C > A	p.(Pro171Leu)	Heterozygous	Stone et al., 2017
FRPN-315[2]	RPN-725	MD/STG	*ABCA4* (NM_000350.3)	**c.6310C > T**	**p.(Gln2104*)**	**Heterozygous**	**This study**
				c.3386G > T	p.(Arg1129Leu)	Heterozygous	Allikmets et al., 1997
FRPN-316[2]	RPN-726	RP	*NRL* (NM_001354768.3)	c.149C > T	p.(Ser50Leu)	Heterozygous	Koyanagi et al., 2019
			ABCA4 (NM_000350.3)	c.5908C > T	p.(Leu1970Phe)	Heterozygous	Rozet et al., 1998
FRPN-318[2]	RPN-728	Joubert syndrome	*CEP290* (NM_025114.4)	c.4966_4967del	p.(Glu1656Asnfs*3)	Heterozygous	Sheck et al., 2018
				c.2817G > T	p.(Lys939Asn)	Heterozygous	Srivastava et al., 2017
FRPN-320[2]	RPN-730	MD/STG	*PRPH2* (NM_000322.5)	c.537G > A	p.(Trp179*)	Heterozygous	Diñeiro et al., 2020
FRPN-322[2]	RPN-732	RP	*PDE6B* (NM_000283.4)	**c.1920 + 1G > A**	**p.?**	**Heterozygous**	**This study**
				c.2470_2478del	**p.(Lys824_Glu826del)**	**Heterozygous**	**This study**
FRPN-323[2]	RPN-733	MD	*PRPH2* (NM_000322.5)	c.421T > C	p.(Tyr141His)	Heterozygous	Diñeiro et al., 2020
			ABCA4 (NM_000350.3)	c.5908C > T	p.(Leu1970Phe)	Heterozygous	Rozet et al., 1998
FRPN-324[2]	RPN-734	MD/CD	*ABCA4* (NM_000350.3)	c.3113C > T	p.(Ala1038Val)	Heterozygous	Rozet et al., 1998
				c.4539 + 2064C > T	[p.?; p.(= , Arg1514Leufs*36)]	Heterozygous	Zernant et al., 2014; Bauwens et al., 2019
				c.1364T > A	p.(Leu455Gln)	Heterozygous	Salles et al., 2018
FRPN-325[2]	RPN-735	NA	*EYS* (NM_001142800.2)	**c.8854del**	**p.(Thr2973Leufs*23)**	**Heterozygous**	**This study**
				c.1194del	**p.(Gly399Aspfs*22)**	**Heterozygous**	**This study**
			RDH5 (NM_002905.3)	c.712G > T	p.(Gly238Trp)	Heterozygous	Gonzalez-Fernandez et al., 1999
FRPN-328[2]	RPN-737	MD/STG	*PRPH2* (NM_000322.5)	c.641G > A	p.(Cys214Tyr)	Heterozygous	Trujillo et al., 2001
FPRN-327[2]	RPN-738	MD/STG	*BBS1* (NM_024649.4)	c.1169T > G	p.(Met390Arg)	Homozygous	Nishimura et al., 2010
FRPN-335[2]	RPN-745	RP	*RPGR* (NM_001034853.2)	c.935-2A > G	p.?	Hemizygous	Koyanagi et al., 2019
			ABCA4 (NM_000350.3)	c.5908C > T	p.(Leu1970Phe)	Heterozygous	Rozet et al., 1998
			PDE6A (NM_000440.3)	**c.2144T > C**	**p.(Met715Thr)**	**Heterozygous**	**This study**
FRPN-337[2]	RPN-747	RP	*RHO* (NM_000539.3)	**c.670G > A**	**p.(Gly224Arg)**	**Heterozygous**	**This study**
FRPN-339[2]	RPN-749	STG	*ABCA4* (NM_000350.3)	c.3386G > T	p.(Arg1129Leu)	Heterozygous	Allikmets et al., 1997
				c.3210_3211dup	p.(Ser1071Cysfs*14)	Heterozygous	Nasonkin et al., 1998
				c.560G > A	p.(Arg187His)	Heterozygous	Cornelis et al., 2017
$FRPN-340[2]	RPN-750	LCA	*CEP290* (NM_025114.4)	c.2991 + 1655A > G	p.?	Homozygous	Den Hollander et al., 2006

Novel pathogenic variants are highlighted in bold font.
FRPN, family number; FRPN-"1," families studied with PV1; FRPN-"2," families studied with PV2; $FRPN, families in which segregation analysis was performed; RPN, patient number; RP, retinitis pigmentosa; MD, macular dystrophy; p.?, unknown protein effect; STG, stargardt; LCA, leber congenital amaurosis; BCAMD, benign concentric annular macular dystrophy; CD, cone dystrophy; CRD, cone-rod dystrophy; BVMD, best vitelliform macular dystrophy; NA, not available. The "" symbol corresponds to: stop-codon according to the format of mutations nomenclature from the Human Genome Variation Society (HGVS).*

Duijkers et al., 2018; Cideciyan et al., 2019; Garanto et al., 2019; Sangermano et al., 2019; Xue and MacLaren, 2020).

In our study, *ABCA4* and *USH2A* are the most frequent mutated-genes, similar to other studies (Bernardis et al., 2016; Ezquerra-Inchausti et al., 2018; Jespersgaard et al., 2019). In *ABCA4*, 10% of alleles are reported to be complex (Shroyer et al., 2001; Zhang et al., 2015), a value that increased to 25% in our results. Moreover, we reported the variant c.3386G > T (p.Arg1129Leu) in *ABCA4* in 37.5% of the resolved patients with mutations in this gene (**Table 1**), which was not surprising because this variant appears to be very frequent in the Spanish population as we can observe in a study performed by Del Pozo-Valero et al. (2020). On the other hand, variants with an allelic frequency higher than 1% (MAF < 0.01) are usually ruled out as

TABLE 2 | Patients in which only one pathogenic variant in a recessive gene has been identified.

Family	Patient	Clinic diagnosis	Gene	Nucleotide change	Protein change	Zygosity	References
FRPN-243[1]	RPN-645	RP	*USH2A* (NM_206933.4)	c.2276G > T	p.(Cys759Phe)	heterozygous	Rivolta et al., 2000
			CEP290 (NM_025114.4)	**c.7394_7395del**	**p.(Glu2465Valfs*2)**	**heterozygous**	**This study**
FRPN-272[1]	RPN-678	STG	*ABCA4* (NM_000350.3)	c.288C > A	p.(Asn96Lys)	heterozygous	Stenirri et al., 2004
			USH2A (NM_206933.4)	c.754G > T	p.(Gly252Cys)	heterozygous	Bravo-Gil et al., 2016
FRPN-283[1]	RPN-691	RP Punctata albensces	*CDHR1* (NM_033100.3)	c.783G > A	(p.Pro261 =)	heterozygous	Glockle et al., 2014
			POC1B (NM_172240.3)	**c.1079_1080del**	**p.(Pro360Argfs*8)**	**heterozygous**	**This study**
FRPN-287[1]	RPN-695	NA	*ABCA4* (NM_000350.3)	c.6089G > A	p.(Arg2030Gln)	heterozygous	Lewis et al., 1999
FRPN-288[1]	RPN-696	NA	*ABCA4* (NM_000350.3)	c.6148G > C	p.(Val2050Leu)	heterozygous	Allikmets et al., 1997
FRPN-304[1]	RPN-712	RP	*RPGRIP1* (NM_020366.3)	**c.3339 + 5G > C**	**p.?**	**heterozygous**	**This study**
FRPN-305[1]	RPN-713	RP	*SAG* (NM_000541.5)	c.577C > T	p.(Arg193*)	heterozygous	Maw et al., 1998
			GUCY2D (NM_000180.4)	**c.1991A > G**	**p.(His664Arg)**	**heterozygous**	**This study**
FRPN-308[2]	RPN-717	RP	*ABCA4* (NM_000350.3)	c.6148G > C	p.(Val2050Leu)	heterozygous	Allikmets et al., 1997
FRPN-311[2]	RPN-720	RP (early onset)	*RPGRIP1* (NM_020366.3)	c.767C > G	p.(Ser256*)	heterozygous	Jamshidi et al., 2019
FRPN-313[2]	RPN-722	RP	*RBP3* (NM_002900.3)	c.3238G > A	p.(Asp1080Asn)	heterozygous	den Hollander et al., 2009
FRPN-314[2]	RPN-724	RP	*EYS* (NM_001142800.2)	**c.6882_6883del**	**p.(Gln2294Hisfs*3)**	**heterozygous**	**This study**
FRPN-319[2]	RPN-729	RP	*CNGA3* (NM_001298.3)	**c.673 + 5G > T**	**p.?**	**heterozygous**	**This study**
FRPN-336[2]	RPN-746	MD	*PCARE* (NM_001271441.2)	**c.656_665dup**	**p.(Ala223Argfs*38)**	**heterozygous**	**This study**

Novel pathogenic variants identified are highlighted in bold font.
FRPN, family number; FRPN-"1," families studied with PV1; FRPN-"2," families studied with PV2; RPN, patient number; RP, retinitis pigmentosa; STG, stargardt; NA, not available; p.?, unknown protein effect; SNHL, sensorineural hearing loss; XL, X-linked. The "" symbol corresponds to: stop-codon according to the format of mutations nomenclature from the Human Genome Variation Society (HGVS).*

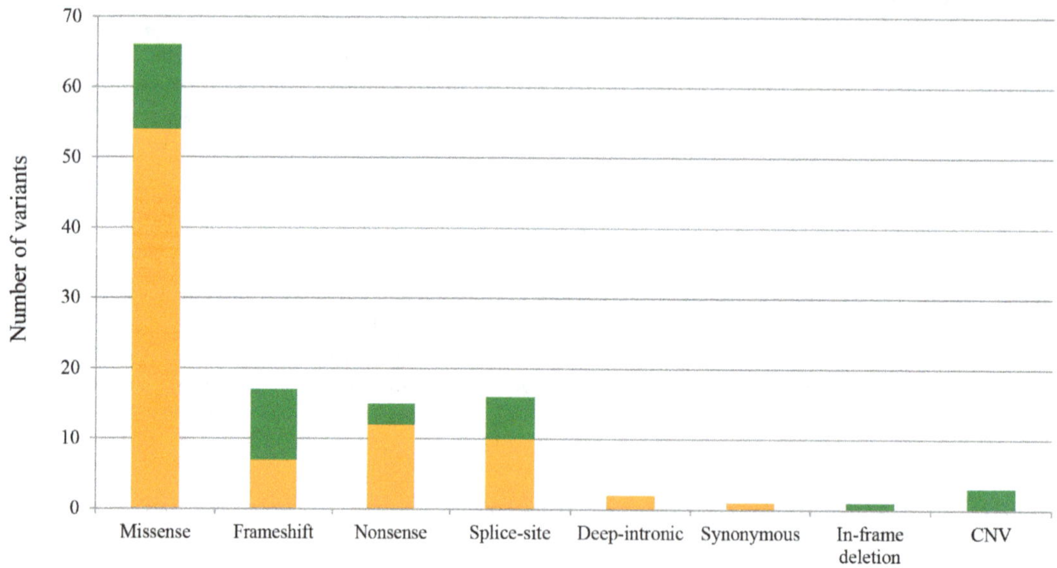

FIGURE 1 | Representation of the total alleles identified in this study classified according to the alteration type. The X-axis refers to the different types of variants identified in this study, and the Y-axis concerns the total allele count for each type of variant. Pathogenic variants identified in this study are represented in green, while those previously described are in orange.

the cause of disease in prioritization analyses; however, in some cases, the frequency of some variants, although > 1%, is higher in patients than in healthy individuals, suggesting that they are causal for the disease. Examples of this have been reported for *ABCA4*. For instance, the variant c.5603A > T (p.Asn1868Ile) was presented in STGD patients four times more frequently than expected (Zernant et al., 2017), and it is a disease-causing variant in 5% of patients when it is in trans with a severe allele in *ABCA4*. This variant was initially considered benign, however, recent studies consider it pathogenic with reduced

TABLE 3 | Criteria considered for the pathogenicity classification of the novel identified variants.

Gene	Mutation		Classification	Frequency (gnomAD Ex)	Pathogenicity scores[a]	Conservation score (GERP)[b]	Reputable source	
	Nucleotide change	Protein change					ClinVar	HGMD[c]
ABCA4 (NM_000350.3)	c.2953G > A	p.(Gly985Arg)	Likely pathogenic	NF	12 of 13	5.7199	NA	NA
	c.4880del	p.(Leu1627Argfs*35)	Pathogenic	0.0000159	NA	5.6399	Pathogenic	NA
	c.5714 + 1G > A	p.?	Pathogenic	0.00000398	NA	4.7399	Likely pathogenic	NA
	c.6310C > T	p.(Gln2104*)	Pathogenic	NF	NA	6.0799	NA	NA
CEP290 (NM_025114.4)	c.7394_7395del	p.(Glu2465Valfs*2)	Pathogenic	0.000598	NA	5.42	NA	NA
CNGA3 (NM_001298.3)	c.673 + 5G > T	p.?	Likely pathogenic	0.0000199	NA	5.09	NA	NA
RPGRIP1 (NM_020366.3)	c.3339 + 5G > C	p.?	Likely pathogenic	NF	2 of 2	NA	Likely pathogenic	NA
CNGB1 (NM_001297.5)	c.2492 + 2T > G	p.?	Pathogenic	NF	NA	5.4499	NA	NA
CRB1 (NM_201253.3)	c.481G > A	p.(Ala161Thr)	Likely pathogenic	NF	12 of 13	5.5199	Uncertain significance	NA
PCARE (NM_001271 441.2)	c.656_665dup	p.(Ala223Argfs*38)	Likely pathogenic	0.0000579	NA	1.8514	NA	NA
EYS (NM_0011 42800.2)	c.1194del	p.(Gly399Aspfs*22)	Pathogenic	NF	NA	6.07	NA	NA
	c.6882_6883del	p.(Gln2294Hisfs*3)	Pathogenic	NF	NA	5.38	NA	NA
	c.7736_7742del	p.(Thr2579Lysfs*36)	Pathogenic	0.0000127	NA	4.01	Likely pathogenic	NA
	c.8854del	p.(Thr2952Leufs*23)	Pathogenic	NF	NA	4.57	NA	NA
GUCY2D (NM_000180.4)	c.1991A > G	p.(His664Arg)	Likely pathogenic	NF	11 of 12	5.35	NA	NA
GUCA1A (NM_000409.5)	c.66C > A	p.(Tyr22*)	Likely pathogenic	0.00000795	NA	5.75	Uncertain significance	NA
OTX2 (NM_001 270525.2)	c.638T > A	p.(Leu213*)	Pathogenic	NF	NA	5.53	NA	NA
PDE6A (NM_000440.3)	c.2144T > C	p.(Met715Thr)	Likely pathogenic	0.000231	12 of 13	5.32	Uncertain significance	NA
PDE6B (NM_000283.4)	c.1920 + 1G > A	p.?	Pathogenic	NF	NA	4.19	NA	NA
	c.2470_2478del	p.(Lys824_Glu826del)	Uncertain significance	0.000128	NA	4.1599	NA	NA
POC1B (NM_172240.3)	c.1079_1080del	p.(Pro360Argfs*8)	Pathogenic	0.0000145	NA	5.69	NA	NA
PROM1 (NM_006017.2)	exon 11 del	p.?	Pathogenic	NF	NA	NA	NA	NA
PRPH2 (NM_000322.5)	c.440dup	p.(Gly148Trpfs*29)	Pathogenic	NF	NA	5.8699	NA	NA
	c.647C > A	p.(Pro216His)	Likely pathogenic	NF	12 of 13	5.0999	NA	NA
RHO (NM_000539.3)	c.670G > A	p.(Gly224Arg)	Likely pathogenic	0.0000159	12 of 13	5.0399	NA	NA
RPGR (NM_001 034853.2)	c.1366del	p.(Gln456Lysfs*20)	Pathogenic	NF	NA	4.73	NA	NA
USH2A (NM_206933.4)	c.4955C > T	p.(Pro1652Leu)	Likely pathogenic	0.000016	10 of 13	5.21	NA	NA
	c.6957 + 1G > C	p.?	Pathogenic	NF	NA	5.8099	NA	NA
	c.13894C > T	p.(Pro4632Ser)	Likely pathogenic	0.00000797	8 of 13	5.21	NA	NA

Column "Classification" refers to classification according to AMCG. [a]Pathogenicity Scores from https://varsome.com/for missense variants (accessed November 2020) (BayesDel_addAF, DANN, DEOGEN2, EIGEN, FATHMM-MKL, LIST-S2, M-CAP, MVP, MutationAssessor, MutationTaster, PrimateAI, REVEL, and SIFT). Represent predictors supporting the pathogenic effect against the total of available predictors. [b]GERP conservation score based on the reduction in the number of substitutions in the multi-species sequence alignment compared to the neutral expectation using the genomes of 35 mammals. Range: -12.3 to 6.17 (most conserved). [c]HGMD public version (accessed November 2020). p.?, unknown protein effect; NF, no found; NA, not applicable. The "" symbol corresponds to: stop-codon according to the format of mutations nomenclature from the Human Genome Variation Society (HGVS).*

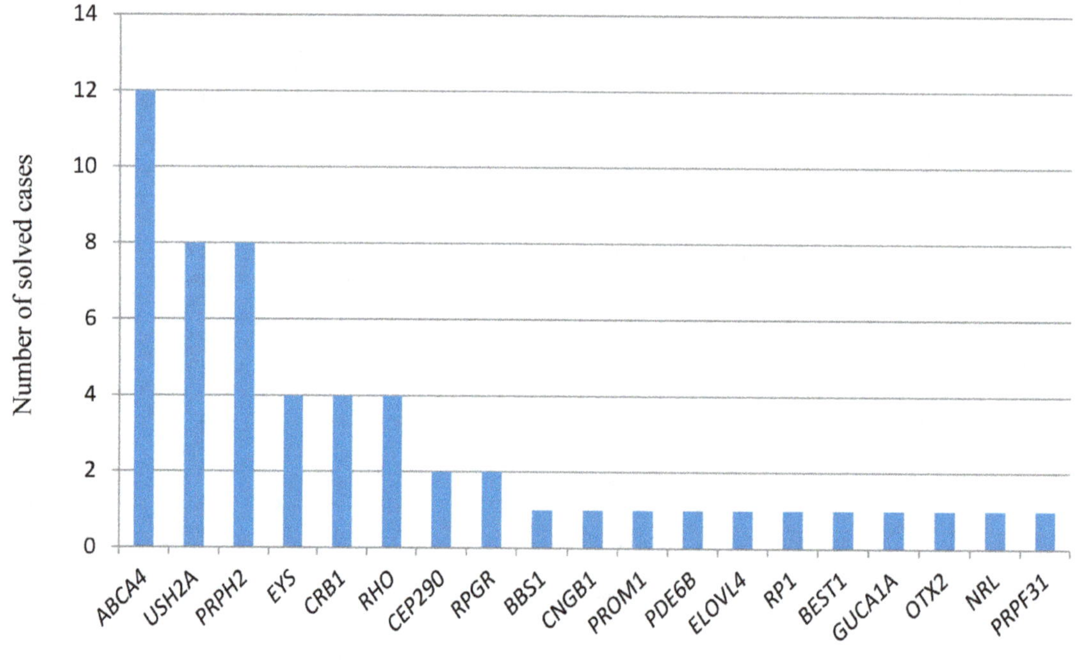

FIGURE 2 | Number of solved cases with mutations in the different disease-causing genes. The X-axis refers to the responsible genes for each solved case, and the Y-axis to the number of solved cases for each disease-causing gene. Only genes responsible for the disease are represented. For patient RPN-670 (FRPN-265), the three different possible responsible genes for the IRD are represented.

penetrance (Zernant et al., 2017; Cremers et al., 2018; Runhart et al., 2018). For autosomal dominant cases, *PRPH2* was found to be responsible for 14.8% of the resolved cases (**Table 1**), whilst a prevalence of 10.3% in *PRPH2* was the highest obtained thus far (Manes et al., 2015).

Concerning the patients who carry mutations in more than one IRD gene (**Table 1**), it is estimated that 2.7 billion individuals worldwide (36%) are carriers of an IRD disease-causing mutation, whereas 5.5 million are expected to be affected (Hanany et al., 2020). In this study, we diagnosed patient RPN-670, who was a carrier of disease-causing variants in *RP1*, *PRPH2*, and *USH2A* (**Table 1**). Despite the fact that any relative displays any symptoms, we cannot confirm that *PRPH2* and *RP1* variants are *de novo*, as DNA from family members was not available for segregation analysis. Incomplete penetrance can also be suggested, since it has been described for patients carrying pathogenic variants in *PRPH2* and *RP1* (Dietrich, 2002; Boon et al., 2008; Thiadens et al., 2012; Coco-Martin et al., 2020). It is important to remark that the fact of being a carrier of pathogenic variants in more than one gene can have a major impact on the reproductive choices for IRD patients, as well as impact their eligibility for gene-specific genetic therapies. This finding outstands the significance of achieving an exhaustive diagnosis.

The *OTX2* gene is associated with syndromic diseases, such as microphthalmia and retinal degeneration with or without pituitary dysfunction (OMIM: 610125; 610125). In this study, we also identified a nonsense variant in the *OTX2* gene in a family (FRPN-300) (**Table 1**) with an autosomal dominant mode of inheritance but only retinal symptoms. Similarly, two autosomal dominant families with heterozygous pathogenic variants in *OTX2* with only retinal degeneration patterns were previously reported (Vincent et al., 2014). Eleven truncating and two missense pathogenic variants have been described in this gene (LOVD accessed on April 7, 2021) and both type of variants have been associated with both syndromic and non-syndromic cases (Vincent et al., 2014; Slavotinek et al., 2015; Ellingford et al., 2016; Wang et al., 2016; Bryant et al., 2017; Patel et al., 2018; Sanchez-Navarro et al., 2018). Thus, a correlation between the type of mutation and the clinical diagnosis cannot be assessed.

A clear difference of the use of PV1 or PV2 concerning the solved cases (57.1% with the PV1 and 58.6% with PV2) did not exist. Strikingly, the rate of partially solved cases is almost half for the PV1 (11.1%) when compared to the PV2 (19.35%). It would be expected that the number of partially solved cases would be lower with a panel that includes all the deep-intronic mutations reported to date for *ABCA4* and *USH2A*. In our opinion, this could be due to the lower sample size analyzed with the PV2.

In general, custom panel designs remain an excellent option for the genetic diagnosis of IRD. However, due to the rapid increase of the number of genes involved, some groups prefer to use alternative approaches, such as WES (Lee et al., 2015; Riera et al., 2017; Zhang et al., 2018). Both sequencing strategies have their pros and cons. A specific panel of genes will allow the study of known IRD at a high time/effectiveness ratio regardless of the clinical diagnosis, which is an advantage in those cases in which the clinical diagnosis is not well defined or overlaps between different clinical entities. Furthermore, it allows not only the possibility of including a greater number of probes in repetitive regions such as ORF15 of the *RPGR* gene, which is highly involved in X-linked IRD cases (Vervoort et al., 2000; Megaw et al., 2015; Chiang et al., 2018; Charng et al., 2019), but also reported deep-intronic pathogenic variants (González-del Pozo et al., 2018; Di Scipio et al., 2020). On the other hand, WES made it possible to find mutations in novel IRD-related genes without updating the panel in low prevalent genes not included for the sake of increasing the depth of coverage or to identify novel IRD genes. The price reduction for high throughput sequencing has made the costs between the panels and WES quite even, so, it does not make the difference between the panels and WES. Taking this into account, the choice between both depends on the preferences of the clinician/researcher in terms of comprehensiveness, accuracy, and time consumption.

Currently, there is no significant difference between the panels and WES concerning the diagnostic rates, as the WES rate did not reach > 70% (Lee et al., 2015; Riera et al., 2017; Wang et al., 2018; Zhang et al., 2018; Liu et al., 2020). Therefore, further studies, including introns, other non-coding regions and epigenetics, are needed to achieve a comprehensive molecular diagnosis of IRD.

ETHICS STATEMENT

The studies involving human participants were reviewed and approved by the Hospital La Fe Ethics Committee. Written informed consent to participate in this study was provided by the participants' legal guardian/next of kin.

AUTHOR CONTRIBUTIONS

EA, JM, and GG: conceptualization. BG and AR: methodology. BG, AR, EA, and TJ: resources. BG: writing—original draft preparation. BG, AR, EA, TJ, GG, and JM: writing—review and editing. GG and JM: supervision. JM: funding acquisition. All authors have read and agreed to the published version of the manuscript.

ACKNOWLEDGMENTS

We sincerely acknowledge the patients for their voluntary participation and the Association Retina-Comunidad Valenciana.

REFERENCES

Allikmets, R., Singh, N., Sun, H., Shroyer, N. F., Hutchinson, A., Chidambaram, A., et al. (1997). A photoreceptor cell-specific ATP-binding transporter gene (ABCR) is mutated in recessive Starqardt macular dystrophy. *Nat. Genet.* 15, 236–246. doi: 10.1038/ng0397-236

Antiñolo, G., Sánchez, B., Borrego, S., Rueda, T., Chaparro, P., and Cabeza, J. C. (1994). Identification of a new mutation at codon 171 of rhodopsin gene causing autosomal dominant retinitis pigmentosa. *Hum. Mol. Genet.* 3, 1421–1421. doi: 10.1093/hmg/3.8.1421

Ávila-Fernández, A., Cantalapiedra, D., Aller, E., Vallespín, E., Aguirre-Lambán, J., Blanco-Kelly, F., et al. (2010). Mutation analysis of 272 Spanish families affected by autosomal recessive retinitis pigmentosa using a genotyping microarray. *Mol. Vis.* 16, 2550–2558.

Ayuso, C., and Millan, J. M. (2010). Retinitis pigmentosa and allied conditions today: a paradigm of translational research. *Genome Med.* 2:34. doi: 10.1186/gm155

Bauwens, M., De Zaeytijd, J., Weisschuh, N., Kohl, S., Meire, F., Dahan, K., et al. (2015). An augmented ABCA4 screen targeting noncoding regions reveals a deep intronic founder variant in belgian stargardt patients. *Hum. Mutat.* 36, 39–42. doi: 10.1002/humu.22716

Bauwens, M., Garanto, A., Sangermano, R., Naessens, S., Weisschuh, N., De Zaeytijd, J., et al. (2019). ABCA4-associated disease as a model for missing heritability in autosomal recessive disorders: novel noncoding splice, cis-regulatory, structural, and recurrent hypomorphic variants. *Genet. Med.* 21, 1761–1771. doi: 10.1038/s41436-018-0420-y

Baux, D., Larrieu, L., Blanchet, C., Hamel, C., Ben Salah, S., Vielle, A., et al. (2007). Molecular and in silico analyses of the full-length isoform of usherin identify new pathogenic alleles in Usher type II patients. *Hum. Mutat.* 28, 781–789. doi: 10.1002/humu.20513

Baux, D., Vaché, C., Blanchet, C., Willems, M., Baudoin, C., Moclyn, M., et al. (2017). Combined genetic approaches yield a 48% diagnostic rate in a large cohort of French hearing-impaired patients. *Sci. Rep.* 7:16783. doi: 10.1038/s41598-017-16846-9

Bax, N. M., Sangermano, R., Roosing, S., Thiadens, A. A. H. J., Hoefsloot, L. H., van den Born, L. I., et al. (2015). Heterozygous deep-intronic variants and deletions in ABCA4 in persons with retinal dystrophies and one exonic ABCA4 variant. *Hum. Mutat.* 36, 43–47. doi: 10.1002/humu.22717

Bernardis, I., Chiesi, L., Tenedini, E., Artuso, L., Percesepe, A., Artusi, V., et al. (2016). Unravelling the complexity of inherited retinal dystrophies molecular testing?: added value of targeted next-generation sequencing. *Biomed Res. Int.* 2016:6341870. doi: 10.1155/2016/6341870

Besnard, T., García-García, G., Baux, D., Vaché, C., Faugère, V., Larrieu, L., et al. (2014). Experience of targeted Usher exome sequencing as a clinical test. *Mol. Genet. Genomic Med.* 2, 30–43. doi: 10.1002/mgg3.25

Boon, C. J. F., den Hollander, A. I., Hoyng, C. B., Cremers, F. P. M., Klevering, B. J., and Keunen, J. E. E. (2008). The spectrum of retinal dystrophies caused by mutations in the peripherin/RDS gene. *Prog. Retin. Eye Res.* 27, 213–235. doi: 10.1016/j.preteyeres.2008.01.002

Braun, T. A., Mullins, R. F., Wagner, A. H., Andorf, J. L., Johnston, R. M., Bakall, B. B., et al. (2013). Non-exomic and synonymous variants in ABCA4 are an important cause of Stargardt disease. *Hum. Mol. Genet.* 22, 5136–5145. doi: 10.1093/hmg/ddt367

Bravo-Gil, N., Méndez-Vidal, C., Romero-Pérez, L., González-Del Pozo, M., Rodríguez-De La Rúa, E., Dopazo, J., et al. (2016). Improving the management of Inherited Retinal Dystrophies by targeted sequencing of a population-specific gene panel. *Sci. Rep.* 6:23910. doi: 10.1038/srep23910

Bryant, L., Lozynska, O., Maguire, A., Aleman, T., and Bennett, J. (2017). Prescreening whole exome sequencing results from patients with retinal degeneration for variants in genes associated with retinal degeneration. *Clin. Ophthalmol.* 12, 49–63. doi: 10.2147/OPTH. S147684

Burke, T. R., Fishman, G. A., Zernant, J., Schubert, C., Tsang, S. H., Theodore Smith, R., et al. (2012). Retinal phenotypes in patients homozygous for the G1961E mutation in the ABCA4 gene. *Invest. Ophthalmol. Vis. Sci.* 53, 4458–4467. doi: 10.1167/iovs.11-9166

Carss, K., Arno, G., Erwood, M., Stephens, J., Sanchis-Juan, A., Hull, S., et al. (2017). Comprehensive rare variant analysis via whole-genome sequencing to determine the molecular pathology of inherited retinal disease. *Am. J. Hum. Genet.* 100, 75–90. doi: 10.1016/j.ajhg.2016.12.003

Charng, J., Cideciyan, A. V., Jacobson, S. G., Sumaroka, A., Schwartz, S. B., Swider, M., et al. (2019). Variegated yet non-random rod and cone photoreceptor disease patterns in RPGR-ORF15-associated retinal degeneration. *Hum. Mol. Genet.* 28, 175–175. doi: 10.1093/hmg/ddy342

Chiang, J. P. W., Lamey, T. M., Wang, N. K., Duan, J., Zhou, W., McLaren, T. L., et al. (2018). Development of high-throughput clinical testing of RPGR ORF15 using a large inherited retinal dystrophy cohort. *Invest. Opthalmol. Vis. Sci.* 59:4434. doi: 10.1167/iovs.18-24555

Cideciyan, A. V., Jacobson, S. G., Drack, A. V., Ho, A. C., Charng, J., Garafalo, A. V., et al. (2019). Effect of an intravitreal antisense oligonucleotide on vision in Leber congenital amaurosis due to a photoreceptor cilium defect. *Nat. Med.* 25, 225–228. doi: 10.1038/s41591-018-0295-0

Coco-Martin, R. M., Sanchez-Tocino, H. T., Desco, C., Usategui-Martín, R., and Tellería, J. J. (2020). PRPH2-Related retinal diseases: broadening the clinical spectrum and describing a new mutation. *Genes (Basel)* 11:773. doi: 10.3390/genes11070773

Collin, R. W. J., Littink, K. W., Klevering, B. J., van den Born, L. I., Koenekoop, R. K., Zonneveld, M. N., et al. (2008). Identification of a 2 Mb human ortholog of *Drosophila* eyes shut/spacemaker that is mutated in patients with retinitis pigmentosa. *Am. J. Hum. Genet.* 83, 594–603. doi: 10.1016/j.ajhg.2008.10.014

Coppieters, F., Casteels, I., Meire, F., De Jaegere, S., Hooghe, S., van Regemorter, N., et al. (2010). Genetic screening of LCA in Belgium: predominance of CEP290 and identification of potential modifier alleles in AHI1 of CEP290-related phenotypes. *Hum. Mutat.* 31, E1709–E1766. doi: 10.1002/humu.21336

Cornelis, S. S., Bax, N. M., Zernant, J., Allikmets, R., Fritsche, L. G., den Dunnen, J. T., et al. (2017). In silico functional meta-analysis of 5,962 ABCA4 variants in 3,928 retinal dystrophy cases. *Hum. Mutat.* 38, 400–408. doi: 10.1002/humu.23165

Corton, M., Tatu, S. D., Avila-Fernandez, A., Vallespín, E., Tapias, I., Cantalapiedra, D., et al. (2013). High frequency of CRB1 mutations as cause of Early-Onset Retinal Dystrophies in the Spanish population. *Orphanet J. Rare Dis.* 8:20. doi: 10.1186/1750-1172-8-20

Cremers, F. (1998). Autosomal recessive retinitis pigmentosa and cone-rod dystrophy caused by splice site mutations in the Stargardt's disease gene ABCR. *Hum. Mol. Genet.* 7, 355–362. doi: 10.1093/hmg/7.3.355

Cremers, F. P. M., Cornelis, S. S., Runhart, E. H., and Astuti, G. D. N. (2018). Author response: penetrance of the ABCA4 p.Asn1868Ile allele in stargardt disease. *Invest. Opthalmol. Vis. Sci.* 59:5566. doi: 10.1167/iovs.18-25944

Del Pozo-Valero, M., Riveiro-Alvarez, R., Blanco-Kelly, F., Aguirre-Lamban, J., Martin-Merida, I., Iancu, I.-F., et al. (2020). Genotype–Phenotype correlations in a Spanish cohort of 506 families With biallelic ABCA4 pathogenic variants. *Am. J. Ophthalmol.* 219, 195–204. doi: 10.1016/j.ajo.2020.06.027

Den Hollander, A. I., Koenekoop, R. K., Yzer, S., Lopez, I., Arends, M. L., Voesenek, K. E. J., et al. (2006). Mutations in the CEP290 (NPHP6) gene are a frequent cause of leber congenital amaurosis. *Am. J. Hum. Genet.* 79, 556–561. doi: 10.1086/507318

den Hollander, A. I., McGee, T. L., Ziviello, C., Banfi, S., Dryja, T. P., Gonzalez-Fernandez, F., et al. (2009). A homozygous missense mutation in the IRBP gene (RBP3) associated with autosomal recessive retinitis pigmentosa. *Invest. Ophthalmol. Vis. Sci.* 50, 1864–1872. doi: 10.1167/iovs.08-2497

den Hollander, A. I., ten Brink, J. B., de Kok, Y. J. M., van Soest, S., van den Born, L. I., van Driel, M. A., et al. (1999). Mutations in a human homologue of *Drosophila* crumbs cause retinitis pigmentosa (RP12). *Nat. Genet.* 23, 217–221. doi: 10.1038/13848

Di Resta, C., Spiga, I., Presi, S., Merella, S., Pipitone, G. B., Manitto, M. P., et al. (2018). Integration of multigene panels for the diagnosis of hereditary retinal disorders using Next Generation Sequencing and bioinformatics approaches. *Electron. J. Int. Fed. Clin. Chem. Lab. Med.* 29, 15–25.

Di Scipio, M., Tavares, E., Deshmukh, S., Audo, I., Green-Sanderson, K., Zubak, Y., et al. (2020). Phenotype driven analysis of whole genome sequencing identifies deep intronic variants that cause retinal dystrophies by aberrant exonization. *Invest. Opthalmol. Vis. Sci.* 61:36. doi: 10.1167/iovs.61.10.36

Dietrich, K. (2002). A novel mutation of the RP1 gene (Lys778ter) associated with autosomal dominant retinitis pigmentosa. *Br. J. Ophthalmol.* 86, 328–332. doi: 10.1136/bjo.86.3.328

Diñeiro, M., Capín, R., Cifuentes, G. Á, Fernández–Vega, B., Villota, E., Otero, A., et al. (2020). Comprehensive genomic diagnosis of inherited retinal and optical nerve disorders reveals hidden syndromes and personalized therapeutic options. *Acta Ophthalmol.* 98, e1034–e1048. doi: 10.1111/aos.14479

Dryja, T. P., Hahn, L. B., Kajiwara, K., and Berson, E. L. (1997). Dominant and digenic mutations in the peripherin/RDS and ROM1 genes in retinitis pigmentosa. *Invest. Ophthalmol. Vis. Sci.* 38, 1972–1982.

Duijkers, L., van den Born, L., Neidhardt, J., Bax, N., Pierrache, L., Klevering, B., et al. (2018). Antisense oligonucleotide-based splicing correction in individuals with leber congenital amaurosis due to compound heterozygosity for the c.2991+1655A>G mutation in CEP290. *Int. J. Mol. Sci.* 19:753. doi: 10.3390/ijms19030753

Ellingford, J. M., Barton, S., Bhaskar, S., O'Sullivan, J., Williams, S. G., Lamb, J. A., et al. (2016). Molecular findings from 537 individuals with inherited retinal disease. *J. Med. Genet.* 53, 761–767. doi: 10.1136/jmedgenet-2016-103837

Ezquerra-Inchausti, M., Anasagasti, A., Barandika, O., Garai-Aramburu, G., Galdós, M., López de Munain, A., et al. (2018). A new approach based on targeted pooled DNA sequencing identifies novel mutations in patients with Inherited Retinal Dystrophies. *Sci. Rep.* 8:15457. doi: 10.1038/s41598-018-33810-3

Fadaie, Z., Khan, M., Del Pozo-Valero, M., Cornelis, S. S., Ayuso, C., Cremers, F. P. M., et al. (2019). Identification of splice defects due to noncanonical splice site or deep-intronic variants in ABCA4. *Hum. Mutat.* 40, 2365–2376. doi: 10.1002/humu.23890

Farrar, G. J., Carrigan, M., Dockery, A., Millington-Ward, S., Palfi, A., Chadderton, N., et al. (2017). Toward an elucidation of the molecular genetics of inherited retinal degenerations. *Hum. Mol. Genet.* 26, R2–R11. doi: 10.1093/hmg/ddx185

Fishman, G. A. (2003). ABCA4 gene sequence variations in patients with autosomal recessive cone-rod dystrophy. *Arch. Ophthalmol.* 121:851. doi: 10.1001/archopht.121.6.851

Fowler, A., Mahamdallie, S., Ruark, E., Seal, S., Ramsay, E., Clarke, M., et al. (2016). Accurate clinical detection of exon copy number variants in a targeted NGS panel using DECoN. *Wellcome Open Res.* 1:20. doi: 10.12688/wellcomeopenres.10069.1

Garanto, A., Duijkers, L., Tomkiewicz, T. Z., and Collin, R. W. J. (2019). Antisense oligonucleotide screening to optimize the rescue of the splicing defect caused by the recurrent deep-intronic ABCA4 Variant c.4539+2001G>A in stargardt disease. *Genes (Basel)* 10:452. doi: 10.3390/genes10060452

Gerber, S., Rozet, J. M., van de Pol, T. J. R., Hoyng, C. B., Munnich, A., Blankenagel, A., et al. (1998). Complete exon–intron structure of the retina-specific ATP binding transporter gene (ABCR) allows the identification of novel mutations underlying stargardt disease. *Genomics* 48, 139–142. doi: 10.1006/geno.1997.5164

Glockle, N., Kohl, S., Mohr, J., Scheurenbrand, T., Sprecher, A., Weisschuh, N., et al. (2014). Panel-based next generation sequencing as a reliable and efficient technique to detect mutations in unselected patients with retinal dystrophies. *Eur. J. Hum. Genet.* 22, 99–104. doi: 10.1038/ejhg.2013.72

González-del Pozo, M., Borrego, S., Barragán, I., Pieras, J. I., Santoyo, J., Matamala, N., et al. (2011). Mutation screening of multiple genes in Spanish patients with autosomal recessive retinitis pigmentosa by targeted resequencing. *PLoS One* 6:27894. doi: 10.1371/journal.pone.0027894

González-del Pozo, M., Martín-Sánchez, M., Bravo-Gil, N., Méndez-Vidal, C., Chimenea, Á, Rodríguez-de la Rúa, E., et al. (2018). Searching the second hit in patients with inherited retinal dystrophies and monoallelic variants in ABCA4, USH2A and CEP290 by whole-gene targeted sequencing. *Sci. Rep.* 8:13312. doi: 10.1038/s41598-018-31511-5

Gonzalez-Fernandez, F., Kurz, D., Bao, Y., Newman, S., Conway, B. P., Young, J. E., et al. (1999). 11-cis retinol dehydrogenase mutations as a major cause of the congenital night-blindness disorder known as fundus albipunctatus. *Mol. Vis.* 5:41.

Hanany, M., Rivolta, C., and Sharon, D. (2020). Worldwide carrier frequency and genetic prevalence of autosomal recessive inherited retinal diseases. *Proc. Natl. Acad. Sci. U.S.A.* 117, 2710–2716. doi: 10.1073/pnas.1913179117

Hu, F., Gao, F., Li, J., Xu, P., Wang, D., Chen, F., et al. (2020). Novel variants associated with Stargardt disease in Chinese patients. *Gene* 754:144890. doi: 10.1016/j.gene.2020.144890

Jacobson, S. G., Cideciyan, A. V., Iannaccone, A., Weleber, R. G., Fishman, G. A., Maguire, A. M., et al. (2000). Disease expression of RP1 mutations causing autosomal dominant retinitis pigmentosa. *Invest. Ophthalmol. Vis. Sci.* 41, 1898–1908.

Jamshidi, F., Place, E. M., Mehrotra, S., Navarro-Gomez, D., Maher, M., Branham, K. E., et al. (2019). Contribution of noncoding pathogenic variants to RPGRIP1-mediated inherited retinal degeneration. *Genet. Med.* 21, 694–704. doi: 10.1038/s41436-018-0104-7

Jespersgaard, C., Fang, M., Bertelsen, M., Dang, X., Jensen, H., Chen, Y., et al. (2019). Molecular genetic analysis using targeted NGS analysis of 677 individuals with retinal dystrophy. *Sci. Rep.* 9:1219. doi: 10.1038/s41598-018-38007-2

Kajiwara, K., Berson, E., and Dryja, T. (1994). Digenic retinitis pigmentosa due to mutations at the unlinked peripherin/RDS and ROM1 loci. *Science* 264, 1604–1608. doi: 10.1126/science.8202715

Khan, M., Cornelis, S. S., Khan, M. I., Elmelik, D., Manders, E., Bakker, S., et al. (2019). Cost-effective molecular inversion probe-based ABCA4 sequencing reveals deep-intronic variants in Stargardt disease. *Hum. Mutat.* 40, 1749–1759. doi: 10.1002/humu.23787

Kinnick, T. R., Mullins, R. F., Dev, S., Leys, M., Mackey, D. A., Kay, C. N., et al. (2011). Autosomal recessive vitelliform macular dystrophy in a large cohort of vitelliform macular dystrophy patients. *Retina* 31, 581–595. doi: 10.1097/IAE.0b013e318203ee60

Kohl, S., Christ-Adler, M., Apfelstedt-Sylla, E., Kellner, U., Eckstein, A., Zrenner, E., et al. (1997). RDS/peripherin gene mutations are frequent causes of central retinal dystrophies. *J. Med. Genet.* 34, 620–626. doi: 10.1136/jmg.34.8.620

Koyanagi, Y., Akiyama, M., Nishiguchi, K. M., Momozawa, Y., Kamatani, Y., Takata, S., et al. (2019). Genetic characteristics of retinitis pigmentosa in 1204 Japanese patients. *J. Med. Genet.* 56, 662–670. doi: 10.1136/jmedgenet-2018-105691

Le Quesne Stabej, P., Saihan, Z., Rangesh, N., Steele-Stallard, H. B., Ambrose, J., Coffey, A., et al. (2012). Comprehensive sequence analysis of nine Usher syndrome genes in the UK National Collaborative Usher Study. *J. Med. Genet.* 49, 27–36. doi: 10.1136/jmedgenet-2011-100468

Lee, K., Berg, J. S., Milko, L., Crooks, K., Lu, M., Bizon, C., et al. (2015). High diagnostic yield of whole exome sequencing in participants with retinal dystrophies in a clinical ophthalmology setting. *Am. J. Ophthalmol.* 160, 354–363.e9. doi: 10.1016/j.ajo.2015.04.026

Lenassi, E., Vincent, A., Li, Z., Saihan, Z., Coffey, A. J., Steele-Stallard, H. B., et al. (2015). A detailed clinical and molecular survey of subjects with nonsyndromic USH2A retinopathy reveals an allelic hierarchy of disease-causing variants. *Eur. J. Hum. Genet.* 23, 1318–1327. doi: 10.1038/ejhg.2014.283

Lewis, R. A., Shroyer, N. F., Singh, N., Allikmets, R., Hutchinson, A., Li, Y., et al. (1999). Genotype/Phenotype analysis of a photoreceptor-specific ATP-Binding cassette transporter gene, ABCR, in stargardt disease. *Am. J. Hum. Genet.* 64, 422–434. doi: 10.1086/302251

Liquori, A., Vaché, C., Baux, D., Blanchet, C., Hamel, C., Malcolm, S., et al. (2016). Whole USH2A gene sequencing identifies several new deep intronic mutations. *Hum. Mutat.* 37, 184–193. doi: 10.1002/humu.22926

Littink, K. W., Pott, J.-W. R., Collin, R. W. J., Kroes, H. Y., Verheij, J. B. G. M., Blokland, E. A. W., et al. (2010). A novel nonsense mutation in CEP290 induces exon skipping and leads to a relatively mild retinal phenotype. *Invest. Opthalmol. Vis. Sci.* 51, 3646. doi: 10.1167/iovs.09-5074

Liu, X. Z., Li, Y. Y., and Yang, L. P. (2020). [Comparison study of whole exome sequencing and targeted panel sequencing in molecular diagnosis of inherited retinal dystrophies]. *Beijing Da Xue Xue Bao* 52, 836–844.

Lotery, A. J. (2001). Mutations in the CRB1 gene cause leber congenital amaurosis. *Arch. Ophthalmol.* 119:415. doi: 10.1001/archopht.119.3.415

Manes, G., Guillaumie, T., Vos, W. L., Devos, A., Zeitz, C., Marquette, V., et al. (2015). High prevalence of PRPH2 in autosomal dominant retinitis pigmentosa in france and characterization of biochemical and clinical features. *Am. J. Ophthalmol.* 159, 302–314. doi: 10.1016/j.ajo.2014.10.033

Maw, M., Kumaramanickavel, G., Kar, B., John, S., Bridges, R., and Denton, M. (1998). Two Indian siblings with Oguchi disease are homozygous for an arrestin mutation encoding premature termination. *Hum. Mutat.* 11, S317–S319. doi: 10.1002/humu.1380110199

Megaw, R. D., Soares, D. C., and Wright, A. F. (2015). RPGR: its role in photoreceptor physiology, human disease, and future therapies. *Exp. Eye Res.* 138, 32–41. doi: 10.1016/j.exer.2015.06.007

Nasonkin, I., Illing, M., Koehler, M. R., Schmid, M., Molday, R. S., and Weber, B. H. F. (1998). Mapping of the rod photoreceptor ABC transporter (ABCR) to 1p21-p22.1 and identification of novel mutations in Stargardt's disease. *Hum. Genet.* 102, 21–26. doi: 10.1007/s004390050649

Neveling, K., den Hollander, A. I., Cremers, F. P. M., and Collin, R. W. J. (2012). "Identification and analysis of inherited retinal disease genes," in *Retinal Degeneration. Methods in Molecular Biology (Methods and Protocols)*, Vol. 935, eds B. Weber, and T. LANGMANN (Totowa, NJ: Humana Press), 3–23. doi: 10.1007/978-1-62703-080-9_1

Nishimura, D. Y., Baye, L. M., Perveen, R., Searby, C. C., Avila-Fernandez, A., Pereiro, I., et al. (2010). Discovery and functional analysis of a retinitis pigmentosa gene, C2ORF71. *Am. J. Hum. Genet.* 86, 686–695. doi: 10.1016/j.ajhg.2010.03.005

Parmeggiani, F., Sorrentino, F. S., Ponzin, D., Barbaro, V., Ferrari, S., and Di Iorio, E. (2011). Retinitis pigmentosa: genes and disease mechanisms. *Curr. Genomics* 12, 238–249. doi: 10.2174/138920211795860107

Patel, N., Khan, A. O., Alsahli, S., Abdel-Salam, G., Nowilaty, S. R., Mansour, A. M., et al. (2018). Genetic investigation of 93 families with microphthalmia or posterior microphthalmos. *Clin. Genet.* 93, 1210–1222. doi: 10.1111/cge.13239

Payne, A. M., Downes, S. M., Bessant, D. A. R., Bird, A. C., and Bhattacharya, S. S. (1998). Founder effect, seen in the british population, of the 172 Peripherin/RDS mutation—and further refinement of genetic positioning of the Peripherin/RDS gene. *Am. J. Hum. Genet.* 62, 192–195. doi: 10.1086/301679

Perea-Romero, I., Gordo, G., Iancu, I. F., Del Pozo-Valero, M., Almoguera, B., Blanco-Kelly, F., et al. (2021). Genetic landscape of 6089 inherited retinal dystrophies affected cases in Spain and their therapeutic and extended epidemiological implications. *Sci. Rep.* 11:1526. doi: 10.1038/s41598-021-81093-y

Richards, S., Aziz, N., Bale, S., Bick, D., Das, S., Gastier-Foster, J., et al. (2015). Standards and guidelines for the interpretation of sequence variants: a joint consensus recommendation of the American College of Medical Genetics and Genomics and the Association for Molecular Pathology. *Genet. Med.* 17, 405–423. doi: 10.1038/gim.2015.30

Riera, M., Navarro, R., Ruiz-Nogales, S., Méndez, P., Burés-Jelstrup, A., Corcóstegui, B., et al. (2017). Whole exome sequencing using Ion Proton system enables reliable genetic diagnosis of inherited retinal dystrophies. *Sci. Rep.* 7:42078. doi: 10.1038/srep42078

Rivolta, C., Berson, E. L., and Dryja, T. P. (2002). Paternal uniparental heterodisomy with partial isodisomy of chromosome 1 in a patient with retinitis pigmentosa without hearing loss and a missense mutation in the Usher syndrome type II gene USH2A. *Arch. Ophthalmol.* 120, 1566–1571.

Rivolta, C., Sweklo, E. A., Berson, E. L., and Dryja, T. P. (2000). Report missense mutation in the USH2A gene: association with recessive retinitis pigmentosa without hearing loss. *Am. J. Hum. Genet* 66, 1975–1978. doi: 10.1086/302926

Rodríguez-Muñoz, A., Aller, E., Jaijo, T., González-García, E., Cabrera-Peset, A., Gallego-Pinazo, R., et al. (2020). Expanding the clinical and molecular heterogeneity of nonsyndromic inherited retinal dystrophies. *J. Mol. Diagnostics* 22, 532–543. doi: 10.1016/j.jmoldx.2020.01.003

Rozet, J. M., Gerber, S., Souied, E., Perrault, I., Châtelin, S., Ghazi, I., et al. (1998). Spectrum of ABCR gene mutations in autosomal recessive macular dystrophies. *Eur. J. Hum. Genet.* 6, 291–295. doi: 10.1038/sj.ejhg.5200221

Runhart, E. H., Sangermano, R., Cornelis, S. S., Verheij, J. B. G. M., Plomp, A. S., Boon, C. J. F., et al. (2018). The common ABCA4 Variant p.Asn1868Ile shows nonpenetrance and variable expression of stargardt disease when present in trans with severe variants. *Invest. Opthalmol. Vis. Sci.* 59, 3220. doi: 10.1167/iovs.18-23881

Sahel, J. A., Marazova, K., and Audo, I. (2015). Clinical characteristics and current therapies for inherited retinal degenerations. *Cold Spring Harb. Perspect. Med.* 5, 1–25. doi: 10.1101/cshperspect.a017111

Salles, M. V., Motta, F. L., Martin, R., Filippelli-Silva, R., Dias da Silva, E., Varela, P., et al. (2018). Variants in the ABCA4 gene in a Brazilian population with Stargardt disease. *Mol. Vis.* 24, 546–559.

Salmaninejad, A., Motaee, J., Farjami, M., Alimardani, M., Esmaeilie, A., and Pasdar, A. (2019). Next-generation sequencing and its application in diagnosis of retinitis pigmentosa. *Ophthalmic Genet.* 40, 393–402. doi: 10.1080/13816810.2019.1675178

Sanchez-Navarro, R. J. I, da Silva, L., Blanco-Kelly, F., Zurita, O., Sanchez-Bolivar, N., Villaverde, C., et al. (2018). Combining targeted panel-based resequencing and copy-number variation analysis for the diagnosis of inherited syndromic retinopathies and associated ciliopathies. *Sci. Rep.* 8:5285. doi: 10.1038/s41598-018-23520-1

Sanchis-Juan, A., Stephens, J., French, C., Gleadall, N., Mégy, K., Penkett, C., et al. (2018). Complex structural variants resolved by short-read and long-read whole genome sequencing in mendelian disorders. *BioRxiv* [preprint] doi: 10.1101/281683 281683

Sangermano, R., Garanto, A., Khan, M., Runhart, E. H., Bauwens, M., Bax, N. M., et al. (2019). Deep-intronic ABCA4 variants explain missing heritability in Stargardt disease and allow correction of splice defects by antisense oligonucleotides. *Genet. Med.* 21, 1751–1760. doi: 10.1038/s41436-018-0414-9

Schulz, H. L., Grassmann, F., Kellner, U., Spital, G., Rüther, K., Jägle, H., et al. (2017). Mutation spectrum of the ABCA4 gene in 335 stargardt disease patients from a multicenter german cohort—impact of selected deep intronic variants and common SNPs. *Invest. Opthalmol. Vis. Sci.* 58:394. doi: 10.1167/iovs.16-19936

Schwartz, S. B., Aleman, T. S., Cideciyan, A. V., Windsor, E. A. M., Sumaroka, A., Roman, A. J., et al. (2005). Disease expression in usher syndrome caused by VLGR1 gene mutation (USH2C) and comparison with USH2A phenotype. *Invest. Opthalmol. Vis. Sci.* 46:734. doi: 10.1167/iovs.04-1136

Sheck, L., Davies, W. I. L., Moradi, P., Robson, A. G., Kumaran, N., Liasis, A. C., et al. (2018). Leber congenital amaurosis associated with mutations in CEP290, clinical phenotype, and natural history in preparation for trials of novel therapies. *Ophthalmology* 125, 894–903. doi: 10.1016/j.ophtha.2017.12.013

Shroyer, N. F., Lewis, R. A., Yatsenko, A. N., and Lupski, J. R. (2001). Null missense ABCR (ABCA4) mutations in a family with stargardt disease and retinitis pigmentosa. *Invest. Ophthalmol. Vis. Sci.* 42, 2757–2761.

Slavotinek, A. M., Garcia, S. T., Chandratillake, G., Bardakjian, T., Ullah, E., Wu, D., et al. (2015). Exome sequencing in 32 patients with anophthalmia/microphthalmia and developmental eye defects. *Clin. Genet.* 88, 468–473. doi: 10.1111/cge.12543

Slijkerman, R. W., Vaché, C., Dona, M., García-García, G., Claustres, M., Hetterschijt, L., et al. (2016). Antisense oligonucleotide-based splice correction for USH2A-associated Retinal degeneration caused by a frequent deep-intronic mutation. *Mol. Ther. Nucleic Acids* 5:e381. doi: 10.1038/mtna.2016.89

Srivastava, S., Ramsbottom, S. A., Molinari, E., Alkanderi, S., Filby, A., White, K., et al. (2017). A human patient-derived cellular model of Joubert syndrome reveals ciliary defects which can be rescued with targeted therapies. *Hum. Mol. Genet.* 26, 4657–4667. doi: 10.1093/hmg/ddx347

Stenirri, S., Fermo, I., Battistella, S., Galbiati, S., Soriani, N., Paroni, R., et al. (2004). Denaturing HPLC profiling of the ABCA4 gene for reliable detection of allelic variations. *Clin. Chem.* 50, 1336–1343. doi: 10.1373/clinchem.2004.033241

Stone, E. M., Andorf, J. L., Whitmore, S. S., DeLuca, A. P., Giacalone, J. C., Streb, L. M., et al. (2017). Clinically focused molecular investigation of 1000 consecutive families with inherited retinal disease. *Ophthalmology* 124, 1314–1331. doi: 10.1016/j.ophtha.2017.04.008

Tatour, Y., and Ben-Yosef, T. (2020). Syndromic inherited retinal diseases: genetic, clinical and diagnostic aspects. *Diagnostics* 10:779. doi: 10.3390/diagnostics10100779

Thiadens, A. A. H. J., Phan, T. M. L., Zekveld-Vroon, R. C., Leroy, B. P., Van Den Born, L. I., Hoyng, C. B., et al. (2012). Clinical course, genetic etiology, and visual outcome in cone and cone-rod dystrophy. *Ophthalmology* 119, 819–826. doi: 10.1016/j.ophtha.2011.10.011

To, K., Adamian, M., and Berson, E. L. (2004). Histologic study of retinitis pigmentosa due to a mutation in the RP13 gene (PRPC8): comparison with rhodopsin Pro23His, Cys110Arg, and Glu181Lys. *Am. J. Ophthalmol.* 137, 946–948. doi: 10.1016/j.ajo.2003.10.047

Trujillo, M. J., Martinez-Gimeno, M., Gimenez, A., Lorda, I., Bueno, J., Garcia-Sandoval, B., et al. (2001). Two novel mutations (Y141H; C214Y) and previously published mutation (R142W) in the RDS-peripherin gene in autosomal dominant macular dystrophies in Spanish families. *Hum. Mutat.* 17:80.

Vaché, C., Besnard, T., le Berre, P., García-García, G., Baux, D., Larrieu, L., et al. (2012). Usher syndrome type 2 caused by activation of an USH2A pseudoexon: implications for diagnosis and therapy. *Hum. Mutat.* 33, 104–108. doi: 10.1002/humu.21634

Vervoort, R., Lennon, A., Bird, A. C., Tulloch, B., Axton, R., Miano, M. G., et al. (2000). Mutational hot spot within a new RPGR exon in X-linked retinitis pigmentosa. *Nat. Genet.* 25, 462–466. doi: 10.1038/78182

Vincent, A., Forster, N., Maynes, J. T., Paton, T. A., Billingsley, G., Roslin, N. M., et al. (2014). OTX2 mutations cause autosomal dominant pattern dystrophy of the retinal pigment epithelium. *J. Med. Genet.* 51, 797–805. doi: 10.1136/jmedgenet-2014-102620

Wang, L., Zhang, J., Chen, N., Wang, L., Zhang, F., Ma, Z., et al. (2018). Application of whole exome and targeted panel sequencing in the clinical molecular diagnosis of 319 Chinese families with inherited retinal dystrophy and comparison study. *Genes (Basel)* 9, 1–11. doi: 10.3390/genes9070360

Wang, S., Zhang, Q., Zhang, X., Wang, Z., and Zhao, P. (2016). Clinical and genetic characteristics of Leber congenital amaurosis with novel mutations in known genes based on a Chinese eastern coast Han population. *Graefes Arch. Clin. Exp. Ophthalmol.* 254, 2227–2238. doi: 10.1007/s00417-016-3428-5

Webb, T. R., Parfitt, D. A., Gardner, J. C., Martinez, A., Bevilacqua, D., Davidson, A. E., et al. (2012). Deep intronic mutation in OFD1, identified by targeted genomic next-generation sequencing, causes a severe form of X-linked retinitis pigmentosa (RP23). *Hum. Mol. Genet.* 21, 3647–3654. doi: 10.1093/hmg/dds194

Xue, K., and MacLaren, R. E. (2020). Antisense oligonucleotide therapeutics in clinical trials for the treatment of inherited retinal diseases. *Expert Opin. Invest. Drugs* 29, 1163–1170. doi: 10.1080/13543784.2020.1804853

Zaneveld, J., Siddiqui, S., Li, H., Wang, X., Wang, H., Wang, K., et al. (2015). Comprehensive analysis of patients with Stargardt macular dystrophy reveals new genotype–phenotype correlations and unexpected diagnostic revisions. *Genet. Med.* 17, 262–270. doi: 10.1038/gim.2014.174

Zenteno, J. C., García-Montaño, L. A., Cruz-Aguilar, M., Ronquillo, J., Rodas-Serrano, A., Aguilar-Castul, L., et al. (2020). Extensive genic and allelic heterogeneity underlying inherited retinal dystrophies in Mexican patients molecularly analyzed by next-generation sequencing. *Mol. Genet. Genomic Med.* 8, 1–17. doi: 10.1002/mgg3.1044

Zernant, J., Lee, W., Collison, F. T., Fishman, G. A., Sergeev, Y. V., Schuerch, K., et al. (2017). Frequent hypomorphic alleles account for a significant fraction of ABCA4 disease and distinguish it from age-related macular degeneration. *J. Med. Genet.* 54, 404–412. doi: 10.1136/jmedgenet-2017-104540

Zernant, J., Schubert, C., Im, K. M., Burke, T., Brown, C. M., Fishman, G. A., et al. (2011). Analysis of the ABCA4 gene by next-generation sequencing. *Invest. Ophthalmol. Vis. Sci.* 52, 8479–8487. doi: 10.1167/iovs.11-8182

Zernant, J., Xie, Y. A., Ayuso, C., Riveiro-Alvarez, R., Lopez-Martinez, M.-A., Simonelli, F., et al. (2014). Analysis of the ABCA4 genomic locus in Stargardt disease. *Hum. Mol. Genet.* 23, 6797–6806. doi: 10.1093/hmg/ddu396

Zhang, L., Sun, Z., Zhao, P., Huang, L., Xu, M., Yang, Y., et al. (2018). Whole-exome sequencing revealed HKDC1 as a candidate gene associated with autosomal-recessive retinitis pigmentosa. *Hum. Mol. Genet.* 27, 4157–4168. doi: 10.1093/hmg/ddy281

Zhang, N., Tsybovsky, Y., Kolesnikov, A. V., Rozanowska, M., Swider, M., Schwartz, S. B., et al. (2015). Protein misfolding and the pathogenesis of ABCA4-associated retinal degenerations. *Hum. Mol. Genet.* 24, 3220–3237. doi: 10.1093/hmg/ddv073

6

Evaluation of the Genetic Variation Spectrum Related to Corneal Dystrophy in a Large Cohort

Wei Li[1,2,3†], Ning Qu[4†], Jian-Kang Li[5†], Yu-Xin Li[1,2,6], Dong-Ming Han[1,2], Yi-Xi Chen[7], Le Tian[1,2,6], Kang Shao[5], Wen Yang[5], Zhuo-Shi Wang[3,8], Xuan Chen[9], Xiao-Ying Jin[10], Zi-Wei Wang[1,2], Chen Liang[6], Wei-Ping Qian[4], Lu-Sheng Wang[5*] and Wei He[3,8*]*

[1] BGI Education Center, University of Chinese Academy of Sciences, Shenzhen, China, [2] College of Life Sciences, University of Chinese Academy of Sciences, Beijing, China, [3] Shenyang Industrial Technology Institute of Ophthalmology, Shenyang, China, [4] Department of Reproductive Medicine, Peking University Shenzhen Hospital, Shenzhen, China, [5] City University of Hong Kong Shenzhen Research Institute, Shenzhen, China, [6] School of Basic Medicine, Qingdao University, Qingdao, China, [7] School of Biology and Biological Engineering, South China University of Technology, Guangzhou, China, [8] He Eye Specialists Hospital, He University, Shenyang, China, [9] College of Plant Protection, Hunan Agricultural University, Changsha, China, [10] College of Informatics, HuaZhong Agricultural University, Wuhan, China

***Correspondence:**
Wei-Ping Qian
qianweipingsz@126.com
Lu-Sheng Wang
cswangl@cityu.edu.hk
Wei He
hewei@huh.edu.cn

†These authors share first authorship

Aims: To characterize the genetic landscape and mutation spectrum of patients with corneal dystrophies (CDs) in a large Han ethnic Chinese Cohort with inherited eye diseases (IEDs).

Methods: Retrospective study. A large IED cohort was recruited in this study, including 69 clinically diagnosed CD patients, as well as other types of eye diseases patients and healthy family members as controls. The 792 genes on the Target_Eye_792_V2 chip were used to screen all common IEDs in our studies, including 22 CD-related genes.

Results: We identified 2334 distinct high-quality variants on 22 CD-related genes in a large IEDs cohort. A total of 21 distinct pathogenic or likely pathogenic mutations were identified, and the remaining 2313 variants in our IED cohort had no evidence of CD-related pathogenicity. Overall, 81.16% (n = 56/69) of CD patients received definite molecular diagnoses, and transforming growth factor-beta-induced protein (*TGFBI*), *CHTS6*, and *SLC4A11* genes covered 91.07, 7.14, and 1.79% of the diagnosed cases, respectively. Twelve distinct disease-associated mutations in the *TGFBI* gene were identified, 11 of which were previously reported and one is novel. Four of these *TGFBI* mutations (p.D123H, p.M502V, p.P501T, and p.P501A) were redefined as likely benign in our Han ethnic Chinese IED cohort after performing clinical variant interpretation. These four *TGFBI* mutations were detected in asymptomatic individuals but not in CD patients, especially the previously reported disease-causing mutation p.P501T. Among 56 CD patients with positive detected mutations, the recurrent *TGFBI* mutations were p.R124H, p.R555W, p.R124C, p.R555Q, and p.R124L, and the proportions were 32.14, 19.64, 14.29, 10.71, and 3.57%, respectively. Twelve distinct pathogenic or likely pathogenic mutations of *CHTS6* were detected in 28 individuals. The recurrent mutations were p.Y358H, p.R140X, and p.R205W, and the proportions were 25.00, 21.43, and 14.29%, respectively. All individuals associated with *TGFBI* were missense mutations; 74.19% associated with *CHTS6* mutations were missense mutations, and 25.81% were non-sense mutations. Hot regions were located in exons 4 and 12 of *TGFBI* individuals and located in exon 3 of *CHTS6* individuals. No *de novo* mutations were identified.

Conclusion: For the first time, our large cohort study systematically described the variation spectrum of 22 CD-related genes and evaluated the frequency and pathogenicity of all 2334 distinct high-quality variants in our IED cohort. Our research will provide East Asia and other populations with baseline data from a Han ethnic population-specific level.

Keywords: corneal dystrophy, NGS-panel, mutation spectrum, population-specific level, baseline data

INTRODUCTION

Corneal dystrophies (CDs) are genetically heterogeneous disorders characterized by the gradual accumulation of deposits within different corneal layers, resulting in changes in corneal transparency and refractive index (Bron, 1990).

Clinically, these diseases are divided into anatomical categories according to the specific corneal layer involved. According to the current International Committee for Classification of Corneal Dystrophies (IC3D), CDs can be divided into 4 categories and 22 subcategories. CDs can classify into one of the following anatomical categories (Weiss et al., 2008, 2015): (a) epithelial and subepithelial CDs; (b) epithelial–stromal transforming growth factor-beta-induced protein (*TGFBI*) CDs; (c) stromal CDs; and (d) endothelial CDs. At present, corneal transplants are the most effective method for the treatment of CDs. Due to lack of clinical symptoms, some patients may be misdiagnosed before phototherapeutic keratectomy (PTK) treatment or neglected before refractive surgery, which highlights the urgent need to understand the disease mechanism of CDs (Zeng et al., 2017).

Genetically, CDs are autosomal dominant, autosomal recessive or X-linked modes. Autosomal dominant inheritance accounts for most cases and is accompanied by a high degree of penetrance (Pieramici and Afshari, 2006). To date, studies have identified disease-causing mutations in 18 genes associated with CDs, many of which have established genotype–phenotype associations. For example, mutations in six genes (*CHST6*, OMIM 605294; *UBIAD1*, OMIM 611632; *SLC4A11*, OMIM 610206; *PIKFYVE*, OMIM 609414; *TACSTD2*, OMIM 137290; *DCN*, and OMIM 125255) have found a direct genetic association with macular corneal dystrophies (MCD), Schnyder CD (SCD), congenital hereditary endothelial dystrophy (CHED), fleck CD (FCD), gelatinous drop-like CD (GDLD), and congenital stromal CD (CSCD), respectively, (Zhang et al., 2013). At the same time, there are significant heterogeneities in distinct mutations of the same gene. For instance, according to the second edition of IC3D, five distinct *TGFBI* mutations (p.R124H, p.R555W, p.R124C, p.R555Q, and p.R124L) cause different types of CDs, including Granular corneal dystrophy, type 2; Granular corneal dystrophy, type 1; Lattice corneal dystrophy, type 1 (LCD1); Thiel-Behnke corneal dystrophy (TBCD); and Reis-Bücklers corneal dystrophy, respectively, (Weiss et al., 2008, 2015).

Panel-based targeted exon sequencing has proven to have excellent performance in the molecular diagnosis of heterogeneous genetic diseases. Studies have confirmed that targeted enrichment based on multi-gene panels are highly sensitive, accurate, and reproducible (Adams and Eng, 2018). A comprehensive overview of the genetic landscape associated with the CD phenotype have been provided based on sequencing hundreds of potentially related disease-causing genes. In this study, we conducted a comprehensive CD-related genetic mutation spectrum evaluation on a large IED group, including 69 patients with clinically diagnosed CDs. Our results can provide an accurate and reliable diagnosis, and comprehensively describe the detection and carrying of disease-causing mutations in the Chinese population. These findings provide a useful reference for the pre-clinical diagnosis and treatment of patients with suspected CDs, as well as carrier screening before PKT treatment or refractive surgery.

MATERIALS AND METHODS

Subjects and Ethics Statement

The Ethics Committee of the He Eye Specialists Hospital of He University approved the study, and the studies complied with the tenets of the Declaration of Helsinki. A large IED group and their available family members were recruited from the genetic department between July 2016 and December 2019, including 69 CD patients from 50 unrelated families diagnosed in the He Eye Specialists Hospital (**Figure 1A**). All members participating in the study collected 5 ml of peripheral blood and signed informed consent forms.

Clinical Assessment

Corneal dystrophies are initially classified according to their corneal phenotypic characteristics and anatomical invasion and then combined with genetic testing results to obtain a more accurate diagnosis. According to the second edition of IC3D classification, individuals who meet the diagnostic criteria of CDs were included in this study (Weiss et al., 2015). All participants received comprehensive, detailed clinical examinations and obtained a family history, previous surgical history, and a description of the patient's symptoms. Clinical examination includes the following categories: best-corrected

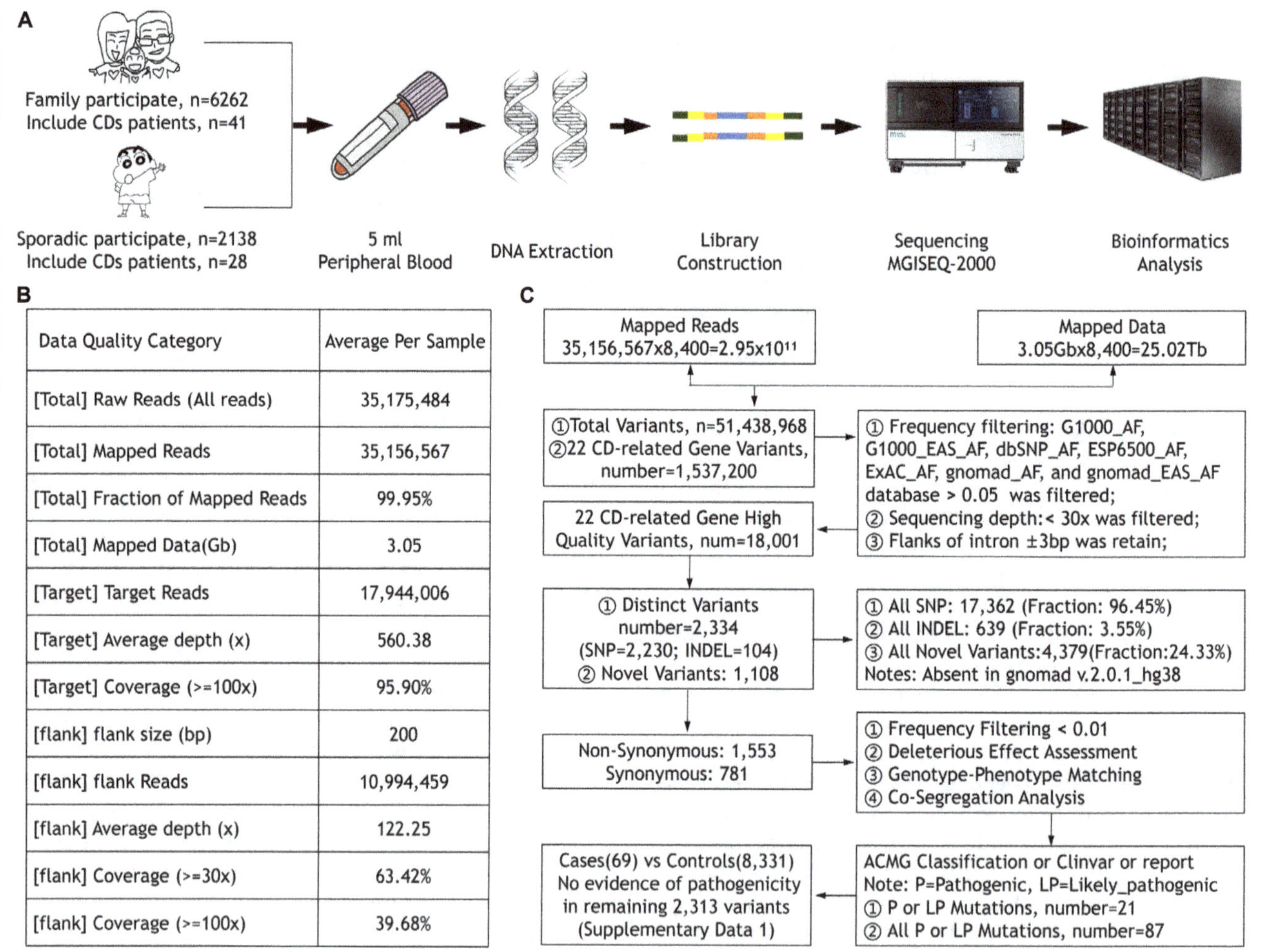

Data Quality Category	Average Per Sample
[Total] Raw Reads (All reads)	35,175,484
[Total] Mapped Reads	35,156,567
[Total] Fraction of Mapped Reads	99.95%
[Total] Mapped Data(Gb)	3.05
[Target] Target Reads	17,944,006
[Target] Average depth (x)	560.38
[Target] Coverage (>=100x)	95.90%
[flank] flank size (bp)	200
[flank] flank Reads	10,994,459
[flank] Average depth (x)	122.25
[flank] Coverage (>=30x)	63.42%
[flank] Coverage (>=100x)	39.68%

FIGURE 1 | (A) The sample collection, DNA extraction and detection, library construction, and sequencing process. **(B)** The quality of the data. **(C)** The workflow of data processing and analysis.

visual acuity, slit-lamp biomicroscopic, intraocular pressure (IOP, Goldmann tonometry), fundus autofluorescence, full-field electroretinography, typical *in vivo* confocal microscopy, and spectral-domain optical coherence tomography images recorded.

The classification of CD subtypes was based on phenotypic appearance and anatomical location, and the precise diagnostic criteria referred to the second edition of IC3D (Weiss et al., 2015). Patients with extraocular somatic cell defects or other ocular or developmental abnormalities were excluded from this study, and 69 patients with suspected congenital CDs were included.

Genetic Analysis

All participants' blood were collected and DNA were extracted using the FlexiGene DNA Kit (Qiagen, Venlo, Netherlands) according to the manufacturer's protocol. Our high-throughput targeted enrichment method analyzes 792 genes. **Supplementary Table 1A** lists 792 genes used for common inherited eye diseases (IEDs). A custom-made capture panel (Target_Eye_792_V2 chip) was designed and produced by Beijing Genomics Institute (Shenzhen, China). The panel covers the exon-capture region of 792 genes associated with common IEDs and its flank ± 200 bp. Overall, the average depth of target region was more than 560.38×, that of the flank region was 122.25×, and the coverage of the target region greater than 100× was close to 96% using the MGISEQ-2000 (DNBSEQ-G400) platform (MGI, Inc., BGI-Shenzhen, China; **Figure 1B**). We used the Burrows–Wheeler aligner version 0.7.10 (BWA-MEM) to align sequence reads to the reference human genome (UCSC hg 38). Previously reported variants were determined using the Human Gene Mutation Database (HGMD; professional version 2019.3), ClinVar, and locus-specific databases. As previously reported (Richards et al., 2015), according to the American Medical Genetics and Genomics guidelines (ACMG), mutations were classified as pathogenic, likely pathogenic, and uncertain of significance. We used Sanger sequencing to verify whether clinically uncertain novel variants that passed the initial filtration were co-segregated among members of the same family. **Figure 1C** presents the workflow of data processing and analysis. **Supplementary Table 1B** lists 22 CD-related genes on the Target_Eye_792_V2 chip and their clinical significance.

RESULTS

Cohort Characteristics

A total of 8400 individuals were included in this cohort, including 69 clinically diagnosed CD patients, as well as 8331 other types of eye disease patients and healthy family members as controls. All patients were classified into three subgroups according to different clinical characteristics: anterior segment disorders (ASDs, *n* = 1001), posterior segment disorders (PSDs, *n* = 3390), and other phenotypes (*n* = 462). The ASD subgroup includes three types of phenotypic abnormalities of the lens (*n* = 892), the cornea (*n* = 69), and iris (*n* = 40). The PSD subgroup includes choroid dystrophy (*n* = 40), retina dystrophy (*n* = 2,570), glaucoma (*n* = 173), optic neurophenotypes (*n* = 382), retinoblastoma (*n* = 40), and vitreoretinopathy (*n* = 185). All IEDs that do not meet the above two groups are divided into other phenotypes, including myopia, nystagmus, and microphthalmia. Based on these IEDs studies, we collected 69 patients with clinically definite diagnosed CDs, including two patients from two unrelated families with atypical corneal signs but positive family history, and *TGFBI* mutation was detected. These CD patients come from 50 unrelated families (total patients: 69, total participants: 91). The average age of diagnosis was 44.72 ± 19.97 (range: 3–83, median: 44), and the ratio of male patients was 49.3%.

Diagnostic Yield

Collectively, 81.16% (56/69) of patients with a clinical diagnosis of CD received a definite molecular diagnosis, and the detection rate of genetically confirmed diagnosis in families (77.27%, *n* = 17/22) did not differ greatly from sporadic cases (75%, *n* = 21/28). *TGFBI* mutations were most frequently detected. Eight distinct pathogenic mutations account for 91.07% (51/56) of the cases. Five distinct *CHTS6* pathogenic or likely pathogenic mutations were detected in 7.14% (4/56) of the cases, including three compound heterozygous mutations (p.D203Y/p.R211W, p.D203Y/p.W232X, and p.R140X/p.R205W) and one homozygous mutation (p.R205W). A homozygous mutation (p.E170K) in the *SLC4A11* gene was detected in 1.79% (1/56) of the cases (**Figure 2A**). No mutations of interest were detected in the remaining 13 cases.

Genetic Spectrum

Overall, 2334 distinct high-quality variants on 22 CD-related genes in 8400 individuals were identified. 21 distinct pathogenic or likely pathogenic mutations were detected, and the remaining 2313 variants in our IED cohort had no evidence of CD-related pathogenicity (**Supplementary Data 1**). Of them, 8 had *TGFBI* mutations, 12 had *CHTS6* mutations, and 1 had *SLC4A11* mutation. The collective explanation rate in our study was 81.16% (*n* = 56/69; **Table 1**). Pathogenic variants in *TGFBI* individuals were distributed across exons 4, 12, 13, and 14; 90.20% of mutations were distributed across exons 4 (55%, 28/51) and 12 (35%, 18/51; **Figure 2B**). All CHTS6 mutations were located in exon 3. Eight *TGFBI* pathogenic mutations were detected in 51 CD patients, and 12 *CHTS6* pathogenic or likely pathogenic mutations were detected in 4 CD patients and 24 heterozygous carriers. The frequency of each pathogenic or likely pathogenic mutation is shown in **Figures 2C,D**.

The transforming growth factor-beta-induced protein (*TGFBI*; OMIM 601692, also known as βig-H3, and keratoepithelin) is a 68-kD extracellular matrix protein. It has an *N*-terminal signal peptide (SP), *N*-terminal cysteine-rich (EMI) domain, four homologous FAS1 domains, and *C*-terminal arg-gly-asp (RGD) motif. It is autosomal dominant (Ivanov et al., 2008). According to previous reports (Ha et al., 2003b; Zenteno et al., 2009; Groppe, 2013), four *TGFBI* disease-associated mutations (p.D123H, p.M502V, p.P501T, and p.P501A) were classified as likely benign in this cohort after performing clinical variant interpretation. All these four *TGFBI* mutations occurred in individuals without clinical symptoms of CDs, especially the previously reported disease-causing mutation p.P501T that was detected in 71 individuals, which include both IEDs and healthy family members without CD symptoms. Most *TGFBI* mutations (88.25%, 45/51) identified in 51 CD patients were in one of the two recurrent mutations of the first FAS1 domain codon p.R124 or the fourth FAS1 domain p.R555 (**Figure 3A**). Fifty-one patients with *TGFBI* corneal dystrophy were detected, including 8 patients with p.R124C, 18 patients with p.R124H (15 patients with heterozygous mutations and 3 patients with homozygous mutations), 2 patients with p.R124L, 1 patient with p.T538R, 11 patients with p.R555W, 6 patients with p.R555Q, 2 patients with p.L565H, and 3 patients with p.H626R. Among them, the heterozygous and homozygous mutations of recurrent p.R124H were detected in 16 individuals and 3 individuals, respectively, and only 1 heterozygous individual showed a normal phenotype. The results indicate that the penetrance of heterozygous carriers of p.R124H mutation was 93.75% (15/16). The other four recurrent mutations (p.R555W, p.R124C, p.R555Q, and p.R124L) were all heterozygous, and the penetrance was 100%. Of the five individuals who carried the heterozygous p.L565H mutation, 3 showed a normal phenotype, indicating that the penetrance of the mutation is 40% in this IED cohort. p.T538R and p.H626R were not detected in individuals with normal phenotype. The p.R124H homozygous mutation was detected in three CD patients.

The Carbohydrate Sulfotransferase 6 protein (*CHST6*; OMIM 605294) encodes an enzyme that mediates keratin sulfate in the cornea and plays a role in maintaining corneal transparency. The defects in *CHST6* can cause MCD (OMIM 217800), an autosomal recessive genetic disease characterized by bilateral progressive stromal opacity and loss of vision, which ultimately requires corneal transplantation. A total of 12 distinct pathogenic mutations were detected in 28 individuals, including 10 missense, and 2 non-sense mutations. The recurrent mutations were p.Y358H (*n* = 7), p.R140X (*n* = 6), p.R205W (*n* = 4), which represent 25.00, 21.43, and 14.29%, respectively, (**Figure 3B**). Among 28 individuals with detected *CHTS6* mutation, there were 4 CDs patients and 24 heterozygous carriers with non-CD phenotype or normal phenotype. Among these four clinically diagnosed CD patients, three had compound heterozygous mutations p.D203Y and p.R211W, p.R140X and p.R205W, p.D203Y and p.W232X, and one had compound mutation

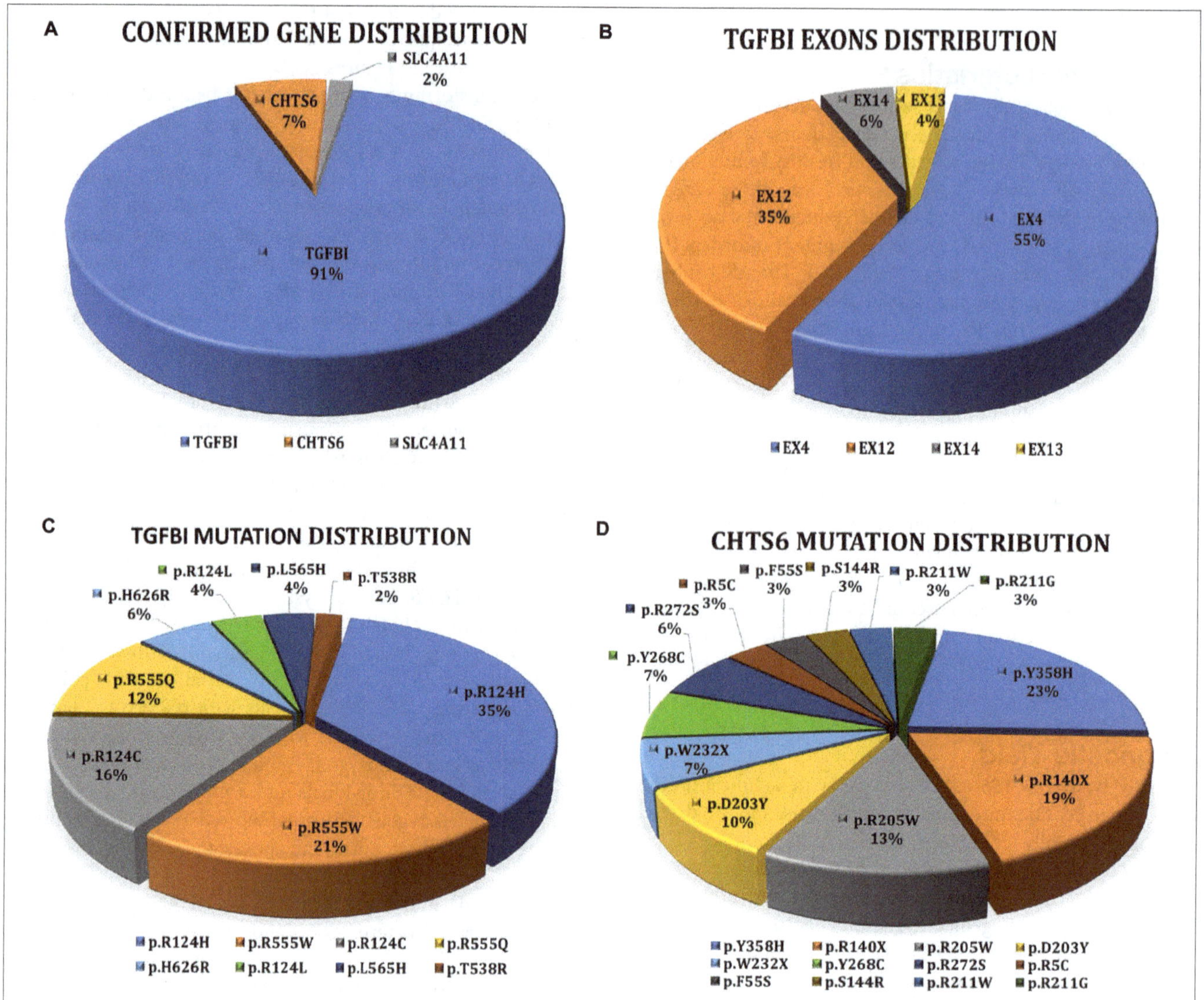

FIGURE 2 | (A) Interpretation rate of three genes detected in 56 clinically diagnosed CD patients with clear molecular diagnosis. 51 patients with *TGFBI*, four patients with *CHST6*, and one patient with *SLC4A11*. **(B)** Distribution of TGFBI pathogenic mutations in exons. **(C)** Proportion of eight *TGFBI* distinct pathogenic mutations detected in 51 CD patients. **(D)** Proportion of 12 *CHST6* distinct pathogenic or likely pathogenic mutations identified in four patients and 24 heterozygous carriers.

p.R205W. In this IED cohort, the proportion of carriers of *CHTS6* pathogenic mutations is 0.39%, so we speculate that the prevalence of *CHTS6* pathogenic mutations in the Han ethnic Chinese general population is less than 1.5/100,000.

The Solute Carrier Family 4 Member 11 protein (*SLC4A11*; OMIM 610206) encodes the membrane transport protein of the basolateral corneal endothelium, causing CHED and Fuchs endothelial corneal dystrophy (FECD). In this study, we detected an *SLC4A11* homozygous mutation in one case, and no carrier was detected.

All mutations associated with *TGFBI* are missense mutations; 74.19% (23/31) with *CHTS6* mutations are missense mutations, and 25.81% (8/31) are non-sense mutations. Moreover, of the four patients with *CHTS6* mutations, 2 (50%) had missense + missense mutation (M + M), and 2 (50%) had missense + non-sense mutation (M + N). Furthermore, 5.35% (n = 2) of the CD patients who received molecular diagnoses had refinement in the initial clinical diagnoses. These cases showed atypical clinical symptoms, but had positive family history of *TGFBI* mutations. The remaining 95.65% received definite genetic subtypes of CDs.

Supplementary Data 1 shows the result of 2334 distinct high-quality variants on 22 CD-related genes, including 2230 SNPs and 104 indels, with the total number of variants being 18,001. A total of 781 synonymous mutations and 1553 non-synonymous variants were discovered, of which 1108 novel variants that do not exist in the gnomad database (v.2.0.1.hg38) were discovered in this study. After frequency filtering, deleterious effect assessment, genotype–phenotype matching, and co-segregation analysis, 21 pathogenic mutations were found through ACMG classification, ClinVar, and or were previously reported. The remaining 2313 variants in our IED cohort had no evidence of CD-related

TABLE 1 | Variations included in HGMD or ClinVar or previously reported were identified in this study.

Gene Refseq ID	Mut_Name	Amino_Acid_Change	Exon/ intron ID	Chrs:por:mut	Mutation type	*In silico* prediction	ACMG classification	References	Zygote (number of carriers/number of CD patients)
TGFBI NM_000358	c.367G > C	p.Asp123His| p.D123H	EX4	chr5:136046403:G > C	Missense	D,D,D,D	Likely_benign	Ha et al., 2003b	Het (6/0)
	c.370C > T	p.Arg124Cys| p.R124C	EX4	chr5:136046406:C > T	Missense	D,D,D,D	Pathogenic	Munier et al., 1997	Het (8/8)
	c.371G > A	p.Arg124His| p.R124H	EX4	chr5:136046407:G > A	Missense	D,D,D,D	Pathogenic	Munier et al., 1997	Het (16/15); Hom (3/3)
	c.371G > T	p.Arg124Leu| p.R124L	EX4	chr5:136046407:G > T	Missense	D,D,D,D	Pathogenic	Okada et al., 1998	Het (2/2)
	c.1504A > G	p.Met502Val| p.M502V	EX11	chr5:136055773:A > G	Missense	T,N,P,D	Likely_benign	Zenteno et al., 2009	Het (4/0)
	c.1501C > A	p.Pro501Thr| p.P501T	EX11	chr5:136055770:C > A	Missense	D,D,D,T	Likely_benign	Yamamoto et al., 1998	Het (71/0)
	c.1501C > G	p.Pro501Ala| p.P501A	EX11	chr5:136055770:C > G	Missense	T,D,D,T	Likely_benign	Novel	Het (2/0)
	c.1613C > G	p.Thr538Arg| p.T538R	EX12	chr5:136056730:C > G	Missense	D,D,D,D	Pathogenic	Munier et al., 1997	Het (1/1)
	c.1663C > T	p.Arg555Trp| p.R555W	EX12	chr5:136056780:C > T	Missense	D,D,D,D	Pathogenic	Munier et al., 1997	Het (11/11)
	c.1664G > A	p.Arg555Gln| p.R555Q	EX12	chr5:136056781:G > A	Missense	T,D,D,D	Pathogenic	El-Ashry et al., 2005	Het (6/6)
	c.1694T > A	p.Leu565His| p.L565H	EX13	chr5:136059105:T > A	Missense	D,D,D,D	Pathogenic	Zhang et al., 2013	Het (5/2)
	c.1877A > G	p.His626Arg| p.H626R	EX14	chr5:136060907:A > G	Missense	D,D,D,D	Pathogenic	Stewart et al., 2015	Het (3/3)
CHST6 NM_021615	c.13C > T	p.Arg5Cys| p.R5C	EX3	chr16:75479816:G > A	Missense	D,D,P,D	Likely_pathogenic	Dudakova et al., 2014	Het (1/0)
	c.164T > C	p.Phe55Ser| p.F55S	EX3	chr16:75479665:A > G	Missense	D,D,D,D	Likely_pathogenic	Zhang et al., 2013	Het (1/0)
	c.418C > T	p.Arg140Ter| p.R140X	EX3	chr16:75479411:G > A	Non-sense	–,D,D,–	Pathogenic	Liu et al., 2006	Het (6/1)
	c.432C > G	p.Ser144Arg| p.S144R	EX3	chr16:75479397:G > C	Missense	T,D,D,D	Likely_pathogenic	Wang et al., 2017	Het (1/0)
	c.607G > T	p.Asp203Tyr| p.D203Y	EX3	chr16:75479222:C > A	Missense	D,D,D,D	Pathogenic	Birgani et al., 2009	Het (3/2)
	c.613C > T	p.Arg205Trp| p.R205W	EX3	chr16:75479216:G > A	Missense	D,D,D,D	Pathogenic	Park et al., 2015	Het (3/1); Hom (1/1)
	c.631C > T	p.Arg211Trp| p.R211W	EX3	chr16:75479198:G > A	Missense	D,D,D,D	Pathogenic	Liu et al., 2006	Het (1/1)
	c.631C > G	p.Arg211Gly| p.R211G	EX3	chr16:75479198:G > C	Missense	D,D,D,D	Pathogenic	Zhang et al., 2019	Het (1/0)
	c.696G > A	p.Trp232Ter| p.W232X	EX3	chr16:75479133:C > T	Non-sense	–,N,D,–	Pathogenic	Ha et al., 2003a	Het (2/1)
	c.803A > G	p.Tyr268Cys| p.Y268C	EX3	chr16:75479026:T > C	Missense	D,D,D,D	Pathogenic	Thanh et al., 2003	Het (2/0)
	c.814C > A	p.Arg272Ser| p.R272S	EX3	chr16:75479015:G > T	Missense	D,D,D,D	Pathogenic	Liu et al., 2010	Het (2/0)
	c.1072T > C	p.Tyr358His| p.Y358H	EX3	chr16:75478757:A > G	Missense	D,D,D,D	Pathogenic	Dang et al., 2009	Het (7/0)
SLC4A11 NM_001174090	c.508G > A	p.Glu170Lys| p.E170K	EX5	chr20:3234227:C > T	Missense	D,D,D,T	Pathogenic	Ramprasad, 2010	Hom (1/1)

D, damaging; T, tolerant; N, Neutral; and P, polymorphism. In silico prediction was performed by SIFT, LRT, Mutation Taster, and FATHMM. EX, exon.

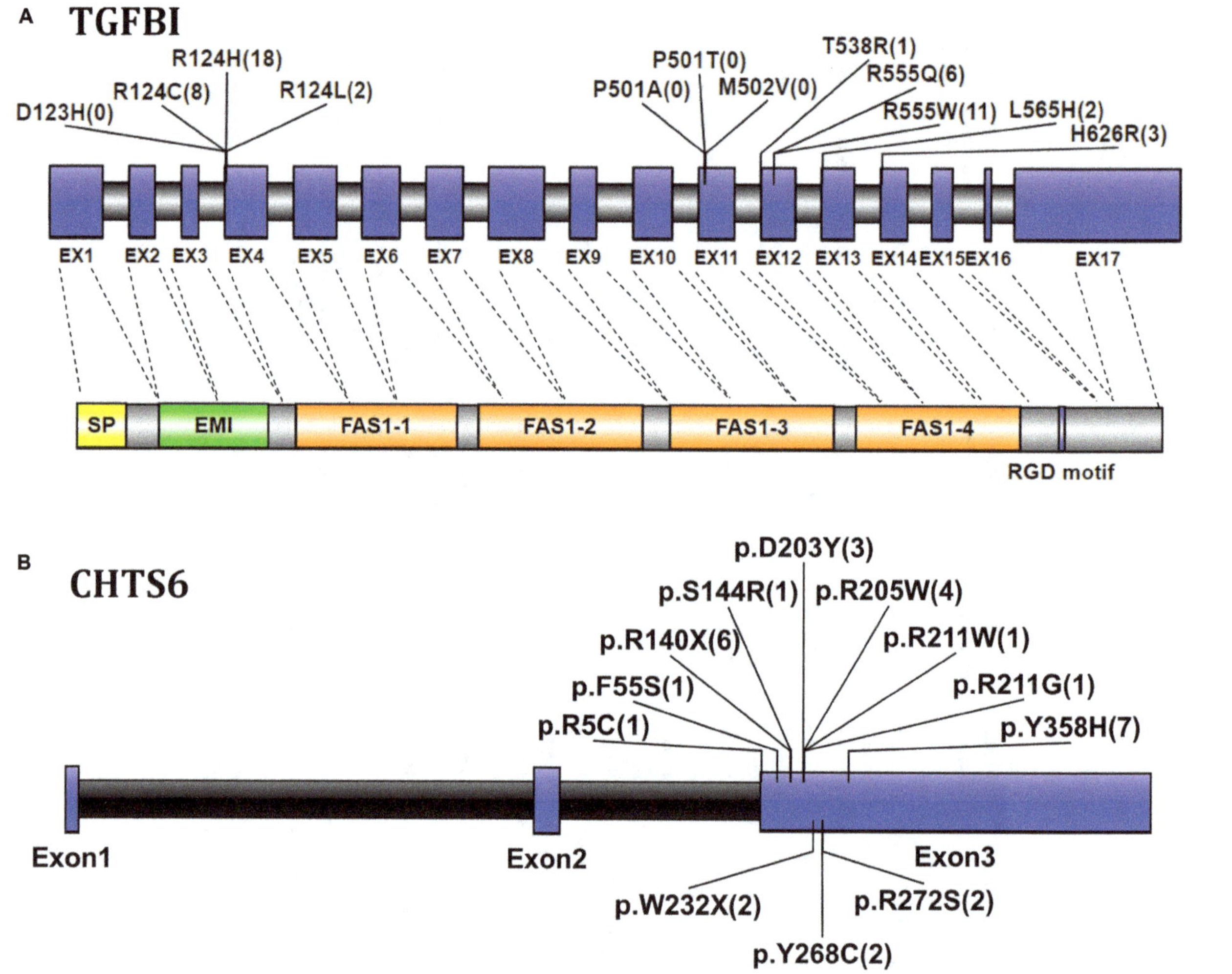

FIGURE 3 | (A) Graphical representation of the *TGFBI* gene and protein structure, showing the position of the detected mutation exon and the corresponding domain. The numbers in parentheses represent the number of CD patients with mutations detected. Exons are drawn to scale; introns are not drawn to scale, indicating exon–intron boundaries. Transcript NM_000358. **(B)** The location and number of CHTS6 mutations detected in the IED population, the numbers in parentheses represent the number of individuals with mutations detected, including 4 CD patients and 24 individuals with non-CD phenotype. Transcript NM_021615.

pathogenicity. Part of the variants included in HGMD with the symbol "DM or DM?," or in ClinVar with "likely_pathogenic or pathogenic," was reported to cause other non-CD phenotype eye disease, but there is no evidence of CD-related pathogenicity in this cohort. Moreover, 111 distinct variants of *TGFBI* were identified in 919 individuals, and only 8 distinct pathogenic mutations were determined to cause CD disease in 51 individuals. 83 distinct variants of *CHST6* were identified in 235 individuals, and only 12 distinct pathogenic or likely pathogenic mutations were detected in 4 CD patients and 24 heterozygous carriers. The allele homogeneity of nine recurrent mutations was evaluated, the frequency of alleles obtained from the gnomAD database (v.2.1.0), and their ethnic group distribution was determined through published literature. Six hotspot mutations and three founder mutations were identified, including two novel suspected founder mutations and one novel suspected hotspot mutation (**Table 2**).

DISCUSSION

To our knowledge, this is the first mutation spectrum study that focuses on genes associated with CDs in a large IED cohort. The customized panel design contains 792 genes associated with IEDs, which provides us with an accurate molecular diagnosis for identifying cases with overlapping phenotypes. Quick and accurate genetic testing can be used for the early detection and diagnosis of different types of CDs. Considering the correlation between the type of CDs and treatment options, it is essential to perform genetic testing before refractive surgery or PTK. Comprehensive molecular screening might contribute to higher overall mutation detection rate (81.16% n = 56/69) and will contribute to better general understanding of the population carriers of autosomal recessive genetic disease-causing mutations (less than 1.5/100,000). According to the IC3D classification, there are up to 22 distinct clinical classifications of CDs

TABLE 2 | The allele homogeneity of nine recurrent mutations was evaluated in this study.

Gene	Mut_Name	Amino_Acid_ Change	gnomAD_AF[#]	AFR_AF	AMR_AF	ASJ_AF	EAS_AF	FIN_AF	NFE_AF	OTH_AF	SAS_AF	Ratio*	Ethnic group distribution (references)	Founder mutation or hot spot mutation? (references)
CHST6	c.1072T > C	p.Y358H	0	0	0	0	0	0	0	0	0	0	China, South Korea (Liu et al., 2010; Park et al., 2015; Wang et al., 2017)	Founder mutation (Wang et al., 2017)
CHST6	c.418C > T	p.R140*	8.058E-06	0	0	0	0	0	1.795E-05	0	0	0	China, British, American (Liu et al., 2005; Sultana et al., 2005; Wang et al., 2017)	Hot spot mutation, this study
CHST6	c.613C > T	p.R205W	8.274E-06	0	0	0	1.117E-04	0	0	0	0	13.50	China, South Korea (Liu et al., 2010; Park et al., 2015; Wang et al., 2017)	Founder mutation, this study
TGFBI	c.370C > T	p.R124C	4.014E-06	0	0	0	0	0	8.857E-06	0	0	0	World Widely dispersed (Fukuoka et al., 2010)	Hot spot mutation (Kheir et al., 2019)
TGFBI	c.371G > A	p.R124H	4.015E-05	0	0	0	5.007E-04	0	8.860E-06	0	0	12.47	World Widely dispersed (Fukuoka et al., 2010)	Hot spot mutation (Kheir et al., 2019)
TGFBI	c.371G > T	p.R124L	0	0	0	0	0	0	0	0	0	0	World Widely dispersed (Fukuoka et al., 2010)	Hot spot mutation (Kheir et al., 2019)
TGFBI	c.1663C > T	p.R555W	0	0	0	0	0	0	0	0	0	0	World Widely dispersed (Fukuoka et al., 2010)	Hot spot mutation (Kheir et al., 2019)
TGFBI	c.1664G > A	p.R555Q	0	0	0	0	0	0	0	0	0	0	World Widely dispersed (Fukuoka et al., 2010)	Hot spot mutation (Kheir et al., 2019)
TGFBI	c.1694T > A	p.L565H	0	0	0	0	0	0	0	0	0	0	China (Zhang et al., 2013)	Founder mutation, this study

The allele frequencies in the respective ethnic group was determined from gnomAD database (v.2.1.0).

[#]gnomAD_AFR_AF: African/African American; gnomAD_AMR_AF: American Admixed/Latino; gnomAD_ASJ_AF: Ashkenazi Jewish; gnomAD_EAS_AF: East Asian; gnomAD_FIN_AF: Finnish; gnomAD_NFE_AF: Non-Finnish European; gnomAD_SAS_AF: South Asian; gnomAD_OTH_AF: Individuals were classified as "OTHER" (OTH) if they did not unambiguously cluster with the major populations in a principal component analysis (PCA).

**Ratio=gnomAD_EAS_AF/gnomAD_AF.*

with overlapping clinical manifestations, and a small number of patients displaying no apparent clinical symptoms. These ambiguities pose a huge challenge for clinicians to accurately diagnose patients (Weiss et al., 2008, 2015).

The Han ethnic group accounts for 91.51% of China's population and are also the dominant ethnic group in Taiwan, Hong Kong, and Singapore. Accounting for a total population of about 1.5 billion in the world, they are about 19% of the global population (Groppe, 2013). The World Health Organization (WHO) released the first version of the World Report on Vision in October 2019, indicating that moderate to severe distance vision impairment or blindness due to corneal opacities is estimated to be at least 4.2 million worldwide (Bourne et al., 2017; Flaxman et al., 2017; Fricke et al., 2018). Due to clinical manifestations varying widely between the different categories, whenever corneal transparency is lost or corneal opacity occurs spontaneously, especially in two corneas, or in offspring with a positive family history or consanguineous marriage, CD should be suspected. The most common causes of corneal opacity were injuries, vitamin A deficiency, and measles infection (Song P. et al., 2017). Existing data cannot provide accurate statistics on the global prevalence of CD. A retrospective histopathological analysis was performed on the corneal specimens of 3112 patients in China. Among the 637 specimens of non-infectious corneal diseases, 7.85% (50/637) of the cases were caused by CD (Li et al., 2014). Another study analyzed 2068 prospective cases of candidates for refractive surgery. Slit-lamp examinations of four cases with corneal opacity in both eyes and one case without corneal opacity were detected with heterozygous p.R124H mutation of *TGFBI*. The prevalence rate was 0.24% (5/2068 = 24.2/10,000; Song Y. et al., 2017). Analysis of commercial test data used for pre-refractive surgery screening from 600,000 samples from around the world, most of which are from Korea and Japan, demonstrated that the detection rate of TGFBI CDs in Korea is approximately 15/10,000, which is similar to the previously reported detection rate in the Korean population, which is about 11.5/10,000, and higher than the detection rate in the Japanese population 3/10,000 (Lee et al., 2010; Chao-Shern et al., 2019). In another United States study, almost 8 million eye care visit records in the national managed-care network were analyzed. A total of 27,372 unique individuals have received two or more diagnoses records of some type of corneal dystrophy, and the overall prevalence of corneal dystrophy is 8.97/10,000 (Møller and Sunde, 2013). Considering that our research group focuses on IED, the detection rate is relatively higher, and the overall prevalence is 66.7/10,000 (56/8400). The essential reason for the difference observed in prevalence across different groups is due to different countries' adoption of different genetic screening strategies. In Korea and Japan, genetic tests are part of the practice guidelines for refractive surgery in clinics/hospitals and are used for screening purposes. In the United States, when performing refractive surgery, some clinics/hospitals use genetic testing for screening, while other clinics/hospitals confirm the clinical diagnosis or exclude *TGFBI* mutations in individuals with the abnormal cornea. European clinics mainly perform clinical diagnosis (Chao-Shern et al., 2019).

The overall detection rate of molecular diagnoses was 81.16% (56/69), which was obviously higher than the previous study, with a mutation detection rate of 59.2% (42/71; Zhang et al., 2013). There was no significant difference between the two subgroups of family (77.27%, n = 17/22) and sporadic (75%, n = 21/28) cases. A total of 21 distinct pathogenic or likely pathogenic mutations were detected in our IED cohort, including 8 *TGFBI* mutations, 12 *CHTS6* mutations, and 1 *SLC4A11* mutation. Moreover, three previously reported disease-associated mutations (p.D123H, p.M502V, and p.P501T) and one novel multiple allele mutation (p.P501A) was detected but was defined as likely_benign mutations in this IED cohort (Ha et al., 2003b; Zenteno et al., 2009; Groppe, 2013). Among them, the p.P501T mutation was detected in 71 individuals with non-CD phenotype or normal phenotype; however, this mutation was found in all 18 patients with Lattice Corneal Dystrophies Type IIIA (LCDIIIA) examined in Japan. LCDIIIA accounts for 11.0% of corneal dystrophy in Japan, while only a few cases of LCDIIIA have been reported in Western countries. Interestingly, the p.P501T mutation was detected in individuals with non-CD phenotype or normal phenotype in China, but not in CD patients, indicating that the pathogenicity may vary between different races (Yamamoto et al., 1998; Tsujikawa et al., 2010; Kheir et al., 2019). Twelve distinct *CHTS6* mutations were detected in 28 individuals, including 3 CD patients with M + M mutation, 1 CD patient with M + N mutation, and the remaining 24 heterozygous carriers with non-CD phenotype or normal phenotypes.

We further verified and clarified the distribution of gene mutations for the Han ethnic Chinese population in three genes: *TGFBI*, *CHTS6*, and *SLC4A11* genes, which account for 91.07% (51/56), 7.14% (4/56), and 1.79% (1/56) of diagnosed cases, respectively. No pathogenic mutations in other 19 CD-related genes were found in this IED cohort. The frequency and pathogenicity of all 2334 distinct high-quality variants in our IED cohort of 8400 individuals were evaluated on 22 CD-related genes, of which 2313 variants had no evidence of CD-related pathogenicity. However, in recent studies of the Chinese Han ethnic, the distribution of gene mutations was mainly observed in five genes: *TGFBI*, *CHTS6*, *SLC4A11*, *AGBL1*, and *COL17A1* and the proportions were 52.38% (22/42), 30.95% (13/42), 9.52% (4/42), 4.76% (2/42), and 2.38% (1/42), respectively, (Zhang et al., 2013). In our study, *TGFBI* mutations were found in 51 CDs patients, and most of these patients (88.23%, 45/51) harbored mutations in one of two recurrent codons: p.Arg124 of the first FAS1 domain or p.Arg555 of the fourth FAS1 domain. These results are similar to previous studies in the Han ethnic Chinese population (81.82%, 18/22; Zhang et al., 2013). *CHST6* mutation is considered to be the most critical genetic factor in MCD (Zhang et al., 2019). In our group of IEDs, we found that the incidence of *CHTS6* pathogenic mutations in the general population is less than 1.5/100,000, so this is consistent with our conclusion that *CHTS6* mutations account for less than one-tenth of confirmed cases. The *CHTS6* mutation has a low incidence in the Han ethnic, despite having a high prevalence in India, Saudi Arabia, and Iceland (Aggarwal et al., 2018). In our study, the proportion of *TGFBI* (91.07%, 51/56) in confirmed cases is significantly higher than the *CHTS6* gene (7.14%, 4/56). It may be due to differences in the types of CDs of recruited patients, and the number of patients with different types of CDs.

Allelic homogeneity is the main factor leading to TGFBI-related corneal dystrophy. It occurs when a few different alleles within the same gene cause similar phenotypic expression (Tsujikawa et al., 2007, 2010). The homogeneity of alleles is explained by two different mechanisms: mutation hotspot and founder mutation. Allelic heterogeneity is a typical feature of CHST6-related corneal dystrophy, which occurs when tens or even hundreds of different alleles within the same gene cause similar phenotypes. A total of 189 distinct disease-causing mutations were found in 375 MCD patients worldwide, including 134 missense mutations, 18 non-sense mutations, and 37 indels (Safari et al., 2020). We evaluated the allele homogeneity of nine recurrent mutations, two novel suspected founder mutations, and one novel hot spot mutation. The p.R124H mutation of the *TGFBI* gene is significantly higher in East Asian populations than other populations, but it is widely reported by various ethnic groups in the world (Fukuoka et al., 2010). We speculate that it had originated in East Asia and spread to all parts of the world over many years.

In conclusion, our results reveal the mutational spectrum of 22 CD-related genes in a large cohort of IEDs. Our large reference study systematically described the variation spectrum of 22 genes relevant to CD and evaluated the frequency and pathogenicity of all 2334 distinct high-quality variants in our IED cohort of 8,400 individuals. Our research will provide East Asia and other populations with baseline data from a Han ethnic population-specific level. We believe that our work not only provides theoretical guidance and frequent genotype profiles for Han ethnic Chinese population but also provides an effective reference for genetic counseling and accurate and early diagnosis of CD patients.

ETHICS STATEMENT

The studies involving human participants were reviewed and approved by The Ethics Committee of the He Eye Specialists Hospital of He University. The patients/participants provided their written informed consent to participate in this study.

AUTHOR CONTRIBUTIONS

WL, NQ, J-KL, W-PQ, L-SW, and WH: conception and design. WL, NQ, W-PQ, WH, and Z-SW: clinical examinations and interpretation. WL, NQ, J-KL, Y-XL, D-MH, Z-WW, Y-XC, LT, XC, X-YJ, and CL: acquisition of data. WL, KS, and WY: analysis and interpretation of data. WL, NQ, and J-KL: writing, review, and revision of the manuscript. All authors contributed to the article and approved the submitted version.

ACKNOWLEDGMENTS

We sincerely thank all of the patients and families who agreed to participate in this study. In addition, we would like to thank BGI Shenzhen for their technical support and the staff at He Eye Specialists Hospital of He University for their assistance. We also acknowledge the English language revision assistance provided by David Cao (Biomedical Engineering, Harvard College). Finally, we are grateful to WH, L-SW, and W-PQ for their invaluable contributions to this work.

REFERENCES

Adams, D. R., and Eng, C. M. (2018). Next-Generation sequencing to diagnose suspected genetic disorders. *N. Eng. J. Med.* 379, 1353–1362. doi: 10.1056/NEJMra1711801

Aggarwal, S., Peck, T., Golen, J., and Karcioglu, Z. A. (2018). Macular corneal dystrophy: a review. *Survey Ophthalmol.* 63, 609–617. doi: 10.1016/j.survophthal.2018.03.004

Birgani, S. A., Salehi, Z., Houshmand, M., Mohamadi, M. J., Promehr, L. A., Mozafarzadeh, Z., et al. (2009). Novel mutations of CHST6 in Iranian patients with macular corneal dystrophy. *Mol. Vis.* 15, 373–377.

Bourne, R. R. A., Flaxman, S. R., Braithwaite, T., Cicinelli, M. V., Das, A., Jonas, J. B., et al. (2017). Magnitude, temporal trends, and projections of the global prevalence of blindness and distance and near vision impairment: a systematic review and meta-analysis. *Lancet Global Health.* 5, e888–e897. doi: 10.1016/S2214-109X(17)30293-0

Bron, A. J. (1990). The corneal dystrophies. *Curr. Opin. Ophthalmol.* 1, 333–346. doi: 10.1097/00055735-199008000-00003

Chao-Shern, C., Dedionisio, L. A., Jang, J. H., Chan, C., Thompson, V., Christie, K., et al. (2019). Evaluation of TGFBI corneal dystrophy and molecular diagnostic testing. *Eye* 33, 874–881. doi: 10.1038/s41433-019-0346-x

Dang, X., Zhu, Q., Wang, L., Su, H., Lin, H., Zhou, N., et al. (2009). Macular corneal dystrophy in a Chinese family related with novel mutations of CHST6. *Mol. Vis.* 15, 700–705.

Dudakova, L., Palos, M., Svobodova, M., Bydzovsky, J., Huna, L., Jirsova, K., et al. (2014). Macular corneal dystrophy and associated corneal thinning. *Eye* 28:1201. doi: 10.1038/eye.2014.164

El-Ashry, M. F., Abd El-Aziz, M. M., Hardcastle, A. J., Bhattacharya, S. S., and Ebenezer, N. D. (2005). A clinical and molecular genetic study of autosomal-dominant stromal corneal dystrophy in British population. *Ophthalmic Res.* 37, 310–317. doi: 10.1159/000087791

Flaxman, S. R., Bourne, R. R. A., Resnikoff, S., Ackland, P., Braithwaite, T., Cicinelli, M. V., et al. (2017). Global causes of blindness and distance vision impairment 1990–2020: a systematic review and meta-analysis. *Lancet Global Health* 5, e1221–e1234. doi: 10.1016/S2214-109X(17)30393-5

Fricke, T. R., Tahhan, N., Resnikoff, S., Papas, E., Burnett, A., Ho, S. M., et al. (2018). Global prevalence of presbyopia and vision impairment from uncorrected presbyopia: systematic review, meta-analysis, and modelling. *Ophthalmology* 125, 1492–1499. doi: 10.1016/j.ophtha.2018.04.013

Fukuoka, H., Kawasaki, S., Yamasaki, K., Matsuda, A., Fukumoto, A., Murakami, A., et al. (2010). Lattice corneal dystrophy type IV (p.Leu527Arg) is caused by a founder mutation of the TGFBI gene in a single Japanese ancestor. *Invest. Ophthalmol. Visual Sci.* 51:4523. doi: 10.1167/iovs.10-5343

Groppe, A. (2013). Critical han studies: the history, representation, and identity of China's majority. *Asian Ethnicity* 14, 483–491. doi: 10.1080/14631369.2013.759770

Ha, N. T., Chau, H. M., Cung, L. X., Thanh, T. K., Fujiki, K., Murakami, A., et al. (2003a). Identification of novel mutations of the CHST6 gene in vietnamese families affected with macular corneal dystrophy in two generations. *Cornea* 22:508. doi: 10.1097/00003226-200308000-00004

Ha, N. T., Cung le, X., Chau, H. M., Thanh, T. K., Fujiki, K., Murakami, A., et al. (2003b). A novel mutation of the TGFBI gene found in a vietnamese family with atypical granular corneal dystrophy. *Jpn. J. Ophthalmol.* 47, 246–248. doi: 10.1016/S0021-5155(03)00019-4

Ivanov, S. V., Ivanova, A. V., Salnikow, K., Timofeeva, O., Subramaniam, M., and Lerman, M. I. (2008). Two novel VHL targets, TGFBI (BIGH3) and its transactivator KLF10, are up-regulated in renal clear cell carcinoma and other tumors. *Biochem. Biophys. Res. Commun.* 370, 536–540. doi: 10.1016/j.bbrc.2008.03.066

Kheir, V., Cortés-González, V., Zenteno, J. C., and Schorderet, D. F. (2019). Mutation update: TGFBI pathogenic and likely pathogenic variants in corneal dystrophies. *Hum. Mutat.* 40, 675–693. doi: 10.1002/humu.23737

Lee, J. H., Cristol, S. M., Kim, W. C., Chung, E. S., Tchah, H., Kim, M. S., et al. (2010). Prevalence of Granular Corneal Dystrophy Type 2 (Avellino Corneal Dystrophy) in the Korean Population. *Ophthalmic Epidemiol.* 17, 160–165. doi: 10.3109/09286581003624939

Li, X., Wang, L., Dustin, L., and Wei, Q. (2014). Age distribution of various corneal diseases in china by histopathological examination of 3112 surgical specimens. *Invest. Ophthalmol. Vis.* 55, 3022–3028. doi: 10.1167/iovs.13-13805

Liu, N. P., Bao, W., Smith, C. F., Vance, J. M., and Klintworth, G. K. (2005). Different mutations in carbohydrate sulfotransferase 6 (CHST6) gene cause macular corneal dystrophy types I and II in a single sibship. *Am. J. Ophthalmol.* 139, 1118–1120. doi: 10.1016/j.ajo.2004.11.054

Liu, N. P., Smith, C. F., Bowling, B. L., Jonasson, F., and Klintworth, G. K. (2006). Macular corneal dystrophy types I and II are caused by distinct mutations in the CHST6 gene in Iceland. *Mol. Vis.* 12, 1148–1152.

Liu, Z., Tian, X., Iida, N., Fujiki, K., Xie, P., Wang, W., et al. (2010). Mutation analysis of CHST6 gene in chinese patients with macular corneal dystrophy. *Cornea* 29, 883–888. doi: 10.1097/ICO.0b013e3181ca2e74

Møller, H. U., and Sunde, L. (2013). Prevalence of corneal dystrophies in the united states: estimates from claims data. *Invest. Ophthalmol. Vis. Sci.* 54:387. doi: 10.1167/iovs.12-11211

Munier, F. L., Korvatska, E., Djema, A., Le Paslier, D., Zografos, L., Pescia, G., et al. (1997). Kerato-epithelin mutations in four 5q31-linked corneal dystrophies. *Nat. Genet.* 15, 247–251. doi: 10.1038/ng0397-247

Okada, M., Yamamoto, S., Watanabe, H., Inoue, Y., Tsujikawa, M., Maeda, N., et al. (1998). Granular corneal dystrophy with homozygous mutations in the kerato-epithelin gene. *Am. J. Ophthalmol.* 129, 411–412. doi: 10.1016/S0002-9394(98)00075-0

Park, S. H., Ahn, Y. J., Chae, H., Kim, Y., Kim, M. S., Kim, M., et al. (2015). Molecular analysis of the CHST6 gene in Korean patients with macular corneal dystrophy: identification of three novel mutations. *Mol. Vis.* 21, 1201–1209.

Pieramici, S. F., and Afshari, N. A. (2006). Genetics of corneal dystrophies: the evolving landscape. *Curr. Opin. Ophthalmol.* 17, 361–366. doi: 10.1097/01.icu.0000233955.94347.84

Ramprasad, V. L. (2010). Novel SLC4A11 mutations in patients with recessive congenital hereditary endothelial dystrophy (CHED2). Mutation in brief #958. Online. *Hum. Mutat.* 28, 522–523. doi: 10.1002/humu.9487

Richards, S., Aziz, N., Bale, S., Bick, D., Das, S., Gastier-Foster, J., et al. (2015). Standards and guidelines for the interpretation of sequence variants: a joint consensus recommendation of the American College of Medical Genetics and Genomics and the Association for Molecular Pathology. *Genet. Med.* 17, 405–424. doi: 10.1038/gim.2015.30

Safari, I., Baradaran-Rafii, A., Issazadeh-Navikas, S., and Elahi, E. (2020). CHST6 mutations identified in Iranian MCD patients and CHST6 mutations reported worldwide identify targets for gene editing approaches including the CRISPR/Cas system. *Int. Ophthalmol.* 40, 2223–2235. doi: 10.1007/s10792-020-01401-9

Song, P., Wang, J., Wei, W., Chang, X., Wang, M., and An, L. (2017). The prevalence of vitamin a deficiency in chinese children: a systematic review and bayesian meta-analysis. *Nutrients* 9:1285. doi: 10.3390/nu9121285

Song, Y., Sun, M., Wang, N., Zhou, X., Zhao, J., Wang, Q., et al. (2017). Prevalence of transforming growth factor β-induced gene corneal dystrophies in Chinese refractive surgery candidates. *J. Cataract Refract. Surg.* 43, 1489–1494. doi: 10.1016/j.jcrs.2017.07.038

Stewart, H. S., Ridgway, A. E., Dixon, M. J., Bonshek, R., Parveen, R., Black, G., et al. (2015). Heterogeneity in granular corneal dystrophy: identification of three causative mutations in the TGFBI (BIGH3) gene—Lessons for corneal amyloidogenesis. *Hum. Mutat.* 14, 126–132. doi: 10.1002/(SICI)1098-1004(1999)14:2<126::AID-HUMU4>3.0.CO;2-W

Sultana, A., Sridhar, M. S., Klintworth, G. K., Balasubramanian, D., and Kannabiran, C. (2005). Allelic heterogeneity of the carbohydrate sulfotransferase-6 gene in patients with macular corneal dystrophy. *Clin. Genet.* 68, 454–460. doi: 10.1111/j.1399-0004.2005.00517.x

Thanh, H. N., Minh, C. H., Xuan, C. L., Thanh, T. K., Fujiki, K., Murakami, A., et al. (2003). Mutation analysis of the carbohydrate sulfotransferase gene in vietnamese with macular corneal dystrophy. *Invest. Ophthalmol. Visual Sci.* 44:3310. doi: 10.1167/iovs.03-0031

Tsujikawa, K., Tsujikawa, M., Watanabe, H., Maeda, N., Inoue, Y., Fujikado, T., et al. (2007). Allelic homogeneity in Avellino corneal dystrophy due to a founder effect. *J. Hum. Genet.* 52, 92–97. doi: 10.1007/s10038-006-0083-4

Tsujikawa, K., Tsujikawa, M., Yamamoto, S., Maeda, N., Inoue, Y., Fujikado, T., et al. (2010). Allelic homogeneity due to a founder mutation in Japanese patients with lattice corneal dystrophy type IIIA. *Am. J. Med. Genet.* 113, 20–22. doi: 10.1002/ajmg.10709

Wang, L., Tang, X., Lv, X., Sun, E., Wu, D., Wang, C., et al. (2017). CHST6 mutation screening and endoplasmatic reticulum stress in macular corneal dystrophy. *Oncotarget* 8, 96301–96312. doi: 10.18632/oncotarget.22028

Weiss, J. S., Møller, H. U., Aldave, A. J., Seitz, B., Bredrup, C., Kivelä, T., et al. (2015). IC3D classification of corneal dystrophies-edition 2. *Cornea* 34, 117–159. doi: 10.1097/ICO.0000000000000307

Weiss, J. S., Møller, H. U., Lisch, W., Kinoshita, S., Aldave, A. J., Belin, M. W., et al. (2008). The IC3D classification of the corneal dystrophies. *Cornea* 27, S1–S42. doi: 10.1097/ICO.0b013e31817780fb

Yamamoto, S., Okada, M., Tsujikawa, M., Shimomura, Y., Nishida, K., Inoue, Y., et al. (1998). A kerato-epithelin (betaig-h3) mutation in lattice corneal dystrophy type IIIA. *Am. J. Hum. Genet.* 62, 719–722. doi: 10.1086/301765

Zeng, L., Zhao, J., Chen, Y., Zhao, F., Li, M., Chao-Shern, C., et al. (2017). TGFBI gene mutation analysis of clinically diagnosed granular corneal dystrophy patients prior to PTK: a pilot study from Eastern China. *Sci. Rep.* 7:596. doi: 10.1038/s41598-017-00716-5

Zenteno, J. C., Correa-Gomez, V., Santacruz-Valdez, C., Suarez-Sanchez, R., and Villanueva-Mendoza, C. (2009). Clinical and genetic features of TGFBI-linked corneal dystrophies in Mexican population: description of novel mutations and novel genotype-phenotype correlations. *Exp. Eye Res.* 89, 172–177. doi: 10.1016/j.exer.2009.03.004

Zhang, J., Wu, D., Li, Y., Fan, Y., Chen, H., Hong, J., et al. (2013). Novel mutations associated with various types of corneal dystrophies in a han chinese population. *Front. Genet.* 10:881. doi: 10.3389/fgene.2019.00881

Zhang, J., Wu, D., Li, Y., Fan, Y., Dai, Y., and Xu, J. (2019). A comprehensive evaluation of 181 reported CHST6 variants in patients with macular corneal dystrophy. *Aging (Albany NY)* 11, 1019–1029. doi: 10.18632/aging.101807

7

Discovery of Novel Genetic Risk Loci for Acute Central Serous Chorioretinopathy and Genetic Pleiotropic Effect with Age-Related Macular Degeneration

Lei Feng[1], Si Chen[1,2], Huatuo Dai[3,4], Rajkumar Dorajoo[5], Jianjun Liu[5,6], Jinfeng Kong[1], Xianyong Yin[7] and Yunqing Ren[3,4]**

[1] Eye Center, The Second Affiliated Hospital of Zhejiang University School of Medicine, Hangzhou, China, [2] Department of Ophthalmology, Jinshan Branch of Shanghai Sixth People's Hospital, Shanghai, China, [3] Department of Dermatology, The Children's Hospital, Zhejiang University School of Medicine, National Clinical Research Center for Child Health, Hangzhou, China, [4] Department of Dermatology, The Second Affiliated Hospital of Zhejiang University School of Medicine, Hangzhou, China, [5] Genome Institute of Singapore, Agency for Science, Technology and Research, Singapore, Singapore, [6] Department of Medicine, Yong Loo Lin School of Medicine, National University of Singapore, Singapore, Singapore, [7] Department of Biostatistics and Center for Statistical Genetics, University of Michigan School of Public Health, Ann Arbor, MI, United States

***Correspondence:**
Yunqing Ren
yqren@zju.edu.cn
Xianyong Yin
xianyongyin@gmail.com

Background: Central serous chorioretinopathy (CSC) is a severe and heterogeneous chorioretinal disorder. Shared clinical manifestations between CSC and age-related macular degeneration (AMD) and the confirmation of CFH as genetic risk locus for both CSC and AMD suggest possible common pathophysiologic mechanisms between two diseases.

Methods: To advance the understanding of genetic susceptibility of CSC and further investigate genetic pleiotropy between CSC and AMD, we performed genetic association analysis of 38 AMD-associated single nucleotide polymorphisms (SNPs) in a Chinese CSC cohort, consisting of 464 patients and 548 matched healthy controls.

Results: Twelve SNPs were found to be associated with CSC at nominal significance ($p < 0.05$), and four SNPs on chromosomes 1, 4, and 15 showed strong associations whose evidences surpassed Bonferroni (BF)-corrected significance [rs1410996, odds ratios (OR) = 1.47, $p = 2.37 \times 10^{-5}$; rs1329428, $OR = 1.40$, $p = 3.32 \times 10^{-4}$; rs4698775, $OR = 1.45$, $p = 2.20 \times 10^{-4}$; and rs2043085, $OR = 1.44$, $p = 1.91 \times 10^{-4}$]. While the genetic risk effects of rs1410996 and rs1329428 (within the well-established locus CFH) are correlated (due to high LD), rs4698775 on chromosome 4 and rs2043085 on chromosome 15 are novel risk loci for CSC. Polygenetic risk score (PRS) constructed by using three independent SNPs (rs1410996, rs4698775, and rs2043085) showed highly significant association with CSC ($p = 2.10 \times 10^{-7}$), with the top 10% of subjects with high PRS showing 6.39 times higher risk than the bottom 10% of subjects with lowest PRS. Three SNPs were also found to be associated with clinic manifestations of CSC patients. In addition, by comparing the genetic effects (ORs) of these 38 SNPs between CSC and AMD, our study revealed significant, but complex genetic pleiotropic effect between the two diseases.

Conclusion: By discovering two novel genetic risk loci and revealing significant genetic pleiotropic effect between CSC and AMD, the current study has provided novel insights into the role of genetic composition in the pathogenesis of CSC.

Keywords: central serous chorioretinopathy, gene, association, pleiotropic effect, risk loci, age-related macular degeneration

INTRODUCTION

Central serous chorioretinopathy (CSC) is a common chorioretinal disorder characterized by serous sensorial retinal detachment (Balaratnasingam et al., 2016). It is now recognized as the fourth most incident eye disorder after age-related macular degeneration (AMD), diabetic retinopathy, and branch retinal vein occlusion among non-surgical retinopathies (Wang et al., 2008). CSC occurs most frequently in midlife, and the prevalence in men is nearly six times higher than in women (Wang et al., 2008; Liew et al., 2013). The etiology of CSC remains unclear, but several factors have been implicated in the disease development including administration of corticosteroids, hypercortisolism, stress, altered plasma cytokine levels, and genetic risk factors (Daruich et al., 2015; Karska-Basta et al., 2020, 2021a,b). CSC patients cluster in families (Oosterhuis, 1996; Weenink et al., 2001), and the prevalence of CSC varies in different ethnic populations, with higher prevalence in Asians than in Caucasians and African Americans (Desai et al., 2003; How and Koh, 2006; Kitzmann et al., 2008; Tsai et al., 2013), suggesting that genetic compositions may contribute to the risk of CSC.

Two main subtypes of CSC, acute and chronic CSC, show distinct clinical presentations in terms of the episode duration, extent of retinal abnormalities, and final vision recovery (Daruich et al., 2015). In comparison with chronic CSC, patients with acute CSC characteristically show a sudden onset of obvious visual deterioration and relatively short course within 6 months (Daruich et al., 2017). In multivariate regression analyses, age of onset, duration of disease, and hyperopia were positively associated with the risk of chronic disease rather than acute CSC (Ersoz et al., 2018). Although most of acute CSC patients have been described to be self-limiting, some patients still suffer recurrences or progress to a chronic condition, indicating interindividual variation of risk and clinical course in acute CSC. These clinical differences suggest that some aspects of underlying molecular pathogenesis might be different between acute and chronic CSCs.

Genetic association studies have identified several genetic variants that are significantly associated with CSC, including single nucleotide polymorphisms (SNPs) in the complement factor H (CFH), solute carrier family 7 member 5 (SLC7A5), age-related maculopathy susceptibility 2 (ARMS2), nuclear receptor subfamily 3 group C member 2 (NR3C2), cadherin 5 (CDH5), and TNF receptor superfamily member 10a (TNFRSF10A) gene, as well as copy number variations in the complement C4B gene (Miki et al., 2014, 2018; Schubert et al., 2014; Breukink et al., 2015; de Jong et al., 2015; van Dijk et al., 2017; Schellevis et al., 2018; Hosoda et al., 2019). However, previous studies focused primarily on chronic CSC, and mainly in western and Japanese populations (van Dijk et al., 2017; Miki et al., 2018; Schellevis et al., 2018). The genetic association study in acute CSC may help to identify genetic factors responsible for clinical variability between acute and chronic CSC, and among acute CSC patients. In addition, the diverse prevalence of CSC across different regions and countries also suggests a possible variation of genetic susceptibility across different ethnic backgrounds (Desai et al., 2003; Tsai et al., 2013). As a result, study in Chinese populations would have the potential to identify novel genetic risk loci and elucidate the genetic heterogeneity of CSC across different populations.

Notably, CFH gene, as a well-established AMD susceptibility gene, is the only genetic association locus for CSC that has been replicated in multiple independent studies so far (Miki et al., 2014; de Jong et al., 2015; Schellevis et al., 2018; Karkhaneh et al., 2021). Interestingly, several manifestations of CSC, such as retinal pigment epithelium (RPE) disruption and neurosensory retinal detachment in macula, are also frequently observed in AMD patients. Those eyes with CSC were documented to be at higher risk of developing AMD even after spontaneous resolution of CSC (Hosoda et al., 2018). Together, these suggest that CSC and AMD may share some common genetic and pathophysiologic background. To investigate AMD-associated genetic risk variants in CSC patients by a genetic association analysis is a good strategy to elucidate genetic susceptibility for CSC and to explore genetic pleiotropic effect between CSC and AMD.

Here, we performed a genetic study to evaluate the association of 38 known AMD-associated SNPs with the risk of acute CSC in a Chinese population. We further investigated the impact of significantly associated risk variants on the clinical manifestations in CSC patients and compared the genetic effects of these loci between CSC and AMD. These findings shed light on the genetic susceptibility of CSC in Chinese populations as well as genetic pleiotropic effect between CSC and AMD.

MATERIALS AND METHODS

Study Participants

A total of 464 Chinese patients were recruited, all of whom had their first episode of idiopathic acute CSC. All patients were enrolled from the Eye Center, the Second Affiliated Hospital, School of Medicine, Zhejiang University, China, between January 2014 and April 2017. Each patient underwent an extensive ophthalmologic examination including fundoscopy, spectral-domain optical coherence tomography (SD-OCT, Zeiss Cirrus OCT 5000, Germany), fundus fluorescein angiography (FFA, Spectralis HRA-II, Germany), and indocyanine green angiography (ICGA, Spectralis HRA-II, Germany). Inclusion criteria in our study were initial presentation of less than 20 days after eye symptoms onset, the presence of subretinal fluid (SRF) in OCT, focal leakage spot on FFA and corresponding hyperfluorescence on ICGA, and without any atrophic RPE changes. Consensus diagnosis of acute CSC was performed by two senior ophthalmologists (LF and SC). We excluded chronic CSC patients that were diagnosed with chronic SRF leakage, with extensive multifocal atrophic RPE changes and/or disease duration of more than 3 months. In addition, we excluded patients with any evidence of AMD, polypoidal choroidal vasculopathy, retinal vascular diseases, diabetic retinopathy, spherical error higher than 3D, intraocular surgery, and laser history. A total of 548 healthy controls were included in the study. Any participants were excluded from the controls if they were (1) with any clinical manifestations of visual impairment, visual distortion, and dyslexia; (2) with any early AMD symptoms in fundus examination, such as pigmentation disorder and atrophy in macular area; (3) with CSC manifestations detected by OCT and FFA; (4) with other ocular and systemic diseases. All the study subjects were of Chinese origin. Each participant provided written informed consent. This study was approved by the Ethics Committee of Zhejiang University School of Medicine and was conducted according to the Declaration of Helsinki.

DNA Isolation and Genotyping

Ethylenediamine tetracetic acid (EDTA)-anticoagulated venous blood samples were collected from each participant, and then genomic DNA from peripheral blood leukocytes were extracted by standard procedures using AxyPrep-96 Blood Genomic DNA Kits (Axygen, Union City, CA, United States). We selected 47 SNPs that have been previously reported for the risk of AMD through manual literature review (**Supplementary Table 1**) and genotyped them in 464 acute CSC patients and 548 controls by SNaPshot Multiplex Kit (Applied Biosystems Co., San Francisco, CA, United States). All procedures were performed according to the manufacturer's instructions.

Quality Control and Statistical Analysis

Three SNPs with minor allele frequency (MAF) <1%, or Hardy-Weinberg disequilibrium in the controls ($p < 10^{-6}$, $n = 6$ SNPs) were excluded from further analysis. In addition, six samples were excluded due to low genotyping call rates (i.e., call rate < 90%). We tested the single-variant association with the risk of CSC using logistic regression with gender and age as covariates in Plink v1.90 (Chang et al., 2015). $p < 0.001$ (0.05/38) was adopted as the significance threshold after Bonferroni correction for multiple testing. We also evaluated the association between the significant risk variants and clinical manifestations relevant to FFA (FFA-traits) and OCT diagnoses (OCT-traits) in the CSC patients through logistic regression (FFA) or linear regression (OCT) in Plink v1.90. We included three covariates, including gender, eye, and age at recruitment, in FFA-traits association analysis, while adjusting an additional covariate of OCT equipment in OCT-traits association tests. To evaluate the cumulative effect of genetic variants on CSC risk, we computed a polygenic risk score (PRS) for each participant through adding up their genotypes for the three independently significant SNPs which were weighted by their corresponding association effect sizes. We then grouped the subjects into four quartiles by their PRSs in healthy controls. The cumulative risk effects were assessed by estimating the odd ratios against the first quartile through logistic regression test.

For the gene ontology (GO) term enrichment analysis, known genes within the 10-kb regions of 12 SNPs shared between CSC and AMD were mapped using the SNP2GENE function in Functional Mapping and Annotation of Genome Wide Association Studies (FUMA) (Watanabe et al., 2017). Gene-set enrichments in GO terms were subsequently performed for the genes using the GENE2FUNC function in FUMA. In gene-set enrichments, tests for overrepresentation of the genes were performed using hypergeometric tests. All gene-set enrichment p-values were adjusted using Benjamini-Hochberg (B-H) correction for multiple tests.

RESULTS

Characteristics of Study Subjects

In our study, 464 acute CSC patients and 548 controls were recruited. The cases (average age = 44.45 ± 7.04 years) and controls (average age = 46.80 ± 14.53 years) were matched on age, but there is a moderate difference in gender ratio between the cases (81.03% being males) and controls (62.22% being males). The clinical features of acute CSC patients are shown in **Figure 1**. The averages of horizontal and vertical dimensions of SRF were 280.06 ± 139.52 μm and 290.90 ± 146.98 μm, respectively. The averages of central subfield thickness and volume were 451.27 ± 146.46 μm and 11.56 ± 1.78 μm, respectively. FFA imaging characteristics varied among patients (**Figure 1**): 1 leakage point in 319 eyes (69.96%), 2 leakage points in 137 eyes (30.04%), inkblot-like leakage in 360 eyes (78.95%), and smokestack leakage in 96 eyes (21.05%).

Association Analysis of AMD Loci in Acute CSC

We tested single-variant association between 38 known AMD-risk SNPs and the risk of CSC in 459 cases and 547 controls. Of the 38 SNPs tested, 12 SNPs showed association at nominal significance ($p < 0.05$; **Table 1** and **Supplementary Table 1**), and 4 SNPs on chromosomes 1, 4, and 15 showed strong association with Bonferroni (BF)-corrected significance (Chr 1: rs1410996, $OR = 1.47$, $p = 2.37 \times 10^{-5}$; Chr 1: rs1329428, $OR = 1.40$, $p = 3.32 \times 10^{-4}$; Chr 4: rs4698775, $OR = 1.45$, $p = 2.20 \times 10^{-4}$; and Chr 15: rs2043085, $OR = 1.44$, $p = 1.91 \times 10^{-4}$). Rs1410996 and rs1329428 on chromosome 1 are in strong linkage disequilibrium ($r^2 = 0.94$); the association at SNP rs1329428 diminished after conditioning on rs1410996 ($p > 0.05$). Pairwise

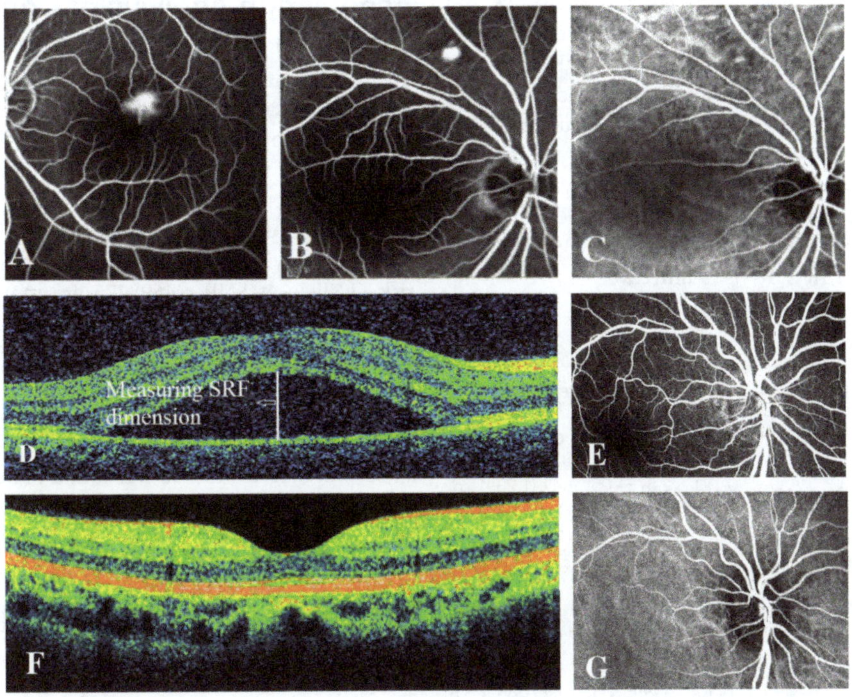

FIGURE 1 | Examples of fundus fluorescein angiography (FFA), indocyanine green (ICG) angiography, and spectral-domain optical coherence tomography (SD-OCT) in individuals with acute CSC and controls. **(A)** The left eye of an individual with a typical smokestack leakage point on FFA. **(B)** The right eye of an individual with a typical inkblot-like leakage point on FFA. **(C)** The ICGA image of the same individual as in panel **(B)**, showing choroidal vascular dilatation. **(D)** An obvious central subretinal fluid (SRF) between retinal neurepithelium layer and retinal pigment epithelium layer on OCT. **(E)** The FFA image of one of the controls showing no leakage point. **(F)** The OCT image of one of the controls showing no subretinal fluid. **(G)** The normal ICGA image of one of the controls.

TABLE 1 | Association results for 12 AMD-known SNPs with nominal significance in acute CSC in Han Chinese population.

SNP	CHR	BP	Gene	A1/A2[a]	EAF		SE	*P*-value	OR-CSC	OR-AMD
					Case	Control				
rs1410996	1	196,696,933	*CFH*	A/G	0.52	0.41	0.09	2.37E−05	1.47	0.37 (Yu et al., 2011)
rs1329428	1	196,702,810	*CFH*	T/C	0.52	0.43	0.09	3.32E−04	1.40	0.36 (Kopplin et al., 2010)
rs2043085	15	58,680,954	*LIPC*	A/G	0.55	0.46	0.10	1.91E−04	1.44	1.15 (Fritsche et al., 2016)
rs4698775	4	110,590,479	*MCUB-PLA2G12A-CFI*	G/T	0.29	0.21	0.10	2.20E−04	1.45	1.14 (Fritsche et al., 2013)
rs429358	19	45,411,941	*APOE*	C/T	0.03	0.06	0.24	8.39E−03	0.53	0.70 (Fritsche et al., 2016)
rs10507047	12	95,604,290	*FGD6*	C/T	0.34	0.29	0.10	1.85E−02	1.26	0.87 (Cheng et al., 2015)
rs1142	7	104,756,326	*KMT2E, SRPK2*	T/C	0.33	0.29	0.10	2.30E−02	1.26	1.11 (Fritsche et al., 2016)
rs4420638	19	45,422,946	*APOE*	G/A	0.08	0.11	0.16	2.56E−02	0.70	0.77 (Fritsche et al., 2013)
rs1713985	4	57,786,450	*NOA1, REST, IGFBP7, POLR2B*	G/T	0.23	0.27	0.11	2.86E−02	0.79	1.30 (Arakawa et al., 2011)
rs10781182	9	76,617,720	*RORB*	G/T	0.29	0.24	0.11	4.11E−02	1.26	0.90 (Fritsche et al., 2016)
rs3812111	6	116,443,735	*COL10A1*	A/T	0.25	0.19	0.11	4.12E−02	1.24	0.91 (Fritsche et al., 2013)
rs2740488	9	107,661,742	*ABCA1*	C/A	0.26	0.22	0.12	4.98E−02	1.26	0.90 (Fritsche et al., 2016)

SNP, single nucleotide polymorphism; CHR, chromosome; BP, base pair in hg19; EAF, effective allele frequency; OR, odds ratio; SE, standard error; CSC, central serous chorioretinopathy; AMD, age-related macular degeneration; CFH, complement factor H; LIPC, hepatic lipase; MCUB, mitochondrial calcium uniporter dominant negative subunit beta; PLA2G12A, phospholipase A2 group XIIA; CFI, Complement factor I; APOE, apolipoprotein E; FGD6, FYVE, RhoGEF, and PH domain containing 6; KMT2E, lysine methyltransferase 2E; SRPK2, SRSF protein kinase 2; NOA1, nitric oxide associated 1; REST, RE1 silencing transcription factor; IGFBP7, insulin-like growth factor-binding protein 7; POLR2B, RNA polymerase II subunit B; RORB, RAR-related orphan receptor B; COL10A1, collagen type X alpha 1 chain; ABCA1, ATP-binding cassette subfamily A member 1.

[a] *A1/A2, effective allele and alternative allele.*

interaction analyses among the three SNPs were also conducted using logistic regression. We only detected interaction between rs1410996 and rs4698775 (p = 0.038), which is, however, not statistically significant after correction for multiple pair-wise interaction testing, suggesting that the genetic association effects at these SNPs are largely additive. Our results also suggested that the genetic association effects at rs1410996, rs4698775, and rs2043085 followed a recessive mode of inheritance (**Table 2**). Next, these three SNPs were used to calculate a PRS for each subject. The PRS showed a highly significant association with CSC ($p = 2.10 \times 10^{-7}$), with the top 10% of subjects with highest PRS showing 6.39 times higher risk than the bottom 10% of subjects with lowest PRS. In comparison with the first quartile, the second, third, and fourth quartiles of PRS conferred significant cumulative risk effect ($OR = 1.10$, $p = 0.03$; $OR = 1.11$, $p = 0.02$; $OR = 1.33$, $p = 4.18 \times 10^{-11}$; **Figure 2**).

TABLE 2 | Association results for the three SNPs under three different models.

CHR	SNP	BP	A1/A2[a]	Model	*P*-value	OR (95% CI)
1	rs1410996	196,696,933	A/G	ADD	2.37E–05	1.47 (1.23–1.75)
				DOM	3.22E–02	1.36 (1.03–1.79)
				REC	7.98E–07	2.19 (1.60–3.00)
4	rs4698775	110,590,479	G/T	ADD	2.20E–04	1.45 (1.19–1.76)
				DOM	3.23E–02	1.33 (1.03–1.72)
				REC	2.91E–06	3.08 (1.92–4.93)
15	rs2043085	58,680,954	A/G	ADD	1.91E–04	1.44 (1.18–1.75)
				DOM	4.62E–02	1.37 (1.00–1.87)
				REC	5.90E–05	1.87 (1.37–2.56)

CHR, chromosome; SNP, single nucleotide polymorphism; BP, base pair; ADD, DOM, REC, additive, dominant, and recessive mode of inheritance, respectively; P, the genetic association p-values under each mode of inheritance; OR, odds ratio; 95% CI, 95% confidence interval.

[a]A1/A2, effective allele and alternative allele.

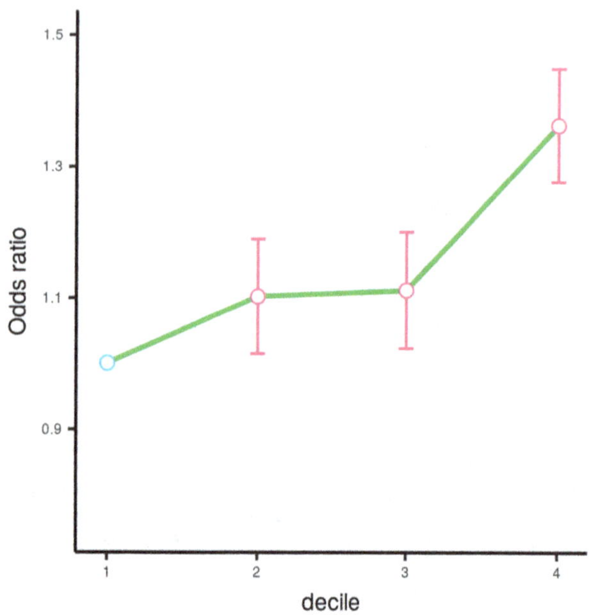

FIGURE 2 | Odds ratios (OR) by the quartile of polygenic risk score estimated based on the top three SNPs. The circle denotes the estimated value of odds ratio. The error bar represents the 95% confidence interval for the odds ratio estimation. The circle is colored in pink ($p < 0.05$) and blue ($p > 0.05$) according to its corresponding respective *p*-value.

Association Analysis of Confirmed CSC Loci With Clinical Phenotypes

To evaluate whether these three risk variants have any effect on the clinical manifestations of the disease, we tested the associations of the three SNPs with FFA- and OCT-traits in CSC patients, including the shape, amount and location of fluid leakage, the central subfield thickness and volume, the maximum horizontal and vertical dimensions of SRF. We found that the patients carrying the risk A allele at SNP rs2043085 or the risk G allele at SNP rs4698775 are more likely to exhibit the smokestack shape of fluid leakage than inkblot-like leakage on FFA in acute CSC patients ($OR = 1.61$, $p = 3.83 \times 10^{-3}$; $OR = 1.39$, $p = 2.34 \times 10^{-2}$, respectively; **Table 3**). Consistently, the PRS also showed significant association with a smokestack shape of fluid leakage ($p = 6.99 \times 10^{-4}$; **Figure 3**). In addition, the risk allele G of SNP rs1410996 was found to be associated with larger central subfield thickness ($\beta = 0.15$, $p = 2.26 \times 10^{-2}$), increased horizontal dimension ($\beta = 0.14$, $p = 3.78 \times 10^{-2}$), and increased vertical dimension of SRF ($\beta = 0.18$, $p = 7.84 \times 10^{-3}$; **Table 4**).

Comparison of the Genetic Effects Between CSC and AMD

To further investigate genetic pleiotropic effect between CSC and AMD, we compared the estimated genetic effects (ORs) of these 38 SNPs on CSC (estimated from the current study) and the previously published ones on AMD. Of the 12 SNPs that achieved nominal associations in CSC ($p < 0.05$), 7 SNPs had opposite effects between CSC and AMD, while 5 SNPs showed the consensus effects between CSC and AMD (**Figure 4**). Of the five SNPs with the same direction of effect, four SNPs showed stronger effect in CSC than AMD. Only rs4420638 at *APOE* locus showed consistent effect between CSC ($OR = 0.70$) and AMD ($OR = 0.77$). In addition, we also performed GO term enrichment analysis of these 12 SNPs using FUMA. No significant GO term enrichments were identified for the seven SNPs that showed opposite effects (data not shown). For the 5 SNPs with consistent effects, the analysis revealed 13 significant enriched GO terms (B-H adj $p < 0.05$). These biological pathways and processes are largely driven by the *APOE* and *APOC1* genes and seem to be related to lipid metabolism (**Figure 5**).

DISCUSSION

In the current study, the associations of 38 AMD-associated SNPs with the risk of acute CSC were investigated in a large Chinese cohort, consisting of 464 acute CSC patients and 548 healthy controls. Three genetic risk loci (rs1410996 on chromosome 1, rs4698775 on chromosome 4, and rs2043085 on chromosome 15) were identified for CSC with solid evidence that surpass the threshold of statistical significance after Bonferroni correction. Of the three loci, the *CFH* locus on chromosome 1 is a well-established genetic risk locus for CSC, and the other two are novel genetic risk loci for CSC. The top 10% of subjects with highest PRS value showed 6.39 times higher risk than the bottom 10% of subjects with lowest PRS, suggesting that the genetic

TABLE 3 | Stratified association analysis of three SNPs with shape of fluid leakage on FFA.

CHR	SNP	BP	A1/A2[a]	OR (95% CI)	*P*-value	Trait
15	rs2043085	58,680,954	G/A	0.62 (0.44–0.87)	3.83E−03	Shape of fluid leakage
4	rs4698775	110,590,479	G/T	1.39 (1.04–1.87)	2.34E−02	Shape of fluid leakage
1	rs1410996	196,696,933	G/A	0.77 (0.57–1.03)	7.78E−02	Shape of fluid leakage

FFA, fundus fluorescein angiography; CHR, chromosome; SNP, single nucleotide polymorphism; BP, base pair; OR, odds ratio; 95% CI, 95% confidence interval.
[a]A1/A2, effective allele and alternative allele.

risk effects of these three risk loci have the potential to identify subjects with high risk of developing acute CSC. These genetic risk variants were also found to impact on the clinic symptoms in CSC patients, further confirming their association with CSC development. To our best knowledge, this is the first genetic association study of acute CSC and the first genetic association study of CSC in Chinese population.

The most significantly association signal was observed at the intronic SNP rs1410996 within the *CFH* gene on chromosome 1. The association of *CFH* genetic variants with chronic CSC has been well-demonstrated by several independent studies (Miki et al., 2014; de Jong et al., 2015; Schellevis et al., 2018). Recently, Mohabati et al. (2019) also confirmed the association between the variants in the *CFH* gene and acute CSC development. The most significant SNP rs1329428 reported in the study of Mohabati et al. (2019) is in strong LD with rs1410996 which was detected in our current study result. Interestingly, we cannot detect any association evidence for rs1061170, although the

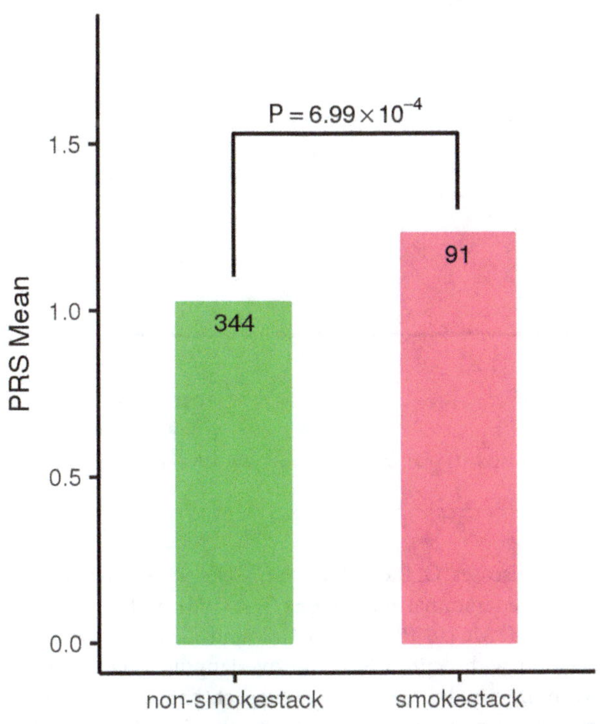

FIGURE 3 | Individuals with classic smoke stack shape of fluid leakage show higher polygenic risk score (PRS) for the top three SNPs.

samples of our current study provided sufficient statistical power for detecting the reported association effect at rs1061170. In addition, SNP rs1061170 are not in LD ($r^2 < 0.04$) with the two SNPs detected in our current study in our study samples. While it is assuring to see the confirmation of this well-established locus in our Chinese cohort of CSC, our study also revealed the ethnic difference of the *CFH* locus (allelic heterogeneity) between Chinese and Caucasian populations. In addition, for the first time, our study discovered the association of the *CFH* variants with the clinical characteristics of CSC, including shape of fluid leakage, the central subfield thickness, and the horizontal and vertical dimensions of SRF. The *CFH* gene encodes complement factor H, which is a key regulator of complement activation. It has been suggested that it could affect choroidal hemodynamics activities and may lead to RPE damage and dysfunction, which has been proposed to contribute to the pathogenesis of CSC (Guyer et al., 1994; Dorner et al., 2003; de Jong et al., 2015). Together with previous findings, our study has highlighted the potentials of the *CFH* gene variants in terms of acute CSC classification and prediction in future.

We have discovered two novel loci for acute CSC. The first novel locus is SNP rs4698775 that is located in an intron of mitochondrial calcium uniporter dominant negative subunit beta (*MCUB*) gene on chromosome 4. It encodes the protein MCUB, but its function and role in disease development has not been well-studied. Based on the information from GTEx database (Gamazon et al., 2018), rs4698775 showed significant expression quantitative trait loci (eQTL) effect for phospholipase A2 group XIIA (*PLA2G12A*, $p = 1.20 \times 10^{-6}$ in esophagus mucosa and 4.10×10^{-5} in transformed fibroblasts) and *MCUB* ($p = 1.50 \times 10^{-6}$ in visceral adipose tissue). *PLA2G12A* encodes phospholipase A2 Group XIIA enzyme that is involved in lipid metabolism. It is notable that SNP rs4698775 is proximal to the *CFI* gene. The *CFI* gene encodes complement factor I, with a catalytic serine protease domain that mediates cleavage of C3 protein. C3 is an acute phase protein and highly expressed in the choroid, which may play an important role in the pathogenesis of CSC (Imamura et al., 2009). The second novel locus is SNP rs2043085 on chromosome 15 that is next to *LIPC* gene. Rs2043085 is significantly correlated with LIPC expression level in the GTEx. *LIPC* encodes a hepatic triglyceride lipase that has been shown to be involved in triglyceride hydrolysis and high-density lipoprotein cholesterol (HDL) metabolism and the progression of AMD (Neale et al., 2010). Moreover, our current study also revealed a suggestive association at the *APOE* gene (rs429358, $p = 8.39 \times 10^{-3}$), which encodes a lipid transport protein. These results suggest that lipid metabolism may play

TABLE 4 | Association of rs1410996 with OCT manifestation.

CHR	SNP	BP	A1/A2[a]	β[b]	SE	*P*-value	Trait
1	rs1410996	196,696,933	G/A	−0.149	0.065	2.26E−02	Central subfield thickness
1	rs1410996	196,696,933	G/A	−0.140	0.067	3.78E−02	Horizontal dimension of SRF
1	rs1410996	196,696,933	G/A	−0.182	0.068	7.84E−03	Vertical dimension of SRF

OCT, optical coherence tomography; CHR, chromosome; SNP, single nucleotide polymorphism; BP, base pair in hg19; SE, standard error; SRF, subretinal fluid.
[a]Effective allele and alternative allele.
[b]Effect size of the effective allele on the risk of the related trait.

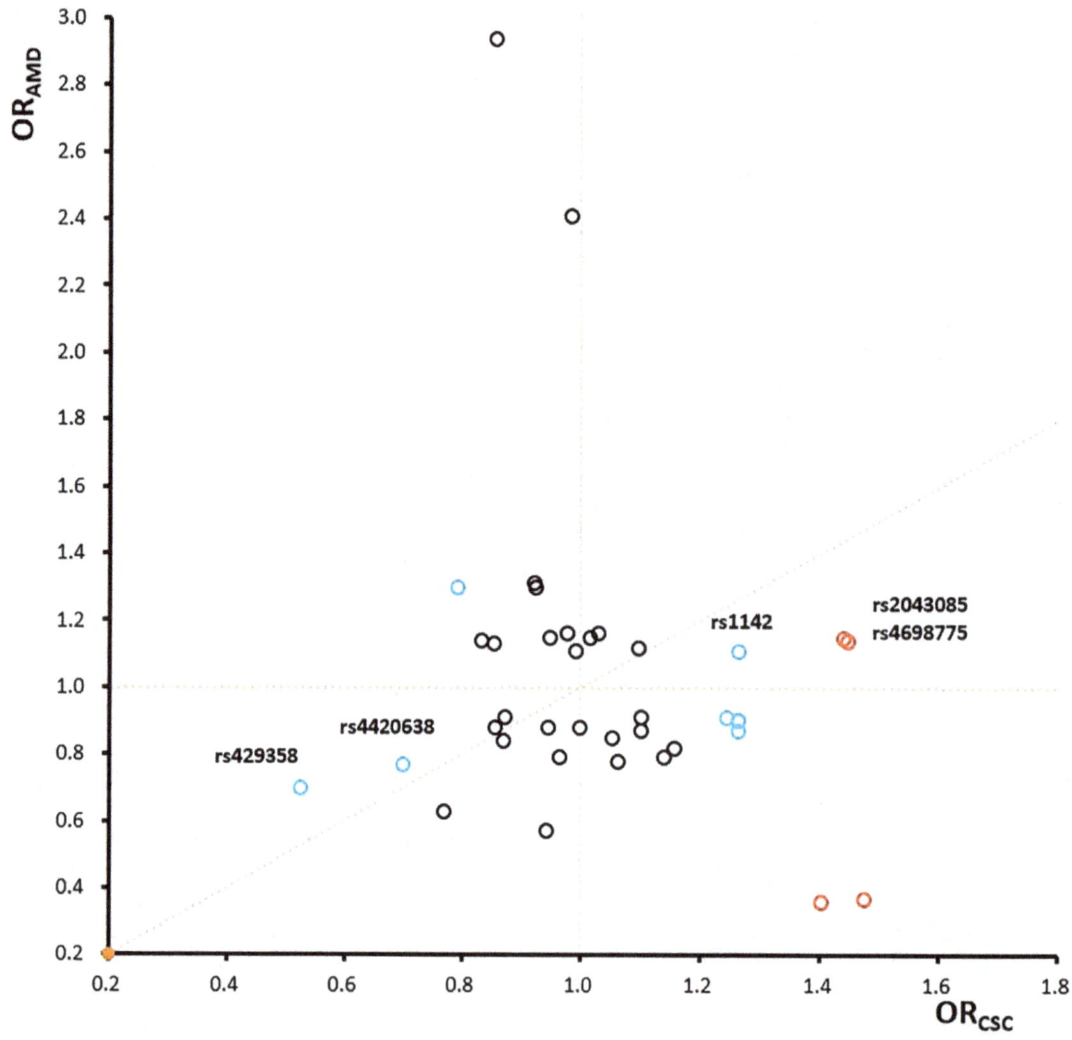

FIGURE 4 | The comparison of odds ratios between CSC and AMD. The four significant SNPs are labeled in red, other eight SNPs with achieved nominal association significance ($p < 0.05$) are labeled in blue, and the remaining ones are in black.

an important role in the development of CSC. The discovery of these two novel loci has advanced the biological understanding of CSC development by not only highlighting the important role of complement system and innate immunity but also revealing the involvement of lipid metabolism in CSC development.

By comparing the genetic risk effects of 38 SNPs for CSC (estimated from the current study) and the previously published ones for AMD, we investigated the genetic pleiotropy between these two diseases. Of the 38 known AMD risk-associated SNPs, 8 SNPs showed nominal associations ($p < 0.05$), and 4 SNPs within 3 loci (*CFH*, *MCUB-PLA2G12A-CFI*, and *LIPC*) showed strong association with acute CSC. The overlapping genetic risk loci between the two diseases strongly suggest that these two diseases share some genetic and pathogenic mechanism. Of the 12 SNPs showing nominal associations in CSC, 7 SNPs showed opposite directions of effects, and 5 SNPs had consistent directions of

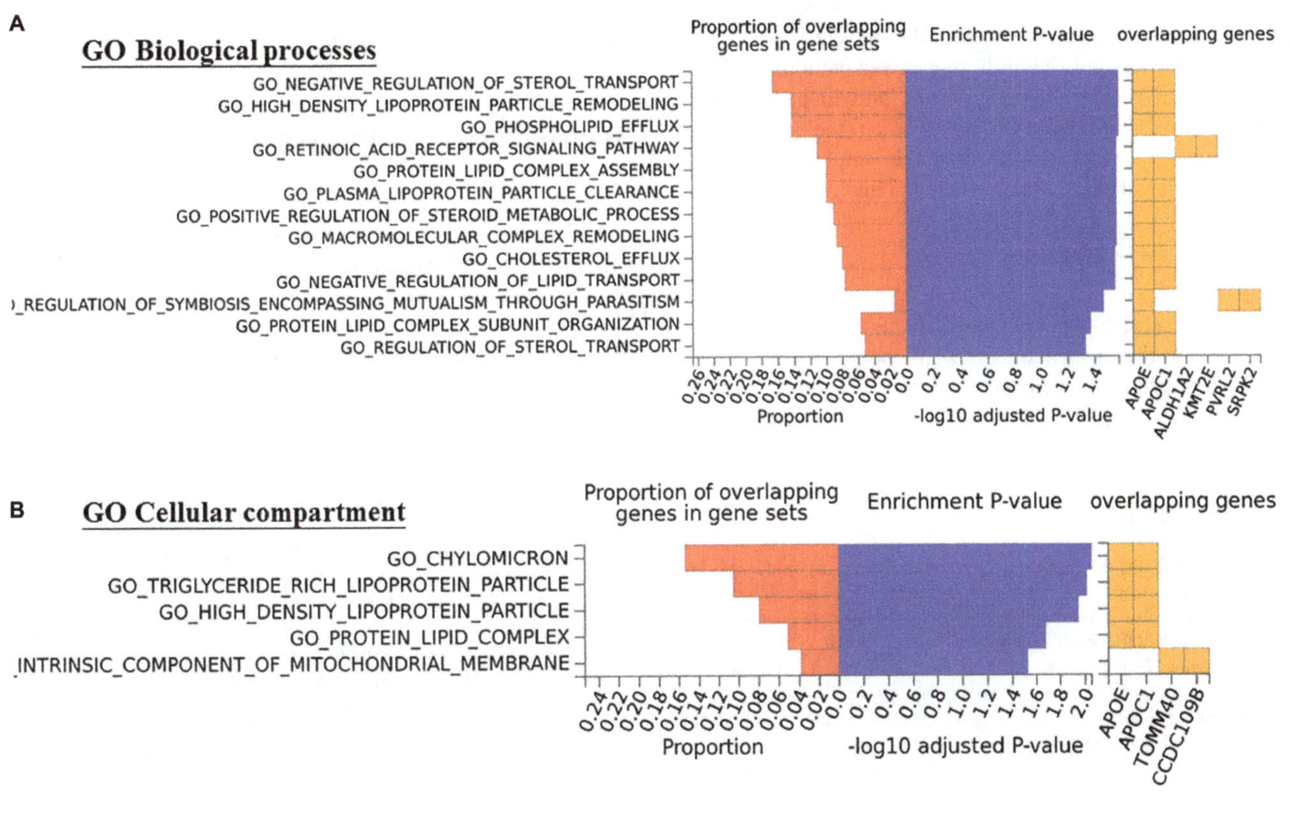

FIGURE 5 | The five SNPs with consistent effects between CSC and AMD show enrichment with Gene Ontology **(A)** Biological processes and **(B)** Cellular compartment terms (mainly related in lipid metabolism, B-H adj $p < 0.05$).

effects between CSC and AMD. For example, the A allele of rs1410996 and the T allele of rs1329428 within the CFH locus showed protective effects for AMD, but both are risk alleles for acute CSC. In contrast, the C allele of rs1061170 conferred risk for AMD but showed protective effect for CSC. However, the missense mutation Y402H (rs1061170) of *CFH*, which is a strong risk variant for AMD (Zareparsi et al., 2005; Yu et al., 2011) did not show any association effect in our CSC cohort, although our samples provide sufficient statistical power (>80%) for detecting the AMD-associated genetic effect. Interestingly, while we did not see any pathway enrichment for the seven SNPs that showed opposite effects, we did observe the significant enrichment of lipid metabolism (B-H adj $p < 0.05$, mainly driven by *APOE* and *APOC1*) for five SNPs that showed consistent effects between CSC and AMD. Therefore, our study has not only indicated some shared pathophysiologic mechanisms between two diseases but also highlighted the diverse and complex roles of these mechanistic processes in CSC and AMD. In particular, our study suggests that lipid metabolism may play a similar pathogenic role in CSC and AMD, which need to be validated by further functional investigations.

In recent years, several genetic variants have been reported consistently for chronic CSC, mainly in European and Japanese populations (Miki et al., 2014, 2018; Schubert et al., 2014; Breukink et al., 2015; de Jong et al., 2015; van Dijk et al., 2017; Schellevis et al., 2018). Among these studies, the association of the *CFH* gene is consistently replicated for the risk of chronic CSC. In the present study, we validated a significant association of the *CFH* gene for acute CSC, but we were not able to find several other associations that have been found for chronic CSC. For example, SNP rs10490924 within the *ARMS2* gene that has been implicated for the risk of chronic CSC had no significant effect on the risk of acute CSC in our study, which is consistent with previous report (Mohabati et al., 2019). However, because the current study focused on the analysis of AMD-associated risk variants, many previously reported genetic risk loci for chronic CSC were not evaluated. As a limitation, our current study could not investigate potential genetic heterogeneity between chronic and acute CSC. A more thorough investigation, such as an unbiased GWAS would be ideal for novel genetic discovery for acute CSC.

CONCLUSION

In conclusion, we have identified three genetic risk loci (i.e., *CFH*, *MCUB-PLA2G12A-CFI*, and *LIPC*) for acute CSC in Chinese population, and *MCUB-PLA2G12A-CFI* and *LIPC* are novel risk loci for CSC. Besides confirming the important role of complement systems and innate immunity, our discovery of novel loci has also suggested the involvement of lipid metabolism in CSC. By demonstrating a good number of shared genetic risk loci between two diseases with both opposite and consistent genetic effects, our study has indicated shared pathophysiological processes with complex functionalities, and in particular, the similar role of lipid metabolism, between the two diseases. Further studies are required to validate the implications of these findings in clinical practice and functional investigations.

ETHICS STATEMENT

The studies involving human participants were reviewed and approved by the institutional review board of the Second Affiliated Hospital of Zhejiang University School of Medicine. The patients/participants provided their written informed consent to participate in this study.

AUTHOR CONTRIBUTIONS

YR and LF conceived and designed the experiments. LF, SC, and YR conducted the sample recruitment and quality control. YR, HD, and LF performed the experiments. SC, XY, RD, and JK undertook the data processing and statistical analysis. LF, YR, XY, and JL interpreted the results and wrote the manuscript. All authors contributed to the article and approved the submitted version.

REFERENCES

Arakawa, S., Takahashi, A., Ashikawa, K., Hosono, N., Aoi, T., Yasuda, M., et al. (2011). Genome-wide association study identifies two susceptibility loci for exudative age-related macular degeneration in the Japanese population. *Nat. Genet.* 43, 1001–1004. doi: 10.1038/ng.938

Balaratnasingam, C., Freund, K. B., Tan, A. M., Mrejen, S., Hunyor, A. P., Keegan, D. J., et al. (2016). Bullous variant of central serous chorioretinopathy: expansion of phenotypic features using multimethod imaging. *Ophthalmology* 123, 1541–1552. doi: 10.1016/j.ophtha.2016.03.017

Breukink, M. B., Schellevis, R. L., Boon, C. J., Fauser, S., Hoyng, C. B., den Hollander, A. I., et al. (2015). Genomic copy number variations of the complement component C4B Gene are associated with chronic central serous chorioretinopathy. *Invest. Ophthalmol. Vis. Sci.* 56, 5608–5613. doi: 10.1167/iovs.15-17343

Chang, C. C., Chow, C. C., Tellier, L. C., Vattikuti, S., Purcell, S. M., and Lee, J. J. (2015). Second-generation PLINK: rising to the challenge of larger and richer datasets. *Gigascience* 4:7. doi: 10.1186/s13742-015-0047-8

Cheng, C. Y., Yamashiro, K., Chen, L. J., Ahn, J., Huang, L., Huang, L., et al. (2015). New loci and coding variants confer risk for age-related macular degeneration in East Asians. *Nat. Commun.* 6:6063. doi: 10.1038/ncomms7063

Daruich, A., Matet, A., Dirani, A., Bousquet, E., Zhao, M., Farman, N., et al. (2015). Central serous chorioretinopathy: recent findings and new physiopathology hypothesis. *Prog. Retin. Eye Res.* 48, 82–118. doi: 10.1016/j.preteyeres.2015.05.003

Daruich, A., Matet, A., Marchionno, L., De Azevedo, J. D., Ambresin, A., Mantel, I., et al. (2017). ACUTE CENTRAL SEROUS CHORIORETINOPATHY: factors influencing episode duration. *Retina* 37, 1905–1915. doi: 10.1097/IAE.0000000000001443

de Jong, E. K., Breukink, M. B., Schellevis, R. L., Bakker, B., Mohr, J. K., Fauser, S., et al. (2015). Chronic central serous chorioretinopathy is associated with genetic variants implicated in age-related macular degeneration. *Ophthalmology* 122, 562–570. doi: 10.1016/j.ophtha.2014.09.026

Desai, U. R., Alhalel, A. A., Campen, T. J., Schiffman, R. M., Edwards, P. A., and Jacobsen, G. R. (2003). Central serous chorioretinopathy in African Americans. *J. Natl. Med. Assoc.* 95, 553–559.

Dorner, G. T., Garhofer, G., Huemer, K. H., Golestani, E., Zawinka, C., Schmetterer, L., et al. (2003). Effects of adrenomedullin on ocular hemodynamic parameters in the choroid and the ophthalmic artery. *Invest. Ophthalmol. Vis. Sci.* 44, 3947–3951.

Ersoz, M. G., Arf, S., Hocaoglu, M., Sayman Muslubas, I., and Karacorlu, M. (2018). Patient characteristics and risk factors for central serous chorioretinopathy: an analysis of 811 patients. *Br. J. Ophthalmol.* 103, 725–729. doi: 10.1136/bjophthalmol-2018-312431

Fritsche, L. G., Chen, W., Schu, M., Yaspan, B. L., Yu, Y., Thorleifsson, G., et al. (2013). Seven new loci associated with age-related macular degeneration. *Nat. Genet.* 45, 433–439. doi: 10.1038/ng.2578

Fritsche, L. G., Igl, W., Bailey, J. N., Grassmann, F., Sengupta, S., Bragg-Gresham, J. L., et al. (2016). A large genome-wide association study of age-related macular degeneration highlights contributions of rare and common variants. *Nat. Genet.* 48, 134–143. doi: 10.1038/ng.3448

Gamazon, E. R., Segre, A. V., van de Bunt, M., Wen, X., Xi, H. S., Hormozdiari, F., et al. (2018). Using an atlas of gene regulation across 44 human tissues to inform complex disease- and trait-associated variation. *Nat. Genet.* 50, 956–967. doi: 10.1038/s41588-018-0154-4

Guyer, D. R., Yannuzzi, L. A., Slakter, J. S., Sorenson, J. A., Ho, A., and Orlock, D. (1994). Digital indocyanine green videoangiography of central serous chorioretinopathy. *Arch. Ophthalmol.* 112, 1057–1062.

Hosoda, Y., Miyake, M., Schellevis, R. L., Boon, C. J. F., Hoyng, C. B., Miki, A., et al. (2019). Genome-wide association analyses identify two susceptibility loci for pachychoroid disease central serous chorioretinopathy. *Commun. Biol.* 2:468. doi: 10.1038/s42003-019-0712-z

Hosoda, Y., Yoshikawa, M., Miyake, M., Tabara, Y., Ahn, J., Woo, S. J., et al. (2018). CFH and VIPR2 as susceptibility loci in choroidal thickness and pachychoroid disease central serous chorioretinopathy. *Proc. Natl. Acad. Sci. U.S.A.* 115, 6261–6266. doi: 10.1073/pnas.1802212115

How, A. C., and Koh, A. H. (2006). Angiographic characteristics of acute central serous chorioretinopathy in an Asian population. *Ann. Acad. Med. Singapore* 35, 77–79.

Imamura, Y., Fujiwara, T., Margolis, R., and Spaide, R. F. (2009). Enhanced depth imaging optical coherence tomography of the choroid in central serous chorioretinopathy. *Retina* 29, 1469–1473. doi: 10.1097/IAE.0b013e3181be0a83

Karkhaneh, R., Toufighi, M., Amirfiroozy, A., Ahmad-Raji, A., Ahmadzadeh, O., Mahdavi, A., et al. (2021). Association of central serous chorioretinopathy with single nucleotide polymorphisms in complement factor H gene in Iranian population. *Eye* doi: 10.1038/s41433-021-01579-x [Epub ahead of print].

Karska-Basta, I., Pociej-Marciak, W., Chrząszcz, M., Kubicka-Trząska, A., Dębicka-Kumela, M., Gawęcki, M., et al. (2021a). Imbalance in the levels of Angiogenic factors in patients with acute and chronic central serous Chorioretinopathy. *J. Clin. Med.* 10:1087. doi: 10.3390/jcm10051087

Karska-Basta, I., Pociej-Marciak, W., Chrząszcz, M., Kubicka-Trząska, A., Romanowska-Dixon, B., and Sanak, M. (2021b). Altered plasma cytokine levels in acute and chronic central serous chorioretinopathy. *Acta Ophthalmol.* 99, e222–e231. doi: 10.1111/aos.14547

Karska-Basta, I., Pociej-Marciak, W., Chrzaszcz, M., Wilanska, J., Jager, M. J., Markiewicz, A., et al. (2020). Differences in anti-endothelial and anti-retinal antibody titers: implications for the pathohysiology of acute and chronic central serous chorioretinopathy. *J. Physiol. Pharmacol.* 71, 235–242. doi: 10.26402/jpp.2020.2.07

Kitzmann, A. S., Pulido, J. S., Diehl, N. N., Hodge, D. O., and Burke, J. P. (2008). The incidence of central serous chorioretinopathy in Olmsted County, Minnesota, 1980-2002. *Ophthalmology* 115, 169–173. doi: 10.1016/j.ophtha.2007.02.032

Kopplin, L. J., Igo, R. P. Jr., Wang, Y., Sivakumaran, T. A., Hagstrom, S. A., Peachey, N. S., et al. (2010). Genome-wide association identifies SKIV2L and MYRIP as protective factors for age-related macular degeneration. *Genes Immun.* 11, 609–621. doi: 10.1038/gene.2010.39

Liew, G., Quin, G., Gillies, M., and Fraser-Bell, S. (2013). Central serous chorioretinopathy: a review of epidemiology and pathophysiology. *Clin. Exp. Ophthalmol.* 41, 201–214. doi: 10.1111/j.1442-9071.2012.02848.x

Miki, A., Kondo, N., Yanagisawa, S., Bessho, H., Honda, S., and Negi, A. (2014). Common variants in the complement factor H gene confer genetic susceptibility to central serous chorioretinopathy. *Ophthalmology* 121, 1067–1072. doi: 10.1016/j.ophtha.2013.11.020

Miki, A., Sakurada, Y., Tanaka, K., Semba, K., Mitamura, Y., Yuzawa, M., et al. (2018). Genome-wide association study to identify a new susceptibility locus for central serous chorioretinopathy in the Japanese population. *Invest. Ophthalmol. Vis. Sci.* 59, 5542–5547. doi: 10.1167/iovs.18-25497

Mohabati, D., Schellevis, R. L., van Dijk, E. H. C., Altay, L., Fauser, S., Hoyng, C. B., et al. (2019). Genetic risk factors in acute central serous chorioretinopathy. *Retina* 39, 2303–2310. doi: 10.1097/IAE.0000000000002333

Neale, B. M., Fagerness, J., Reynolds, R., Sobrin, L., Parker, M., Raychaudhuri, S., et al. (2010). Genome-wide association study of advanced age-related macular degeneration identifies a role of the hepatic lipase gene (LIPC). *Proc. Natl. Acad. Sci. U.S.A.* 107, 7395–7400. doi: 10.1073/pnas.0912019107

Oosterhuis, J. A. (1996). Familial central serous retinopathy. *Graefes Arch. Clin. Exp. Ophthalmol.* 234, 337–341.

Schellevis, R. L., van Dijk, E. H. C., Breukink, M. B., Altay, L., Bakker, B., Koeleman, B. P. C., et al. (2018). Role of the complement system in chronic central serous chorioretinopathy: a genome-wide association study. *JAMA Ophthalmol.* 136, 1128–1136. doi: 10.1001/jamaophthalmol.2018.3190

Schubert, C., Pryds, A., Zeng, S., Xie, Y., Freund, K. B., Spaide, R. F., et al. (2014). Cadherin 5 is regulated by corticosteroids and associated with central serous chorioretinopathy. *Hum. Mutat.* 35, 859–867. doi: 10.1002/humu.22551

Tsai, D. C., Chen, S. J., Huang, C. C., Chou, P., Chung, C. M., Huang, P. H., et al. (2013). Epidemiology of idiopathic central serous chorioretinopathy in Taiwan, 2001-2006: a population-based study. *PLoS One* 8:e66858. doi: 10.1371/journal.pone.0066858

van Dijk, E. H. C., Schellevis, R. L., van Bergen, M. G. J. M., Breukink, M. B., Altay, L., Scholz, P., et al. (2017). Association of a haplotype in the NR3C2 gene, encoding the mineralocorticoid receptor, with chronic central serous chorioretinopathy. *JAMA Ophthalmol.* 135:446. doi: 10.1001/jamaophthalmol.2017.0245

Wang, M., Munch, I. C., Hasler, P. W., Prunte, C., and Larsen, M. (2008). Central serous chorioretinopathy. *Acta Ophthalmol.* 86, 126–145. doi: 10.1111/j.1600-0420.2007.00889.x

Watanabe, K., Taskesen, E., van Bochoven, A., and Posthuma, D. (2017). Functional mapping and annotation of genetic associations with FUMA. *Nat. Commun.* 8:1826. doi: 10.1038/s41467-017-01261-5

Weenink, A. C., Borsje, R. A., and Oosterhuis, J. A. (2001). Familial chronic central serous chorioretinopathy. *Ophthalmologica* 215, 183–187. doi: 10.1159/000050855

Yu, Y., Bhangale, T. R., Fagerness, J., Ripke, S., Thorleifsson, G., Tan, P. L., et al. (2011). Common variants near FRK/COL10A1 and VEGFA are associated with advanced age-related macular degeneration. *Hum. Mol. Genet.* 20, 3699–3709. doi: 10.1093/hmg/ddr270

Zareparsi, S., Branham, K. E., Li, M., Shah, S., Klein, R. J., Ott, J., et al. (2005). Strong association of the Y402H variant in complement factor H at 1q32 with susceptibility to age-related macular degeneration. *Am. J. Hum. Genet.* 77, 149–153. doi: 10.1086/431426

8

Different Phenotypes in Pseudodominant Inherited Retinal Dystrophies

Imen Habibi[1], Yosra Falfoul[2], Hoai Viet Tran[3], Khaled El Matri[2], Ahmed Chebil[2], Leila El Matri[2] and Daniel F. Schorderet[1,4,5]*

[1] IRO-Institute for Research in Ophthalmology, Sion, Switzerland, [2] Oculogenetic Laboratory LR14SP01, Faculty of Medicine of Tunis, Hedi Rais Institute of Ophthalmology (Department B), Tunis El Manar University, Tunis, Tunisia, [3] Hôpital Ophtalmique Jules-Gonin, Unité d'oculogénétique, Lausanne, Switzerland, [4] Faculty of Biology and Medicine, University of Lausanne, Lausanne, Switzerland, [5] Faculty of Life Sciences, Ecole Polytechnique Fédérale de Lausanne, Lausanne, Switzerland

***Correspondence:**
Imen Habibi
habibiimen@hotmail.com

Retinal dystrophies (RD) are a group of Mendelian disorders caused by rare genetic variations leading to blindness. A pathogenic variant may manifest in both dominant or recessive mode and clinical and genetic heterogeneity makes it difficult to establish a precise diagnosis. In this study, families with autosomal dominant RD in successive generations were identified, and we aimed to determine the disease's molecular origin in these consanguineous families. Whole exome sequencing was performed in the index patient of each family. The aim was to determine whether these cases truly represented examples of dominantly inherited RD, or whether another mode of inheritance might be applicable. Six potentially pathogenic variants in four genes were identified in four families. In index patient with enhanced S-cone syndrome in F1, we identified a new digenetic combination: a heterozygous variant p.[G51A];[=] in *RHO* and a homozygous pathogenic variant p.[R311Q];[R311Q] in *NR2E3.* Helicoid subretinal fibrosis associated with recessive *NR2E3* variant p.[R311Q];[R311Q] was identified in F2. A new frameshift variant c.[105delG];[105delG] in *RDH12* was found in F3 with cone-rod dystrophy. In F4, the compound heterozygous variants p.[R964*];[W758*] were observed in *IMPG2* with a retinitis pigmentosa (RP) phenotype. We showed that both affected parents and the offspring, were homozygous for the same variants in all four families. Our results provide evidence that in consanguineous families, autosomal recessive can be transmitted as pseudodominant inheritance in RD patients, and further extend our knowledge of pathogenic variants in RD genes.

Keywords: retinal dystrophies, whole exome sequencing, pathogenic variants, pseudodominant inheritance, retinitis pigmentosa

INTRODUCTION

Retinal dystrophies (RD), a group of heterogeneous hereditary diseases, are caused by perturbed photoreceptor function. It presents significant genetic heterogeneity and contribute notably to the etiology of blindness around the world (den Hollander et al., 2010). To date, more than 300 disease associated genes have been implicated in the pathogenesis of the disease, most of which are involved in the development and normal function of photoreceptor and cells from the retinal pigment epithelium (RPE) (den Hollander et al., 2008, 2010). Clinical symptoms vary widely among different RD subtypes and disease genes (Ellingford et al., 2016). RD are generally classified based on the type of photoreceptor cells affected, i.e., rods or cones, and thus on the location, macula or peripheral retina (Nash et al., 2015).

The described modes of inheritance in RD are recessive (ar) or dominant (ad) and autosomal or X-linked. A few rare cases of RD exist, in which mitochondrial mutations, digenic inheritance, and pseudodominant transmission have been documented (Lewis et al., 1999; Liu et al., 2019).

In this study, we used whole exome sequencing (WES) and Sanger sequencing to investigate four consanguineous families with several members affected by RD, inherited in an apparent ad pattern. We aimed to identify potential gene variants underlining these cases and described the genotypic and phenotypic findings in these complicated RD pedigrees. Distinct inheritance patterns and disease-causing variants were identified in all families.

MATERIALS AND METHODS

Ethical Compliance

This study was approved by the Local Ethics Committee of the Hedi Rais Institute in Tunisia. Informed consent was obtained from all participants in the study. Analyses were done in accordance with local guidelines.

Clinical Investigations

Our study contains four Tunisian families with non-syndromic RD (**Table 1**). All patients underwent detailed clinical examinations and their family history was collected. A comprehensive ophthalmological examination was performed at the Department B of Hedi Rais Institute of Ophthalmology, Tunis (Tunisia), including best-corrected visual acuity (BCVA), slit lamp, dilated fundus examination, and full-field electroretinography according to the International Society for Clinical Electrophysiology of Vision (ISCEV) standards (Métrovision, France), swept source optical coherence

TABLE 1 | Clinical data of four families with gene-associated RD.

Family	Patient	Gender	Age [years]	Age of onset	Visual acuity OD/OS/OU	Ophthalmoscopy	Optical coherence tomography	Full-field ERG (OU)	Diagnosis
F1	II.2	F	19	6	1/20 OU	Mid-peripheral nummular pigment clumping and atrophy	Diffuse macular cystoids edema	Similar waveforms under photopic and scotopic conditions	Enhanced S-cone SD
	I.1	F	68	Infancy	LP LP	Diffuse retinal atrophy	Macular atrophy	Extinct response	Enhanced S-cone SD
F2	II.1	M	13	Infancy	3/10 OU	Circumferential fibrosis on the PP	Macular cysts	Similar responses under scotopic and photopic stimulations	Enhanced S-cone SD
	I.1	M	51	10	1/10 OU	Circumferential fibrosis on the PP	Macular cystoid edema	-	Enhanced S-cone SD
F3	II.1	F	13	Under 5	1/10 OU	Macular atrophy, peripheral spicule déposits	-	-	Cone-rod dystrophy
	I.2	F	37	Infancy	LP LP	Diffuse macular and peripheral deposits	-	-	Cone-rod dystrophy
F4	II.1	F	37	Second decade	5/10 OU	Preserved PP, peripheral spicule deposits	Normal	Reduced rod responses Preserved cone response	RP
	II.2	F	32		7/10 OD 6/10 OS		Normal	-	RP
	II.3	F	28		6/10 OU		Normal	-	RP
	II.4	F	25		9/10 OU		Normal	-	RP
	I.2	F	63		1/10	Macular atrophy Spicule deposits	Macular atrophy	-	Advanced RP

OD, right eye; OS, left eye; OU, both eyes; RP, retinitis pigmentosa; F, female; M, male; PP, posterior pole.

TABLE 2 | Classification of the identified variants.

Variant ID	Evidence of pathogenicity	Class
RHO: p.G51AS	BS1, BS2, BP2	Likely benign
NR2E3: p.R311Q	PS3, PM1, PP5, BS1	Likely pathogenic
RDH12:c.105delG	PVS1, PM1, PM2, PM3, PP1	Pathogenic
IMPG2:p.R964*	PVS1, PM2, PP3, PP5	Likely pathogenic
IMPG2:p.W758*	PVS1, PM2, PP3, PP5	Likely pathogenic

tomography (SS-OCT, Topcon, Swept Source DRI-OCT Triton, Japan), and fundus autofluorescence (FAF) imaging (Heidelberg, HRA 2 Spectralis, Germany).

Genetic Analysis

Peripheral blood samples were obtained from 4 index patients and 13-related individuals, including parents and affected siblings. DNA was extracted from leukocytes according to the salting-out method (Miller et al., 1988).

We sequenced the exome in the index patient, then variants were confirmed by Sanger sequencing and segregation was established in all families.

Whole Exome Sequencing (WES)

Next-generation sequencing was done at Sophia Genetics (SOPHiA GENETICS SA, Saint-Sulpice, Switzerland) using the clinical exome solution v.2 (CES2). The complete list of genes analyzed in CES2 can be obtained at www.sophiagenetics.com. ~98.95% of target regions were covered at least 25×.

Variant Assessment

All variants were first filtered against several public databases for the minor allele frequency (MAF) of <1%. dbSNP database served as a reference to exclude any known frequent variants occurring in coding (missense) and regulatory regions including splice site and promoter regions. **Table 2** lists the criteria to classify the variants described here.

A variant was considered novel if it has not been described in the medical literature or was not present in the Human Mutation Database (www.hgmd.cf.ac.uk/ac). The variant frequency in the control population was evaluated using gnomAD (http://gnomad.broadinstitute.org/).

Sanger Sequencing

All variants were confirmed by Sanger sequencing. PCR reactions and amplification conditions were performed using the following primers in **Table 3**.

TABLE 3 | Primers.

Primers	Forward	Reverse
RHO exon 1	TCA TCC AGC TGG AGC CCT GAG T	AAC ATT GAC AGG ACA GGA GAA GG
NR2E3 exon 6	TCT GAG CCT CTG GCT GAT GTC A	AGA AGG GAG TCC AGC CTC AC
IMPG2 exon13	TGC CCA TCT TCG CAG ATA CT	TCC AAA CTC TCT CTG ATT CTG G
IMPG2 exon14	GGA AAA GTG AGG CAG GGT CT	TGG GTA GAG AAA GGA ATG GAG G
RDH12 exon4	CTT AGT GTG AGC TCG TGA AGG A	TTG GAC TTG AAT CCC AGG TT

RESULTS

Clinical Diagnosis

Family 1

The index patient is a 19-year-old girl from consanguineous marriage with the diagnosis of enhanced S-cone syndrome. She had nyctalopia since the age of 6 years along with visual impairment. Her BCVA was limited to 1/20 in both eyes (OU). On fundus examination, she had mid-peripheral nummular pigment clumping, atrophy and cystoid macular edema better visualized on SS-OCT. FAF showed hyper FAF dots in the posterior pole (**Figures 1A–C**). In full-field ERG, reduced cone and rod responses with similar waveforms under photopic and scotopic conditions were detected (**Figure 2**). Affected mother had severe visual impairment with cataract and diffuse retinal atrophy (**Figures 1D,E**).

Family 2

The index patient was a 13-year-old boy from consanguineous marriage presenting with retinal dystrophy. His BCVA was limited to 3/10 OU. On fundus examination, he had circumferential fibrosis, nummular pigment clumping on the posterior pole and peripheral spicule deposits with preserved macular region (**Figures 1F,G**). In full-field ERG, there were similar cone and rod responses under photopic and scotopic conditions with markedly reduced flicker, which allowed us to retain the diagnosis of enhanced S-cone syndrome (**Figure 2**). Affected father had similar retinal phenotype with bilateral cataract (**Figure 1H**).

Family 3

The index patient is a 13-year-old girl with impaired visual acuity (BCVA: 1/10 OU) and nyctalopia since her first decade of life. She had cone-rod dystrophy with macular atrophy and spicule deposits in the mid peripheral retina (**Figure 3A**). In full-field ERG, there were reduced cone and rod responses. Her mother had similar phenotype with BCVA limited to light perception and diffuse spicule deposits in fundus examination (**Figure 3B**).

Family 4

The index patient is a 38-year-old male diagnosed with familial retinitis pigmentosa (RP). BCVA was 5/10 s. On fundus examination, there were peripheral spicule migrations and preserved posterior pole (**Figures 3C–E**). The same phenotype was present in three-affected sisters. The mother, had BCVA

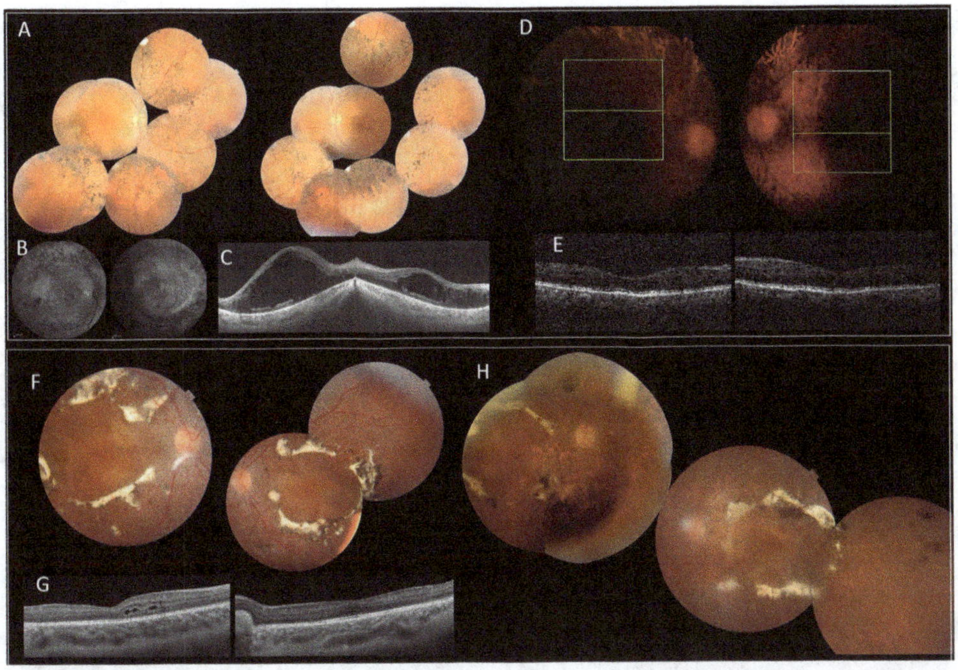

FIGURE 1 | Clinical and imaging features of patients with *NR2E3* mutations. F1 **(A–E)**. **(A)** FP of the index patient with peripheral nummular spicule deposits and atrophy. **(B)** FAF with peripheral hypo-autofluorescence spots and heterogeneous autofluorescence of the posterior pole. **(C)** SS-OCT. Bilateral cystoid macular edema. **(D,E)** Diffuse retinal atrophy. F2 **(F–H)**. **(F,H)** FP of the index patient (II.1) **(F)** and his father (I.1) **(H)** with circumferential fibrosis and nummular pigment clumping and peripheral spicule deposits. **(G)** SS-OCT. intraretinal cysts (II.1). FP, Fundus photography.

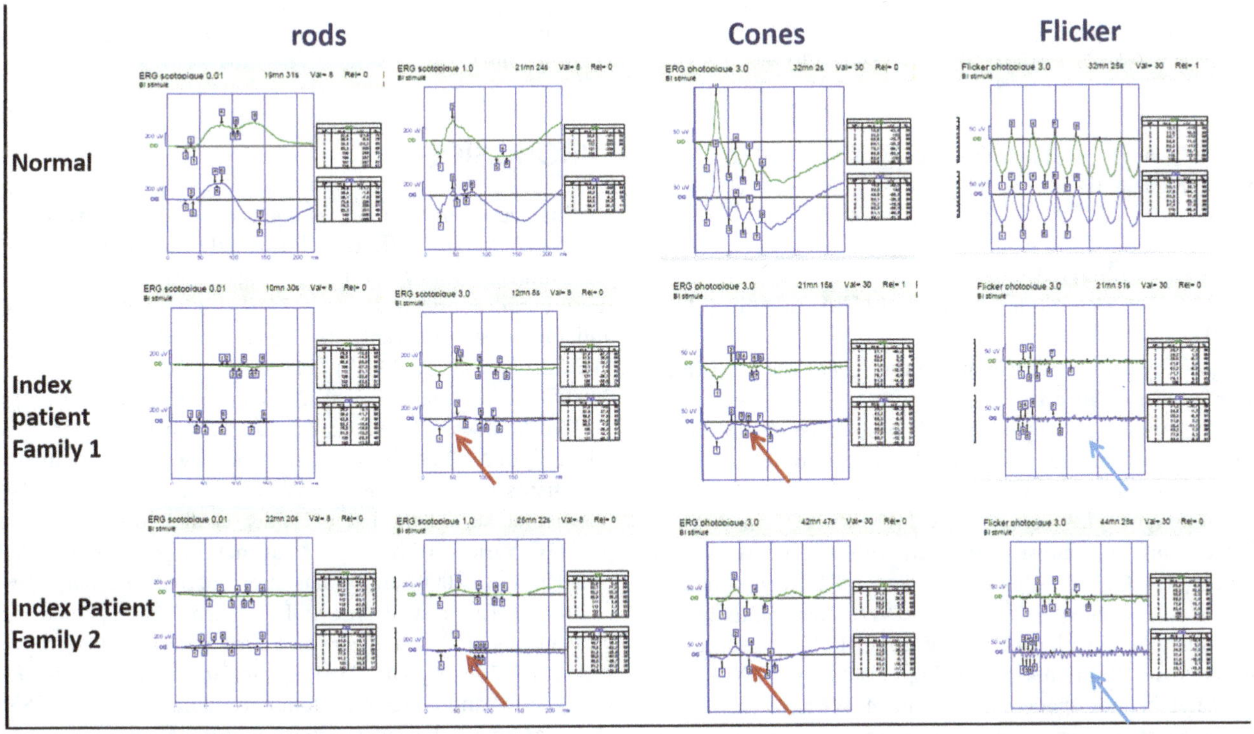

FIGURE 2 | Full-field ERG findings in enhanced-S cone syndrome patients from families 1 and 2 showing similar waveforms in both scotopic and photopic conditions (red arrow) with markedly reduced flicker (blue arrow).

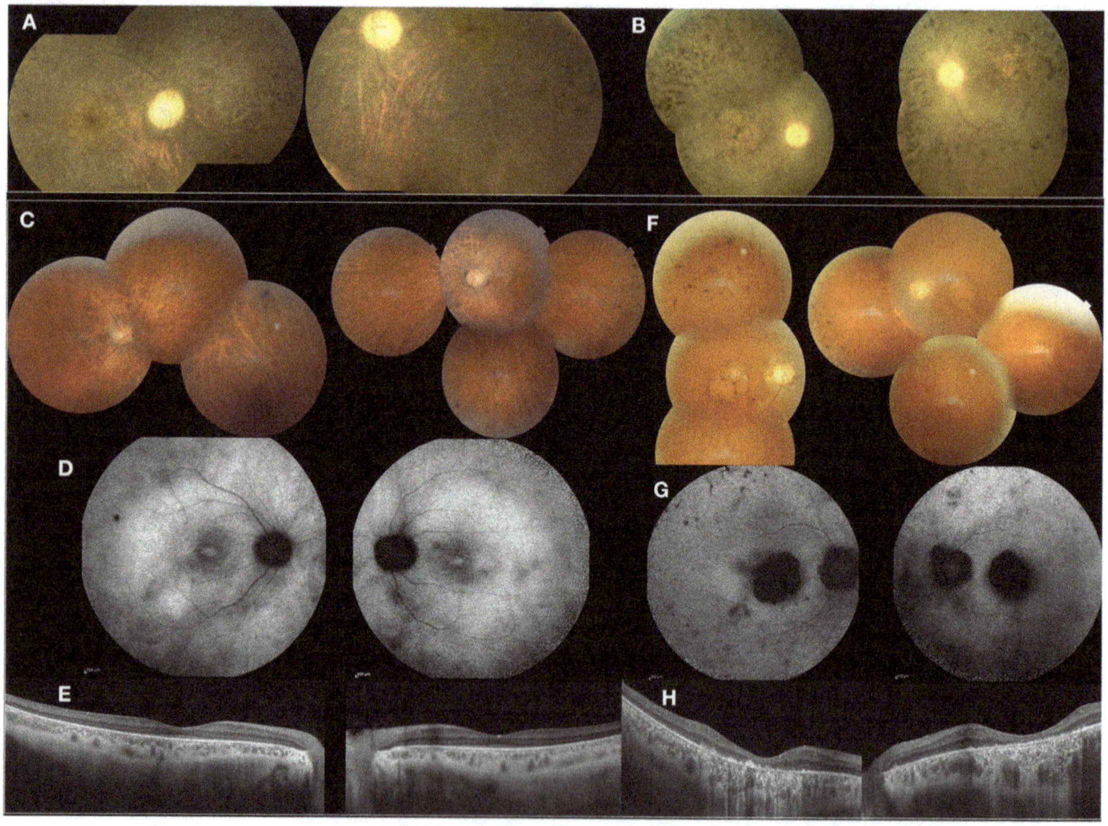

FIGURE 3 | Clinical and imaging features of affected patients from F3 and F4, F3 **(A,B)**. FP of the index patient (II.1) and her mother (I.2) showed cone-rod dystrophy with macular atrophy and spicule deposits in the mid peripheral retina. F4 **(C–H)**. **(C)** FP of the index patient (II.2) with peripheral spicule migrations and preserved posterior pole. **(D)** Foveolar hyperautofluorescence, peripheral hypo-autofluorescence spots. **(E)** SS-OCT. Preserved retinal macular layers. **(F)** FP of the mother (I.2) showing macular atrophy and peripheral spicule deposits. **(G)** FAF with lack of autofluorescence in the macula. **(H)** SS-OCT. Severe and diffuse macular atrophy.

limited to 1/20 OU with macular atrophy and peripheral spicule deposits (**Figures 3F–H**).

Molecular Diagnosis

Identified Pathogenic (P) and Likely Pathogenic (LP) Variants

Six potentially pathogenic variants in four genes were identified in four families (**Figure 4**).

In the index patient with enhanced S-cone syndrome in F1, we identified, a new digenetic combination: a heterozygous likely benign variant p.[G51A];[=] in *RHO* and homozygous LP variant p.[R311Q];[R311Q] in *NR2E3*. Helicoid subretinal fibrosis associated with a recessive *NR2E3* variant p.[R311Q];[R311Q] was identified in F2. New frameshift P variant c.[105delG];[105delG] in *RDH12* was found in the index patient of F3 with cone-rod dystrophy (CRD). Compound heterozygous LP variants p.[R964*];[W758*] in *IMPG2* were observed in the index patient with RP in F4. We have shown that both, the affected parents and the offspring, are homozygous for the same variant in the four families. These variants are classified as pathogenic according to the American College of Medical Genetics (ACMG) guidelines.

DISCUSSION

In this report, molecular testing revealed the coexistence of pathogenic variants affecting distinct RD causing genes in four RD families. Among the five pathogenic variants identified in these families, one was novel (*RDH12* c.105delG, p.Q36Sfs*6) and four were recurrent (*RHO* p.G51A, *NR2E3* p.R311Q and *IMPG2* p.W758*, p.R964*) (Macke et al., 1993; Haider et al., 2000; Bandah-Rozenfeld et al., 2010; Patel et al., 2016).

Two families, F1 and F2, carried the most frequent variant p.R311Q in *NR2E3*. Gerber et al. have previously identified this in patients who may have Enhanced S-cone syndrome (ESCS) (Gerber et al., 2000). Later, Haider et al. reported the same p.R311Q variant with 44.8% frequency in patients with ESCS (Haider et al., 2000) and it was also reported in a patient with Goldmann-Favre syndrome (GFS) (Bernal et al., 2008). The particularity in F1 is the presence of a second heterozygous variant p.G51A in *RHO*. Two diseases are associated with *RHO* variants, RP and congenital stationary night blindness (CSNB). However, in F1 the index patient presented with ESCS, which is more related to *NR2E3*. Interesting, and although *RHO*: p.G51A has been involved in retinitis pigmentosa (Macke et al., 1993), GnomAD mentions a frequency of 0.1% in the general

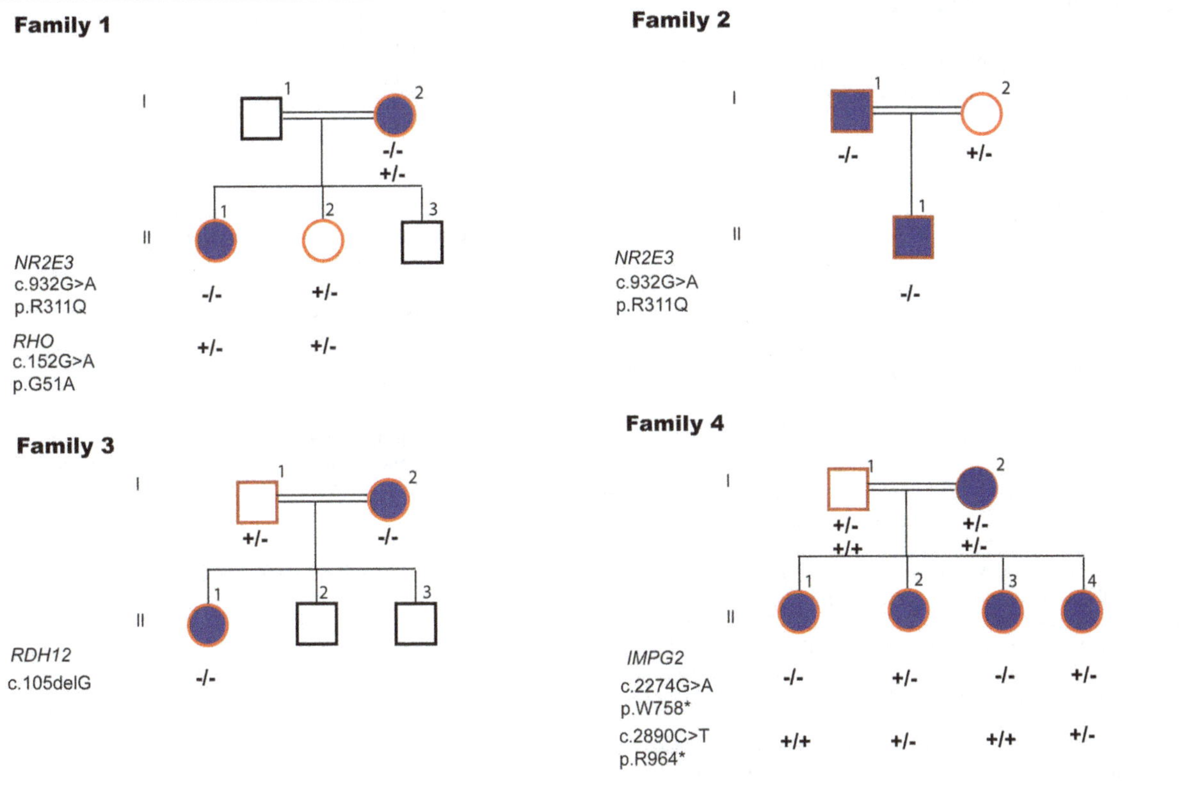

FIGURE 4 | Segregation of the pathogenic variants in four genes identified in four families.

population and ClinVar classifies this variant as benign/likely benign. Family F1 would favor the latter classification.

New pathogenic homozygous variant c.[105delG];[105delG], p.[Q36Sfs*6;[Q36Sfs*6] in *RDH12* was detected in F3. Variants in *RDH12* have been previously linked to Leber congenital amaurosis (LCA) and ad-RP. Retinal pathologies resulting from variants in *RDH12* gene can be inherited in either ad or ar mode (Kumaran et al., 2017; Sarkar et al., 2020). Ar biallelic variants in *RDH12* were first identified in three consanguineous Austrian families with severe retinal dystrophy (Janecke et al., 2004).

F4 harbored compound heterozygous variants p.[W758*];[R964*] in *IMPG2*. This is the first time the association of these two variants is described. Biallelic variants in *IMPG2* have been shown to underlie recessive childhood-onset rod-cone dystrophy with early macular involvement in several families (Khan and Al Teneiji, 2019). At the heterozygous state, *IMPG2* variants have been associated with dominant vitelliform macular dystrophy (Brandl et al., 2017). In F4, the affected mother carried compound likely pathogenic variants, the unaffected father carried a p.W758* heterozygous variant and the affected children a combination of these variants. Pseudodominant inheritance occurs when an individual with a known recessive disorder has a clinically unaffected partner, but then unexpectedly gives birth to children who are affected with the same recessive disorder as the affected parent (Thompson and Thompson, 1986). Although all the parents in the described families were first cousins, each disease followed a dominant pattern of inheritance, with one affected parent and one or several affected children. Molecular analyses allowed us to correctly classify the mode of inheritance as pseudo-dominant, a mode usually associated with a high mutant frequency, like in hemochromatosis.

ETHICS STATEMENT

The studies involving human participants were reviewed and approved by Local Ethics Committee of the Hedi Rais Institute in Tunisia. Written informed consent to participate in this study was provided by the participants' legal guardian/next of kin. Written informed consent was obtained from the individual(s), and minor(s)' legal guardian/next of kin, for the publication of any potentially identifiable images or data included in this article.

AUTHOR CONTRIBUTIONS

DS and LE designed the research protocol. IH and DS performed the analyses. YF, HT, KE, AC, and LE performed the clinical evaluation. IH, YF, LE, and DS wrote the manuscript. All authors reviewed the manuscript.

ACKNOWLEDGMENTS

We thank the family members for their invaluable participation and co-operation. We acknowledge the help provided by the ophthalmologists in this study, and the colleagues who referred patients to us. We thank Denisa Dzulova for reading the manuscript.

REFERENCES

Bandah-Rozenfeld, D., Collin, R. W. J., Banin, E., Van den Born, L. I., Karlien, L. M. C., Siemiatkowska, A. M., et al. (2010). Mutations in IMPG2, encoding interphotoreceptor matrix proteoglycan 2, cause autosomal-recessive retinitis pigmentosa. *Am. J. Hum. Genet.* 1, 199–208. doi: 10.1016/j.ajhg.2010.07.004

Bernal, S., Solans, T., Gamundi, M. J., Hernan, I., de Jorge, L., Carballo, M., et al. (2008). Analysis of the involvement of the NR2E3 gene in autosomal recessive retinal dystrophies. *Clin. Genet.* 73, 360–366. doi: 10.1111/j.1399-0004.2008.00963.x

Brandl, C., Schulz, H. L., Issa, P. C., Birtel, J., Bergholz, R., Lange, C., et al. (2017). Mutations in the genes for interphotoreceptor matrix proteoglycans, IMPG1 and IMPG2, in patients with vitelliform macular lesions. *Genes* 8:170. doi: 10.3390/genes8070170

den Hollander, A. I., Black, A., Bennett, J., and Cremers, F. P. (2010). Lighting a candle in the dark: advances in genetics and gene therapy of recessive retinal dystrophies. *J. Clin. Invest.* 120, 3042–3053. doi: 10.1172/JCI42258

den Hollander, A. I., Roepman, R., Koenekoop, R. K., and Cremers, F. P. (2008). Leber congenital amaurosis: genes, proteins and disease mechanisms. *Prog. Retin. Eye Res.* 27, 391–419. doi: 10.1016/j.preteyeres.2008.05.003

Ellingford, J. M., Barton, S., Bhaskar, S., O'Sullivan, J., Williams, S. G., Lamb, J. A., et al. (2016). Molecular findings from 537 individuals with inherited retinal disease. *J. Med. Genet.* 53, 761–767. doi: 10.1136/jmedgenet-2016-103837

Gerber, S., Rozet, J. M., Takezawa, S. I., dos Santos, L. C., Lopes, L., Gribouval, O., et al. (2000). The photoreceptor cell-specific nuclear receptor gene (PNR) accounts for retinitis pigmentosa in the Crypto-Jews from Portugal (Marranos), survivors from the Spanish Inquisition. *Hum. Genet.* 107, 276–284. doi: 10.1007/s004390000350

Haider, N. B., Jacobson, S. G., Cideciyan, A. V., Swiderski, R., Streb, L. M., Searby, C., et al. (2000). Mutation of a nuclear receptor gene, NR2E3, causes enhanced S cone syndrome, a disorder of retinal cell fate. *Nat. Genet.* 24, 127–131. doi: 10.1038/72777

Janecke, A. R., Thompson, D. A., Utermann, G., Becker, C., Hubner, C. A., Schmid, E., et al. (2004). Mutations in RDH12 encoding a photoreceptor cell retinol dehydrogenase cause childhood-onset severe retinal dystrophy. *Nat. Genet.* 36, 850–854. doi: 10.1038/ng1394

Khan, A. O., and Al Teneiji, A. M. (2019). Homozygous and heterozygous retinal phenotypes in families harbouring IMPG2 mutations. *Ophthalmic Genet.* 40, 247–251. doi: 10.1080/13816810.2019.1627467

Kumaran, N., Moore, A. T., Weleber, R. G., and Michaelides, M. (2017). Leber congenital amaurosis/early-onset severe retinal dystrophy: clinical features, molecular genetics and therapeutic interventions. *Br. J. Ophthalmol.* 101, 1147–1154. doi: 10.1136/bjophthalmol-2016-309975

Lewis, R. A., Shroyer, N. F., Singh, N., Allikmets, R., Hutchinson, A., Li, Y., et al. (1999). Genotype/phenotype analysis of a photoreceptor-specific ATP-binding cassette transporter gene, ABCR, in Stargardt disease. *Am. J. Hum. Genet.* 64, 422–434. doi: 10.1086/302251

Liu, H. Y., Huang, J., Xiao, H., Zhang, M. J., Shi, F. F., Jiang, Y. H., et al. (2019). Pseudodominant inheritance of autosomal recessive congenital stationary night blindness in one family with three co-segregating deleterious GRM6 variants identified by next-generation sequencing. *Mol. Genet. Genomic Med.* 7:e952. doi: 10.1002/mgg3.952

Macke, J. P., Davenport, C. M., Jacobson, S. G., Hennessey, J. C., Gonzalez-Fernandez, F., Conway, B. P., et al. (1993). Identification of novel rhodopsin mutations responsible for retinitis pigmentosa: implications for the structure and function of rhodopsin. *Am. J. Hum. Genet.* 53, 80–89.

Miller, S. A., Dykes, D. D., and Polesky, H. F. (1988). A simple salting out procedure for extracting DNA from human nucleated cells. *Nucleic Acids Res.* 16:1215. doi: 10.1093/nar/16.3.1215

Nash, B. M., Wright, D. C., Grigg, J. R., Bennetts, B., and Jamieson, R. V. (2015). Retinal dystrophies, genomic applications in diagnosis and prospects for therapy. *Transl. Pediatr.* 4, 139–163. doi: 10.3978/j.issn.2224-4336.2015.04.03

Patel, N., Aldahmesh, M. A., and Alkuraya, F. S. (2016). Expanding the clinical, allelic, and locus heterogeneity of retinal dystrophies. *Gene. Med.* 18, 554–562. doi: 10.1038/gim.2015.127

Sarkar, H., Dubis, A. M., Downes, S., and Moosajee, M. (2020). Novel heterozygous deletion in retinol dehydrogenase 12 (RDH12) causes familial autosomal dominant retinitis pigmentosa. *Front. Genet.* 11:335. doi: 10.3389/fgene.2020.00335

Thompson, J. S., and Thompson, M. W. (1986). *Patterns of Single Gene Inheritance in Genetics in Medicine, 4th Edn.* Philadelphia, PA: WB Saunders Co., 44–78.

9

Genetic Screening Revealed Latent Keratoconus in Asymptomatic Individuals

Shihao Chen[1†], Xing-Yong Li[1,2†], Jia-Jia Jin[2], Ren-Juan Shen[2,3], Jian-Yang Mao[2], Fei-Fei Cheng[2], Zhen-Ji Chen[2], Emmanouela Linardaki[4], Stavroula Voulgaraki[5], Ioannis M. Aslanides[1,5] and Zi-Bing Jin[2,3,6‡]*

[1] Center for Refractive Surgery, The Eye Hospital, Wenzhou Medical University, Wenzhou, China, [2] Division of Ophthalmic Genetics, The Eye Hospital, Wenzhou Medical University, National Center for International Research in Regenerative Medicine and Neurogenetics, Wenzhou, China, [3] Beijing Institute of Ophthalmology, Beijing Tongren Eye Center, Beijing Tongren Hospital, Capital Medical University, Beijing Ophthalmology and Visual Sciences Key Laboratory, Beijing, China, [4] DNA Analysis, Molecular Biology and Genetics Center, Heraklion, Greece, [5] Emmetropia Mediterranean Eye Institute, Heraklion, Greece, [6] Beijing Advanced Innovation Center for Big Data-Based Precision Medicine, Beihang University and Capital Medical University, Beijing Tongren Hospital, Beijing, China

***Correspondence:**
Zi-Bing Jin
jinzb@mail.eye.ac.cn

† These authors have contributed equally to this work and share first authorship

***‡ Present address:**
Zi-Bing Jin, Beijing Ophthalmology and Visual Sciences Key Laboratory, Beijing Institute of Ophthalmology, Beijing Tongren Eye Center, Beijing Tongren Hospital, Capital Medical University, Beijing, China

Purpose: To adopt molecular screening in asymptomatic individuals at high risk of developing keratoconus as a combinative approach to prevent subclinical patients from post-refractive surgery progressive corneal ectasia.

Methods: In this study, 79 Chinese and nine Greek families with keratoconus were recruited, including 91 patients with clinically diagnosed keratoconus as well as their asymptomatic but assumptive high-risk first-degree relatives based on underlying genetic factor. Mutational screening of *VSX1*, *TGFBI*, and *ZEB1* genes and full clinical assessment including Pentacam Scheimpflug tomography were carried out in these individuals.

Results: Five variants in *VSX1* and *TGFBI* genes were identified in three Chinese families and one Greek family, and four of them were novel ones. Surprisingly, ultra-early corneal changes in Belin/Ambrosio Enhanced Ectasia Display of Pentacam corneal topography together with co-segregated variants were revealed in the relatives who had no self-reported symptoms.

Conclusions: Variants of *VSX1* and *TGFBI* genes identified in both the clinically diagnosed and subclinical patients may cause the keratoconus through an autosomal dominant inheritance pattern, with different variable expressivity. Combining genetic with Belin/Ambrosio Enhanced Ectasia Display can be used to identify patients with latent keratoconus. This study indicates that genetic testing may play an important supplementary role in re-classifying the disease manifestation and evaluating the preoperative examination of refractive surgery.

Keywords: keratoconus, genetics, latent, asymptomatic, refractive surgery

Abbreviations: ARTmax, Ambrosio relational thickness maximum; BAD, Belin/Ambrosio enhanced ectasia display; BAD-D, total deviation value of Belin/Ambrosio enhanced ectasia display; B.Ele.Th, back elevation at the corneal thinnest location; Da, deviation of Ambrosio relational thickness maximum; Db, deviation of back elevation difference map; Df, deviation of front elevation difference map; Dp, deviation of average pachymetric progression; Dt, deviation of minimum thickness; ExAC, exome aggregation consortium; F.Ele.Th, front elevation at the corneal thinnest location; gnomAD, genome aggregation database; KC, keratoconus; MAF, minor allele frequency; PCA, principal component analysis; PPIavg, pachymetric progression index average; TP, thinnest pachymetry; WES, whole-exome sequencing; 1000G, 1,000 genome.

INTRODUCTION

Keratoconus (KC, OMIM 148300) is a bilateral non-inflammatory ectasia disorder, sometimes asymmetric and characterized by progressive thinning, bulging, and a conical protrusion of the cornea (Krachmer et al., 1984; Rabinowitz, 1998). It is a relatively common disease with a prevalence ranging from 0.3 to 2,300 per 100,000, affecting both genders and diverse populations around the world (Gokhale, 2013), with higher frequency among certain ethnicities such as in Asians and Middle Easterns (Kok et al., 2012; Gokhale, 2013). It has been known that both genetic and environmental factors contribute to the disease occurrence (Gomes et al., 2015). Although most KC cases are sporadic, the incidence of familial aggregation in KC patients ranges from 6 to 23.5%, and first-degree relatives of KC patients have higher prevalence than the general population. High concordance of KC has been reported in studies of monozygotic twins. Most studies suggest an autosomal dominant mode of inheritance with different variable expressivity (Wang et al., 2000; Rabinowitz, 2003; Romero-Jimenez et al., 2010). These findings support the dominant role of a genetic factor in the pathogenesis of KC.

Over the years, many studies have postulated multiple chromosomal regions and genes (e.g., 5q31, 15q22.32-24.2, *VSX1*, *TGFBI*, *ZEB1*, *MIR184*, *SOD1*, and *ZNF469*) to be causative; therefore, KC is suspected to be a genetically heterogeneous disease (Rabinowitz, 2003; Valgaeren et al., 2018). The *VSX1* (OMIM 605020) gene is the most extensively studied gene as a candidate KC gene. An association has been established between *VSX1* gene and the pathogenesis of posterior polymorphous dystrophy (Bykhovskaya et al., 2016). Although the role of *VSX1* gene in KC remains controversial, various *VSX1* gene variants have been identified to be associated with KC in different populations (Shetty et al., 2015; Bykhovskaya et al., 2016; Karolak et al., 2016). It is reported that the expression of *VSX1* has been detected in adult corneas during corneal wound healing (Barbaro et al., 2006). The second candidate KC gene is the *TGFBI* (OMIM 601692) gene, which is responsible for Fuchs endothelial corneal dystrophy. TGFβ1 is reported to be involved in corneal scar formation and fibrosis (Zahir-Jouzdani et al., 2018), and recently, a study found that downregulation of the core elements of the TGF-β pathway influences corneal organization in KC cornea (Kabza et al., 2017). Recently, several mutations in *TGFBI* were identified in Chinese and Polish KC patients, indicating a potential role of *TGFBI* gene in KC pathogenesis (Guan et al., 2012; Bykhovskaya et al., 2016; Karolak et al., 2016). The *ZEB1* (OMIM 189909) gene is also a candidate gene of KC. This gene has been repeatedly reported in corneal dystrophy. Lechner et al. and Mazzotta et al. have identified the same missense variant c.1920G > T of *ZEB1* gene in different patients with KC and other corneal dystrophies, suggesting a potentially significant role of *ZEB1* gene in KC pathogenesis. The above three genes (*VSX1*, *TGFBI*, and *ZEB1*) have been widely studied and have been reported to be related to KC as well as other corneal genetic diseases. Consequently, we selected the above three genes as the target genes for preliminary molecular sequencing, for exploring genetic etiology of KC patients in this study.

In the present study, both genetic and clinical examinations were carried out in clinically diagnosed patients and all relatives. We focused on the genetic etiology and clinical phenotype of asymptomatic relatives, who were at high risk of developing KC, to explore whether molecular screening could be adopted as a combined approach to prevent subclinical patients from post-refractive surgery progressive corneal ectasia.

MATERIALS AND METHODS

This multicenter descriptive cross-sectional study was approved by the Institutional Review Board of The Eye Hospital of Wenzhou Medical University and The Emmetropia Mediterranean Eye Institute. The study adhered to the tenets of the Declaration of Helsinki. Written informed consent was obtained from all subjects prior to this study.

Participant Recruitment

For this study, participants were recruited through patients who were admitted to The Eye Hospital of Wenzhou Medical University or The Emmetropia Mediterranean Eye Institute. A total of 88 families with KC, including 79 Chinese and nine Greek families, were recruited. Each family included a proband with clinically diagnosed KC and first-degree relatives of the proband; the parents of the proband must be included at least, regardless of whether they were asymptomatic or diagnosed as having KC. All the subjects were diagnosed by specialists from China and Greece, respectively. The diagnosis of KC is based on the following criteria: (1) at least one typical clinical feature of KC (e.g., regional stromal thinning, Vogt striae, Fleischer ring, Munson sign); (2) inferior–superior (I-S) index > 1.5, maximum keratometry (Kmax) > 47 D, and the difference in Kmax between the two eyes > 1 D; and (3) abnormal topographic criteria such as asymmetric bow tie, central or inferior steepening (Rabinowitz and McDonnell, 1989).

Mutational Screening

Genomic DNA was isolated from peripheral blood and bidirectional sequencing of all coding regions of *VSX1* (including two additional novel exons) (Hosseini et al., 2008), *TGFBI*, and *ZEB1* genes was screened as previously described (Rao et al., 2017). The primers were designed based on the sequence information from the University of California, Santa Cruz (UCSC) genome browser (**Supplementary Table 1**). Genetic co-segregation of identified variants was confirmed in the families.

Computational Assessment

To assess the functional effect of the identified variants, we employed a series of computational tools as described previously (Huang et al., 2015, 2017; Jin et al., 2017, 2018; Rao et al., 2017), including MutationTaster[1] (Schwarz et al., 2014), Polyphen-2[2] (Adzhubei et al., 2010), and SIFT[3]

[1] http://mutationtaster.org/

[2] http://genetics.bwh.harvard.edu/pph2/

[3] http://sift.jcvi.org/www/SIFT_enst_submit.html

(Kumar et al., 2009). In addition, minor allele frequency (MAF) of variants was obtained from 1,000 Genome (1000G) database, Exome Aggregation Consortium (ExAC) database, and Genome Aggregation Database (gnomAD) (Genomes Project et al., 2010; Lek et al., 2016). To evaluate the conservation of variants, multiple-sequence alignment of *TGFBI* in different species was produced by Clustal X (Version 2.1) and edited by BioEdit (Version 7.2.5.0), and amino acid sequences were obtained from National Center for Biotechnology Information[4]. Furthermore, protein structures of mutant and wild-type proteins of *TGFBI* were modeled by Phyre2[5] and visualized by PyMOL (version 2.7) (Kelley et al., 2015).

Whole-Exome Sequencing

Whole-exome sequencing (WES), as a complementary validation method, was performed on the samples of patients where variants in *VSX1*, *TGFBI*, and *ZEB1* genes were identified by Sanger sequencing. For each individual, at least 3 μg genomic DNA was broken into fragments to generate the Illumina libraries. The whole-exome region libraries were enriched by using an Exome Enrichment V5 Kit (Agilent Technologies, United States) following the manufacturer's protocol and were sequenced by using paired-end 100–300 bp reads on a HiSeq 2000 sequencer (Illumina, United States). After quality control, WES sequence data were mapped to the reference human genome (hg19). Single nucleotide variants and indel variants were identified by GATK and annotated by ANNOVAR. For variant analyses, we summarized 40 candidate genes related to KC (**Supplementary Table 2**), based on several genetics reviews of KC and PubMed database (Bykhovskaya et al., 2016; Loukovitis et al., 2018; Panahi et al., 2019). The pathogenicity of variants in candidate genes with MAF $\leq$ 0.01 in all of the variant databases, including gnomAD, ExAC, and 1,000 Genomes, was compared with that of variants identified by Sanger sequencing.

Corneal Examinations

In case that a candidate variant was identified in a family, the first-degree relatives of the patient were examined by slit-lamp, Pentacam rotating Scheimpflug tomography (software version 1.19r11; Oculus, Wetzlar, Germany), and other routine ophthalmological examinations. Multiple images and parameters were collected from the Pentacam data, based on corneal three-dimensional (3-D) tomography, including the "refractive maps" and the "Belin/Ambrosio Enhanced Ectasia Display (BAD)" maps, which had a good ability to detect the latent changes in early and subclinical stages (Ambrosio et al., 2011; Ruisenor Vazquez et al., 2014), and several parameters from BAD maps: thinnest pachymetry (TP), front and back elevation at the corneal thinnest location (F.Ele.Th and B.Ele.Th), pachymetric progression index average (PPIavg), Ambrosio relational thickness maximum (ARTmax), deviation of front elevation difference map and back elevation difference map (Df and Db), deviation of average pachymetric progression (Dp), deviation of minimum thickness (Dt), deviation of Ambrosio relational thickness maximum (Da), and total deviation value (BAD-D). All clinical data, including corneal signs by slit-lamp and images and parameters by 3-D tomography, were analyzed to compare phenotypic and subclinical phenotypic differences between KC patients and their first-degree relatives, especially the differences between the parents of the KC patient.

Additional Data for Principal Component Analysis

For principal component analysis (PCA), additional 3-D tomography data of BAD maps were obtained from patients who were admitted to the Eye Hospital from November 2016 to October 2017. A total of 332 eyes in 187 patients with KC, 140 eyes in 70 patients with subclinical KC, and 490 eyes in 245 patients with myopia were enrolled. The myopic patients without other ocular diseases served as a control group. The subclinical group included the patients at high risk of developing KC or post-refractive surgery progressive corneal ectasia from refractive surgery candidates; they had at least three or more of the following conditions in at least one eye: (1) the total deviation parameter from BAD map (BAD-D) $\geq$ 1.6; (2) The back elevation at the corneal thinnest location parameter from BAD map (B.Ele.Th) $\geq$ 12; (3) abnormal (red) and/or suspicious (yellow) region(s) found in back elevation difference map from BAD map; (4) thinnest pachymetry < 510 mm; and (5) abnormal pattern in back elevation map from the "refractive maps," such as island shape, tongue shape, or asymmetric hourglass shape. PCA was performed and visualized by Spyder (Version 2.3.8) with Python 2.7.

RESULTS

Clinical Manifestations

In this study, all the 88 families included at least the proband and proband's parents, and the number of participants in these families ranged from three to five. According to the preliminary diagnosis, 91 patients were diagnosed as having KC, including 88 probands in all families and three first-degree relatives in two Greek families (G1, G2). All the rest of first-degree relatives in 88 families were excluded from the diagnosis of clinical KC, without any self-reported complaints or symptoms.

Genetic Variants in Patients With KC

Among the 88 probands with clinical KC, we identified five variants in *VSX1* and *TGFBI* genes. To summarize, a frameshift variant c.758-765delTCAACTCC (p.L253Rfs*18) was found in *VSX1*, and 4 missense variants c.471C > G (p.D157E), c.805C > T (p.L269F), c.1870G > A (p.V624M) and c.1998G > C (p.R666S) were found in *TGFBI* (**Table 1** and **Figure 1A**). Notably, c.805C > T (p.L269F) and c.1998G > C (p.R666S) in *TGFBI* were identified in a single Greek individual (family G1), and other variants were found in different patients from China (F1, F2, and F3).

Identified variants were assessed by computational algorithms and human genome aggregation databases (**Table 1**). All variants

[4]http://www.ncbi.nlm.nih.gov/protein

[5]http://www.sbg.bio.ic.ac.uk/servers/phyre2/html/page.cgi?id=index

TABLE 1 | Bioinformatics data of variants identified by Sanger sequencing of the four probands.

Family	Source	Genotype	Gene	Amino acid change	1000 G	ExAC	gnomAD	Mutationtaster[a]	Polyphen2[b]	SIFT[c]
F1	Maternal	Het	*TGFBI*	c.471C > G:p.D157E	0.0008	0.00009	0.00012	D	P	T
F2	Maternal	Het	*TGFBI*	c.1870G > A:p.V624M	0.001	0.0003	0.00024	D	D	D
F3	Paternal	Het	*VSX1*	c.758-765delTCAACTCC p.L253Rfs*18	NI	0.00013	0.0002	D	NI	NI
G1	Maternal	Het	*TGFBI*	c.805C > T:p.L269F	0.0024	0.0018	0.00165	D	D	D
	Paternal	Het	*TGFBI*	c.1998G > C:p.R666S	0.0008	0.0016	0.00117	A	B	T

Het, heterozygosis; NI, no information.
[a]*MutationTaster: A, known to be deleterious; D, probably deleterious; N, probably harmless; P, known to be harmless.*
[b]*Polyphen2: D, probably damaging; P, possibly damaging; B, benign.*
[c]*SIFT: D, deleterious; T, tolerate.*

were novel except variant c.1998G > C in *TGFBI*, which had been previously reported (Boutboul et al., 2006). All these variants were predicted deleterious, and the MAF of each one was less than 0.005 in gnomAD, ExAC, and 1000G. In addition, all missense variants in the *TGFBI* were highly conserved across different species (**Figure 1B**). Meanwhile, we predicted the three-dimensional structure of mutant proteins and wild-type ones for missense variants in *TGFBI*. Structure models demonstrated that D157E and L269F were located in a β-sheet and V624M in an α-helix, while L269F and R666S had a change in the hydrogen bonds (**Figure 1C**). In summary, we identified five variants in *VSX1* and *TGFBI* genes in four unrelated keratoconic families, four of which are reported for the first time.

Whole-Exome Sequencing

To further verify the pathogenicity of the variants identified in *VSX1* and *TGFBI* genes, WES was performed in the four families (**Supplementary Table 3**). The mean depth of the WES targeted regions was > 60×, and the median coverage reached > 95%. As a result, WES captured the variants successfully, again confirming the variants in the *VSX1* and *TGFBI* genes. In addition, no better explainable variant was found in other known candidate genes responsible for KC, based on a comprehensive analysis of MAF, pathogenicity prediction, and co-segregation. In the absence of further functional studies, these data collectively indicate that the variants identified in both the patients and asymptomatic parents may be major genetic predisposing factors.

Asymptomatic Relatives in the Families With Genetic Variants

We hypothesized that the relatives in the families are at high risk of developing KC even though they did not have self-reported symptoms. To test this hypothesis, we performed mutational screening in the four families with defined variants as mentioned above. Surprisingly, four asymptomatic relatives were found to carry disease-causing variants in an autosomal dominant inheritance pattern (**Figure 1A**).

In Chinese family F1, the asymptomatic mother (F1:I:2) who carried the missense variant c.471C > G in *TGFBI* gene transmitted it to the KC patient (F1:II:1). Clinical examination of the mother showed transverse diffused pigmentations in the central region of the cornea, and topographical examination showed five suspicious parameters (PPIavg, ARTmax, Dp, Da, and BAD-D) in the BAD maps of the right eye. Furthermore, there was a suspicious circular region highlighted in yellow in the "difference elevation map" of the front surface of cornea in the left eye with two suspicious parameters (Dt and BAD-D). The topographic parameters of the unaffected father (F1:I:1) were almost normal except a slightly abnormal BAD-D parameter in both eyes (**Supplementary Figure 1** and **Supplementary Table 4**).

In Chinese family F2, the *TGFBI* variant c.1870G > A was identified in both the KC patient (F2:II:1) and the mother (F2:I:2) who had no self-conscious symptom. The mother was found to have dour suspicious parameters (B.Ele.Th, PPIavg, Dp, and BAD-D) in BAD maps of the right eye, while a yellow region in the back "difference elevation map" with five suspicious parameters (B.Ele.Th, PPIavg, Db, Dp, and BAD-D) was found in the left eye. The father (F2: I:1) was unaffected with KC but had an explicit history of trauma and pterygium in the right eye (**Figure 2**, **Supplementary Figure 2**, and **Supplementary Table 4**).

In the third Chinese family (F3), two siblings (F3:II:2 and F3:II:1) carried the frameshift variant c.758-765delTCAACTCC in *VSX1* gene which was inferably inherited from the asymptomatic father (F3:I:1) who was found to have transverse diffused pigmentations in the inferior region of the cornea in both eyes and a suspicious region in the back "difference elevation map" in the right eye. The father was found to have three suspicious parameters (ARTmax, Da, and BAD-D) and three abnormal parameters (B.Ele.Th, PPIavg, and Dp) in BAD maps of the right eye, while three suspicious parameters (PPIavg, Dp, and BAD-D) were found in the left eye. In the mother (F3:I:2), only a slightly suspicious BAD-D value (1.61) was found in the left eye. The brother (F3:II:1) also had no suspicious clinical finding (**Supplementary Figure 3** and **Supplementary Table 4**).

In the Greek family (G1), the proband (G1:II:2) carried two different heterozygous variants in the same gene *TGFBI*. The variant c.1998G > C was inherited from the affected father (G1:I:1) who had received cross-linking therapy in both eyes, while the variant c.805C > T was shared with the affected brother (G1:II:1), and both inherited from the asymptomatic mother (G1:I:2) who was found to have three suspicious parameters (TP, Dt, and BAD-D) in BAD maps of the right eye and four suspicious parameters (TP, B.Ele.Th, Dt, and BAD-D) in the left eye. The sister (G1:II:3), without detectable variant, had no suspicious clinical finding. In addition, compared to the father and brother,

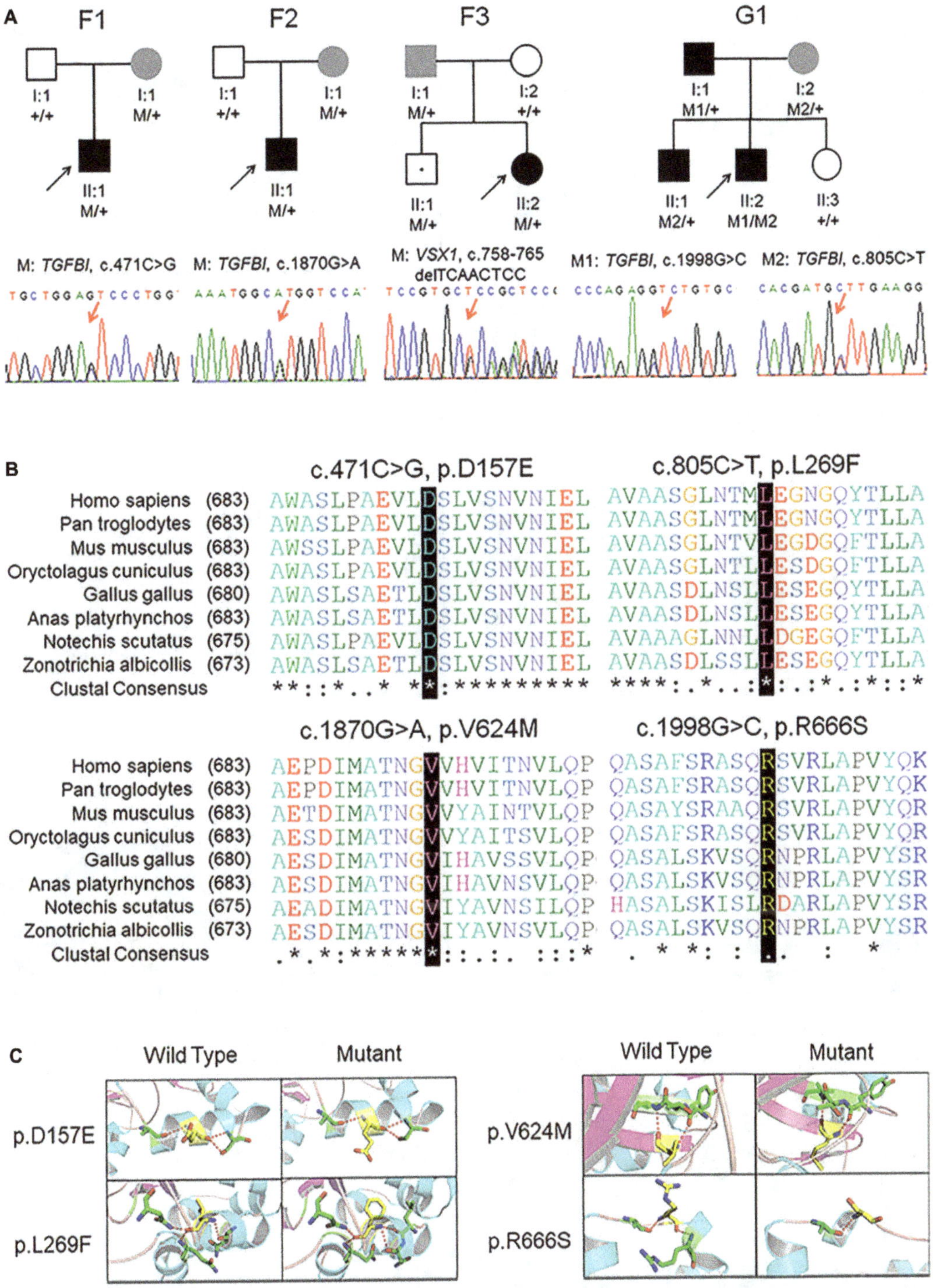

FIGURE 1 | Pedigree, genotype, and clinical data of four probands with keratoconus. **(A)** Pedigree charts. Black symbol indicates affected member, white symbol indicates unaffected individual, gray symbol indicates member with subclinical keratoconus, and dotted symbol denotes variant carrier without any clinical feature. M represents a variant, and + indicates normal allele. The sequence chromatogram with red arrow represents mutant type. **(B)** Conservation analysis revealed evolutionary conservation of the variants. **(C)** Predicted three-dimensional structure of proteins.

the proband had more severe symptoms and earlier onset age of the KC (**Supplementary Figure 4** and **Supplementary Table 4**).

PCA had been employed to compare corneal parameters in BAD maps of the KC group, subclinical group, myopia group, and eight eyes in four subclinical parents in this study (**Figure 3**). We observed that most eyes (6/8) from the four subclinical parents just happen to be in the border region (dotted line area) between myopia group and KC group.

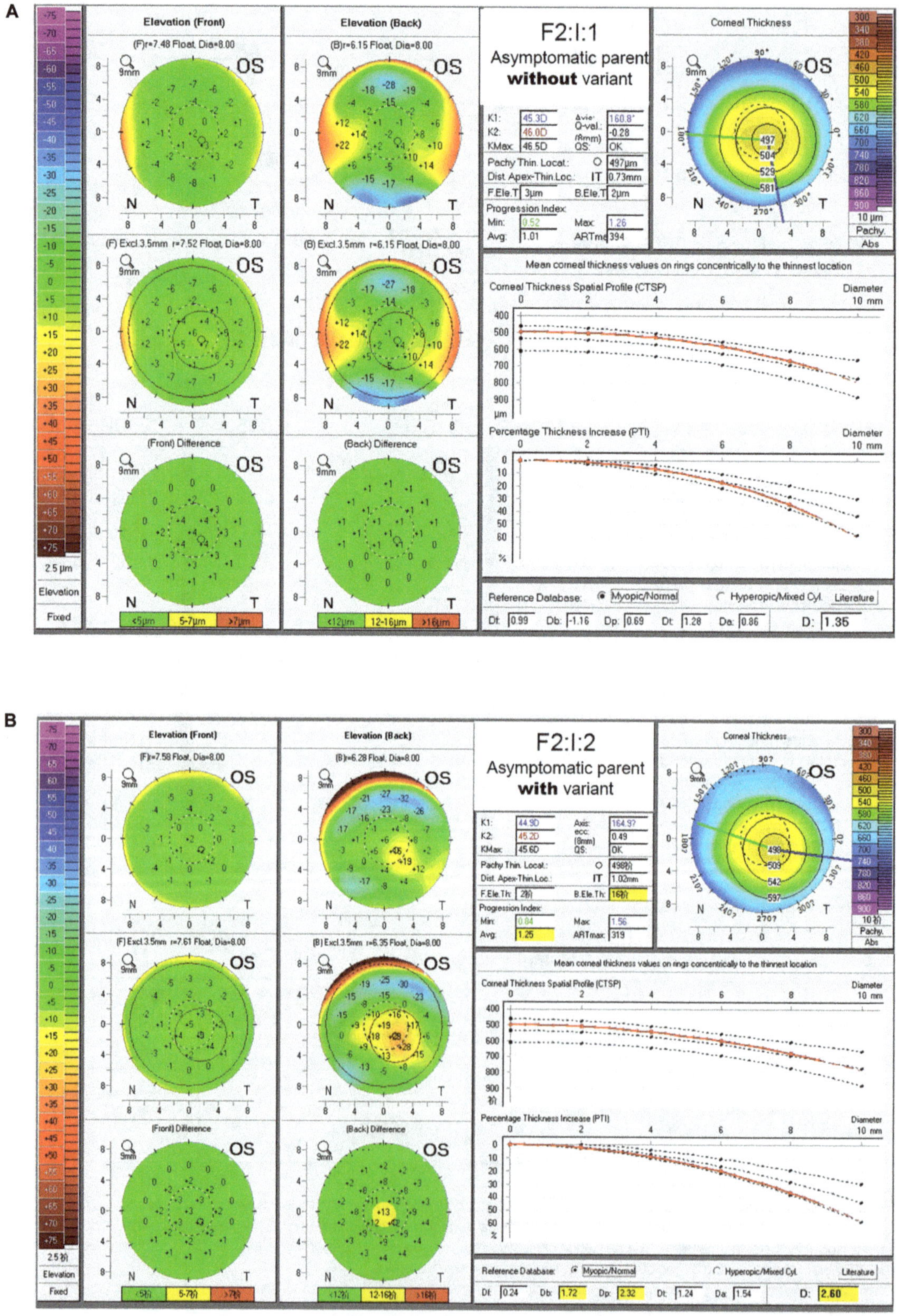

FIGURE 2 | BAD maps of left eye of the asymptomatic parents with different genotypes in an example family. **(A)** Tomographic display from "Belin/Ambrosio Enhanced Ectasia Display (BAD)" maps of the asymptomatic parent without variant (F2:I:1). **(B)** Tomographic display from BAD maps of the asymptomatic parent with variant (F2:I:2). Region highlighted in yellow in the "difference elevation map" indicates suspicious region. OD, right eye; OS, left eye.

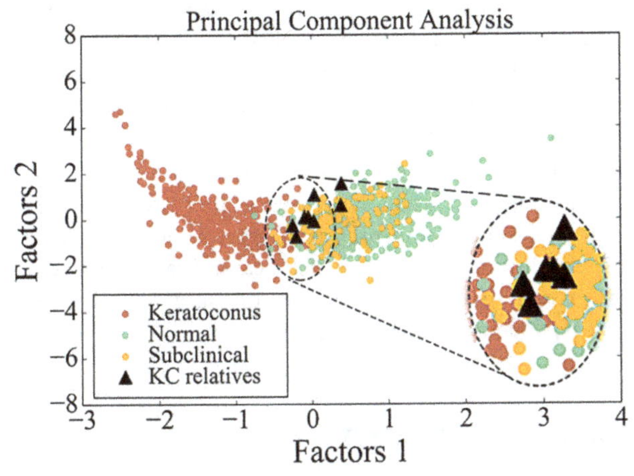

FIGURE 3 | Scatter diagram of data from BAD maps in different groups by principal component analysis. Red circle indicates data from patient with keratoconus, green circle indicates data from control, yellow circle indicates data from subclinical one, and black triangle indicates data from the asymptomatic parent with variant in this study. The image in the upper right corner is a larger image of the dotted line area.

Taken together, genetic variants together with ultra-early corneal topographical changes were found in asymptomatic parents (**Figure 4**), supporting that the relatives in KC families are of higher risk of developing a latent subclinical KC.

DISCUSSION

Patients with KC often exhibit a range of disease manifestations of varying severity (Rabinowitz, 1998). Importantly, post-refractive surgery progressive corneal ectasia had occurred in many patients who did not exhibit any clinical sign of risk factors prior to surgery (Klein et al., 2006). Based on the fact that KC has a clear genetic tendency, previous studies have found a large number of families with dominant inheritance (Paliwal et al., 2011). Given the genetic basis of this disease, we screened the genetic variants in two cohorts from China and Greek. With the identified variants in KC patients by Sanger sequencing and WES, we found the same variants in the asymptomatic parents in these families. Further corneal topographical examination discovered the subclinical abnormalities in these parents.

Most patients with KC were sporadic in previous reports (Romero-Jimenez et al., 2010); however, familial aggregation of KC and high prevalence of first-degree relatives of patients with KC had been widely reported. In addition, several scholars had conducted in-depth studies on the corneal topography of first-degree relatives. Awwad et al. (2019) recruited 183 first-degree relatives aged 6 to 18 years of patients with KC for clinical research. Finally, 32 relatives (17.5%) were revealed as having KC by tomographic evaluation, and the unilateral KC accounted for 37.5%. They concluded that first-degree relatives of KC patients were at high risk of developing KC, and the high rate of unilateral KC suggested a high likelihood of developing KC from normal eyes of first-degree relatives. Kaya et al. (2008) analyzed the corneal topographic features of 72 first-degree relatives of patients with KC and found that eight of them were diagnosed as having KC. Meanwhile, in the remaining 64 asymptomatic relatives, more abnormal corneal parameters could be detected, compared with the control group. Shneor et al. (2020). also found that 18% of first-degree relatives were diagnosed with KC or KC suspect, and 34% had at least one abnormal corneal parameter. Steele et al. (2008) found that KC traits were more likely to appear in the corneal topography of first-degree relatives of patients with KC and suggested an autosomal dominant pattern of inheritance with variable expressivity in some families. Karimian et al. (2008). found that relatives of patients with KC had high incidence of latent KC through topographic evaluation. In our study, we found four parents without self-reported symptoms indeed carry genetic variants in the *VSX1* and *TGFBI* genes. Furthermore, corneal examinations revealed subclinical changes in the cornea. These findings are suggestive of disease predisposition by the same genetic variants with various degrees of disease expressivity and, more importantly, warrant further study on asymptomatic family members and early diagnosis of KC. We speculate that the asymptomatic family members of the KC patients are high-risk

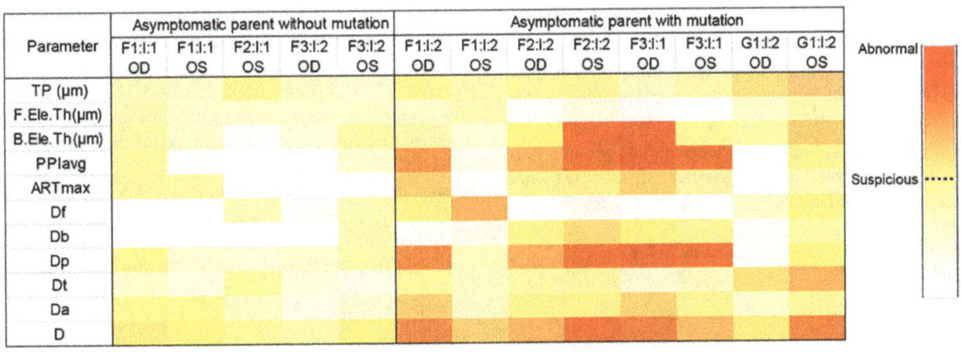

FIGURE 4 | Heatmap of parameters from Pentacam of the parents in the four families. Data visualization was carried out based on the different value range of each parameter, and the darker color represents the higher probability of anomaly. *Data of the right eye of F2: I:1 was excluded from our study because of pterygium, corneal macula, and explicit history of trauma. OD, right eye; OS, left eye.

individuals based on the significant genetic trend of this disease and further hypothesize that there are many similarly high-risk individuals in the population.

From PCA diagram (**Figure 3**), we can observe the continuity between the patient group and the control group, which is consistent with the clinical situation, because there is no clear boundary between KC patients and normal people. In addition, most eyes of the four subclinical parents (6/8) just happen to be in the critical region (dotted line area) between the two groups, as well as many from the subclinical population, so we speculate that many people similar to them may be at potential risk.

With the sharp increase of myopic population globally, there is a huge demand for refractive surgery, which makes a large number of high-risk individuals face the risk of postoperative corneal ectasia after refractive surgery. Post-refractive surgery progressive corneal ectasia is a rare but severe complication of refractive surgery. In the absence of recognized classification system for KC, especially for the subclinical KC, it is important to find a way to accurately screen these high-risk groups. However, despite the rapid development of corneal measurement technology, it is still hard to find a clinical approach with sufficient sensitivity and specificity to identify subclinical KC. Our study supports that genetic screening is important in detecting subclinical KC in extremely early stage or even suspects without any clinical signs.

In conclusion, we performed genetic screening in a large cohort of Chinese and Greek patients with KC and suggested that variants in the *VSX1* and *TGFBI* genes might be responsible for KC through autosomal dominant inheritance pattern with variable expressivity. Further functional studies will be conducted in the future to verify the results of this study. At the same time, the asymptomatic members in keratoconic families were at high risk to carry subclinical KC and should be encouraged to undertake molecular screening and Pentacam Scheimpflug tomography. Our finding suggested that "Belin/Ambrosio Enhanced Ectasia Display" on the Pentacam plays an important role in detecting the latent subclinical changes, and genetic screening is of great value in establishing disease classification system of subclinical and early-stage KC and for the preoperative screening of refractive surgery individuals to prevent postoperative corneal ectasia.

ETHICS STATEMENT

The studies involving human participants were reviewed and approved by Institutional Review Board of The Eye Hospital of Wenzhou Medical University and the Emmetropia Mediterranean Eye Institute. Written informed consent to participate in this study was provided by the participants' legal guardian/next of kin.

AUTHOR CONTRIBUTIONS

Z-BJ designed the experiments and supervised the whole study. SC, X-YL, J-JJ, Z-JC, J-YM, R-JS, EL, SV, and IA performed the experiments. SC, X-YL, F-FC, and IA analyzed the data. SC and X-YL wrote the manuscript. All authors contributed to manuscript revision, read, and approved the submitted version.

REFERENCES

Adzhubei, I. A., Schmidt, S., Peshkin, L., Ramensky, V. E., Gerasimova, A., Bork, P., et al. (2010). A method and server for predicting damaging missense mutations. *Nat. Methods* 7, 248–249.

Ambrosio, R. Jr., Caiado, A. L., Guerra, F. P., Louzada, R., Sinha, R. A., Luz, A., et al. (2011). Novel pachymetric parameters based on corneal tomography for diagnosing keratoconus. *J. Refract. Surg.* 27, 753–758.

Awwad, S. T., Yehia, M., Mehanna, C. J., Fattah, M. A., Saad, A., Hatoum, A., et al. (2019). Tomographic and refractive characteristics of pediatric first-degree relatives of keratoconus patients. *Am. J. Ophthalmol.* 207, 71–76. doi: 10.1016/j.ajo.2019.05.032

Barbaro, V., Di Iorio, E., Ferrari, S., Bisceglia, L., Ruzza, A., De Luca, M., et al. (2006). Expression of VSX1 in human corneal keratocytes during differentiation into myofibroblasts in response to wound healing. *Invest. Ophthalmol. Vis. Sci.* 47, 5243–5250. doi: 10.1167/iovs.06-0185

Boutboul, S., Black, G. C., Moore, J. E., Sinton, J., Menasche, M., Munier, F. L., et al. (2006). A subset of patients with epithelial basement membrane corneal dystrophy have mutations in TGFBI/BIGH3. *Hum. Mutat.* 27, 553–557. doi: 10.1002/humu.20331

Bykhovskaya, Y., Margines, B., and Rabinowitz, Y. S. (2016). Genetics in Keratoconus: where are we? *Eye Vis. (Lond.)* 3:16.

Genomes Project, C., Abecasis, G. R., Altshuler, D., Auton, A., Brooks, L. D., Durbin, R. M., et al. (2010). A map of human genome variation from population-scale sequencing. *Nature* 467, 1061–1073. doi: 10.1038/nature09534

Gokhale, N. S. (2013). Epidemiology of keratoconus. *Indian J. Ophthalmol.* 61, 382–383. doi: 10.4103/0301-4738.116054

Gomes, J. A., Tan, D., Rapuano, C. J., Belin, M. W., Ambrosio, R. Jr., Guell, J. L., et al. (2015). Global consensus on keratoconus and ectatic diseases. *Cornea* 34, 359–369. doi: 10.1097/ico.0000000000000408

Guan, T., Liu, C., Ma, Z., and Ding, S. (2012). The point mutation and polymorphism in keratoconus candidate gene TGFBI in Chinese population. *Gene* 503, 137–139. doi: 10.1016/j.gene.2012.04.061

Hosseini, S. M., Herd, S., Vincent, A. L., and Heon, E. (2008). Genetic analysis of chromosome 20-related posterior polymorphous corneal dystrophy: genetic heterogeneity and exclusion of three candidate genes. *Mol. Vis.* 14, 71–80.

Huang, X. F., Huang, F., Wu, K. C., Wu, J., Chen, J., Pang, C. P., et al. (2015). Genotype-phenotype correlation and mutation spectrum in a large cohort of patients with inherited retinal dystrophy revealed by next-generation sequencing. *Genet. Med.* 17, 271–278. doi: 10.1038/gim.2014.138

Huang, X. F., Mao, J. Y., Huang, Z. Q., Rao, F. Q., Cheng, F. F., Li, F. F., et al. (2017). Genome-Wide detection of copy number variations in unsolved inherited retinal disease. *Invest. Ophthalmol. Vis. Sci.* 58, 424–429. doi: 10.1167/iovs.16-20705

Jin, Z. B., Li, Z., Liu, Z., Jiang, Y., Cai, X. B., and Wu, J. (2018). Identification of de novo germline mutations and causal genes for sporadic diseases using trio-based whole-exome/genome sequencing. *Biol. Rev. Camb. Philos. Soc.* 93, 1014–1031. doi: 10.1111/brv.12383

Jin, Z. B., Wu, J., Huang, X. F., Feng, C. Y., Cai, X. B., Mao, J. Y., et al. (2017). Trio-based exome sequencing arrests de novo mutations in early-onset high myopia. *Proc. Natl. Acad. Sci. U.S.A.* 114, 4219–4224. doi: 10.1073/pnas.1615970114

Kabza, M., Karolak, J. A., Rydzanicz, M., Szczesniak, M. W., Nowak, D. M., Ginter-Matuszewska, B., et al. (2017). Collagen synthesis disruption and downregulation of core elements of TGF-beta, Hippo, and Wnt pathways in keratoconus corneas. *Eur. J. Hum. Genet.* 25, 582–590. doi: 10.1038/ejhg.2017.4

Karimian, F., Aramesh, S., Rabei, H. M., Javadi, M. A., and Rafati, N. (2008). Topographic evaluation of relatives of patients with keratoconus. *Cornea* 27, 874–878. doi: 10.1097/ico.0b013e31816f5edc

Karolak, J. A., Polakowski, P., Szaflik, J., Szaflik, J. P., and Gajecka, M. (2016). Molecular screening of keratoconus susceptibility sequence variants in VSX1, TGFBI, DOCK9, STK24, and IPO5 genes in polish patients and novel TGFBI variant identification. *Ophthalmic Genet.* 37, 37–43.

Kaya, V., Utine, C. A., Altunsoy, M., Oral, D., and Yilmaz, O. F. (2008). Evaluation of corneal topography with Orbscan II in first-degree relatives of patients with keratoconus. *Cornea* 27, 531–534. doi: 10.1097/ico.0b013e318165d110

Kelley, L. A., Mezulis, S., Yates, C. M., Wass, M. N., and Sternberg, M. J. (2015). The Phyre2 web portal for protein modeling, prediction and analysis. *Nat. Protoc.* 10, 845–858. doi: 10.1038/nprot.2015.053

Klein, S. R., Epstein, R. J., Randleman, J. B., and Stulting, R. D. (2006). Corneal ectasia after laser in situ keratomileusis in patients without apparent preoperative risk factors. *Cornea* 25, 388–403. doi: 10.1097/01.ico.0000222479.68242.77

Kok, Y. O., Tan, G. F., and Loon, S. C. (2012). Review: keratoconus in Asia. *Cornea* 31, 581–593. doi: 10.1097/ico.0b013e31820cd61d

Krachmer, J. H., Feder, R. S., and Belin, M. W. (1984). Keratoconus and related noninflammatory corneal thinning disorders. *Surv. Ophthalmol.* 28, 293–322. doi: 10.1016/0039-6257(84)90094-8

Kumar, P., Henikoff, S., and Ng, P. C. (2009). Predicting the effects of coding non-synonymous variants on protein function using the SIFT algorithm. *Nat. Protoc.* 4, 1073–1081. doi: 10.1038/nprot.2009.86

Lek, M., Karczewski, K. J., Minikel, E. V., Samocha, K. E., Banks, E., Fennell, T., et al. (2016). Analysis of protein-coding genetic variation in 60,706 humans. *Nature* 536, 285–291.

Loukovitis, E., Sfakianakis, K., Syrmakesi, P., Tsotridou, E., Orfanidou, M., Bakaloudi, D. R., et al. (2018). Genetic aspects of keratoconus: a literature review exploring potential genetic contributions and possible genetic relationships with comorbidities. *Ophthalmol. Ther.* 7, 263–292. doi: 10.1007/s40123-018-0144-8

Paliwal, P., Tandon, R., Dube, D., Kaur, P., and Sharma, A. (2011). Familial segregation of a VSX1 mutation adds a new dimension to its role in the causation of keratoconus. *Mol. Vis.* 17, 481–485.

Panahi, Y., Azimi, A., Naderi, M., Jadidi, K., and Sahebkar, A. (2019). An analytical enrichment-based review of structural genetic studies on keratoconus. *J. Cell. Biochem.* 120, 4748–4756. doi: 10.1002/jcb.27764

Rabinowitz, Y. S. (1998). Keratoconus. *Surv. Ophthalmol.* 42, 297–319.

Rabinowitz, Y. S. (2003). The genetics of keratoconus. *Ophthalmol. Clin. North Am.* 16, 607–620. vii

Rabinowitz, Y. S., and McDonnell, P. J. (1989). Computer-assisted corneal topography in keratoconus. *Refract. Corneal Surg.* 5, 400–408. doi: 10.3928/1081-597x-19891101-10

Rao, F. Q., Cai, X. B., Cheng, F. F., Cheng, W., Fang, X. L., Li, N., et al. (2017). Mutations in LRP5,FZD4, TSPAN12, NDP, ZNF408, or KIF11 genes account for 38.7% of Chinese patients with familial exudative vitreoretinopathy. *Invest. Ophthalmol. Vis. Sci.* 58, 2623–2629. doi: 10.1167/iovs.16-21324

Romero-Jimenez, M., Santodomingo-Rubido, J., and Wolffsohn, J. S. (2010). Keratoconus: a review. *Cont. Lens Anterior Eye* 33, 157–166; quiz 205.

Ruisenor Vazquez, P. R., Galletti, J. D., Minguez, N., Delrivo, M., Fuentes Bonthoux, F., Pfortner, T., et al. (2014). Pentacam Scheimpflug tomography findings in topographically normal patients and subclinical keratoconus cases. *Am. J. Ophthalmol.* 158, 32–40.e32..

Schwarz, J. M., Cooper, D. N., Schuelke, M., and Seelow, D. (2014). MutationTaster2: mutation prediction for the deep-sequencing age. *Nat. Methods* 11, 361–362. doi: 10.1038/nmeth.2890

Shetty, R., Nuijts, R. M., Nanaiah, S. G., Anandula, V. R., Ghosh, A., Jayadev, C., et al. (2015). Two novel missense substitutions in the VSX1 gene: clinical and genetic analysis of families with Keratoconus from India. *BMC Med. Genet.* 16:33. doi: 10.1186/s12881-015-0178-x

Shneor, E., Frucht-Pery, J., Granit, E., and Gordon-Shaag, A. (2020). The prevalence of corneal abnormalities in first-degree relatives of patients with keratoconus: a prospective case-control study. *Ophthalmic Physiol. Opt.* 40, 442–451. doi: 10.1111/opo.12706

Steele, T. M., Fabinyi, D. C., Couper, T. A., and Loughnan, M. S. (2008). Prevalence of Orbscan II corneal abnormalities in relatives of patients with keratoconus. *Clin. Exp. Ophthalmol.* 36, 824–830. doi: 10.1111/j.1442-9071.2009.01908.x

Valgaeren, H., Koppen, C., and Van Camp, G. (2018). A new perspective on the genetics of keratoconus: why have we not been more successful? *Ophthalmic Genet.* 39, 158–174. doi: 10.1080/13816810.2017.1393831

Wang, Y., Rabinowitz, Y. S., Rotter, J. I., and Yang, H. (2000). Genetic epidemiological study of keratoconus: evidence for major gene determination. *Am. J. Med. Genet.* 93, 403–409. doi: 10.1002/1096-8628(20000828)93:5<403::aid-ajmg11>3.0.co;2-a

Zahir-Jouzdani, F., Soleimani, M., Mahbod, M., Mottaghitalab, F., Vakhshite, F., Arefian, E., et al. (2018). Corneal chemical burn treatment through a delivery system consisting of TGF-beta1 siRNA: in vitro and in vivo. *Drug Deliv. Transl. Res.* 8, 1127–1138. doi: 10.1007/s13346-018-0546-0

10

An Early Diagnostic Clue for *COL18A1*- and *LAMA1*-Associated Diseases: High Myopia with Alopecia Areata in the Cranial Midline

Panfeng Wang[1]*, Xiaoyun Jia[1], Xueshan Xiao[1], Shiqiang Li[1], Yuxi Long[1], Mengchu Liu[1], Yongyu Li[1], Jun Li[1], Yan Xu[1,2] and Qingjiong Zhang[1]*

[1] State Key Laboratory of Ophthalmology, Zhongshan Ophthalmic Center, Sun Yat-sen University, Guangzhou, China,
[2] Guangdong Provincial Key Laboratory of Reproductive Medicine, Reproductive Medicine Center, The First Affiliated Hospital, Sun Yat-sen University, Guangzhou, China

***Correspondence:**
Panfeng Wang
wpf5113@163.com
Qingjiong Zhang
zhangqji@mail.sysu.edu.cn

Background: High myopia with alopecia areata in the occipital region has been observed in patients with Knobloch syndrome caused by *COL18A1* mutations. This study investigated other possible genetic causes of high myopia in patients with alopecia areata in the cranial midline.

Methods: Six patients with early onset high myopia and alopecia areata in the cranial midline were recruited. Targeted high-throughput sequencing was performed on the proband's DNA to detect potential pathogenic variants. Cosegregation analysis was performed for available family members. Minigene assay and RNA Sequencing were used to validate the abnormality of possible splicing change and gross deletion. Ophthalmological and neuroimaging examinations were performed.

Results: Eight novel and one known loss-of-function mutants were detected in all six patients, including a gross deletion detected by RNA sequencing. Four *COL18A1* mutants in three patients with scalp leisure in the occipital region; and five *LAMA1* mutations in three patients with scalp leisure in the parietal region. Further assessments indicated that patients with *COL18A1* mutations had Knobloch syndrome, and the patients with *LAMA1* mutations had Poretti–Boltshauser syndrome.

Conclusion: Our study found that early onset high myopia with midline alopecia areata could be caused not only by mutations of the *COL18A1* gene but also by mutations in the *LAMA1* gene. To our knowledge, we are the first to observe scalp defects in patients with *LAMA1* mutations. High myopia with alopecia areata in the cranial midline could be treated as an early diagnostic clue for ophthalmologists to consider the two kinds of rare diseases.

Keywords: alopecia areata, cranial midline, syndromic high myopia, molecular genetics, diagnostic techniques

INTRODUCTION

Myopia, particularly high myopia, could occur independently or as a feature in hundreds of ocular and systemic syndromes. Myopic syndromes have a wide range of clinical manifestations that affect patients' daily lives in various ways, from mild discomfort to even death shortly after birth or in childhood. The nervous system is one of the most common parts of the body involved in these syndromes in addition to myopia; when affected, it can present with typical signs such as intellectual disability, microcephaly, cerebellar hypoplasia, special facial features, and hearing loss. These syndromes are usually rare and complex and include Coffin–Siris syndrome 1 (OMIM_135900) (Hoyer et al., 2012); Donnai–Barrow syndrome (OMIM_222448) (Kantarci et al., 2007); DOOR syndrome (deafness, onychodystrophy, osteodystrophy, mental retardation and seizures; OMIM_220500) (James et al., 2007); Hamamy syndrome (OMIM_611174) (Hamamy et al., 2007); Knobloch syndrome (KNO; OMIM_267750) (Passos-Bueno et al., 1994; Sertie et al., 2000); muscular dystrophy-dystroglycanopathy (congenital with brain and eye anomalies), type A, 10 (OMIM_615041) (Vuillaumier-Barrot et al., 2012); Pitt–Hopkins syndrome (OMIM_610954) (Whalen et al., 2012); Poretti–Boltshauser syndrome (PBS; OMIM_615960) (Aldinger et al., 2014; Micalizzi et al., 2016); Rubinstein–Taybi syndrome 2 (OMIM_613684) (Bartsch et al., 2010); Schuurs–Hoeijmakers syndrome (OMIM_615009) (Schuurs-Hoeijmakers et al., 2012); Shprintzen–Goldberg syndrome (OMIM_182212) (Doyle et al., 2012); and Temtamy syndrome (OMIM_218340) (Zahrani et al., 2013). Because high myopia might be an early feature in these syndromes or due to unawareness of the atypical manifestations of other signs, it is challenging for ophthalmologists to recognize these myopic syndromes, especially in children under 10 years of age. It would be helpful if certain signs could be obtained by physical examination to help doctors consider myopic syndromes with nervous system involvement, as is possible with Marfan syndrome.

KNO, with a prevalence estimated to be less than 1/1,000,000 (Orphanet, 2020a), is an autosomal recessive developmental disorder characterized by typical eye abnormalities with occipital skull defects. Linkage analysis successfully identified that KNO1 is mainly caused by mutations in the *COL18A1* gene (OMIM_120328) (Sertie et al., 2000), which plays a role in embryonic eye development and neural tube closure (Aikio et al., 2013; Banerjee et al., 2013). The eye abnormalities included high myopia, cataracts, dislocated lenses, vitreoretinal degeneration, and retinal detachment, while the occipital skull defect ranges from encephalocele to occipital bone fenestrae, meningocele, and cutis aplasia. Other rare phenotypes, including nervous system defects and missing nails, have also been reported (Keren et al., 2007; Williams et al., 2008; Ackerman et al., 2012; Abouelhoda et al., 2016). Congenital midline scalp defects have been described for most patients, including small areas of alopecia with a flat, wine-color hemangioma, occipital cutis aplasia (Kliemann et al., 2003), pigmented lesion in the occipital area (Balikova et al., 2020), midline occipital soft tissue swelling and alopecia hypotonia (Mahajan et al., 2010), and hair abnormalities (Williams et al., 2008; Hull et al., 2016). Physical examination of the skin of the scalp could be a fast and convenient way for ophthalmologists to detect signs for considering KNO and *COL18A1* mutations when treating children with high myopia.

In this study, we performed targeted high-throughput sequencing on patients with early onset high myopia with cutis aplasia in the skull to identify possible causative genes. In addition, we sought to determine whether a simple physical examination of the skin of the scalp could provide meaningful clues for further examination for myopic syndrome with nervous system involvement.

METHODS

Patient Selection

This study was approved by the Institutional Review Board of the Zhongshan Ophthalmic Center. Unrelated probands with early onset high myopia were collected from the Zhongshan Ophthalmic Center as part of the project to identify genetic loci and genes for high myopia. Patients presenting with skull defects due to cutis aplasia not only in the occipital region but also extending to the cranial midline were recruited. Informed consent conforming to the tenets of the Declaration of Helsinki was obtained from the involved individuals or their guardians prior to the study. Genomic DNA was prepared from the venous blood of the patients and available family members. Standard ophthalmological examinations including visual acuity, refractive error examination after mydriasis, slit lamp, and fundus photography were performed on all probands and available family members. Electroretinogram (ERG), B-scan, X-ray, CT, and MRI were performed on selected patients when possible. The ERG response was recorded according to the International Society for Clinical Electrophysiology of Vision (ISCEV) standards Marmor et al. (1989).

Mutation Screening and Analyses

Whole-exome sequencing (WES) or targeted exome sequencing (TES) was performed on genomic DNA from six probands to screen genetic defects. The WES or TES data were analyzed through multistep bioinformatics analysis as described previously (Li et al., 2015; Wang et al., 2019). The genes of target panel are listed in **Supplementary Table 1**. The possible influence of splicing change was predicted by software including Human Splicing Finder[1] and Berkeley Drosophilia Genome Project (BDGP)[2]. Potential pathogenic variants (PPVs) were further classified according to the guidelines of the American College of Medical Genetics and Genomics (ACMG) (Richards et al., 2015); and variants of uncertain significance (VUSs), likely benign, and benign variants were ruled out. Sanger sequencing was used to confirm PPVs and to validate their cosegregation in available family members. The PPVs were described according to the nomenclature for sequence variations (Human Genome Variation Society) (den Dunnen and Antonarakis, 2000). The transcript, NM_130444.2, was used to nomenclature variants detected in *COL18A1*; and the transcript, NM_005559.4, was used to nomenclature variants detected in *LAMA1*.

Splicing Change Confirmed by Minigene Assay

Three rounds of PCR were performed using nested primers (**Supplementary Table 2**): the first PCR was performed using

[1] http://www.umd.be/HSF3/
[2] http://www.fruitfly.org

genomic DNA (a total of two sets of DNA) as a template, with two pairs of primers, 49029-COL18A1-F and 51125-COL18A1-R (product length: 2,096 bp), as well as 49321-COL18A1-F and 50763-COL18A1-R (product length: 1,443 bp) with annealing temperature of 57°C, treating the products with size of 1,443 bp as a template. The second PCR was performed to produce human COL18A1 fragment covering exon 35 (145 bp)–intron 35 (79 bp)–exon 36 (74 bp)–intron 36 (406 bp)–exon 37 (129 bp), as follows: pcDNA3.1-COL18A1-*Kpn*I-F and pcDNA3.1-COL18A1-*Bam*HI-R as primers were used to produce pcDNA3.1-wt (wild type) fragment of 833 bp; pcDNA3.1-COL18A1-*Kpn*I-F and COL18A1-MUT-R as primers were used to produce mutant fragment 1; and COL18A1-MUT-F and pcDNA3.1-COL18A1-*Bam*HI-R as primers were used to produce mutant fragment 2. Finally, mutant fragments 1 and 2 were mixed together with ratio of 1:1 and were treated as template to amplify pcDNA3.1-mut (mutant fragment) of 798 bp (c.4259-28_4265del) with primers of pcDNA3.1-COL18A1-*Kpn*I-F and pcDNA3.1-COL18A1-*Bam*HI-R.

The PCR products pcDNA3.1-wt and pcDNA3.1-mut were purified (DNA Gel Extraction Kit, SIMGEN, Hangzhou, China) and inserted into the eukaryotic expression vector pcDNA3.1 using *Kpn*I/*Bam*HI to construct two sets of plasmids: pcDNA3.1-COL18A1-wt and pcDNA3.1-COL18A1-mut. Fragments were verified by Sanger sequencing.

The four kinds of recombinant vectors were transiently transfer into human embryonic kidney cells (HEK-293) and cervical cancer cells (HeLa) according to the manufacturer's

TABLE 1 | Summary of clinical data in high myopia patients with alopecia areata in the cranial midline.

	14410	14518	20204	5176	7856	19618
Gene	*COL18A1*	*COL18A1*	*COL18A1*	*LAMA1*	*LAMA1*	*LAMA1*
Gender	Male	Male	Male	Male	Male	Female
Age at onset of disease (years)	5	2	4	2	0.5	0.4
First complain sigh	Strabismus	Strabismus	Nystagmus Strabismus	Strabismus	Strabismus	Strabismus
Age when examined	6	8	17	3	2.75	3
Visual acuity (R/L)	0.06/0.12	0.06/0.03	0.05/0.05	0.2/0.1	NA	NA
High myopia (R/L)	−10.25/−7.75	−11.50/−11.25	−18.00/−10.25	−11.50/−13.25	−12.25/−10.50	−15.00/−14.00
Anterior segment	(−)	(−)	Cataract OU	(−)	(−)	(−)
Optic disc	Peripapillary atrophy	Peripapillary atrophy	Peripapillary atrophy	Disc pallor	Disc pallor	Disc pallor
Leopard fundus	+++	+++	+++	+	+++	+++
Chorioretinal sclerosis and atrophy	+++	+++	+++	+	+++	+++
Macular atrophy	++	+++	+++	+++	+	+++
Pigment distribution	−	Center++/periphery++	Periphery++	Center+	−	Periphery++
Strabismus	+	+	+	+	+	+
Nystagmus	+	+	+	+	+	NA
Axial length (OD/OSmm)	NA	26.16/26.44	NA	26.32/26.01	NA	NA
ERG	NA	NA	Moderately reduced	Moderately reduced	Severe reduced	Moderately reduced
Scalp defect region	Occipital	Occipital	Occipital	Parietal	Parietal	Parietal
CSF leak	Transient	Transient	Transient	Denied	Denied	Denied
Skull	Normal	Occipital bone defect	Normal	Parietal bone defect	Normal	NA
MRI	Normal	NA	NA	Cerebellar dysplasia with enlarged fourth ventricle; cortical-subcortical cysts	Cerebellar dysplasia with enlarged fourth ventricle	NA
Other system defects	−	−	−	Accessary ear in the left	Motor delay and ataxia	Motor delay and ataxia

NA, not available; ERG, electroretinogram; CSF, cerebrospinal fluid.

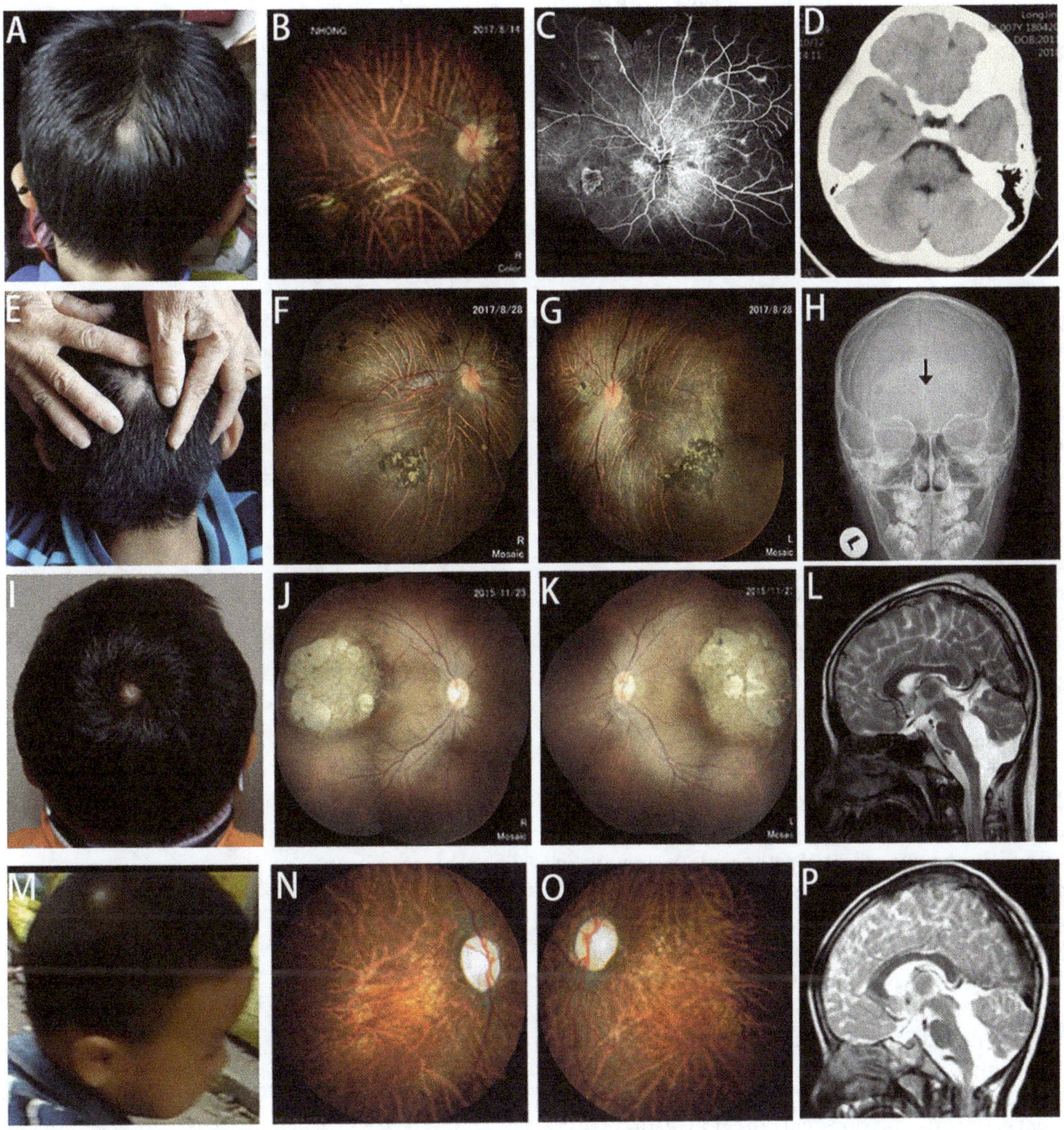

FIGURE 1 | Scalp defects, fundus changes, and neuroimaging in patients with *COL18A1* and *LAMA1* mutations. **(A,E)** Alopecia areata appears in the midline of the occipital region of patients with *COL18A1* mutations. **(I,M)** Alopecia areata appears in the midline of the parietal region (in the center of hair whorl) in patients with *LAMA1* mutations. **(B,C,F,G,J,K,N,O)** In addition to the typical high myopia fundus leopard-like pattern, dysplasia of the papilla, and macular degeneration, characteristic fundus degeneration can be observed for all patients including optic degeneration, chorioretinal sclerosis and atrophy, foveal hypoplasia, atrophic patch with extra bone spicule accumulation, and loss of pigmentation temporal to the macula. **(C)** Fluorescein angiograms reveal vascular leakage in patient 14410. **(D)** MRI reveals a normal brain image for patient 14410. **(H)** Black arrow indicates a small hole in the occipital region of patient 14518 by X-ray. **(L,P)** Cerebellar dysplasia and obvious enlargement of the fourth ventricle are observed in patients 5176 and 7856.

instruction (Rapid Plasmid Mini Kit, SIMGEN). The transfected cells were cultured for 48 h and then collected for transcript expression analysis.

TRIzol method (RNAiso PLUS, TaKaRa, Dalian, China) was used to extract total RNA from HEK-293 cells and HeLa cells. Reverse transcription polymerase chain reaction (RT-PCR) was carried out [HifairTM 1st Strand Cdna Synthesis SuperMix for qPCR (Gdna digester plus), YEASEN, Shanghai, China] to check the splicing method and verified through Sanger sequencing.

RNA Sequencing

RNA sequencing was carried out by commercial company (Shanghai Cino Medical Laboratory Co., Ltd., Shanghai, China). Peripheral blood was collected in PAXgene Blood RNA Tube (BD Biosciences, San Jose, CA, United States), and RNA was isolated by MagMAX for Stabilized Blood Tubes RNA Isolation Kit according to the kit's instruction. All RNA sample were measured for quantity and quality by NanodropOne (Thermo Fisher Scientific, Waltham, MA, United States) and Qseq400 (BiOptic,

New Taipei City, Taiwan). Samples with RNA quality score (RQS) above 7 were proceeded with RNA-seq library preparation by the KAPA RNA HyperPrep Kit (Kapa Biosystems, Inc., Woburn, MA, United States) after depletion of rRNA with the KAPA RNA HyperPrep Kit (Kapa Biosystems). The total RNA input was 1 μg. Sequencing was performed on Illumina HiSeq 2000 instrument with PE150, and 15-G raw data were achieved per sample. The RNA sequencing data were checked for quality using FastQC and mapped and analyzed using the VIPER Snakemake pipeline (Cornwell et al., 2018). Briefly, VIPER aligns the files to the hg19 transcriptome using STAR, followed by differential expression analysis using DESeq2. Visualization and sashimi plot of the *COL18A1* gene were performed by Integrative Genomics Viewer (IGV) (Thorvaldsdottir et al., 2013). The abnormality mRNA of *COL18A1* was further validate by RT-PCR and Sanger sequencing after being amplified with temple of cDNA.

RESULTS

A total of six unrelated probands (five males and one female) were recruited. The first complaint sign of strabismus was noticed in all patients, with an average age of 1.89 years (from 0.4 to 5). The average refractive error was -10.92 ± 1.83, and the best corrected vision was less than 0.2 (**Table 1**). All of them had skull defect from cutis aplasia in the cranial midline, three of which were located in the occipital region, while the rest were located in the parietal region (in the center of the hair whorl) (**Figures 1A,E,I,M**).

Eight novel and one known potential pathogenic mutants were identified in these six probands (**Table 2**). Of these mutations, two were homozygous and one was compound heterozygous in the *COL18A1* gene, including c. [4290_4299del];[4290_4299del][p.(Gly1016Glufs*9)]; [(Gly1016Glufs*9)], c.[4259-28_4265del]; and c.[ex.32-36del] and a known mutation c.[4759_4760del]; [4759_4760del]p.[(Leu1587Valfs*72)]; [(Leu1587Valfs*72)]. The remaining mutations were all located in the *LAMA1* gene, including c.[4579C>T]; [1487dup]p.[(Gln1527*)]; [(Asn496Lysfs*15)], c.[6151C>T];[1494_1504del]p.[(Arg2051*)];[(Gly499Valfs*8)], and c.[4171_4172del]; [4171_4172del]p.[(Arg1391Glyfs*19)]; [(Arg1391Glyfs*19)]. The mutation c.4259-28_4265del was predicted to activate a new cryptic Acceptor site and by HSF, and the confidence scores of the old Acceptor site were diminished from 0.88 to 0 before and after the mutation by FF. All eight mutations were predicted to result in complete loss of function (LOF) for the corresponding proteins. All mutations were confirmed with Sanger sequencing and segregated by disease in the available family members (**Figure 2** and **Table 2**).

A minigene splicing assay was built to validate whether the splicing change detected in *COL18A1*, c.4259-28_4265del, affects splicing products (**Figures 3A–D**). A total of eight samples were harvested after 48 h of transfection. The gel view of the reverse transcription PCR showed that band b (mut) migrated faster than band a (wt), which meant that the mut fragment (274 bp) was smaller than that of wt (348 bp) (**Figure 3B**). DNA sequencing

TABLE 2 | Eight potential pathogenic mutations in *COL18A1* and *LAMA1* genes.

Patient ID	Gene	Position	Transcript	Nucleotide change	Exon	Status	Amino acid change	Effect	Origin	GenomAD-EAS	Sequencing strategy
14410	*COL18A1*	chr21:46925303_46925312	NM_130444.2	c.4290_4299del	E35/41	Hmz	p.(Gly1431Glufs*9)	Frameshift	Parents	None	TES
14518	*COL18A1*	chr21:46925244_46925278	NM_130444.2	c.4259-28_4265del	IVS34/41	Hmz	–	Splice site broken -86.23	Father	None	TES
		?	NM_130444.2	?	E32–E36	Het	Gross deletion		Mother	None	RNA sequencing
20204	*COL18A1*	chr21:46929996_46929997	NM_130444.2	c.4759_4760del	E39/41	Hmz	p.(Leu1587Valfs*72)	Frameshift	Parents	None	TES
5176	*LAMA1*	chr18:6999528	NM_005559.4	c.4579C > T	E32/63	Het	p.(Gln1527*)	Non-sense	Father	0	WES
		chr18:7038885		c.1487dup	E11/63	Het	p.(Asn496Lysfs*15)	Frameshift	Mother	5.45E–05	
7856	*LAMA1*	chr18:6978234	NM_005559.4	c.6151C > T	E43/63	Het	p.(Arg2051*)	Non-sense	Father	5.01E–05	WES
		chr18:7038868_7038878		c.1494_1504del	E11/63	Het	p.(Gly499Valfs*8)	Frameshift	Mother	None	
19618	*LAMA1*	chr18:7007226_7007227	NM_005559.4	c.4171_4172del	E29/63	Hmz	p.(Arg1391Glyfs*19)	Frameshift	Parents	1.50E–04	TES

*TES, targeted exome sequencing; WES, whole-exome sequencing; *, Termination codon.*

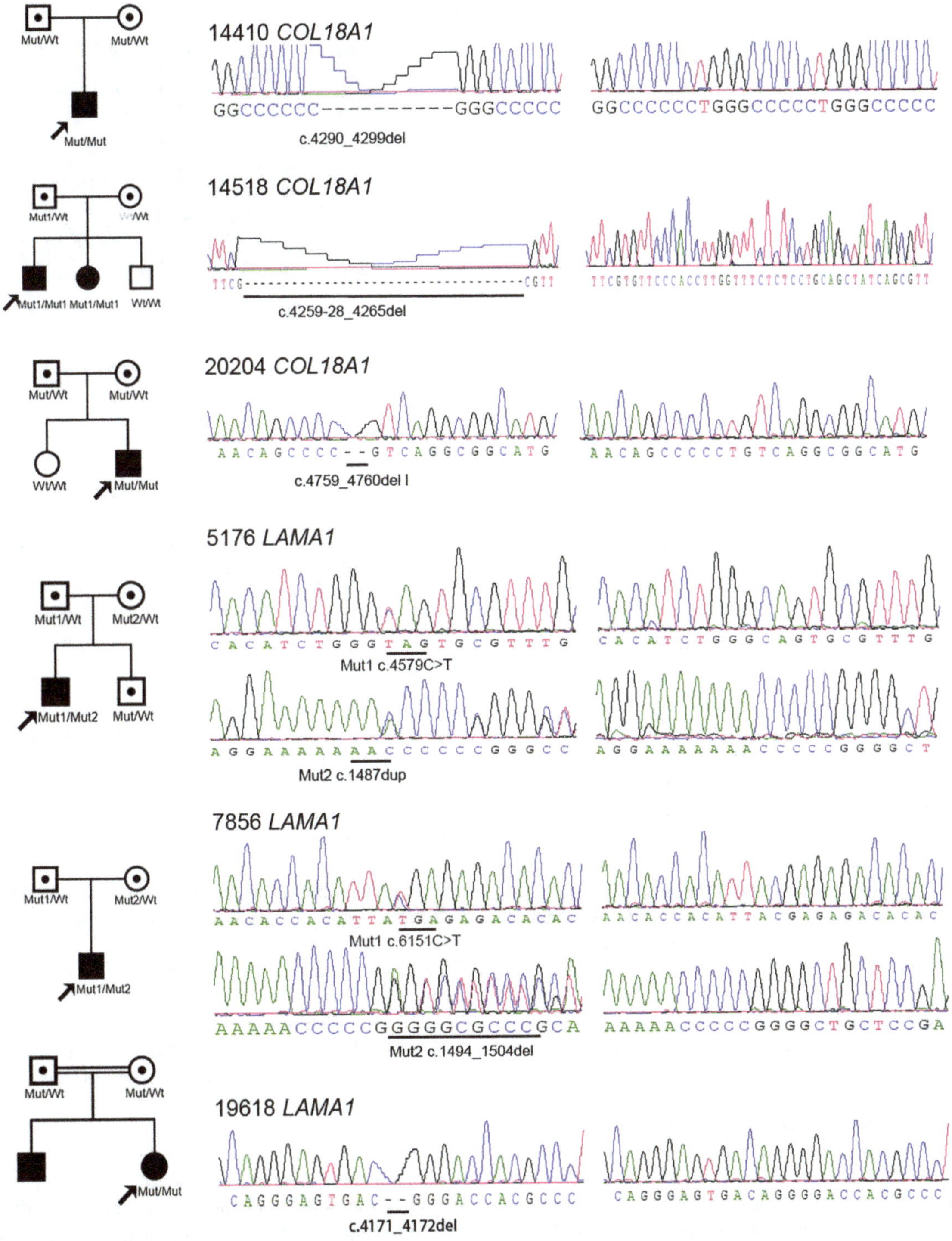

FIGURE 2 | Pedigrees and sequences of eight novel loss-of-function mutations in the *COL18A1* and *LAMA1* genes. The genotypes of all probands and available family members are shown below each individual. The black symbols represent the affected individuals. The white symbols with black points represent carriers. Mut, mutation; wt, wild type. One allele of the wt in the mother of 14518 is marked as gray because it is a pseudo-wild type caused by gross deletion cross missing by Sanger sequencing.

indicated that the wild-type minigene expressed normal mRNA composed of exon 34, exon 35, and exon 36; the mutant type minigene expressed a shorter mRNA composed of exon 34 and exon 36 (**Figures 3C,D**). The mutation c.4259-28_4265del damaged the Acceptor of Exon 35 and resulted in the skipping of exon 35. The result is consistent with the *in silico* prediction.

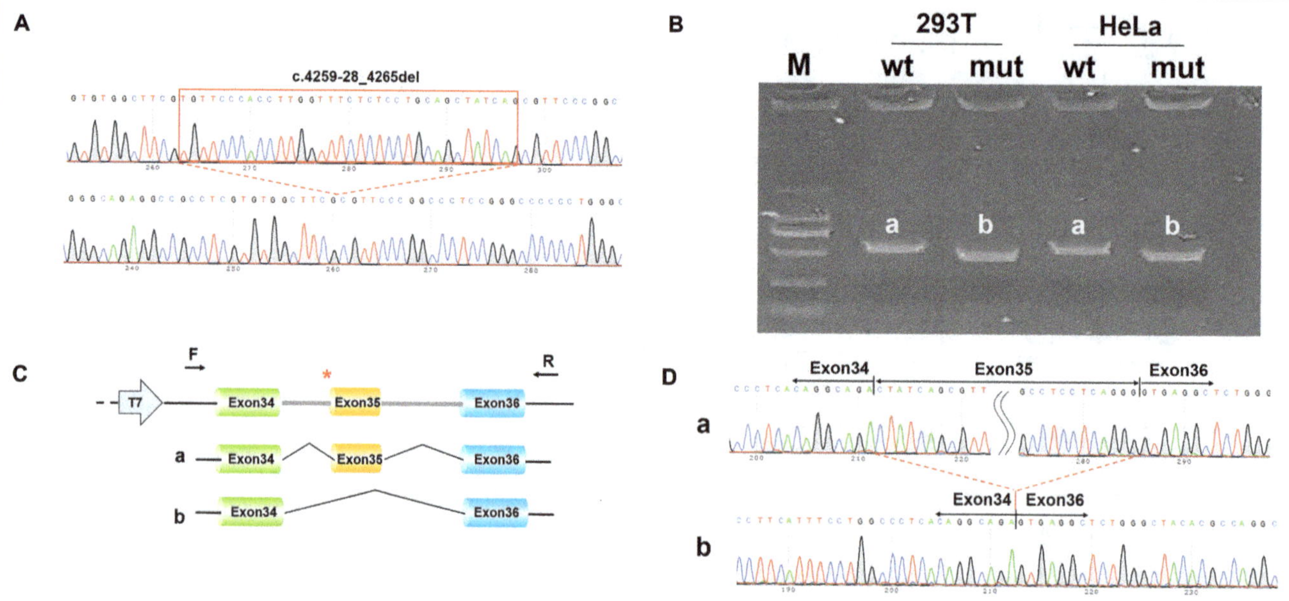

FIGURE 3 | Alternative splicing assays in minigene. **(A)** Sequencing results of pcDNA3.1-wt (wild type) fragment (top) and pcDNA3.1-mut (mutant fragment) with c.4259-28_4265del of *COL18A1* (bottom). **(B)** Gel view of reverse transcription polymerase chain reaction (RT-PCR). The size of expression of pcDNA3.1-COL18A1-wt (band a) is larger than that of pcDNA3.1-COL18A1-mut in both 293T cell and HeLa cell. **(C)** Schematic diagram of minigene construction and schematic diagram of expression. The "a" represents the normal mRNA composed of exon 34, exon 35, and exon 36, while the "b" represents the aberrant mRNA with exon 36 skipped. * indicates the mutation position. **(D)** Sequencing results of the bands in **(B)**.

In family 14518, cosegregation analysis showed that the proband and sister harbored homozygous mutation, c.4259-28_4265del, in *COL18A1*; the father harbored heterozygous mutation, while the mother and youngest brother were normal by Sanger sequencing. Since allele dropout has been ruled out by change amplify primers, it was reasonable to suspect potential heterozygous deletions involving one or more exons in a mother or independent uniparental disomy (UPD) that happened twice in this family from the father. To solve the question, RNA sequencing was performed on all five family members of 14518. By RNA sequencing, we identified a heterozygous intron inclusion event in proband II1 and his father I1 (**Figures 4A,B**). Different from *in silicon* prediction, the Acceptor splice site change variant, c.4259-28_4265del in *COL18A1*, created two splicing-in of the intronic segments of IVS34 and IVS35, leading to an an in-frame pseudoexon. Unexpectedly, another heterozygous aberrant exon deletion in proband II1 and his mother I2 was simultaneously observed (**Figures 4A,B**). The exon of exon 33 to exon 37 of *COL18A1* was skipped besides a normal transcript way. Both events were absent in II3, who is clinically normal. The results were further proved by electrophoresis (**Figure 4C**) and Sanger sequencing (**Figure 4D**). The gross deletion legitimately explained the phenotype that the mother seems normal in c.4259-28_4265del by Sanger sequencing. The proband harbored biallelic different mutants: one was c.4259-28_4265del, which was inherited from the father, and another was a gross deletion crossing exon 32 and exon 36, which was inherited from the mother. A similar situation happened in his younger sister, who also suffered from early onset high myopia and alopecia areata that appeared in the midline of the occipital regions, with encephalocele revealed by MRI when she was 3 months old. Cosegregation supported the pathogenetic biallelic mutants discovered in these families.

The ocular and systemic manifestations of the six probands are summarized in **Table 1**. Congenital cataracts were recorded in one patient (20204) with *COL18A1* mutant. In addition to the typical high myopia fundus characteristics, such as a leopard pattern, dysplasia of the papilla, and macular degeneration, characteristic fundus degeneration was noticed in all patients, including optic degeneration, chorioretinal sclerosis and atrophy, foveal hypoplasia, atrophic patch with extra bone spicule accumulation, and loss of pigmentation temporal to the macula (**Figures 1B,C,F,G,J,K,N,O**). Fluorescein angiograms exhibited vascular leakage in patient 14410 (**Figure 1C**). ERG indicates a moderate-to-severe decrease in cone and rod cells.

Skin thickening in the regions of alopecia areata was observed in all patients. Furthermore, alopecia areata appeared in the midline of the occipital regions of three patients with *COL18A1* mutations (**Figures 1A,E**). A small hole was found in the occipital bone of patient 14518 by X-ray (**Figure 1H**), while the other two had normal occipital bone. Transient leakage of liquid in the region of alopecia areata was reported by the parents of all three patients while they were infants. Normal brain images were exhibited on MRI for patient 14410 (**Figure 1D**). No extra abnormality was noticed in the other systems of all three patients. High myopia, defects in the occipital region, and *COL18A1* mutation supported a diagnosis of KNO for all three patients. For the three patients with *LAMA1* mutations, alopecia areata

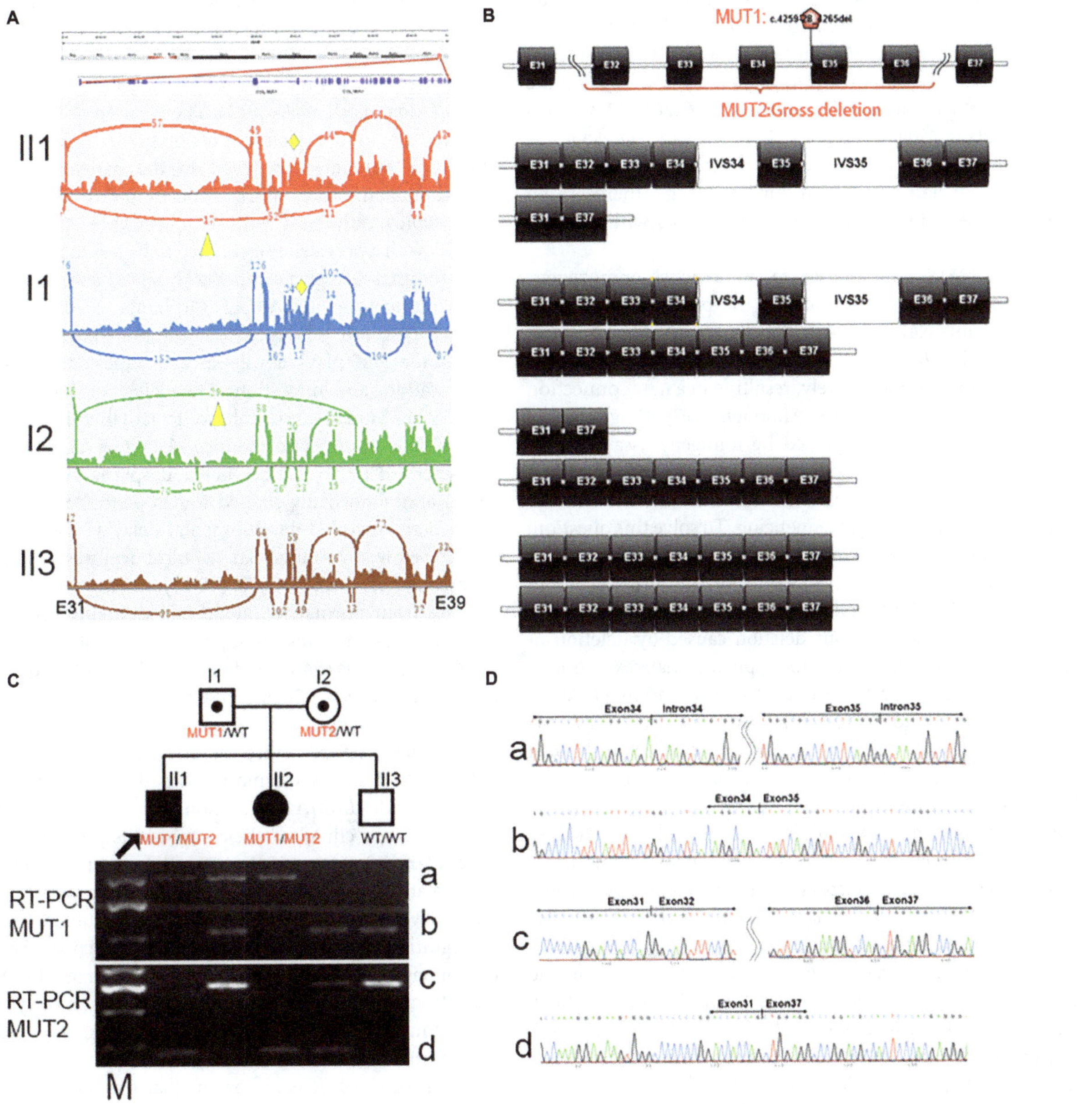

FIGURE 4 | Identification of biallelic mutants for *COL18A1* in family 14518 by RNA sequencing. **(A)** Splicing-in of the pseudoexon, IVS34 and IVS35, is observed in proband II1 and his father I1, indicated by a yellow rhombus. Gross deletion crossing Exon 32 to exon 36 is observed in proband II1 and his mother, indicated by a yellow triangle. **(B)** Schematic diagram of four different kinds of transcript way between Exon 37 to exon 37 of *COL18A1* in proband, carriers, and normal of different genotypes. **(C)** The biallelic mutants is observed in RT-PCR amplicons from family 14518. MUT1: Compare with wildtype of band b with 525bp in II3, the aberrant band a is longer (1010 bp) due to splicing-in of the IVS34 and IVS35 (485 bp). MUT2: Compare with wildtype of band c with 724 bp covering exon 31-37 in II3, the aberrant band d is shorter (192 bp) caused by deletion of exon 32 to 36 (532 bp). **(D)** The aberrant bands are confirmed by Sanger sequencing. M: DL2000 DNA Marker with a brighter fragment at 750 bp.

appeared in the midline of the parietal region (in the center of hair whorl) (**Figures 1I,M**). All parents denied observing transient leakage of liquid in the alopecia areata region. MRI examination was performed on patients 5176 and 7856, and the imaging results, including cerebellar dysplasia and obvious enlargement of the fourth ventricle, supported a diagnosis of PBS for both patients (**Figures 1L,P**). Developmental delay and ataxia were noticed in patients 7856 and 19618. An accessory ear on the left side was observed in patient 5176.

DISCUSSION

In the present study, pathogenic mutations were detected in six early onset high myopia patients with midline alopecia areata, and the causative genes included not only the *COL18A1* gene but also the *LAMA1* gene. RNA sequencing identified biallelic mutants for *COL18A1* including a variant introducing an in-frame pseudoexon, and a gross deletion missed by TES and Sanger sequencing. The patients shared characteristic fundus degeneration, although the systemic abnormalities were different, as they were caused by different genes. The scalp defect in the three patients with *COL18A1* mutations were in the occipital region, which is consistent with previous reports describing the defective area of patients with KNO caused by *COL18A1* mutants (Sertie et al., 2000; Aldahmesh et al., 2011). The scalp defect in the three patients with *LAMA1* mutations was in the parietal region (in the center of hair whorl). To our knowledge, there are no prior reports describing skull defects in humans with *LAMA1* mutations.

In family 14518, initially, we found a novel homozygous splicing change c.4259-28_4265del in the proband. The novel splice site variant (c.4259-28_4265del) is located at the 5' splice site exon 35 of *COL18A1*, and the minigene assay showed that the mutation skipped exon 35 entirely, resulting in a new connection between exon 34 and exon 36. Although the pathogenesis of the splicing change was supported by minigene assay, a fault was observed in cosegregation result, of which the proband inherited this mutant from his father, but his mother seemed normal at this point by Sanger sequencing. To solve this question, RNA sequencing was performed on all five family members of 14518 and identified biallelic abnormality transcript event in *COL18A1* including IVS34 and IVS35 inclusion caused by c.4259-28_4265del, as well as an exons deletion caused by deletion of exon 32 to exon 36. There were four splicing changes and four gross deletions recorded by Human Gene Mutation Database (HGMD) (202002) and addressed as damaged mutation (DM) (Sertie et al., 2000; Keren et al., 2007; Suzuki et al., 2009; Aldahmesh et al., 2011; Retterer et al., 2016; Turro et al., 2020); and most of them were detected by WES or whole-genome sequencing (WGS), but none of them were identified or validated at the transcript level. The novel finding highlights the utility of RNA sequencing for the detection and interpretation of variants missed by the current routine diagnostic approach and provides a basis for genetic diagnosis of KNO.

The HGMD (Professional 202002) lists 33 DMs for the *COL18A1* gene and 35 DMs for the *LAMA1* gene; of these, 88% (29/33) in *COL18A1* and 91% (32/35) in *LAMA1* were nonsense, frameshift, splice site variants, and copy number variations (CNVs), all of which were predicted to result in LOF. In our study, all night mutants we detected were LOF including three frameshifts (c.4290_4299del, c.4759_4760del, and ex.32-36 deletion) and one splice site variant (c.4259-28_4265del) in *COL18A1*, and three frameshifts (c.1487dup, 1494_1504del, and c.4171_4172del) and two non-senses (c.4579C > T and c.6151 C > T) in *LAMA1*. In this study, the *COL18A1* mutations clustered at the C terminal, and the clinical manifestations of the patients with *COL18A1* mutations primarily consist of ocular abnormalities, including high myopia, fundus degeneration, and strabismus, while the system phenotypes were mild, as alopecia areata appeared in the midline of occipital region. The mutation, c.4759_4760del (p.L1172VfsX72) in proband 20204, was one hotspot and has been detected in different patients (Suzuki et al., 2009; Joyce et al., 2010; Aldahmesh et al., 2011; Aldahmesh et al., 2013). The phenotypes of patients with the c.4759_4760del (homozygous) mutations ranged from ocular abnormality without systemic defect (Aldahmesh et al., 2011), ocular abnormality and mild occipital cutis aplasia (Aldahmesh et al., 2013), to visual problems (glaucoma, lens dislocation, and retinal and corneal dystrophy), cerebellar ataxia, and cognitive deficiency (Paisan-Ruiz et al., 2009), to epilepsy without occipital defect (Aldahmesh et al., 2013). The position of mutation cannot explain the mild systemic phenotype in our study. Similar situations were also observed in the patients with *LAMA1* mutation, and more effort is necessary to identify possible phenotypic modifiers.

PBS, with a prevalence estimated to be less than 1/1,000,000, is an autosomal recessive cerebellar dysplasia syndrome caused by biallelic mutations in *LAMA1* (Orphanet, 2020b). The LAMA1 protein (laminin α1) is major component of the basement membrane and plays a role in cell adhesion, differentiation, proliferation, and migration. The defect of *LAMA1* will lead to PBS in human and embryonic lethality in mice because of multiple brain abnormalities (Heng et al., 2011). PBS is characterized by typical cerebellar dysplasia (100%) with cysts (91%) and abnormally shaped fourth ventricle (83%). Most of the patients revealed developmental delay as the first symptom at age below 6 months. The clinical features comprise non-progressive cerebellar ataxia (100%), cognitive function defect ranging from normal to intellectual disability (88%), and eye abnormalities including myopia (67%), ocular motor apraxia (67%), strabismus (54%), and retinopathy (46%) (Aldinger et al., 2014; Micalizzi et al., 2016). Rare phenotypes were also reported including dry skin, brain malformations, hypotonia, retinal vasculopathy, severe arthrogryposis, and tics (**Supplementary Table 3**). In contrast to typical PBS patients, the three unrelated patients with *LAMA1* mutations in our study visited an ophthalmology clinic for their strabismus problems when they were infants (2, 0.5, and 0.4 years old), at which point their high myopia and characteristic fundus degeneration were discovered. Neurodevelopmental deficits, such as motor delay, speech delay, or cognition impairment were mild or negligible. The classical neuroimaging changes in PBS were confirmed by MRI after *LAMA1* mutations were detected. Children with early onset high myopia might harbor other ocular or systemic symptoms despite a full assessment due to unawareness or atypical manifestation of other major signs. It is important that further examinations be performed for children with early onset high myopia to diagnose early possible myopic syndrome.

KNO and PBS are rare and highly clinical heterozygous genetic diseases. The occipital defects of KNO can range from mildly pigmented skin spot on the back of the head to alopecia areata in our study, and encephalocele, which forms part of the classical triad of symptoms. PBS also presents with a wide range of neurodevelopmental features, including non-progressive cerebellar ataxia, intellectual disability, and ocular abnormality. Their unique neuroimaging phenotypes are the gold standard when diagnosing the conditions. Manifestations of both syndromes outside of ocular are non-specific and hence do not provide useful clues of diagnosis, especially at onset. Ideally, a simple physical examination could provide meaningful clues to suggest further examinations for myopic syndrome involving the nervous system. In our study, we collected six patients with early onset high myopia and skull defects from cutis aplasia in the cranial midline, and 100% detected causative gene defects by targeted high-throughput sequencing in all patients. Further assessments indicated that the three patients with *COL18A1* mutations had KNO, and the three patients with *LAMA1* mutations had PBS. Alopecia areata in the occipital region or parietal region of the cranial midline, as observed by simple physical examinations, combined with the ocular abnormalities of early onset high myopia and characteristic fundus degeneration, dramatically delineated the two rare myopia syndromes with nervous system involvement, KNO, and PBS. Although the results were summarized from six unrelated families, the power of the association between the two manifestations and the two syndromes should be further evaluated in a larger cohort. The defects of the scalp could be considered as an early diagnostic clue of KNO or PBS for ophthalmologists when treating children with high myopia and alopecia areata in the cranial midline at eye clinics. Further function study is needed to clarify the pathogenesis between *LAMA1* mutation and alopecia areata in the occipital region or parietal region of the cranial midline.

ETHICS STATEMENT

The studies involving human participants were reviewed and approved by the Institutional Review Board of the Zhongshan Ophthalmic Center. Written informed consent to participate in this study was provided by the participants' legal guardian/next of kin.

AUTHOR CONTRIBUTIONS

PFW participated in the entire process of research, data analysis, and wrote the first draft of the manuscript. XYJ, SQL, and XSX contributed to data collection and implementation of the research. YXL, MCL, YYL, JL, and YX performed the experimental process. QJZ guided the entire process in terms of theory and practice and revised the manuscript. All authors contributed to the article and approved the submitted version.

ACKNOWLEDGMENTS

We thank all probands and their available family members for their participation. A part of this work was presented as an abstract to the Association for Research in Vision and Ophthalmology 2019.

REFERENCES

Abouelhoda, M., Sobahy, T., El-Kalioby, M., Patel, N., Shamseldin, H., Monies, D., et al. (2016). Clinical genomics can facilitate countrywide estimation of autosomal recessive disease burden. *Genet. Med* 18, 1244–1249. doi: 10.1038/gim.2016.37

Ackerman, C., Locke, A. E., Feingold, E., Reshey, B., Espana, K., Thusberg, J., et al. (2012). An excess of deleterious variants in VEGF-A pathway genes in Down-syndrome-associated atrioventricular septal defects. *Am. J. Hum. Genet.* 91, 646–659. doi: 10.1016/j.ajhg.2012.08.017

Aikio, M., Hurskainen, M., Brideau, G., Hagg, P., Sormunen, R., Heljasvaara, R., et al. (2013). Collagen XVIII short isoform is critical for retinal vascularization, and overexpression of the Tsp-1 domain affects eye growth and cataract formation. *Invest. Ophthalmol. Vis. Sci.* 54, 7450–7462. doi: 10.1167/iovs.13-13039

Aldahmesh, M. A., Khan, A. O., Mohamed, J. Y., Alkuraya, H., Ahmed, H., Bobis, S., et al. (2011). Identification of ADAMTS18 as a gene mutated in Knobloch syndrome. *J. Med. Genet.* 48, 597–601. doi: 10.1136/jmedgenet-2011-100306

Aldahmesh, M. A., Khan, A. O., Mohamed, J. Y., Levin, A. V., Wuthisiri, W., Lynch, S., et al. (2013). No evidence for locus heterogeneity in Knobloch syndrome. *J. Med. Genet.* 50, 565–566. doi: 10.1136/jmedgenet-2013-101755

Aldinger, K. A., Mosca, S. J., Tetreault, M., Dempsey, J. C., Ishak, G. E., Hartley, T., et al. (2014). Mutations in LAMA1 cause cerebellar dysplasia and cysts with and without retinal dystrophy. *Am. J. Hum. Genet.* 95, 227–234. doi: 10.1016/j.ajhg.2014.07.007

Balikova, I., Sanak, N. S., Fanny, D., Smits, G., Soblet, J., De Baere, E., et al. (2020). Three cases of molecularly confirmed Knobloch syndrome. *Ophthalmic Genet.* 41, 83–87. doi: 10.1080/13816810.2020.1737948

Banerjee, S., Isaacman-Beck, J., Schneider, V. A., and Granato, M. (2013). A novel role for Lh3 dependent ECM modifications during neural crest cell migration in zebrafish. *PLoS One* 8:e54609. doi: 10.1371/journal.pone.0054609

Bartsch, O., Labonte, J., Albrecht, B., Wieczorek, D., Lechno, S., Zechner, U., et al. (2010). Two patients with EP300 mutations and facial dysmorphism different from the classic Rubinstein-Taybi syndrome. *Am. J. Med. Genet. A* 152A, 181–184. doi: 10.1002/ajmg.a.33153

Cornwell, M., Vangala, M., Taing, L., Herbert, Z., Koster, J., Li, B., et al. (2018). VIPER: visualization pipeline for RNA-seq, a snakemake workflow for efficient and complete RNA-seq analysis. *BMC Bioinformatics* 19:135. doi: 10.1186/s12859-018-2139-9

den Dunnen, J. T., and Antonarakis, S. E. (2000). Mutation nomenclature extensions and suggestions to describe complex mutations: a discussion. *Hum. Mutat.* 15, 7–12. doi: 10.1002/(SICI)1098-1004(200001)15:1<7::AID-HUMU4<3.0.CO;2-N

Doyle, A. J., Doyle, J. J., Bessling, S. L., Maragh, S., Lindsay, M. E., Schepers, D., et al. (2012). Mutations in the TGF-beta repressor SKI cause Shprintzen-Goldberg syndrome with aortic aneurysm. *Nat. Genet.* 44, 1249–1254. doi: 10.1038/ng.2421

Hamamy, H. A., Teebi, A. S., Oudjhane, K., Shegem, N. N., and Ajlouni, K. M. (2007). Severe hypertelorism, midface prominence, prominent/simple ears, severe myopia, borderline intelligence, and bone fragility in two brothers: new syndrome? *Am. J. Med. Genet. A* 143A, 229–234. doi: 10.1002/ajmg.a.31594

Heng, C., Lefebvre, O., Klein, A., Edwards, M. M., Simon-Assmann, P., Orend, G., et al. (2011). Functional role of laminin alpha1 chain during cerebellum development. *Cell Adh. Migr.* 5, 480–489. doi: 10.4161/cam.5.6.19191

Hoyer, J., Ekici, A. B., Endele, S., Popp, B., Zweier, C., Wiesener, A., et al. (2012). Haploinsufficiency of ARID1B, a member of the SWI/SNF-a chromatin-remodeling complex, is a frequent cause of intellectual disability. *Am. J. Hum. Genet.* 90, 565–572. doi: 10.1016/j.ajhg.2012.02.007

Hull, S., Arno, G., Ku, C. A., Ge, Z., Waseem, N., Chandra, A., et al. (2016). Molecular and clinical findings in patients with knobloch syndrome. *JAMA Ophthalmol.* 134, 753–762. doi: 10.1001/jamaophthalmol.2016.1073

James, A. W., Miranda, S. G., Culver, K., Hall, B. D., and Golabi, M. (2007). DOOR syndrome: clinical report, literature review and discussion of natural history. *Am. J. Med. Genet. A* 143A, 2821–2831. doi: 10.1002/ajmg.a.32054

Joyce, S., Tee, L., Abid, A., Khaliq, S., Mehdi, S. Q., and Maher, E. R. (2010). Locus heterogeneity and Knobloch syndrome. *Am. J. Med. Genet. A* 152A, 2880–2881. doi: 10.1002/ajmg.a.33619

Kantarci, S., Al-Gazali, L., Hill, R. S., Donnai, D., Black, G. C., Bieth, E., et al. (2007). Mutations in LRP2, which encodes the multiligand receptor megalin, cause Donnai-Barrow and facio-oculo-acoustico-renal syndromes. *Nat. Genet.* 39, 957–959. doi: 10.1038/ng2063

Keren, B., Suzuki, O. T., Gerard-Blanluet, M., Bremond-Gignac, D., Elmaleh, M., Titomanlio, L., et al. (2007). CNS malformations in Knobloch syndrome with splice mutation in COL18A1 gene. *Am. J. Med. Genet. A* 143A, 1514–1518. doi: 10.1002/ajmg.a.31784

Kliemann, S. E., Waetge, R. T., Suzuki, O. T., Passos-Bueno, M. R., and Rosemberg, S. (2003). Evidence of neuronal migration disorders in Knobloch syndrome: clinical and molecular analysis of two novel families. *Am. J. Med. Genet. A* 119A, 15–19. doi: 10.1002/ajmg.a.20070

Li, J., Gao, B., Guan, L., Xiao, X., Zhang, J., Li, S., et al. (2015). Unique variants in OPN1LW cause both syndromic and nonsyndromic X-linked high myopia mapped to MYP1. *Invest. Ophthalmol. Vis. Sci.* 56, 4150–4155. doi: 10.1167/iovs.14-16356

Mahajan, V. B., Olney, A. H., Garrett, P., Chary, A., Dragan, E., Lerner, G., et al. (2010). Collagen XVIII mutation in Knobloch syndrome with acute lymphoblastic leukemia. *Am. J. Med. Genet. A* 152A, 2875–2879. doi: 10.1002/ajmg.a.33621

Marmor, M. F., Arden, G. B., Nilsson, S. E. G., and Zrenner, E. (1989). Standard for clinical electroretinography. International Standardization Committee. *Arch. Ophthalmol.* 107, 816–819. doi: 10.1001/archopht.1989.01070010838024

Micalizzi, A., Poretti, A., Romani, M., Ginevrino, M., Mazza, T., Aiello, C., et al. (2016). Clinical, neuroradiological and molecular characterization of cerebellar dysplasia with cysts (Poretti-Boltshauser syndrome). *Eur. J. Hum. Genet.* 24, 1262–1267. doi: 10.1038/ejhg.2016.19

Orphanet (2020a). Available online at: https://www.orpha.net/consor/cgi-bin/Disease_Search.php?lng=EN&data_id=1722&Disease_Disease_Search_diseaseGroup=Knobloch-syndrome&Disease_Disease_Search_diseaseType=Pat&Disease(s)/group%20of%20diseases=Knobloch-syndrome&title=Knobloch%20syndrome&search=Disease_Search_Simple (accessed Dec 22, 2020).

Orphanet (2020b). Available online at: https://www.orpha.net/consor/cgi-bin/Disease_Search.php?lng=EN&data_id=22466&Disease_Disease_Search_diseaseGroup=Poretti-Boltshauser-syndrome&Disease_Disease_Search_diseaseType=Pat&Disease(s)/group%20of%20diseases=Ataxia-intellectual-disability-oculomotor-apraxia-cerebellar-cysts-syndrome&title=Ataxia-intellectual%20disability-oculomotor%20apraxia-cerebellar%20cysts%20syndrome&search=Disease_Search_Simple (accessed Dec 22, 2020).

Paisan-Ruiz, C., Scopes, G., Lee, P., and Houlden, H. (2009). Homozygosity mapping through whole genome analysis identifies a COL18A1 mutation in an Indian family presenting with an autosomal recessive neurological disorder. *Am. J. Med. Genet. B Neuropsychiatr. Genet.* 150B, 993–997. doi: 10.1002/ajmg.b.30929

Passos-Bueno, M. R., Marie, S. K., Monteiro, M., Neustein, I., Whittle, M. R., Vainzof, M., et al. (1994). Knobloch syndrome in a large Brazilian consanguineous family: confirmation of autosomal recessive inheritance. *Am. J. Med. Genet.* 52, 170–173. doi: 10.1002/ajmg.1320520209

Retterer, K., Juusola, J., Cho, M. T., Vitazka, P., Millan, F., Gibellini, F., et al. (2016). Clinical application of whole-exome sequencing across clinical indications. *Genet. Med.* 18, 696–704. doi: 10.1038/gim.2015.148

Richards, S., Aziz, N., Bale, S., Bick, D., Das, S., Gastier-Foster, J., et al. (2015). Standards and guidelines for the interpretation of sequence variants: a joint consensus recommendation of the American College of Medical Genetics and Genomics and the Association for Molecular Pathology. *Genet. Med.* 17, 405–424. doi: 10.1038/gim.2015.30

Schuurs-Hoeijmakers, J. H., Oh, E. C., Vissers, L. E., Swinkels, M. E., Gilissen, C., Willemsen, M. A., et al. (2012). Recurrent de novo mutations in PACS1 cause defective cranial-neural-crest migration and define a recognizable intellectual-disability syndrome. *Am. J. Hum. Genet.* 91, 1122–1127. doi: 10.1016/j.ajhg.2012.10.013

Sertie, A. L., Sossi, V., Camargo, A. A., Zatz, M., Brahe, C., and Passos-Bueno, M. R. (2000). Collagen XVIII, containing an endogenous inhibitor of angiogenesis and tumor growth, plays a critical role in the maintenance of retinal structure and in neural tube closure (Knobloch syndrome). *Hum. Mol. Genet.* 9, 2051–2058. doi: 10.1093/hmg/9.13.2051

Suzuki, O., Kague, E., Bagatini, K., Tu, H., Heljasvaara, R., Carvalhaes, L., et al. (2009). Novel pathogenic mutations and skin biopsy analysis in Knobloch syndrome. *Mol. Vis.* 15, 801–809.

Thorvaldsdottir, H., Robinson, J. T., and Mesirov, J. P. (2013). Integrative Genomics Viewer (IGV): high-performance genomics data visualization and exploration. *Brief. Bioinform.* 14, 178–192. doi: 10.1093/bib/bbs017

Turro, E., Astle, W. J., Megy, K., Graf, S., Greene, D., Shamardina, O., et al. (2020). Whole-genome sequencing of patients with rare diseases in a national health system. *Nature* 583, 96–102. doi: 10.1038/s41586-020-2434-2

Vuillaumier-Barrot, S., Bouchet-Seraphin, C., Chelbi, M., Devisme, L., Quentin, S., Gazal, S., et al. (2012). Identification of mutations in TMEM5 and ISPD as a cause of severe cobblestone lissencephaly. *Am. J. Hum. Genet.* 91, 1135–1143. doi: 10.1016/j.ajhg.2012.10.009

Wang, P., Li, S., Sun, W., Xiao, X., Jia, X., Liu, M., et al. (2019). An ophthalmic targeted exome sequencing panel as a powerful tool to identify causative mutations in patients suspected of hereditary eye diseases. *Transl. Vis. Sci. Technol.* 8:21. doi: 10.1167/tvst.8.2.21

Whalen, S., Heron, D., Gaillon, T., Moldovan, O., Rossi, M., Devillard, F., et al. (2012). Novel comprehensive diagnostic strategy in Pitt-Hopkins syndrome: clinical score and further delineation of the TCF4 mutational spectrum. *Hum. Mutat.* 33, 64–72. doi: 10.1002/humu.21639

Williams, T. A., Kirkby, G. R., Williams, D., and Ainsworth, J. R. (2008). A phenotypic variant of Knobloch syndrome. *Ophthalmic Genet.* 29, 85–86. doi: 10.1080/13816810701850041

Zahrani, F., Aldahmesh, M. A., Alshammari, M. J., Al-Hazzaa, S. A., and Alkuraya, F. S. (2013). Mutations in c12orf57 cause a syndromic form of colobomatous microphthalmia. *Am. J. Hum. Genet.* 92, 387–391. doi: 10.1016/j.ajhg.2013.01.008

11

Autosomal Recessive Rod-Cone Dystrophy Associated with Compound Heterozygous Variants in *ARL3* Gene

Leming Fu [1], Ya Li [2], Shun Yao [2], Qingge Guo [2], Ya You [2], Xianjun Zhu [3] and Bo Lei [1,2]*

[1] Henan University People's Hospital, Henan Provincial People's Hospital, Zhengzhou, China, [2] Henan Branch of National Clinical Research Center for Ocular Diseases, Henan Eye Institute/Henan Eye Hospital, People's Hospital of Zhengzhou University, Henan Provincial People's Hospital, Zhengzhou, China, [3] Department of Laboratory Medicine, Sichuan Provincial People's Hospital, School of Medicine, University of Electronic Science and Technology of China, Chengdu, China

***Correspondence:**
Bo Lei
bolei99@126.com*

Purpose: *ARL3* (ADP-ribosylation factor-like 3) variants cause autosomal dominant retinitis pigmentosa (RP) or autosomal recessive Joubert syndrome. We found a family with rod-cone dystrophy (RCD) and verified it was associated with compound heterozygous variants in *ARL3* gene.

Methods: Ophthalmic examinations including optical coherence tomography and electroretinogram (ERG) were performed. Targeted next generation sequencing (NGS) was performed for the proband using a custom designed panel. Sanger sequencing and co-segregation were conducted in the family members. Changes of protein structure mediated by the variants were studied *in vitro*. ARL3 protein stability and its interaction with RP2 protein were assessed by cycloheximide chase assay and co-immunoprecipitation (Co-IP) assay.

Results: Visual acuity of the 18-year-old male proband was 0.25 in the right and 0.20 in the left eye, while his non-consanguineous parents and sister was normal. The proband showed signs of RCD, including nyctalopia, peripheral field loss, bone-spicule deposits in the retina, and reduced ERG responses. The father, aged 50 years old, showed visual acuity of 1.0 in both eyes. Unlike the proband, he presented late onset and mild cone-rod dystrophy (CRD), including macular atrophy, central scotomata, moderate reduction in photopic ERG responses. None of all the family members had hearing abnormality, mental dysplasia or gait instability. We identified two novel compound heterozygous variants (c.91A>G, p.T31A; c.353G>T, p.C118F) in *ARL3* in the proband, while his father only had variant c.91A>G. Bioinformatics analysis indicated amino acid positions of the two variants are highly conserved among species. The *in silico* tools predicted the variants to be harmful. Protein structure analysis showed the two variants had potential to alter the protein structure. Based on the ACMG guidelines, the two variants were likely pathogenic. In addition, the *ARL3* mutations destabilized ARL3 protein, and the mutation c.353G>T disrupted the interaction between ARL3 and RP2 in HEK293T cells.

Conclusions: We showed novel compound heterozygous variants in *ARL3* were associated with early onset of autosomal recessive RCD, while c.91A>G along may be associated with a late onset of dominant CRD. The two variants in *ARL3* could be causative by destabilizing ARL3 protein and impairing its interaction with RP2 protein.

Keywords: ***ARL3*, compound heterozygous variants, rod-cone dystrophy, cone-rod dystrophy, RP2**

INTRODUCTION

Retinitis pigmentosa (RP) is a group of highly heterogeneous inherited retinal diseases, and it is one of the most important causes of blindness worldwide (Narayan et al., 2016). Almost 2.5 million individuals suffered with RP around the world (Hu et al., 2019). RP is typically characterized by night blindness (nyctalopia), progressive constriction of visual field, changes in the fundus and reduced electroretinogram (ERG), and ultimately resulting in complete blindness (Ali et al., 2017). Rod-cone dystrophy (RCD) is a common form of RP due to primary degeneration of rod cells followed by degeneration of cone cells (Pagon, 1988). RP manifests in a syndromic or a non-syndromic form. Non-syndromic RP can be in different traits, including autosomal dominant RP (adRP), autosomal recessive RP (arRP), X-linked recessive form and simplex/sporadic type. Nowadays, around 90 genes were identified to be associated with non-syndromic RP (https://sph.uth.tmc.edu/retnet/). The proteins encoded by RP-associated genes exert different roles in transcription, retina phototransduction, transport processes via the photoreceptor connecting cilium, cell growth, cellular structure, and metabolism of vitamin A (Collin et al., 2011; Bhatia et al., 2019).

Human *ARL3* (ADP-ribosylation factor-like 3; MIM:604695) gene is mapped to chromosome 10q24.32, and contains 6 exons. The encoded protein ARL3 is a small molecule GTP-binding protein belonging to the ADP-ribosylation factor (ARF) family. In the mammalian retina, ARL3 is mainly localized to microtubule structures throughout the retina and is enriched in the connecting cilium of rod and cone photoreceptors (Grayson et al., 2002). ARL3 is crucial for ciliogenesis and axoneme formation, as well as cargo displacement of lipidated proteins in the cilium (Hanke-Gogokhia et al., 2016). Besides, ARL3 also acts as an allosteric factor for the release of lipidated proteins bound to PDE6D (delta subunit of phosphodiesterase) and UNC119A/B in an apparent GTP dependent manner (Hanke-Gogokhia et al., 2018). The activity of ARL3 is regulated by a GTP-exchange factor ARL13B (ADP-ribosylation factor-like protein 13B) (Gotthardt et al., 2015) and a GTPase-activating protein RP2 (Retinitis Pigmentosa 2) (Veltel et al., 2008).

A missense variant in *ARL3* (NM_004311.3) (c.269A>G, p.Tyr90Cys) has previously been reported as a possible cause of non-syndromic autosomal dominant RP in two families (Strom et al., 2016; Holtan et al., 2019). In addition, homozygocity for two different *ARL3* Arg149 missense variants (c.445C>T, p.Arg149Cys; c.446G>A, p.Arg149His) were reported to cause Joubert syndrome (Alkanderi et al., 2018). A most recent report indicated that a homozygous variant in *ARL3* (c.296G>T, p. Arg99Ile) caused cone-rod dystrophy (CRD) in two consanguineous families (Sheikh et al., 2019). In this study, we found a Chinese family with typical rod-cone dystrophy (RCD), which was associated with novel compound heterozygous variants in *ARL3*. In addition, we presumed that one of the variants might be associated with a late onset of dominant CRD. This study expanded both the phenotype and genotype of *ARL3* associated retinal dystrophy. Furthermore, our data suggested that the pathogenicity of the variants were related with destabilizing of ARL3 protein, as well as impairing its interaction with RP2, another protein that is associated with RP.

MATERIALS AND METHODS

Subjects and Clinical Assessment

The study was performed in accordance with the Declaration of Helsinki and approved by the Ethics Committee of Henan Eye Hospital for the release of clinical information, family history, and blood extraction for genetic testing [IRB approval number: HNEECKY-2019 (15)]. Written informed consent was obtained from all participants after the study risks and benefits were thoroughly explained.

All the members were enquired about the family and medical history. Each member was accepted a complete ocular examination, including best corrected visual acuity (BCVA), intraocular pressure (IOP), slit-lamp biomicroscopy, color vision, fundus photography, visual field, swept-source optical coherence tomography (SS-OCT, VG200D SVision Imaging, China), and full-field electroretinogram (ERG).

Targeted Gene Sequencing and Data Analysis

Genomic DNA was extracted from peripheral blood of all family members with the TIANGEN Blood DNA Kit (DP304, TIANGEN, China). Targeted next generation sequencing (NGS) was performed for the proband using a custom designed panel (PS400) containing 376 known genes associated with inherited retinal diseases (Zhu et al., 2021). The Nextseq 500 (Illumina, San Diego, CA, USA) platform was used for paired-end sequencing with read lengths of 150 bp and average sequencing depth of almost 300 X. Raw reads were mapped to the human genome reference (UCSC hg19) using three commercial software including XYGeneRanger 2.0 (Xunyin, Shanghai, China), TGex (LifeMap Sciences, Alameda, CA, USA) and Efficient Genosome Intepration System, EGIS (SierraVast Bio-Medical Technology Co., Ltd, Shanghai, China). Variant-filtering was based on public and in-house SNP databases, including 1000Genome project, HGMD, ExAC and ClinVar, as well as our internal database.

The non-synonymous and splicing variants with MAF < 2% were kept for further analysis. Sanger sequencing and co-segregation analysis were performed for the verification of suspicious disease-relevant gene variants in the available family members. Primer sequences and PCR conditions were shown in **Supplementary Tables 1, 2**, respectively.

In silico Molecular Genetic Analysis and Bioinformatics Analysis

To assess the possible pathogenicity of these mutations, and to predict whether a protein sequence variation affected protein function, the following web applications was used: LRT (Likelihood Ratio Test), PolyPhen-2 (Polymorphism Phenotyping v2), Mutation Taster (Schwarz et al., 2010), SIFT (Sorting Intolerant From Tolerant) (Kumar et al., 2009), FATHMM (Functional Analysis Through Hidden Markov Models) (Rogers et al., 2018), and CADD (Combined Annotation Dependent Depletion) (Kircher et al., 2014). Multiple protein sequence alignment among various species was carried out by Clustal Omega (Sievers and Higgins, 2018). The tertiary structure of protein was predicted by the Swiss-Model workspace (http://swissmodel.expasy.org) (Biasini et al., 2014). CDD online software (https://www.ncbi.nlm.nih.gov/Structure/cdd/wrpsb.cgi) was used to conduct domains analysis. HOPE online software (http://www.cmbi.umcn.nl/hope) was used to analyze the structural effects of mutation. Superimposition of homology models of ARL3 was constructed using PyMOL software (https://pymol.org/2/). The protein stability of *ARL3* mutations was predicted with the online tools MUpro (http://mupro.proteomics.ics.uci.edu/) (Cheng et al., 2006)and I-Mutant v2.0 (http://folding.biofold.org/i-mutant/i-mutant2.0) (Capriotti et al., 2005). All the sources were provided in the public domain.

Cell Culture

HEK293T cell line was purchased from American Type Culture Collection. Cells were cultured in DMEM/HIGH GLUCOSE medium (SH30022.01, Hyclone, USA) containing 10% fetal bovine serum (35-081-CV, Corning, USA) with 100 units/mL penicillin and 100 µg/mL streptomycin at 37°C with 5% CO_2.

Plasmids and Transfection

The wild-type, c.91 A>G (p.T31A), and c.353G>T (p.C118F) CDS sequences of the *ARL3* gene with the Flag tag at the C-terminal were synthesized and subcloned into the pcDNA3.1 (+) expression vector (Invitrogen, USA), respectively. The wild-type *RP2* cDNA with the HA tag at the N-terminal was subcloned into the pcDNA3.1 (+) expression vector. All plasmids were confirmed by DNA sequencing and WB analysis. When cells grow to 80–90% confluence, cell transfection was performed using Lipofectamine 3000 (L3000015, Invitrogen, USA). After transfection, the cells were harvested at 24 h for protein extraction and further analysis.

Western Blots and Antibodies

The primary antibodies used were as follows: the flag antibody (147935, CST, USA), β-actin antibody (200068-8F10, ZENBIO, China), RP2 antibody (ab174840, Abcam, UK). Cells were lysed by RIPA lysis buffer (PC101, EpiZyme, China) with 1% protease inhibitor cocktail (GRF101, EpiZyme, China). The samples were resolved in 12% SDS-PAGE gel and transferred to a polyvinylidene difluoride (PVDF) membrane (IPVH00010, MILLIPORE, Ireland). The membranes were blocked with 5% non-fat dry milk for 1 h and then incubated with the primary antibody overnight at 4°C. After three washes with TBST (containing 1% Tween-20), the membranes were treated with horseradish peroxidase-conjugated secondary antibody at room temperature for 2 h. Then the membranes were exposed to X-ray film after washed for three times.

Protein Stability Assay

Protein stability was assessed by cycloheximide chase assay. Cycloheximide (CHX, 66-81-9, Selleck, USA), a protein synthesis inhibitor, was used. HEK293T cells were transfected with empty vector, wild-type, T31A and C118F mutation *ARL3* vectors for 24 h. The cells were subsequently treated with 100 µg/ml CHX for 1, 3, and 6 h, respectively. The total protein was extracted for Western blot. Wild-type and mutant ARL3 protein levels were detected using flag antibody. The protein levels of β-actin were the endogenous control.

Co-immunoprecipitation (Co-IP) Assay

HEK293T cells were co-transfected with 6.25 µg of HA-RP2-WT plasmid and 6.25 µg of either wild-type or mutant Flag-ARL3 plasmids, and harvested for protein extraction after 24 h. Total protein lysate was extracted by immunoprecipitation buffer (BL509A, Biosharp, China), and the concentration of the supernatants was quantified with a BCA protein assay kit (P0011, Beyotime, China). Total proteins of 300 µg were added with 5× SDS to prepare as the input sample. Total proteins of 500 µg were mixed with 10 µg anti-Flag magnetic beads (HY-K0207, MCE, USA) and shaken for 4 h at 4°C on rotor. The beads were collected by Magnetic Separator and washed three times by immunoprecipitation buffer with 1% protease inhibitor. The beads were mixed with sample loading buffer (1×) and boiled for 10 min. The supernatant was collected and used for western blot analysis.

Statistical Analysis

We normalized the data from each group by dividing the measurement of the tested variant from that of the references. The value of the control was set to one and tested measurement was adjusted accordingly. GraphPad Prism 8.0 was used for the statistical analysis. Student's *t*-test and one-way analysis of variance (ANOVA) were performed with a 95% confidence level to evaluate the differences. *P*-value < 0.05 was considered statistically significant. All quantitative data were displayed as mean ± standard deviation (SD).

RESULTS

Clinical Features

We found a Chinese family with RCD, the pedigree was presented in **Figure 1A**. In this family, the proband showed typical RCD but his father present with a late onset and mild CRD, while

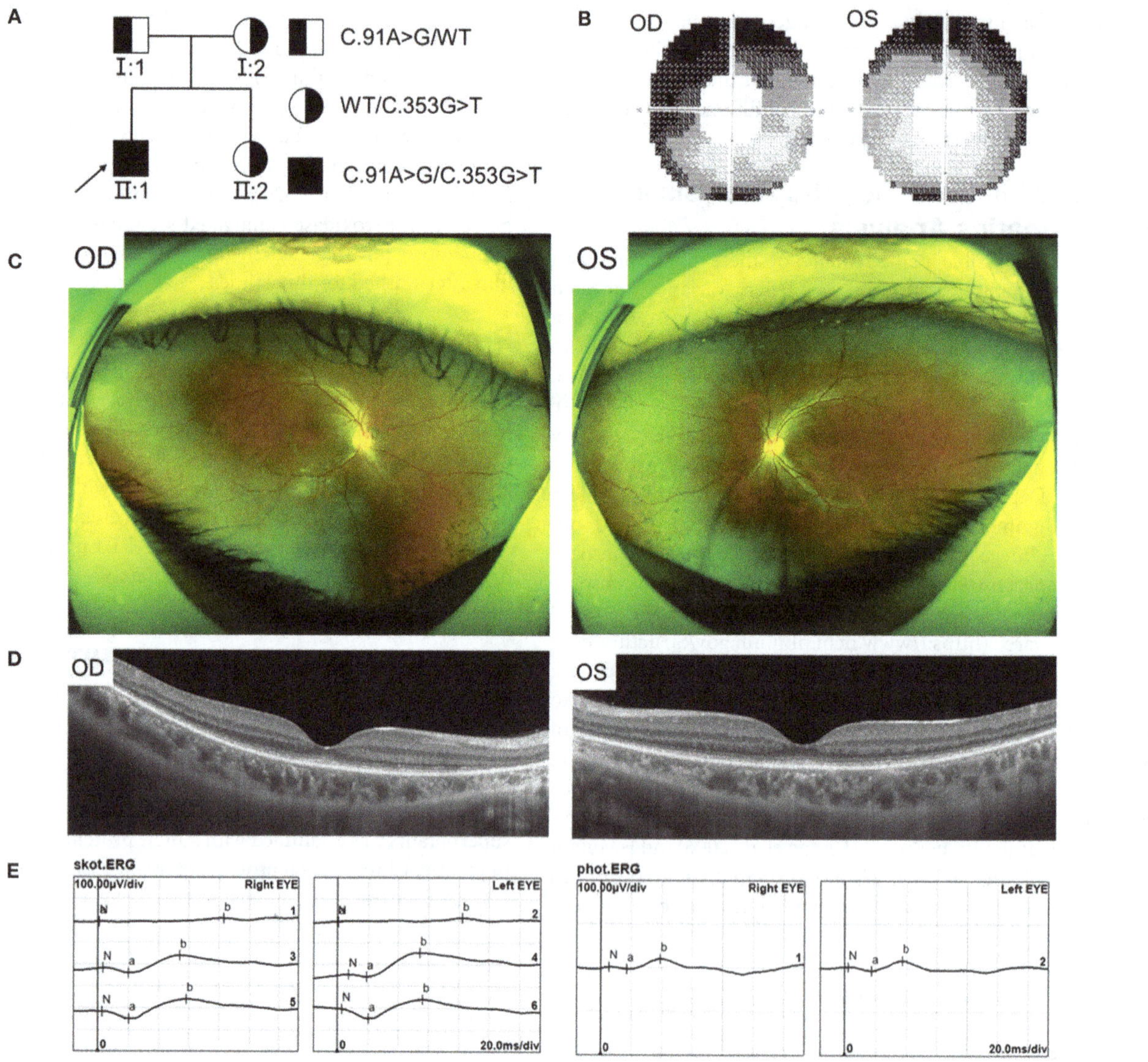

FIGURE 1 | Pedigree and Clinical features of the proband with RCD. **(A)** Pedigree of the family with autosomal recessive RCD. **(B)** Visual field showed tunnel vision. **(C)** Fundus photographs showed peripheral bone spicule pigmentation. **(D)** SS-OCT showed atrophy of the retinal outer layers of the binocular macular area. **(E)** ERG showed severe reduced rod responses and to less extent cone responses.

the mother and sister were unaffected. The proband, a 19-year-old male, had decrease of vision and nyctalopia for 4 years. The BCVA was 0.25 in the right and 0.20 in the left eye. The proband also had dyserythrochloropsia. Visual field testing revealed tunnel visual field (**Figure 1B**). Fundus photography showed peripheral bone spicule pigmentation (**Figure 1C**). SS-OCT presented atrophy of the retinal outer layers of the binocular macular area where the light reflection signal of ellipsoid zone and chimeric zone was weakened, coarse and interrupted. The reflection of RPE/Bruch membrane was rough (**Figure 1D**). ERG showed severe reduction in scotopic ERG responses and to a less extent in photopic ERG responses (**Figure 1E**).

The father, aged 50 years old, showed normal visual acuity of 1.0 in both eyes and had mild dyserythrochloropsia. Unlike the proband, the father's vision field appeared as central scotoma (**Figure 2A**). Fundus examination revealed circular degeneration around macular fovea without pigmentation of the peripheral retina (**Figure 2B**). SS-OCT revealed the binocular outer retinal layers of the macular area was thinned with macular sparing, and the light reflection signal of the ellipsoid zone in the parafovea was weakened and discontinuous (**Figure 2C**). The ERG showed a moderate decrease in the binocular cone and rod systems (**Figure 2D**).

Other examinations including anterior segment and IOP of the proband and his father were normal. Neither the proband's mother nor sister showed any abnormalities in the eyes. None of all the family members, including the proband, presented hearing abnormality, mental dysplasia, or gait instability.

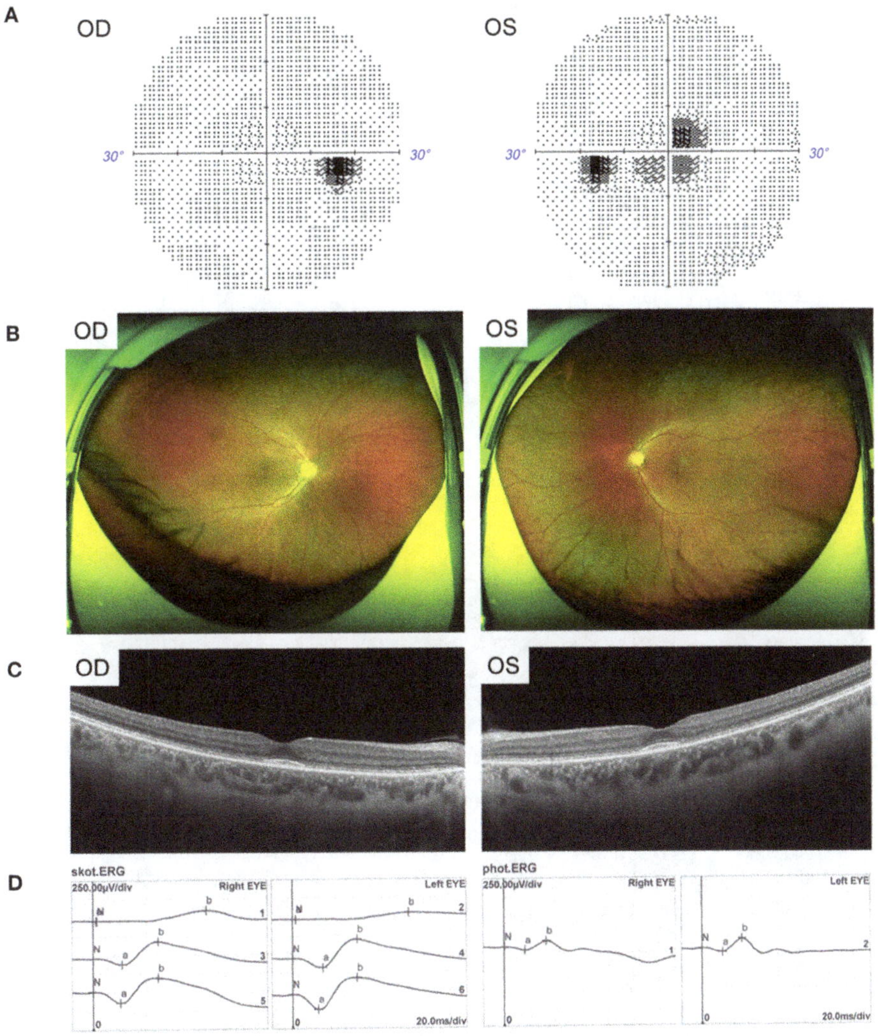

FIGURE 2 | Clinical features of the father with CRD. **(A)** Visual field showed central scotoma. **(B)** Fundus photographs showed circular degeneration around macular fovea. **(C)** SS-OCT revealed the binocular macular area outer retinal was thinned by atrophy. **(D)** ERG showed a moderate decrease in the binocular cone and rod systems.

Two Novel Missense Variants in *ARL3* Were Identified

Targeted NGS identified two novel compound heterozygous variants (c.91A>G, p.T31A; c.353G>T, p.C118F) in *ARL3* in the proband. Sanger sequencing of *ARL3* revealed segregation of the two variants with the RCD phenotype in participating individuals (**Figure 3A**). Neither variant had been reported in the human gene mutation database (HGMD). The reported allele frequency for c.353G>T (p.C118F) was concentrated in the East Asian populations almost 0.0010 in the Genome Aggregation Database (GnomAD), while no record for the c.91A>G (p.T31A) mutation was found. Furthermore, c.353G>T (p.C118F) has not been reported homozygous in GnomAD. Multiple alignments of amino acid sequences of ARL3 protein from different species revealed that Thr31 is evolutionally conserved among species, while Cys118 is only conserved in mammals, but not in zebrafish and yeast (**Figure 3B**). Moreover, both of the variants T31A and C118F were considered "Deleterious" as predicted by LRT, Mutation Taster, SIFT, FATHMM, and CADD, but Polyphen-2 predicted the pathogenicity for the variant C118F benign (**Table 1**).

In addition, other variants in the proband were screened out, including two heterozygous missense variants (c.13491T>A, p.F4497L; c.11197A>G, p.N3733D) in *USH2A* and a heterozygous missense variant (c.2432T>C, p.I811T) in *FBN2* (**Supplementary Table 3**), all of which were inherited from his mother (**Supplementary Figure 1**). These two mutations in *USH2A* were cis-mutations, and the results predicted by *in silico* prediction such as SIFT, Polyphen-2, Mutation Taster, and CADD indicated that these two missense mutations might be benign. Moreover, neither the proband nor his mother showed sensorineural deafness. On the other hand, we noticed

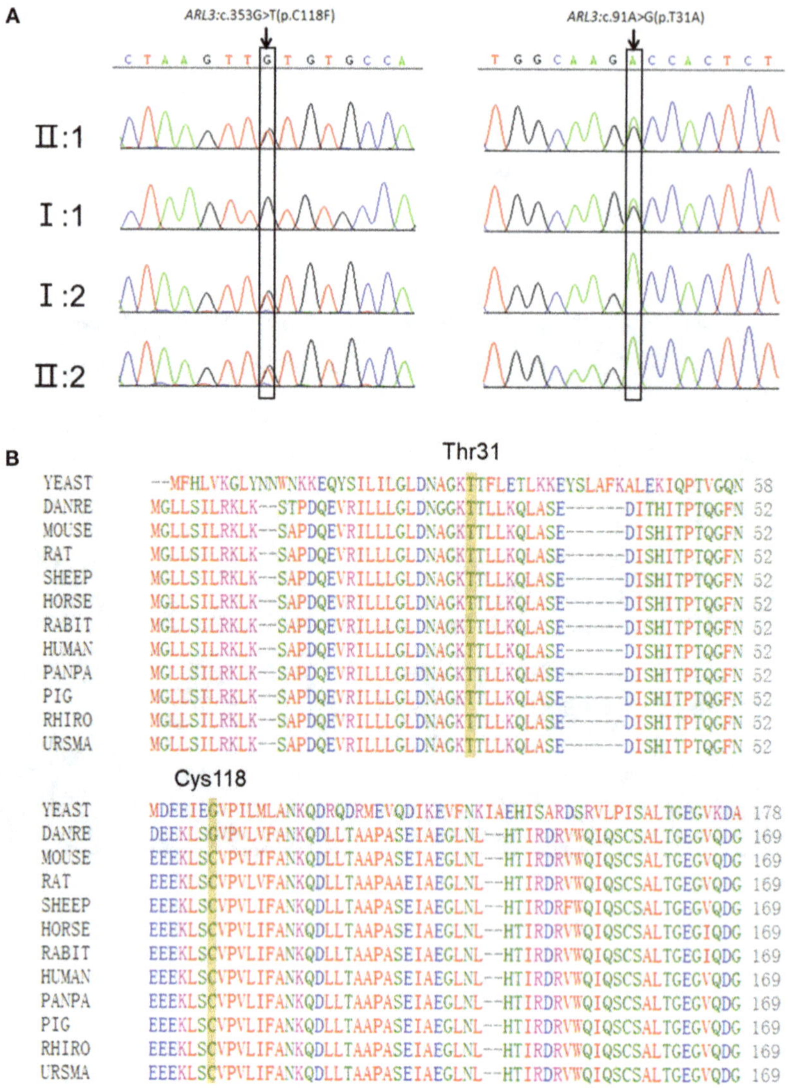

FIGURE 3 | Two novel *ARL3* variants (c.91A>G, p.T31A; c.353G>T, p.C118F) were identified in the RCD family. **(A)** Sanger sequencing in all family numbers. **(B)** Multiple alignments of Thr31 and Cys118 of ARL3 protein from different species. Both variants occurred on the conserved residues of the ARL3 protein.

TABLE 1 | *In silico* pathogenicity prediction.

Algorithm	*ARL3*: c.91A>G (p.T31A)	*ARL3*: c.353G>T (p.C118F)
LRT	0 (Deleterious)	0 (Deleterious)
PolyPhen-2_HDIV	0.99 (Probably damaging)	0.105 (Benign)
PolyPhen-2_HVAR	0.756 (Probably damaging)	0.125 (Benign)
Mutation Taster	1 (Disease-causing)	0.998 (Disease-causing)
SIFT	0.023 (Damaging)	0 (Damaging)
FATHMM	−2.34 (Damaging)	−1.55 (Damaging)
CADD	26.8 (Damaging)	25.4 (Damaging)

Results for the variants c.91A>G (p.T31A) and c.353G>T (p.C118F) in ARL3.

that the variant c.2432T>C in *FBN2* was predicted to be possibly damaging by *in silico* prediction. Variants in *FBN2* have been reported to associated with congenital contractural arachnodactyly (CCA) (Putnam et al., 1995) and early-onset macular degeneration (MD) (Ratnapriya et al., 2014), whereas the proband's mother and sister who carried the heterozygous missense variant (c.2432T>C, p.I811T) in *FBN2* didn't have any phenotypes of CCA or MD.

Protein Structure and Function Prediction

To visualize the structure changes of the protein mediated by p.T31A and p.C118F mutations, we used HOPE online software. The schematic structures of the original and the mutant amino acid were shown in **Figure 4A**. The 3D-structure of wild-type and mutant proteins were shown in **Figure 4B**. Compared with the wild-type residue, the mutant residue at position 31 was smaller and more hydrophobic, while the mutant residue at position 118 was bigger and more hydrophobic. Among the interactors of ARL3 are RP2, ARL13B, UNC119A, who interact with ARL3 in

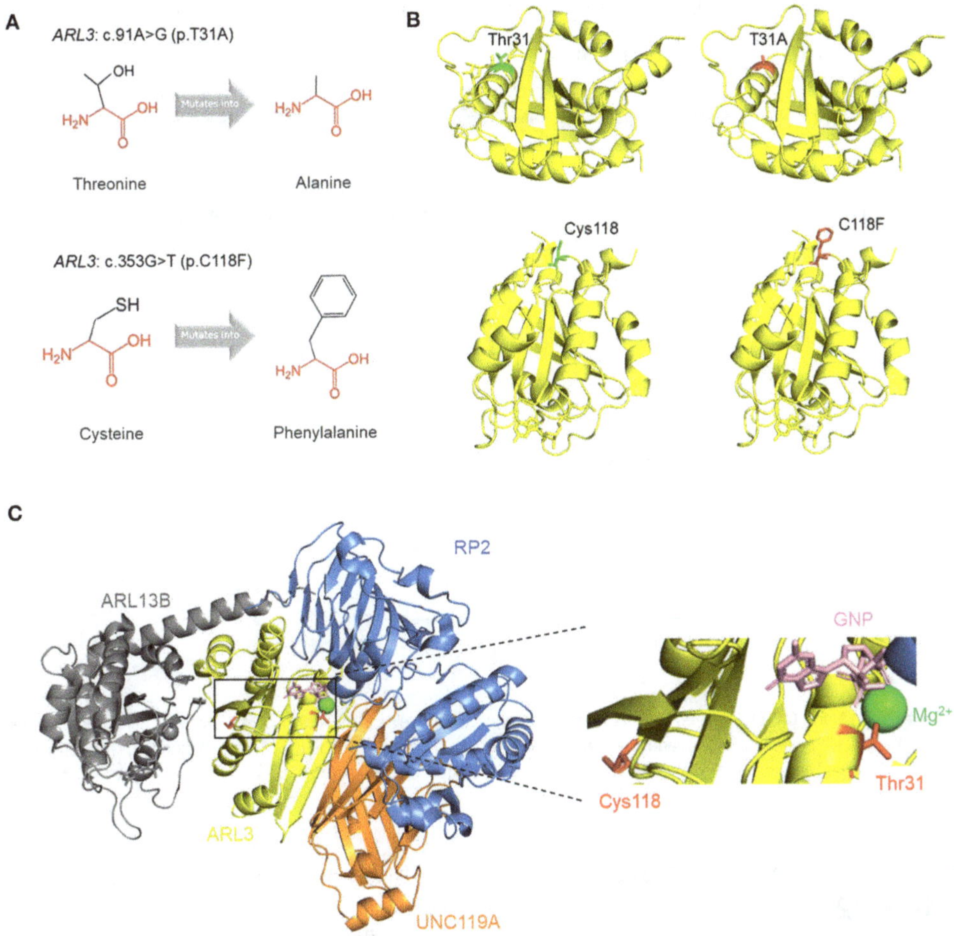

FIGURE 4 | Tertiary structure prediction of mutant proteins. **(A)** The schematic structures of the original and the mutant amino acids. The backbone was colored in red; the side chain was colored in black. **(B)** The 3D-structure of the wild-type and mutant proteins. The main structure of the ARL3 protein was colored in yellow. The side chains of the wild-type and the mutant residues were colored in green and red, respectively. **(C)** Superimposition of the structures of ARL3 (yellow) in complex with its interactors: RP2 (blue; PDB: 3BH6) (Veltel et al., 2008), ARL13B (gray; PDB: 5DI3) (Gotthardt et al., 2015), and UNC119A (orange; PDB: 4GOJ) (Ismail et al., 2012). On the right side is a zoomed-in view of some structures, including GNP (pink), Mg^{2+} (green), and the side chains of Thr31 and Cys118 (red).

a GTP dependent manner. In order to visualize the interactions, we superimposed the known structures of ARL3 in complex with the interactors (**Figure 4C**).

T31A and C118F Mutations Impaired the Stabilities of ARL3 Proteins

The conformational change of protein caused by the change of amino acid properties was closely related to the stability of protein. Thus, we wondered whether *ARL3* T31A and C118F mutations affected the stability of the protein. The online tools MUpro and I-Mutant v2.0 were used to predict protein stability and results suggested that the two mutant ARL3 proteins showed decrease of stability (**Table 2**).

To determine whether *ARL3* T31A and C118F mutations destabilize ARL3 protein, CHX chase assays was performed. HEK293T cells were transfected with empty vector, wild-type and two mutant *ARL3* vectors for 24 h, followed by treatment with cycloheximide (CHX) for 1, 3, and 6 h, respectively. Wild-type and two mutant ARL3 protein levels were analyzed using the flag antibody with Western blot. In **Figure 5**, both the half-lives of ARL3 T31A and ARL3 C118F protein showed a decreasing trend compared with the wild-type ARL3 protein. These results indicated that both T31A and C118F mutations decreased the stability of ARL3 protein.

TABLE 2 | Prediction of the protein stability with online tools.

Online tools	ARL3: c.91A>G (p.T31A)	ARL3: c.353G>T (p.C118F)
Mupro	ΔΔG: −0.19 (DECREASE stability)	ΔΔG: −0.23 (DECREASE stability)
I-Mutant v2.0	ΔΔG: −0.50 (Decrease stability)	ΔΔG: −0.13 (Decrease stability)

ΔΔG: ΔG (mutated protein) −ΔG (wild type protein) in kcal/mol. ΔΔG < 0: decrease stability. ΔΔG > 0: increase stability.

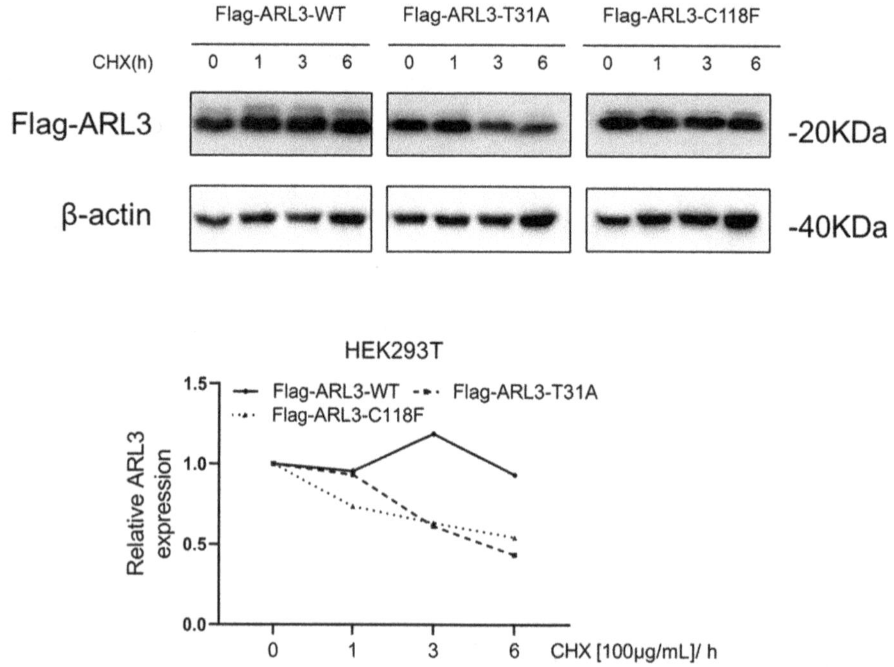

FIGURE 5 | The ARL3 variants T31A and C118F impaired the stabilities of the encoded proteins in HEK293T cells. HEK293T cells were transfected with empty vector, wild-type, *ARL3* T31A and C118F vectors for 24 h and then treated with 100 μg/ml cycloheximide (CHX) for 1, 3, and 6 h, respectively. ARL3 protein levels were detected using the flag antibody. The protein levels of β-actin were used as endogenous control ($n = 1$).

C118F Mutation Disrupted the Protein Interaction With RP2

As a small molecule GTP-binding protein, ARL3 was activated when combined with GTP. But it depends on the presence of functional guanine nucleotide exchange factor, ARL13B (Gotthardt et al., 2015). Protein RP2 could interact with ARL3, and it was identified as a negative regulator by hydrolyzing GTP. In addition, it was reported that the impaired interaction between RP2 and ARL3 induced by RP2 mutation could cause RP (Kuhnel et al., 2006). To investigate whether the novel ARL3 variants affected the interaction between ARL3 and RP2, we conducted co-IP analysis. Plasmid of HA-RP2-WT was co-transfected with Flag-ARL3-WT, Flag-ARL3-T31A, or Flag-ARL3-C118F in HEK293T cells. As in **Figure 6**, RP2 was detected after Flag-ARL3 pull-down, suggesting interaction between ARL3 and RP2 in HEK293T cells. The relative level of RP2 protein was significantly reduced in the C118F mutant group compared with the control group, while there was no significant change in the T31A mutant group. The results demonstrated that *ARL3* mutation C118F inhibited the interaction between ARL3 and RP2 proteins.

DISCUSSION

In this study, we identified two novel variants (c.91A>G, p.T31A; c.353G>T, p.C118F) in *ARL3* gene in a Chinese RCD family. According to the American College of Medical Genetics and Genomics (ACMG) standards and guidelines, the two variants were "likely pathogenic," which was supported by the following evidences. The two variants, (1) were supported by functional tests *in vitro* (PS3); (2) located in an important domain that acts as GTP/Mg2+ binding site and GAP interaction site (PM1); (3) not found in the 200 unrelated health controls and absent from any databases (PM2); (4) The two variants were considered as "Deleterious" by function prediction software, and were highly conserved during evolution (PP3).

The ARL3 Thr31 and Cys118 residues are highly conserved among species, and *in silico* prediction tools suggested that either missense change was likely to be pathogenic. HOPE analysis showed that, compared with the wild-type residues (Threonine and Cysteine), the mutant residue (Alanine) of p.T31A was smaller and more hydrophobic, and the mutant residue (Phenylalanine) of p.C118F was bigger and more hydrophobic. The changes of size and hydrophobicity may cause the loss of hydrogen bonds in the core of the protein, and disturbing protein folding, and then destabilize ARL3 protein. In CHX chase assays, our results revealed that the T31A and C118F protein showed a rapid degradation while the wild-type ARL3 protein was stabilized, indicating the T31A and C118F mutation decreased the stability of ARL3 protein. On the other hand, we noticed that p. Thr31 was central to the P-loop NTPase domain in ARL3, and involved in direct binding of the beta and gamma phosphate moieties of GXP (GTP or GDP) and Mg^{2+} cation (**Figure 4C**). Another substitution at T31, T31N, has been widely used as a synthetic ARL3-GDP conformational mimic. In addition, the

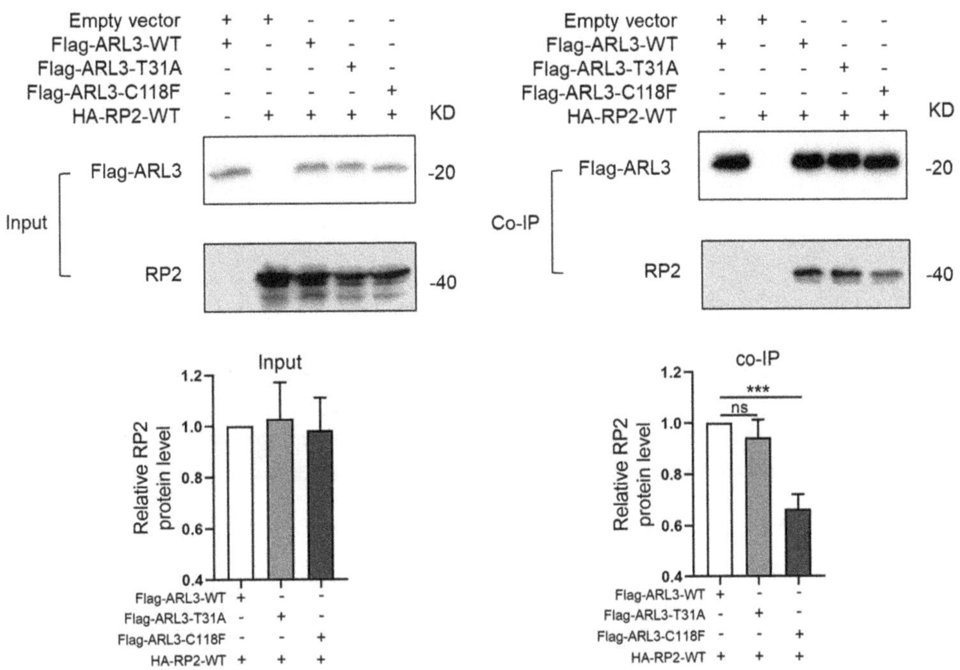

FIGURE 6 | *ARL3* variants T31A and C118F disrupted the combination between ARL3 and RP2. Plasmids of HA-RP2-WT were co-transfected with wild-type or mutant Flag-ARL3 plasmids into HEK293T cells. ARL3 was immunoprecipitated with anti-Flag antibody. Western blotting was performed to detect the specific proteins indicated on the left side of each panel (Error bars indicate means ± SD; $n = 3$, $^{***}p < 0.001$).

known interaction partners of ARL3 mainly include PDE6D, UNC119A/B, RP2 and ARL13B, whose interactions with ARL3 are GTP-dependent. Therefore, the replacement of Threonine with Arginine at residue 31 variant may impact GTP binding or exchange and thereby affected the normal interactions with these molecules or other parts of the protein, which is most likely a loss-of-function mechanism.

In the mammalian retina, ARL3 functions as a cargo displacement factor and plays an important role in the transport of lipidated protein to the outer segment of the photoreceptors. In addition, RP2 and ARL3 co-localize to the ciliary apparatus (Grayson et al., 2002), and RP2 could stimulate the exchange of GTP to GDP on ARL3, stimulating the release of the lipidated proteins bound to PDE6D and UNC119A/B (Hanke-Gogokhia et al., 2018). On the other hand, Arl3 and RP2 regulated the trafficking of specific ciliary tip kinesins, Kif7 and Kif17, independently of lipidated protein trafficking(Schwarz et al., 2017). The well-regulated protein trafficking in photoreceptors is crucial for normal visual function. The connecting cilium is a key player for the vectorial transport of proteins from the endoplasmic reticulum to the outer segment. Unsurprisingly, mutations in several connecting cilium-associated proteins have been shown to be associated with various types of retinal dystrophy like Joubert syndrome-associated RP, dominant RP, X-linked RP and dominant CRD (Liu et al., 2002; Cantagrel et al., 2008; Thomas et al., 2014; Zhang et al., 2019). It indicates that close cooperation of related proteins is necessary for normal operation of protein transport in photoreceptors.

Our co-IP results revealed that C118F mutant showed a reduced affinity for RP2. But it is unknown how C118F mutant contributes to the occurrence and development of RCD. Significantly, the reported allele frequency of c.353G>T (p.C118F) in GnomAD is concentrated in the East Asian population with almost 1:1,000. This allele frequency is borderline as being too common to cause a very rare disease like RCD. Furthermore, C118F is only conserved in mammals, but not in zebrafish and yeast, and not all the *in silico* prediction tools predicted the C118F variant would be pathogenic. Given that the mother and sister who carried the variant of C118F were unaffected, the mutation C118F may not cause disease when it exists alone as a heterozygote.

On the other hand, when T31A was carried by the father as a heterozygote, he showed a late onset and relatively mild phenotype of CRD. Significantly, the proband who carried the compound heterozygous variants of T31A and C118F typically presented with poor visual acuity, nyctalopia and peripheral field loss when he was young. ERG revealed severely reduced rod and cone system functions. We presumed these two variants may work together to promote the occurrence and development of RCD. Thus, compound heterozygous variants T31A and C118F in *ARL3* caused earlier and severer RCD condition. However, considering the limitation of cell

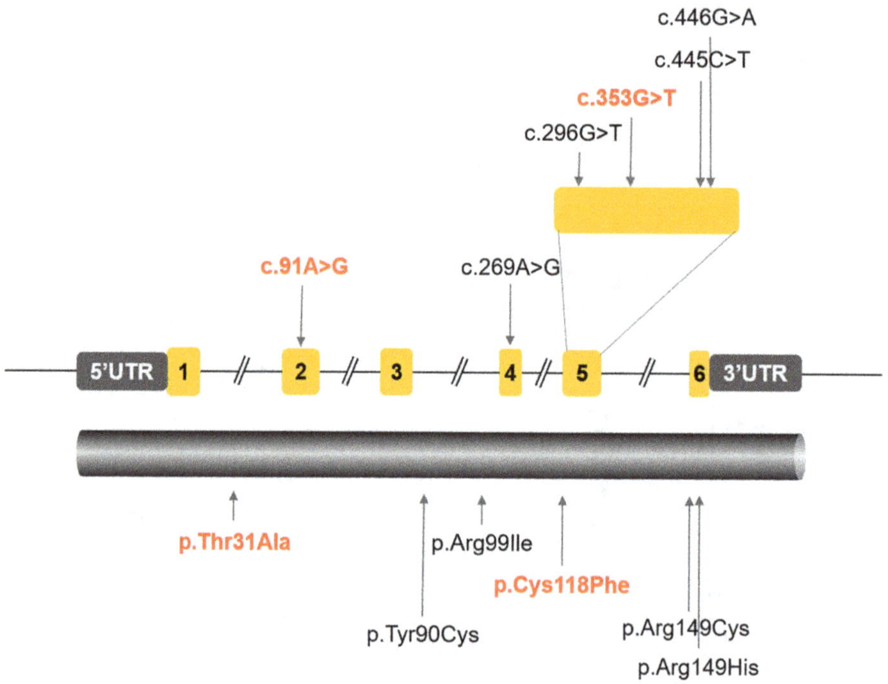

FIGURE 7 | All the reported *ARL3* pathogenic mutations were labeled in the schematic diagram of ARL3 gene and protein. The *ARL3* mutations c.91A>G (p.T31A) and c.353G>T (p.C118F) were indicated in red.

model, the *in vivo* tests of the two variants could not be inferred with confidence at this moment. And it could be helpful to identify whether his father had other gene mutation that caused this phenotype. Further functional studies are still necessary.

So far, four *ARL3* mutations have been identified (**Figure 7**), most of which locate at the important domain, affecting the stability of encoded protein or the affinity with interactors. Previously, two different *ARL3* Arg149 missense variants (c.445C>T, p.Arg149Cys; c.446G>A, p.Arg149His) were reported to cause recessive Joubert syndrome, characterized by hypoplasia of the cerebellar vermis, developmental delay, renal anomalies, and RCD in two families (Alkanderi et al., 2018). The study showed that substitution of arginine at position 149 disrupted the known interaction between ARL3 and ARL13B and thus prevented the correct release of intraciliary cargos. Patients with heterozygous missense variant (c.269A>G, p.Tyr90Cys) in *ARL3* have recently been found to cause non-syndromic autosomal dominant RP, confirming earlier reports of this missense variant causing retinal disease. The missense variant is predicted to disrupt protein folding and compromise GTP binding or exchange. A most recent report indicated that a homozygous variant in *ARL3* (c.296G>T, p. Arg99Ile) caused CRD in two consanguineous families. The study suggested that the mutation p.Arg99Ile may alter the affinity of encoded protein for guanine nucleotides, resulting in a much less stable protein. Thus, although *ARL3* is not a common cause of retinal degeneration in humans, it is a strong prior candidate gene.

In conclusion, our results extended both genotype and phenotype of *ARL3* associated retinal dystrophy. We defined two novel pathogenic variants (c.91A>G, p.T31A; c.353G>T, p.C118F) of *ARL3* in a Chinese family with typical RCD. We presumed that these compound heterozygous variants were associated with the early onset of recessive RCD, while c.91A>G along might be associated with a late onset of dominant CRD. We further found the *ARL3* variants T31A and C118F destabilized ARL3 protein, and the C118F disrupted the interaction with RP2 in HEK293T cells. On the other hand, considering the limitation of cell model and number of patients, the detailed mechanisms that the two *ARL3* variants causing RCD deserve further studies.

ETHICS STATEMENT

The studies involving human participants were reviewed and approved by The Ethics Committee of Henan Eye Hospital. Written informed consent to participate in this study was provided by the participants' legal guardian/next of kin. Written informed consent was obtained from the individual(s), and minor(s)' legal guardian/next of kin, for the publication of any potentially identifiable images or data included in this article.

AUTHOR CONTRIBUTIONS

BL conceptualized and designed the study. YL, QG, and YY collected the clinical samples and clinical data. LF, YL, and YY performed the genetic analysis and bioinformatics evaluations. LF conducted the molecular biology experiments and drafted the manuscript. BL, SY, and XZ interpreted the results. BL and XZ reviewed and edited the draft. All authors agreed to be accountable for the content of the work and approved the final manuscript.

ACKNOWLEDGMENTS

We would like to thank all the patients and their families for participating in this study.

REFERENCES

Ali, M. U., Rahman, M. S. U., Cao, J., and Yuan, P. X. (2017). Genetic characterization and disease mechanism of retinitis pigmentosa; current scenario. *Biotech* 7:251. doi: 10.1007/s13205-017-0878-3

Alkanderi, S., Molinari, E., Shaheen, R., Elmaghloob, Y., Stephen, L. A., Sammut, V., et al. (2018). ARL3 mutations cause Joubert syndrome by disrupting ciliary protein composition. *Am. J. Hum. Genet.* 103, 612–620. doi: 10.1016/j.ajhg.2018.08.015

Bhatia, S., Kaur, N., Singh, I. R., and Vanita, V. (2019). A novel mutation in MERTK for rod-cone dystrophy in a North Indian family. *Can. J. Ophthalmol.* 54, 40–50. doi: 10.1016/j.jcjo.2018.02.008

Biasini, M., Bienert, S., Waterhouse, A., Arnold, K., Studer, G., Schmidt, T., et al. (2014). SWISS-MODEL: modelling protein tertiary and quaternary structure using evolutionary information. *Nucleic Acids Res.* 42, W252–258. doi: 10.1093/nar/gku340

Cantagrel, V., Silhavy, J. L., Bielas, S. L., Swistun, D., Marsh, S. E., Bertrand, J. Y., et al. (2008). Mutations in the cilia gene ARL13B lead to the classical form of Joubert syndrome. *Am. J. Hum. Genet.* 83, 170–179. doi: 10.1016/j.ajhg.2008.06.023

Capriotti, E., Fariselli, P., and Casadio, R. (2005). I-Mutant2.0: predicting stability changes upon mutation from the protein sequence or structure. *Nucleic. Acids Res.* 33, W306–310. doi: 10.1093/nar/gki375

Cheng, J., Randall, A., and Baldi, P. (2006). Prediction of protein stability changes for single-site mutations using support vector machines. *Proteins* 62, 1125–1132. doi: 10.1002/prot.20810

Collin, R. W., van den Born, L. I., Klevering, B. J., de Castro-Miro, M., Littink, K. W., Arimadyo, K., et al. (2011). High-resolution homozygosity mapping is a powerful tool to detect novel mutations causative of autosomal recessive RP in the Dutch population. *Invest. Ophthalmol. Vis. Sci.* 52, 2227–2239. doi: 10.1167/iovs.10-6185

Gotthardt, K., Lokaj, M., Koerner, C., Falk, N., Giessl, A., and Wittinghofer, A. (2015). A G-protein activation cascade from Arl13B to Arl3 and implications for ciliary targeting of lipidated proteins. *Elife* 4:15. doi: 10.7554/eLife.11859.015

Grayson, C., Bartolini, F., Chapple, J. P., Willison, K. R., Bhamidipati, A., Lewis, S. A., et al. (2002). Localization in the human retina of the X-linked retinitis pigmentosa protein RP2, its homologue cofactor C and the RP2 interacting protein Arl3. *Hum. Mol. Genet.* 11, 3065–3074. doi: 10.1093/hmg/11.24.3065

Hanke-Gogokhia, C., Frederick, J. M., Zhang, H., and Baehr, W. (2018). Binary function of ARL3-GTP revealed by gene knockouts. *Adv. Exp. Med. Biol.* 1074, 317–325. doi: 10.1007/978-3-319-75402-4_39

Hanke-Gogokhia, C., Wu, Z., Gerstner, C. D., Frederick, J. M., Zhang, H., and Baehr, W. (2016). Arf-like protein 3 (ARL3) regulates protein trafficking and ciliogenesis in mouse photoreceptors. *J. Biol. Chem.* 291, 7142–7155. doi: 10.1074/jbc.M115.710954

Holtan, J. P., Teigen, K., Aukrust, I., Bragadottir, R., and Houge, G. (2019). Dominant ARL3-related retinitis pigmentosa. *Ophthalmic Genet.* 40, 124–128. doi: 10.1080/13816810.2019.1586965

Hu, Y. S., Song, H., Li, Y., Xiao, Z. Y., and Li, T. (2019). Whole-exome sequencing identifies novel mutations in genes responsible for retinitis pigmentosa in 2 nonconsanguineous Chinese families. *Int. J. Ophthalmol.* 12, 915–923. doi: 10.18240/ijo.2019.06.06

Ismail, S. A., Chen, Y. X., Miertzschke, M., Vetter, I. R., Koerner, C., and Wittinghofer, A. (2012). Structural basis for Arl3-specific release of myristoylated ciliary cargo from UNC119. *EMBO J.* 31, 4085–4094. doi: 10.1038/emboj.2012.257

Kircher, M., Witten, D. M., Jain, P., O'Roak, B. J., Cooper, G. M., and Shendure, J. (2014). A general framework for estimating the relative pathogenicity of human genetic variants. *Nat. Genet.* 46, 310–315. doi: 10.1038/ng.2892

Kuhnel, K., Veltel, S., Schlichting, I., and Wittinghofer, A. (2006). Crystal structure of the human retinitis pigmentosa 2 protein and its interaction with Arl3. *Structure* 14, 367–378. doi: 10.1016/j.str.2005.11.008

Kumar, P., Henikoff, S., and Ng, P. C. (2009). Predicting the effects of coding non-synonymous variants on protein function using the SIFT algorithm. *Nat. Protoc.* 4, 1073–1081. doi: 10.1038/nprot.2009.86

Liu, Q., Zhou, J., Daiger, S. P., Farber, D. B., Heckenlively, J. R., Smith, J. E., et al. (2002). Identification and subcellular localization of the RP1 protein in human and mouse photoreceptors. *Invest. Ophthalmol. Vis. Sci.* 43, 22–32.

Narayan, D. S., Wood, J. P., Chidlow, G., and Casson, R. J. (2016). A review of the mechanisms of cone degeneration in retinitis pigmentosa. *Acta Ophthalmol.* 94, 748–754. doi: 10.1111/aos.13141

Pagon, R. A. (1988). Retinitis pigmentosa. *Surv. Ophthalmol.* 33, 137–177. doi: 10.1016/0039-6257(88)90085-9

Putnam, E. A., Zhang, H., Ramirez, F., and Milewicz, D. M. (1995). Fibrillin-2 (FBN2) mutations result in the Marfan-like disorder, congenital contractural arachnodactyly. *Nat. Genet.* 11, 456–458. doi: 10.1038/ng1295-456

Ratnapriya, R., Zhan, X., Fariss, R. N., Branham, K. E., Zipprer, D., Chakarova, C. F., et al. (2014). Rare and common variants in extracellular matrix gene Fibrillin 2 (FBN2) are associated with macular degeneration. *Hum. Mol. Genet.* 23, 5827–5837. doi: 10.1093/hmg/ddu276

Rogers, M. F., Shihab, H. A., Mort, M., Cooper, D. N., Gaunt, T. R., and Campbell, C. (2018). FATHMM-XF: accurate prediction of pathogenic point mutations via extended features. *Bioinformatics* 34, 511–513. doi: 10.1093/bioinformatics/btx536

Schwarz, J. M., Rodelsperger, C., Schuelke, M., and Seelow, D. (2010). MutationTaster evaluates disease-causing potential of sequence alterations. *Nat. Methods* 7, 575–576. doi: 10.1038/nmeth0810-575

Schwarz, N., Lane, A., Jovanovic, K., Parfitt, D. A., Aguila, M., Thompson, C. L., et al. (2017). Arl3 and RP2 regulate the trafficking of ciliary tip kinesins. *Hum. Mol. Genet.* 26:3451. doi: 10.1093/hmg/ddx245

Sheikh, S. A., Sisk, R. A., Schiavon, C. R., Waryah, Y. M., Usmani, M. A., Steel, D. H., et al. (2019). Homozygous variant in ARL3 causes autosomal recessive cone rod dystrophy. *Invest. Ophthalmol. Vis. Sci.* 60, 4811–4819. doi: 10.1167/iovs.19-27263

Sievers, F., and Higgins, D. G. (2018). Clustal Omega for making accurate alignments of many protein sequences. *Protein Sci.* 27, 135–145. doi: 10.1002/pro.3290

Strom, S. P., Clark, M. J., Martinez, A., Garcia, S., Abelazeem, A. A., Matynia, A., et al. (2016). *De novo* occurrence of a variant in ARL3 and apparent autosomal dominant transmission of retinitis pigmentosa. *PLoS ONE* 11:e0150944. doi: 10.1371/journal.pone.0150944

Thomas, S., Wright, K. J., Le Corre, S., Micalizzi, A., Romani, M., Abhyankar, A., et al. (2014). A homozygous PDE6D mutation in Joubert syndrome impairs targeting of farnesylated INPP5E protein to the primary cilium. *Hum. Mutat.* 35, 137–146. doi: 10.1002/humu.22470

Veltel, S., Gasper, R., Eisenacher, E., and Wittinghofer, A. (2008). The retinitis pigmentosa 2 gene product is a GTPase-activating protein for Arf-like 3. *Nat. Struct. Mol. Biol.* 15, 373–380. doi: 10.1038/nsmb.1396

Zhang, J., Gao, F., Du, C., Wang, J., Pi, X., Guo, W., et al. (2019). A novel RP2 missense mutation Q158P identified in an X-linked retinitis pigmentosa family impaired RP2 protein stability. *Gene* 707, 86–92. doi: 10.1016/j.gene.2019.05.006

Zhu, Q., Rui, X., Li, Y., You, Y., Sheng, X., and Lei, B. (2021). Identification of four novel variants and determination of genotype-phenotype correlations for ABCA4 variants associated with inherited retinal degenerations. *Front. Cell Develop. Biol.* 9:634843. doi: 10.3389/fcell.2021.634843

12

A Novel *ARL3* Gene Mutation Associated with Autosomal Dominant Retinal Degeneration

Rinki Ratnapriya[1,2], Samuel G. Jacobson[3]*, Artur V. Cideciyan[3], Milton A. English[1], Alejandro J. Roman[3], Alexander Sumaroka[3], Rebecca Sheplock[3] and Anand Swaroop[1]*

[1] Neurobiology-Neurodegeneration and Repair Laboratory, National Eye Institute, National Institutes of Health, Bethesda, MD, United States, [2] Department of Ophthalmology, Baylor College of Medicine, Houston, TX, United States, [3] Department of Ophthalmology, Perelman School of Medicine, Scheie Eye Institute, University of Pennsylvania, Philadelphia, PA, United States

***Correspondence:**
Rinki Ratnapriya
RinkiRatna.Priya@bcm.edu
Samuel G. Jacobson
jacobsos@pennmedicine.upenn.edu

Despite major progress in the discovery of causative genes, many individuals and families with inherited retinal degenerations (IRDs) remain without a molecular diagnosis. We applied whole exome sequencing to identify the genetic cause in a family with an autosomal dominant IRD. Eye examinations were performed and affected patients were studied with electroretinography and kinetic and chromatic static perimetry. Sequence variants were analyzed in genes (n = 271) associated with IRDs listed on the RetNet database. We applied a stepwise filtering process involving the allele frequency in the control population, *in silico* prediction tools for pathogenicity, and evolutionary conservation to prioritize the potential causal variant(s). Sanger sequencing and segregation analysis were performed on the proband and other family members. The IRD in this family is expressed as a widespread progressive retinal degeneration with maculopathy. A novel heterozygous variant (c.200A > T) was identified in the *ARL3* gene, leading to the substitution of aspartic acid to valine at position 67. The Asp67 residue is evolutionary conserved, and the change p.Asp67Val is predicted to be pathogenic. This variant was segregated in affected members of the family and was absent from an unaffected individual. Two previous reports of a *de novo* missense mutation in the *ARL3* gene, each describing a family with two affected generations, are the only examples to date of autosomal dominant IRD associated with this photoreceptor gene. Our results, identifying a novel pathogenic variant in *ARL3* in a four-generation family with a dominant IRD, augment the evidence that the *ARL3* gene is another cause of non-syndromic retinal degeneration.

Keywords: chromatic perimetry, ciliopathy, cones, electroretinography, retinal degeneration, rods, whole exome sequencing

INTRODUCTION

Emerging from the era of ungenotyped inherited retinal degenerations (IRDs), we are now aware of the heterogeneous basis of these blinding diseases (Bramall et al., 2010; Wright et al., 2010; Ratnapriya and Swaroop, 2013; Verbakel et al., 2018; Garafalo et al., 2020). From the linkage mapping of disease loci to the identification of causative genes and mutations, there was a steady increase in the number of genes associated with IRDs in the three decades from 1990 onward (RetNet, the Retinal Information Network)[1]. Yet, there remain many IRD patients and families with unknown genetic diagnosis (at least 30%; Birtel et al., 2018; Garafalo et al., 2020; Hejtmancik and Daiger, 2020). The largest percentage of these molecularly unresolved Mendelian IRDs has been the simplex/multiplex or presumed autosomal recessively inherited diseases (Garafalo et al., 2020).

We have been investigating patients and families with non-syndromic retinal degeneration, and whenever a genetic cause for an autosomal dominant IRD was identified, the family was screened for known mutations. In recent years, the next-generation sequencing technologies, especially targeted and whole exome sequencing, have expedited the molecular diagnosis efforts (Booij et al., 2011; O'Sullivan et al., 2012; Ratnapriya and Swaroop, 2013; Beryozkin et al., 2015; Roberts et al., 2016). In the current study, we applied whole exome sequencing to a multi-generation dominant IRD family which was initially screened for known mutations but gave negative results. We analyzed all genes associated with IRDs as reported in the RetNet database and identified a novel, rare, heterozygous variant p.Asp67Val in *ARL3* as a causative mutation. *ARL3* encodes ADP-ribosylation factor, (Arf)-like protein 3. This soluble small GTPase has been localized to photoreceptors, and mutations in the *ARL3* gene are considered to cause retinal ciliopathy (Frederick et al., 2020; Sánchez-Bellver et al., 2021).

A missense variant in *ARL3* has previously been associated with non-syndromic autosomal dominant retinitis pigmentosa (OMIM 604695; Fahim et al., 2000). Specifically, the c.269A > G (p.Tyr90Cys) variant was determined to be a *de novo* mutation in two unrelated families, each with two generations of affected members (Strom et al., 2016; Holtan et al., 2019). *ARL3* has also been implicated as an autosomal recessive cause of Joubert syndrome and non-syndromic retinal degeneration (Alkanderi et al., 2018; Sheikh et al., 2019; Fu et al., 2021).

The identification of causal genes underlying human diseases has clear clinical and research utility, and there has been recent progress toward therapy in dominant forms of IRD (Sudharsan and Beltran, 2019; Kruczek et al., 2021). Further, specifically considering the *ARL3* gene, there are studies in patient-derived cell lines and animal models that can be the foundation for understanding the mechanism and devising the therapeutic strategies (Grayson et al., 2002; Evans et al., 2010; Schwarz et al., 2012; Hanke-Gogokhia et al., 2016; Kruczek and Swaroop, 2020).

MATERIALS AND METHODS

Human Subjects

Patients from a four-generation family with a history of visual impairment were included (**Table 1**). Six family members representing three of the generations underwent a standard ophthalmic examination as well as specialized psychophysical, electrophysiological, and imaging tests. Their clinical visits occurred between 1983 and 2002; molecular studies to identify the causative gene in this family were performed throughout the period from 1992 to 2021.

[1]https://sph.uth.edu/retnet/

TABLE 1 | Clinical characteristics of *ARL3* family.

Patient number/ Sex	Age at first visit (years)	Ages at follow-up (years)	Best corrected visual acuity (first visit)		Refractive error (first visit) as spherical equivalent	
			OD	**OS**	**OD**	**OS**
II-1/M	69	One visit	HM	HM	−0.75	−0.75
III-1/M	47	55	20/300	HM	−3.50	−4.00
III-2/M	41	42, 46, 48, 52	20/20	20/25	−0.50	−1.00
IV-1/F	13	14, 15, 16, 18, 20	20/50	20/40	−9.00	−7.00
IV-2/F	10	12, 15, 18, 21	20/40	20/30	−4.50	−5.00
IV-3/F	8	9, 10, 13, 15, 17, 19, 27	20/30	20/40	−3.25	−2.75

Phenotype Studies

Full Field Electroretinography (ERG)

Techniques, methods of data analysis, and normal results for ERGs have been described (Jacobson et al., 1989; Yagasaki and Jacobson, 1989; Azari et al., 2006; Aleman et al., 2009). After a 45-min period of dark adaptation, full-field ERGs were elicited using scotopically matched blue and red lights followed by a series of blue light flashes with increasing intensities to elicit a rod response. Bright flashes of white light were used to obtain a mixed cone and rod response. To elicit a cone response, single flashes of white light on a steady white background, suppressing the rods, was used. Cone function was also measured by using a series of white light flickering at 30 Hz with increasing intensities on a white background. The relationship of rod b-wave amplitude to cone flicker amplitude was calculated and plotted (Yagasaki and Jacobson, 1989).

To directly assess the function of rod-photoreceptor phototransduction activation and rod-driven post-receptoral signaling in patient III-2 at age 52, photoresponses were elicited with different luminances of blue (Wratten 47A) and red (Wratten 26) flashes in the dark-adapted state as previously described (Cideciyan and Jacobson, 1993, 1996; Cideciyan, 2000). In brief, luminances were selected to provide pairs of scotopically matched waveforms to blue and red flashes which when digitally subtracted gave a cone ERG that was then subtracted from the response to a photopically matched blue flash (double subtraction technique). The resulting rod-isolated ERG was assumed to be the sum of two major underlying components, P3 and P2. P3 is generated by the photoreceptors, and P2 is generated by the inner nuclear layer. The P3 component of the rod-isolated ERG was quantitatively estimated by fitting a physiologically based mathematical model previously developed (Cideciyan and Jacobson, 1996) for the leading edges of the waveforms. Then the rod-driven post-receptoral P2 component was derived by subtracting the P3 estimate from the rod-isolated ERG. The derived P2 component was normalized by the maximum size of the P3 component to facilitate comparison between the different amplitudes of patients and normal subjects.

Perimetry

Goldmann kinetic perimetry was performed with V-4e and I-4e test targets. Static perimetry was performed with a modified automated perimeter (Humphrey Field Analyzer 750i) as previously described (Jacobson et al., 1986; Roman et al., 2005). Two-color (500 and 650 nm) dark-adapted function and light-adapted function (600 nm) were measured at 2° intervals across the central visual field (central 60° along horizontal and vertical meridians) and at 12° intervals throughout the visual field. Photoreceptor mediation under dark-adapted conditions was determined by the sensitivity difference between 500- and 650-nm stimuli (Jacobson et al., 1986; Roman et al., 2005).

Imaging

Color fundus photographs were obtained using camera systems available at the time of examinations. In one family member, cross-sectional retinal reflectivity profiles were obtained with optical coherence tomography (OCT; Zeiss Humphrey Instruments, Dublin, CA, United States). Our OCT techniques have been published (e.g., Jacobson et al., 2003; Sumaroka et al., 2019). For the current work, data were acquired with first-generation (time-domain) OCT1 with a theoretical axial resolution in retinal tissue of ~10 μm. Scans were composed of 100 longitudinal reflectivity profiles (LRPs). Five overlapping segments of linear scans (repeated two times each of 4.5-mm length) located along the horizontal and vertical meridian, centered on the anatomical fovea and extending to 9 mm in either direction, were acquired. Post-acquisition processing of OCT data was performed with custom programs (MATLAB R2020b; MathWorks, Natick, MA, United States). LRPs making up the OCT scans were aligned by straightening the major RPE reflection, and scans from the same eccentricities were averaged.

Molecular Studies

Whole Exome Sequencing Analysis

Genomic DNA was extracted from the peripheral blood using standard methods and quantified using the Promega QuantiFluor® dsDNA system (Promega, Madison, WI, United States), according to the manufacturer's instructions. Targeted exome capture was performed using genomic DNA from the proband using the Agilent SureSelect Human All exon 50 Mb kit (Agilent Technologies, Santa Clara, CA, United States), following the manufacturer's instructions. Captured libraries were amplified and converted to clusters using Illumina Cluster Station, and paired-end 126 bp sequencing was performed on Illumina GAIIx (Illumina, Inc., San Diego, CA, United States).

Primary Bioinformatics Analysis

FastQC (available at http://www.bioinformatics.babraham.ac.uk/projects/fastqc/) was used to confirm the quality of sequencing, and adapter indexes were removed using Trimmomatic (Bolger et al., 2014). Sequence reads were mapped against the hg38/GRCh38 human reference genome sequence build using BWA. Aligned reads were processed to mark

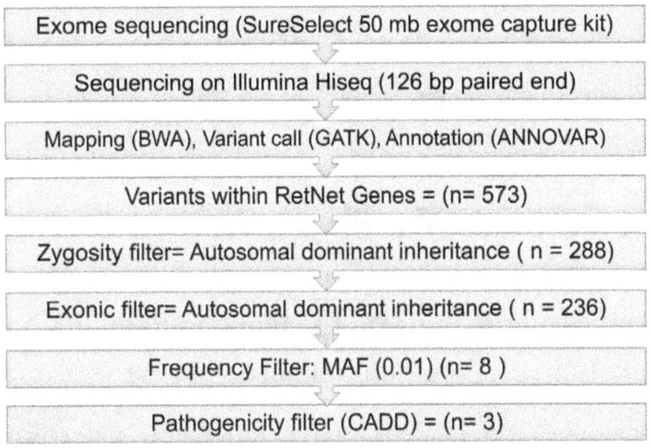

FIGURE 1 | Analysis and filtering pipeline for RetNet genes.

duplicates using Picard[2]. The Genome Analysis Toolkit (GATK) recommendations for best practices were applied for variant calling, local realignment, base quality recalibration, and variant recalibration (DePristo et al., 2011). The annotation of variants was performed with ANNOVAR (Wang et al., 2010). As a part of ANNOVAR annotations, alternate allele frequencies of the variants in non-Finnish European (NFE) populations were obtained from the Exome Aggregation Consortium (ExAC), which constituted data from 33,370 individuals.

Variant Filtering and Prioritization

To identify pathogenic variants, we applied a stepwise filtering process on sequence variants identified in genes listed on the RetNet database (in the public domain; accessed July 2020)[3] (**Figure 1**). First, we retained only functional coding variants (non-synonymous, stop gain, stop loss, splicing, and frameshift insertions/deletions). Next, we excluded variants with a minor allele frequency (MAF) of >0.01 in the ExAC as they were deemed not disease causing because of their prevalence in the apparently normal population. The variants were subsequently selected based on an additional predictive causality filter to focus on the 1% most deleterious variants in the human genome (CADD score ≥ 20).

Confirmation of Candidate Variants by Sanger Sequencing

Candidate variant in *ARL3* identified by whole exome sequencing was validated by Sanger sequencing in the proband and five additional family members (four affected and one unaffected) using an ABI PRISM 3730xl Genetic Analyzer (Applied Biosystems; Thermo Fisher Scientific, Waltham, MA, United States). The primers used to amplify the *ARL3* DNA fragment containing Asp67Val variant were ARL3-F-5′-TCACAACAAATCATTTTCAGCA-3′ and ARL3-R-5′-CTGAGCGACAGCAAAACATC-3′.

[2]http://picard.sourceforge.net

[3]https://sph.uth.edu/Retnet/sum-dis.htm

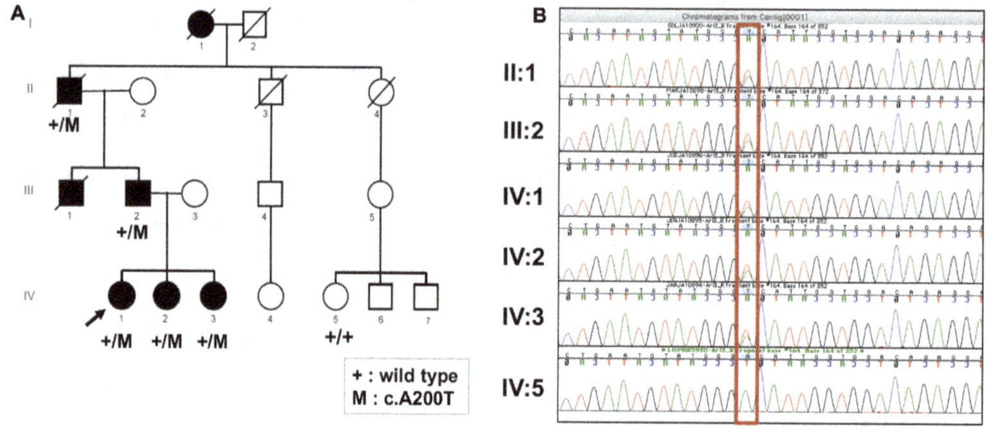

FIGURE 2 | (A) Pedigree of the family, showing members affected and unaffected by the IRD. The segregation of the *ARL3* variant c.A200T is shown where mutation is indicated by "+/M," and its absence is indicated by "+/+." **(B)** Sanger sequencing electropherogram of the available family members confirming the exome sequencing results, as all affected are heterozygous (A/T) and the unaffected is homozygous for the wild-type allele (A/A) (shown in red rectangle).

Conservation of Asp67Val Across Species

We next analyzed the evolutionary conservation of the variant as it is a strong indicator of the deleteriousness of any change. Multiple species protein sequence alignment to assess evolutionary conservation of residue was performed using the UCSC Genome Browser[4].

Protein–Protein Interaction Prediction

To understand the effects of p.Asp67Val mutation, we took advantage of the ARL3 interaction structural information in predicting the impact of this substitution on the affinity of protein–protein complexes. We used mCSM-PPI2 (Rodrigues et al., 2019), which is a machine-learning method that relies on graph-based signatures to evaluate the structure-based prediction of the impact of missense mutations on protein-protein interaction. p.Asp67Val was modeled with mCSM-PPI2 on the structures 3BH6 (RP2), 4GOJ (UNC119A), and 5DI3 (ARL13B).

RESULTS

Phenotype Studies

Clinical Features of the IRD in This Family

The four-generation Ashkenazi-Jewish family with a history of progressive visual loss in some members but no other systemic disease manifestations (**Figure 2A** and **Table 1**) was studied to determine the ocular-retinal phenotype. From the examination of the oldest affected member (PII/1, age 69), it was evident that the retinal disease expression could be severe at this age; night vision losses were recalled by the patient in his third decade of life, and then there was progression to peripheral and central vision loss over subsequent decades. Posterior subcapsular cataracts (PSCs) were present at age 69. The fundus appearance was one of widespread pigmentary retinopathy and chorioretinal atrophy as well as waxy disk pallor and attenuated vessels. An ERG was non-detectable; and kinetic visual fields were not measurable. PIII-1 at age 47 years also had a severe disease expression; central and night vision disturbances were present from the second decade of life. Peripheral vision loss prompted mobility training in his early fourth decade. Acuities were 20/300 with hand motions at first examination (**Table 1**), and only a small central island of visual field was present. ERGs were not detectable at age 47.

In contrast to the severe disease expression of PII-1 and PIII-1, PIII-2 was asymptomatic early in his fifth decade of life. The three daughters of PIII-2 were all examined late in their first or early in their second decades of life. Two (PIV-2 and -3) of the three were asymptomatic while PIV-1 already had complaints of night vision disturbances. Serial visual acuities of five of the affected family members are shown (**Supplementary Figure 1**).

Fundus photographs of affected members were taken on certain visits in the era before other imaging modalities were available. A fundus feature of many of the family members was a parafoveal (bull's eye-like) macular lesion (Krill, 1977). For example, at age 46, PIII-2 had normal-appearing retinal vessels and no peripheral pigmentary changes, but in both maculae, there was a ring of apparent depigmentation surrounding a central area (**Figure 3A**). Acuities in the two eyes were 20/20 (OD) and 20/70 (OS). A daughter, PIV-2, at age 12, had a parafoveal lesion in each eye and no symptoms. Acuities were OD 20/40 and OS, 20/30. Vessel caliber was normal but there was some depigmentation and sparse bone spicule-like pigment in the superior retina (**Figure 3B**). PIII-1 at age 47 had features of retinal degeneration throughout the fundus and there were macular pigmentary disturbances (**Figure 3C**).

Cross-sectional imaging was performed on one of the family members, PIV-3, at age 27 (**Figure 3D**). Unlike the normal OCT showing typical laminar architecture across the central 50 degrees of retina (upper panels), PIV-3 has severely reduced outer nuclear layer (ONL) thickness in the fovea and across the sampled region (lower panels). There is no foveal bulge (foveal cone outer segments), and acuities are reduced; the outer

[4]http://genome.ucsc.edu

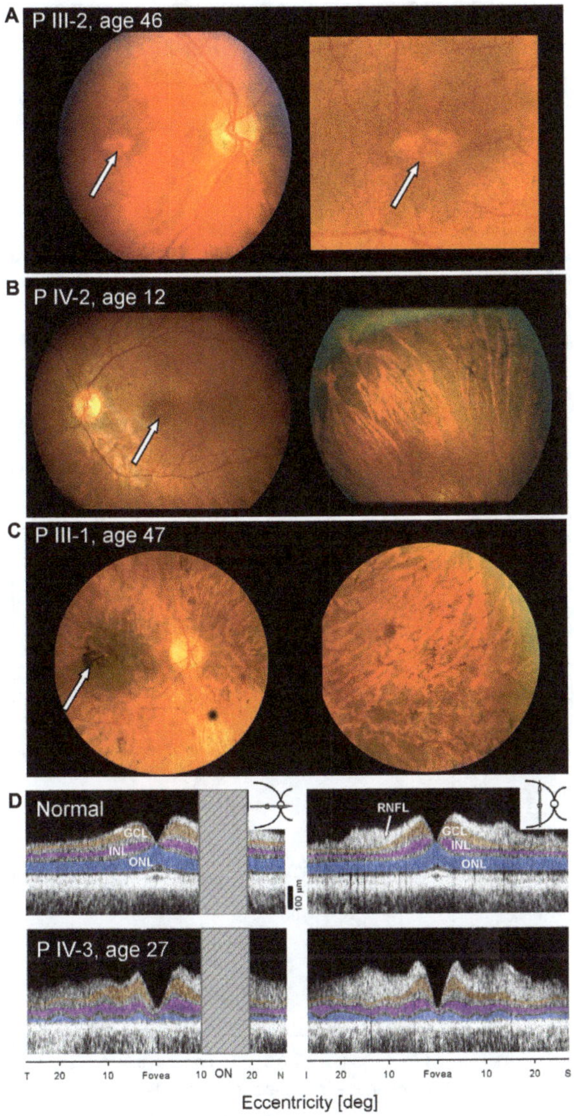

FIGURE 3 | Maculopathy at all stages of the IRD. **(A–C)** Fundus photographs of PIII-2, PIV-2, and PIII-1. Arrows point to maculopathy. **(D)** OCTs of normal subject (upper panels) compared with scans of PIV-3 (lower panels) along horizontal and vertical meridians (insets, upper right). Hatched bar shows the location of the optic nerve head in the horizontal scans. ONL, outer nuclear layer, highlighted in blue; INL, inner nuclear layer, purple; GCL, ganglion cell layer, orange; and RNFL, retinal nerve fiber layer, arrow. T, temporal; N, nasal; I, inferior, S, superior retina.

retinal laminar appearance suggests both rod and cone inner and outer segment losses across the macula (consistent with loss of rod and cone sensitivity noted with chromatic perimetry). Foveal ONL thickness in PIV-3 is 12 μm (defined as average measurement under the foveal pit in horizontal and vertical scans) or 12.1% of the average normal value at this location (98.6 μm, n = 15; age range, 8–62 years, SD = 11.1 μm). At a rod rich area (15° superior retina), ONL is 17.3 μm or 31% of average normal value (56.0 μm; n = 15; age range, 8–62 years, SD = 6.1 μ m).

Retina-Wide Rod and Cone Dysfunction by Electroretinography

All family members studied (n = 6) had abnormally reduced ERGs (**Figure 4C**); rod and cone signals in PII-1 and PIII-1 were non-detectable. Waveforms from two members, PIV-3 and PIII-2, separated in age by 30 years illustrate that there was variable expressivity of disease (**Figure 4A**). PIV-3 at age 18 shows reduced but measurable rod and cone signals. The father, PIII-2, has larger amplitude rod and cone signals but, of interest, the b/a-wave ratio to the maximum white flash that normally produces a mixed cone-rod ERG is reduced (normal mean b/a-wave ratio, 1.6; SD, 0.2; n = 96). This "negative ERG" was present in PIII-2 on three recordings (ages 41, 46, and 48).

At age 52 in PIII-2, there was an opportunity to record specialized ERG photoresponses (**Figure 4B**). The rod component of the mixed rod and cone ERGs to high intensity blue flashes was isolated by the double subtraction technique. The leading edges of the rod-isolated waveforms in a normal subject and in PIII-2 are shown. The phototransduction activation model (gray smooth lines) has been fitted to the responses from an intensity series (small symbols and lines). Normalized rod P2 components from four normal subjects are compared to that of PIII-2; the latter appears smaller than the normal result suggestive of an abnormality at the first synapse of photoreceptors or in rod bipolar cells.

The presence of bull's eye-like maculopathy in many of the family members and the association of this maculopathy with cone and cone-rod diseases (Thiadens et al., 2012) suggested the value of calculating the relationship between rod and cone ERGs to determine if there was a pattern in these data (Yagasaki and Jacobson, 1989; **Figure 4D**). The results indicated that dysfunction equally affected rod and cone systems by these ERG parameters, like one of the patterns previously associated with some cone-rod dystrophies (Yagasaki and Jacobson, 1989).

Kinetic and Chromatic Static Perimetry

Kinetic and static chromatic fields from three family members illustrate variable expressivity: there are comparable degrees of loss in a father and daughter separated in age by 35 years (PIII-2, age 48 and PIV-3, age 13) and there is also a major difference in severity of the two brothers (PIII-1 and PIII-2) at almost the same age (**Figures 5A–C**). PIII-2 has a normal extent of field with the V-4e target but a reduced extent with I-4e. In contrast, PIII-1 has just a small central island of vision remaining. Static perimetry maps of sensitivity in PIII-2 and in his daughter, PIV-3 (at ages 48 and 13, respectively), are similar. Peripheral field sensitivity (defined as loci ≥ 24° eccentricity) is far more reduced than the more central field (48° diameter) sensitivity. Both rod- and cone-mediated sensitivity follow the same general pattern across the field. Serial fields in PIV-3 spanning an interval of 14 years in the second and third decades of life show the development of superior, nasal, and inferior mid-peripheral scotomas by age 27; more function is retained temporally. Only rare loci in the periphery had detectable rod function, and the more

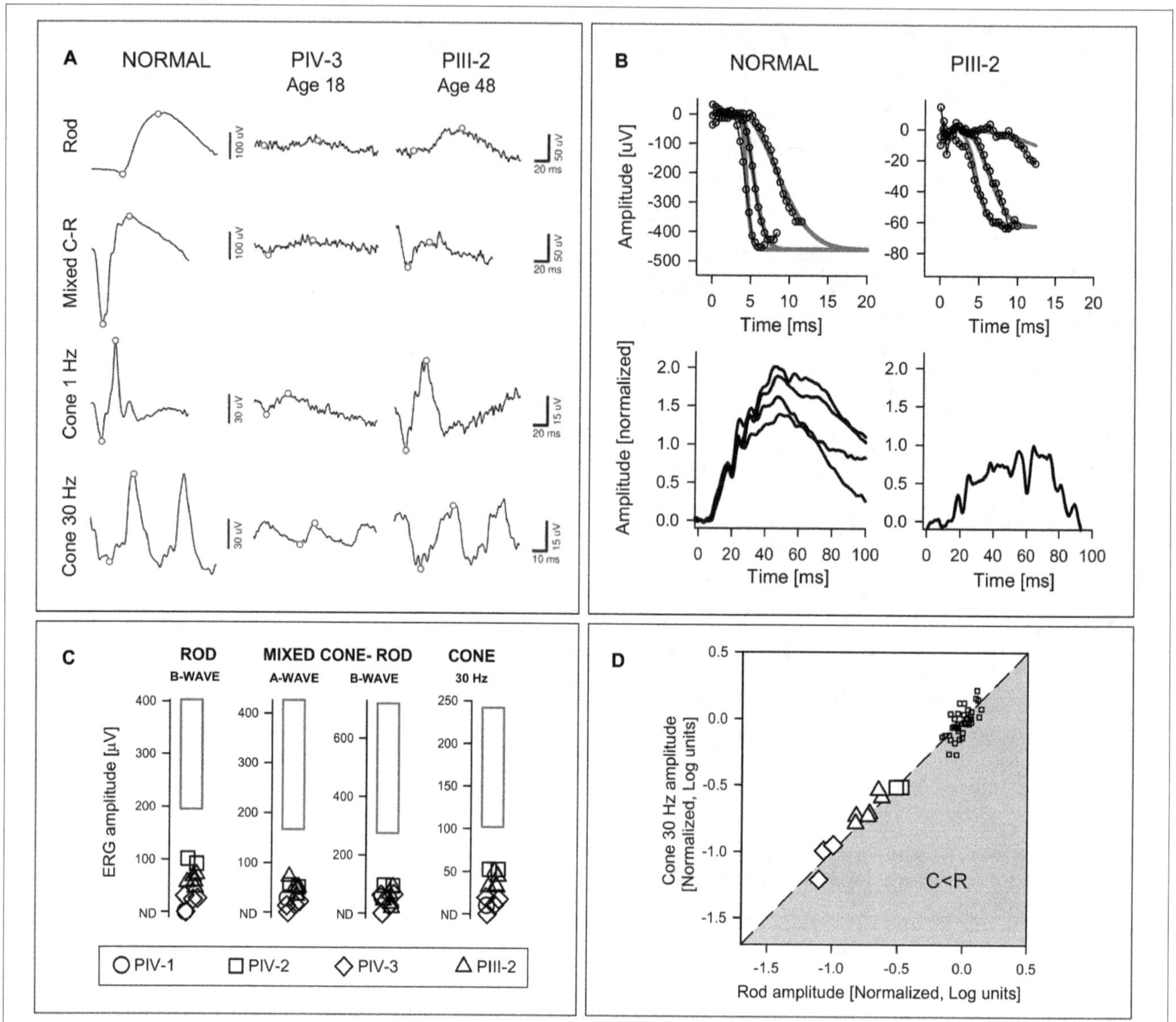

FIGURE 4 | Electroretinography in the *ARL3* family members. **(A)** Rod, mixed (maximum white flash) cone-rod (C-R), and cone ERGs from a subject with normal vision, PIV-3 (age 18) and PIII-2 (age 48). Note the different vertical scales for Normal and Patients. There are larger amplitudes, albeit abnormal, in the father (PIII-2) and the mixed C-R waveform is "negative." **(B)** P2 and P3 component analyses of rod-isolated ERG photoresponses. (Upper) Rod-isolated a-waves to different stimulus intensities in a normal subject and PIII-2. The smooth curves represent a family of functions describing phototransduction activation best fit to the leading edges of the intensity series. (Lower) Normalized rod P2 components in response to the 3.9 log scot·td·s intensity stimulus in four normal subjects, and in PIII-2. **(C)** ERG results from four family members compared with normal limits (rectangle: ±2SD from the mean). **(D)** Relationship of rod b-wave amplitude to cone flicker amplitude. Amplitudes are normalized to mean normal values and expressed in log units. Line describes equal reduction of rod and cone amplitudes; gray zone represents greater cone than rod amplitude reduction (C < R). Patient data are larger symbols and small squares are data from normal subjects for comparison.

central (superior-temporal quadrant only) loci had further reduction in sensitivity compared to the results at the earlier age. Cone sensitivity in the periphery was mainly not detectable; centrally, a few loci (superior-temporally) had detectable but reduced function.

Consistent with the results of the larger field sensitivity maps, rod-, and cone-mediated function could be at the lower limit of normal across a relatively wide expanse of the central field (**Figures 5D–G**). This is illustrated in the dark-adapted two-color horizontal profiles of PIII-2 at age 48 (**Figure 5D**), and his two daughters (PIV-2 and PIV-3) who are ~30 years younger (**Figures 5E,F**). Disease progression in PIV-3 over 14 years (**Figure 5F**) is notable; nasal field rod function becomes barely detectable, and there is reduction at and near the foveal locus. Patches of rod function remain on both nasal and temporal sides of the optic nerve head. PIV-1, another sister, has greater rod losses at a comparable age to PIV-2 and PIV-3 and progression is notable over the next 3 years. Rod-and mixed-mediated loci lose sufficient rod function to become mostly cone-mediated (**Figure 5G**).

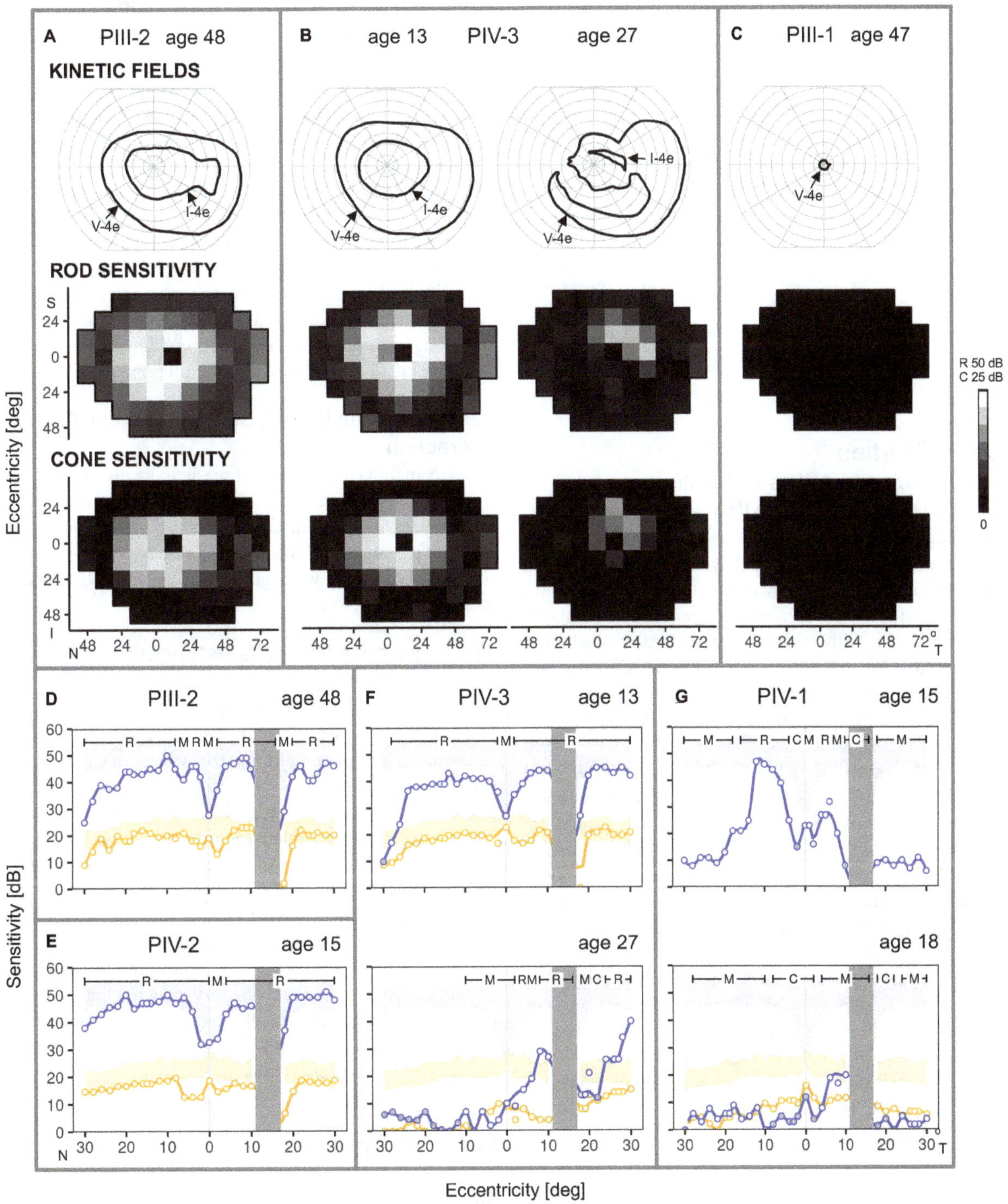

FIGURE 5 | Kinetic and chromatic static perimetry in the family members. **(A)** Full kinetic fields to V-4e but reduced to I-4e test targets in PIII-2 at age 48. Static perimetry shows rod and cone sensitivity is mildly reduced in a large region of central field but there is greater peripheral reduction. **(B)** Serial maps in PIV-3 at age 13 are comparable in pattern to those of PIII-2, but over the subsequent 14 years, there is loss of function in regions of the central field. **(C)** PIII-1, at a similar age to the sibling, PIII-2, has only a small residual central island of vision. **(D–G)** Rod and cone perimetric profiles across the horizontal meridian provide more detail of the central function. **(D,E)** PIII-2 and PIV-2, despite different ages at the visit, show rod and cone sensitivities at the lower limit of normal for most of the central 50°, but there is a decline of function at greater eccentricities. **(F)** PIV-3, at ages 13 and 27, show a sequence of change from central field rod and cone sensitivities at the lower limit of normal to loss of rod and cone function extending from the fovea into the nasal field but some retained peripapillary sensitivities. **(G)** PIV-1 from ages 15–18 shows impaired rod function at the earlier age to barely measurable rod function at the later age. Cone sensitivity was measured at age 18 only and it was abnormally reduced across the horizontal meridian. Blue: 500 nm target, dark-adapted; orange: 600 nm, light-adapted (10 cd.m^{-2} white background); N, nasal; T, temporal; S, superior; I, inferior visual field; R, C, M, rod-, cone- and mixed (rod and cone) -mediated. Shaded areas: normal range (±2SD).

TABLE 2 | Annotations of p.Asp67Val variant in *ARL3*.

Feature	Prediction
MAF(ExAC_NFE)	Not observed
CADD score	32
PolyPhen prediction	Damaging
SHIFT prediction	Damaging
LRT prediction	Damaging
MutationTaster prediction	Damaging
MutationAssessor prediction	Harmful
FATHMM prediction	Damaging
PROVEAN prediction	Damaging
MetaSVM prediction	Damaging
MetaLR prediction	Damaging

Molecular Studies

Exome Sequencing Identifies *ARL3* Missense Mutation Segregating With the IRD

Exome sequencing of the proband, PIV-1, identified a total of 573 variants in the 271 RetNet genes. After selecting heterozygous variants consistent with the autosomal dominant pattern observed in the family, we retained 288 variants in 118 genes associated with retinal diseases. After excluding the variants that did not meet our filtering criteria (see section "Materials and Methods") (**Figure 1**), we identified three variants: ARL3:NM_004311:exon3:c.A200T:p.D67V, TRPM1:NM_001252020:exon17:c.G2200C:p.A734P, and ALMS1:NM_015120:exon11: c.C9712T:p.R3238C. We deemed the Asp67Val variant in *ARL3* as most likely the causal mutation as this variant was never observed in the normal population and was predicted to be pathogenic across all prediction algorithms (SIFT, PolyPhen2-HDIV, PolyPhen2-HVAR, LRT, MutationTaster, MutationAssessor, FATHMM, MetaSVM, and MetaLR) (**Table 2**). Additionally, this variant also had high CADD score of 32. The variant in *ALMS1* was predicted to be not pathogenic across multiple predictors and had a low CADD score. Additionally, dominant mutations are not associated with the *ALMS1* and *TRPM1* genes. *ALMS1* mutations cause autosomal recessive Alström syndrome whereas *TRPM1* mutations are associated with recessive congenital stationary night blindness. Thus, we did not pursue these variants for further investigations.

ARL3 Missense Variant Segregates With the Disease Phenotype

We performed Sanger sequencing to confirm the p.Asp67Val variant in the proband. To further strengthen the evidence of *ARL3* being the causal gene, we obtained samples from five additional family members of which four were affected and one was unaffected. Sanger sequencing analysis showed that the rare heterozygous variant was segregating with the disease phenotype in the family and was absent from the unaffected member (**Figure 2B**).

ARL3 Missense Variant Is Highly Conserved

Multi-species comparisons of genetic variants are a powerful tool for accessing their functional relevance. Thus, we used multi-species alignment from the UCSC genome browser to evaluate the conservation of D67 residue in *ARL3*. The *ARL3* D67 residue is highly conserved across human, rhesus, mouse, dog, elephant, chicken, X_tropicalis, and zebrafish at the amino acid and nucleotide levels (**Figure 6**). D67 is also conserved in ARL1 and ARL2 (data not shown). Protein coding sequences are highly functionally constrained and thus change very slowly during evolution. The conservation of Asp67 residue across species that diverged from a common ancestor around 40–80 million years ago, such as humans and mice, suggest that this variant is functionally important and mutation/alteration at this position will have an adverse effect on gene function.

ARL3 Missense Variant Disrupts Protein–Protein Interaction

In silico analysis of p.Asp67Val predicted a decrease in the ARL3 interactions with three of its interactors, RP2, ARL13B, and UNC119A. All three interactions show decreased affinity as a result of p.Asp67Val substitution (**Table 3**). We therefore predict that ARL3 mutation will significantly impair ARL3 binding with its known interactors.

ARL3 Missense Variant Is Pathogenic

We used population, computational, and segregation data as evidence in the pathogenicity analysis. Based on the guidelines for classification of pathogenic or likely pathogenic variants by Consensus Recommendation of the American College of Medical Genetics and Genomics and the Association for Molecular Pathology (Richards et al., 2015), the p.Asp67Val variant has "moderate" evidence of pathogenicity based on its absence from control subjects. Evidence of pathogenicity is "supporting" based on co-segregation with the disease in multiple affected family members in a gene known to cause the disease, multiple lines of computational evidence to support a deleterious effect on the gene or gene product (conservation and evolutionary), and patient's phenotype or family history, which is highly specific for a disease with a single genetic etiology. These observations support the conclusion that p.Asp67Val is pathogenic and causal for the IRD phenotype present in the family.

DISCUSSION

More than 270 genes have been identified as the cause of IRDs so far (Retinal Information Network, 2021). However, new gene identification has not plateaued for IRDs. A considerable number of yet unknown mutations and IRD genes remain to be identified. Here we report a novel mutation in *ARL3*, which is a ubiquitous small GTPase expressed in ciliated cells of plants and animals and is crucial for ciliogenesis and axoneme formation. The role of *ARL3* in retinal disease was first noticed when it was identified as an RP2 interacting protein (Bartolini et al., 2002; Grayson et al., 2002). Subsequent work showed that mice lacking *Arl3* exhibited photoreceptor degeneration and other ciliary

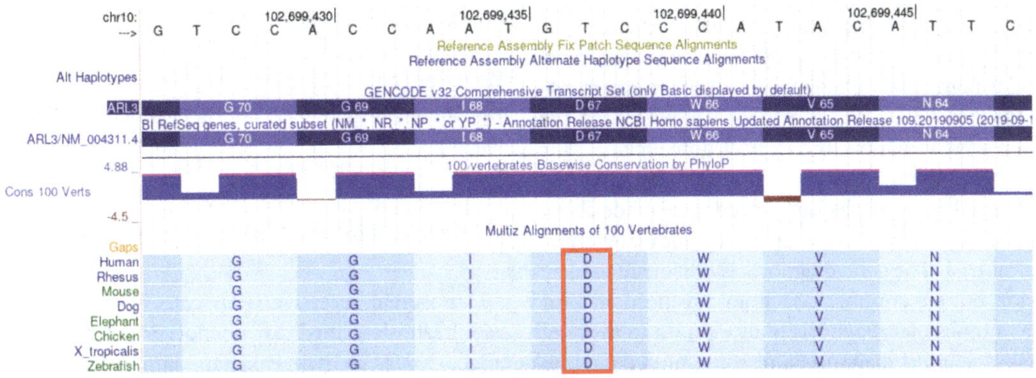

FIGURE 6 | Alignment of ARL3 amino acids surrounding the location corresponding to the D67V mutation in sequences from multiple species. The Asp (D) at residue 67 is indicated by the red rectangle and is conserved across all of the species shown, including human, rhesus, mouse, dog, elephant, chicken, X_tropicalis, and zebrafish. The sequences were aligned with use of the UCSC genome browser.

TABLE 3 | Prediction of the protein stability using mCSM-PPI2.

Protein–protein complex	PDB id	Organism	Predicted Affinity Change ($\Delta\ \Delta\ G^{Affinity}$) *kcal/mol*	mCSM-PPI2 prediction
Arl3-RP2	3BH6	*Mus musculus, Homo sapiens*	−0.534	Decreasing affinity
Arl3GppNHp-UNC119a	4GOJ	*Mus musculus, Homo sapiens*	−0.889	Decreasing affinity
Arl3-Arl13B	5DI3	*Chlamydomonas reinhardtii*	−0.356	Decreasing affinity

phenotypes affecting renal, hepatic, and pancreatic epithelial tubule structures (Schrick et al., 2006). Homozygous mutation in *ARL3* was identified as a cause of autosomal recessive Joubert syndrome, a neurodevelopmental disorder that may include retinal dystrophy, in two unrelated families (Alkanderi et al., 2018). A role for *ARL3* in non-syndromic autosomal recessive IRDs has also been reported (Sheikh et al., 2019; Fu et al., 2021). Two consanguineous Pakistani families with common ancestry both had affected members with a homozygous c.296 > T (p.Arg99Ile) variant (Sheikh et al., 2019). Novel compound heterozygous *ARL3* variants (c.91A > G, p.Thr31Ala; c.353G > T, p.Cys118Phe) were associated with IRD in a Chinese family (Fu et al., 2021).

The role of *ARL3* in dominant IRDs was first suggested based on the identification of a rare, coding heterozygous p.Tyr90Cys variant in a small family (four available members) of European Caucasian descent (Strom et al., 2016). The same variant was later reported in a Norwegian family of four (two affected and two unaffected) (Holtan et al., 2019). In both families, the variant appeared to be *de novo* in origin as the parents of the proband were homozygous for the wild-type allele. p.Tyr90Cys was predicted to be pathogenic and had low population frequency. Here, we report a different mutation in *ARL3* (p.Asp67Val) segregating in an Ashkenazi Jewish family with a dominant IRD. This variant has never been observed in the normal population and is predicted to be pathogenic across all *in silico* prediction tests. The mutation, p.Asp67Val is located in the ARL3 switch 2 region, which is involved in ARL3 conformation changes upon GDP/GTP exchange (Hanke-Gogokhia et al., 2016). The region between switch 1 and switch 2 is known as the interswitch region, which is involved in the binding of PDEδ, RP2, and UNC119 paralogs (Hanke-Gogokhia et al., 2016). Our *in silico* analyses show that substitution of Asp at position 67 is predicted to disrupt the known interactions of ARL3 with RP2, ARL13B, and UNC119A. Arl13B acts as a guanine nucleotide exchange factor for activation of Arl3 within cilia, and this interaction is needed for the release of intra-ciliary cargos (Gotthardt et al., 2015). ARL3 interaction with its effector Unc119 is critical for the allosteric release of ciliary cargo from UNC119 (Ismail et al., 2012). RP2, on the other hand, functions as a GTPase activating protein specific for ARL3 (Veltel et al., 2008), and disruption of the RP2-ARL3 interaction is likely to lead to dysregulation of the trafficking of the specific kinesin to the cilia tips. It has been also shown that constitutive activation of a dominant form of ARL3 leads to disrupted trafficking of prenylated protein trafficking in rod cells leading to progressive photoreceptor degeneration (Wright et al., 2016, 2018). Thus, we speculate that this mutation is likely to disrupt the GDP/GTP exchange, which could affect the precision at which intra-ciliary cargos are released in the photoreceptor outer segment leading to a retinal degeneration phenotype. Our results present independent genetic evidence of *ARL3* as a cause of dominant IRD.

Is there an *ARL3* retinal phenotype? Prior to the current era of molecular diagnoses, clinicians specializing in retinal degenerations agreed that it was important to subclassify IRD patients based on details of phenotype (Marmor et al., 1983; Pagon, 1988). At disease stages when rod and cone ERGs are detectable, the disorders would be labeled by degree of rod versus cone dysfunction across the retina: rod > cone (RCD, or the more general term RP) or cone > rod (CRD) dystrophies (Marmor et al., 1983). Descriptions of phenotype, however, became less rigorous as more attention was paid to genotype.

Patient symptoms of night vision disturbances (nyctalopia) and some extramacular pigmentary retinopathy by funduscopy or fundus photography tended to qualify as RP, while reduced visual acuity and macular pigmentary change without other symptoms became a diagnosis of CRD. When evidence is presented for pathogenicity of a gene mutation, the clinical nomenclature for the disease becomes incorporated into various databases. Full circle has been reached now that decisions need to be made about which patients with what disease features are candidates for a gene-based clinical trial. The gene diagnosis is obviously the key inclusion criterion but we are not at such an advanced state of therapeutics that a molecular diagnosis is all we need to proceed to a clinical trial. A clinical diagnosis and some understanding of the disease phenotype and its natural history are helpful to determine the feasibility or value (to the patient) of a trial and design its outcomes; and to decide if an animal model used for preclinical work is a faithful mimic of the human disease.

The affected family members with dominant *ARL3* p.Asp67Val in the current study manifested equal rod and cone dysfunction by ERG (**Figure 4D**; Yagasaki and Jacobson, 1989), maculopathy in the form of bull's eye changes even at early stages, and late stage loss of macular and peripheral vision with retina-wide pigmentary retinopathy. Bull's eye maculopathy is not specific and has been associated with toxic disorders as well as IRDs but especially cone dystrophy and CRD (Krill, 1977; Michaelides et al., 2007; Thiadens et al., 2012). One family member had a negative ERG, suggesting inner retinal dysfunction (Audo et al., 2008); whether this human phenotypic feature relates to the finding of abnormal rod cell migration in an ARL3 murine mutant requires further study (Wright et al., 2016). Rather than tabulating or trying to describe similarities and differences between the ARL3 phenotype and the extensive list of genetically defined diseases now known to cause IRDs (e.g., see Verbakel et al., 2018; **Table 2**), we compared disease features with those previously reported as associated with *ARL3* mutations. In one dominant family with the p.Tyr90Cys *ARL3* variant (Strom et al., 2016), the mother at age 58 years had modest acuity reduction (20/60 and 20/80). Fundi were described as having "classic" midperipheral pigmentation. A 27-year-old daughter had reduced visual acuities of 20/80 and 20/60. Fundi were said to have "bone-spicules" in the periphery. A 30-year-old son had near normal acuities (20/20, 20/25) and cystoid macular edema. Both siblings were said to have peripheral vision losses. No ERG results or fundus images were shown. The disease was discussed as RP but the main focus of the report was the association of this IRD with the *ARL3* variant. The limited phenotypic data make it difficult to compare these 3 patients with those of the family we report herein.

In the second dominant p.Tyr90Cys family, an affected male member recalled nyctalopia in the first decade of life and 20/80 acuities at age 38, further reducing to 20/125, 20/200 at age 52. The ERG at age 39 was reported as not detectable. Retina-wide pigmentary retinopathy was present at age 57. Central atrophy was present by multiple imaging modalities. The affected son had modestly reduced acuities at age 16 (20/32 and 20/50); a rod ERG was not detectable and cone ERGs were reported to be reduced. Pigmentary retinopathy was shown on fundus photographs, and there was central atrophy by OCT and autofluorescence imaging. Macular atrophy in both family members at early and later stages accompanies the retina-wide pigmentary retinopathy. This is neither "typical RP" nor clearly CRD. The disease expression with peripheral retinal degeneration and maculopathy is interestingly similar to that in *ARL3* family members of the current study.

Autosomal recessive IRDs caused by *ARL3* mutations have also been described by phenotype (Sheikh et al., 2019; Fu et al., 2021). In two Pakistani families that shared the same homozygous pathogenic *ARL3* variant (p.Arg99Ile; Sheikh et al., 2019), there was imaging evidence of maculopathy (whether atrophy or bull's eye changes) in the second to the fourth decades of life and reduced acuities. Visual fields are reported as not showing peripheral vision loss, but no details are provided. It is not clear if color vision is affected—textual reference is made to it being normal but a table indicates abnormalities in some patients. ERGs, albeit using skin electrodes leading to a limited range of amplitude (Bradshaw et al., 2004), had a rod and cone signal relationship that suggested cone > rod dysfunction, unlike the equal cone and rod ERG dysfunction in the present study. From the information provided, the disease expression due to this homozygous *ARL3* variant may be that of a CRD or a maculopathy in these myopic patients. The proband of the Chinese family with a compound *ARL3* heterozygote (p.Thr31Ala, p.Cys118Phe; age 19, male) had reduced acuities and color vision abnormalities. Visual fields are reported as a "tunnel" but only midperipheral fields are shown: a superior temporal abnormality corresponds to the pigmentary changes in the inferior nasal retina. The ERGs are not readily interpretable as shown (without normal data for reference) but are said to be reduced for rod and cone responses. OCTs have abnormalities in outer retinal layers, but there appears to be a well-preserved outer nuclear layer in the scans. The heterozygous father (p.Thr31Ala), the only other family member with a phenotype, is described as having normal visual acuity, a central scotoma, color vision abnormalities, OCT with foveal area preservation but para- and peri-central outer retinal layer abnormalities, and possibly a bull's eye maculopathy ("circular degeneration around macular fovea"; Fu et al., 2021). Both family members seem to show a widespread rod and cone degeneration with different severities.

A conclusion from our report taken together with the other published data of *ARL3* disease is that both rod and cone photoreceptors are affected across the retina and maculopathy tends to be present even at early stages. Forcing the phenotype into a simplified binary clinical classification of RCD (RP) versus CRD may only lead to another molecular disease being labeled as showing phenotypic variability. A more general description for now should open the door for more detailed observations in future patients identified with non-syndromic *ARL3* mutations.

ETHICS STATEMENT

The studies involving human participants were reviewed and approved by the University of Pennsylvania. Written informed consent to participate in this study was provided by the participants or the participants' legal guardian/next of kin. Written informed consent was obtained from the individual(s), and minor(s)' legal guardian/next of kin, for the publication of any potentially identifiable images or data included in this article.

AUTHOR CONTRIBUTIONS

SJ and AC designed and supervised the clinical aspects of the study. RR, ME, and ASw performed and interpreted the molecular results. AR, ASu, and RS analyzed and managed the data from phenotyping. All authors contributed to the article and approved the submitted version.

REFERENCES

Aleman, T. S., Soumittra, N., Cideciyan, A. V., Sumaroka, A. M., Ramprasad, V. L., Herrera, W., et al. (2009). CERKL mutations cause an autosomal recessive cone-rod dystrophy with inner retinopathy. *Invest. Ophthalmol. Vis. Sci.* 50, 5944–5954. doi: 10.1167/iovs.09-3982

Alkanderi, S., Molinari, E., Shaheen, R., Elmaghloob, Y., Stephen, L. A., Sammut, V., et al. (2018). ARL3 mutations cause joubert syndrome by disrupting ciliary protein composition. *Am. J. Hum. Genet.* 103, 612–620. doi: 10.1016/j.ajhg.2018.08.015

Audo, I., Robson, A. G., Holder, G. E,, and Moore, A. T. (2008). The negative ERG: clinical phenotypes and disease mechanisms of inner retinal dysfunction. *Surv. Ophthalmol.* 53, 16–40. doi: 10.1016/j.survophthal.2007.10.010

Azari, A. A., Aleman, T. S., Cideciyan, A. V., Schwartz, S. B., Windsor, E. A., Sumaroka, A., et al. (2006). Retinal disease expression in bardet-biedl syndrome-1 (BBS1) is a spectrum from maculopathy to retina-wide degeneration. *Invest. Ophthalmol. Vis. Sci.* 47, 5004–5010. doi: 10.1167/iovs.06-0517

Bartolini, F., Bhamidipati, A., Thomas, S., Schwahn, U., Lewis, S. A., and Cowan, N. J. (2002). Functional overlap between retinitis pigmentosa 2 protein and the tubulin-specific chaperone cofactor C. *J. Biol. Chem.* 277, 14629–14634. doi: 10.1074/jbc.M200128200

Beryozkin, A., Shevah, E., Kimchi, A., Mizrahi-Meissonnier, L., Khateb, S., Ratnapriya, R., et al. (2015). Whole exome sequencing reveals mutations in known retinal disease genes in 33 out of 68 Israeli families with inherited retinopathies. *Sci. Rep.* 5:13187. doi: 10.1038/srep13187

Birtel, J., Gliem, M., Mangold, E., Müller, P. L., Holz, F. G., Neuhaus, C., et al. (2018). Next-generation sequencing identifies unexpected genotype-phenotype correlations in patients with retinitis pigmentosa. *PloS One* 13:e0207958. doi: 10.1371/journal.pone.0207958

Bolger, A. M., Lohse, M., and Usadel, B. (2014). Trimmomatic: a flexible trimmer for illumina sequence data. *Bioinformatics* 30, 2114–2120. doi: 10.1093/bioinformatics/btu170

Booij, J. C., Bakker, A., Kulumbetova, J., Moutaoukil, Y., Smeets, B., Verheij, J., et al. (2011). Simultaneous mutation detection in 90 retinal disease genes in multiple patients using a custom-designed 300-kb retinal resequencing chip. *Ophthalmology* 118, 160–167. doi: 10.1016/j.ophtha.2010.04.022

Bradshaw, K., Hansen, R., and Fulton, A. (2004). Comparison of ERGs recorded with skin and corneal-contact electrodes in normal children and adults. *Doc. Ophthalmol.* 109, 43–55. doi: 10.1007/s10633-004-1751-3

Bramall, A. N., Wright, A. F., Jacobson, S. G., and McInnes, R. R. (2010). The genomic, biochemical, and cellular responses of the retina in inherited photoreceptor degenerations and prospects for the treatment of these disorders. *Ann. Rev. Neurosci.* 33, 441–472. doi: 10.1146/annurev-neuro-060909-153227

Cideciyan, A. V. (2000). In vivo assessment of photoreceptor function in human diseases caused by photoreceptor-specific gene mutations. *Methods Enzymol.* 316, 611–626. doi: 10.1016/s0076-6879(00)16753-9

Cideciyan, A. V., and Jacobson, S. G. (1993). Negative electroretinograms in retinitis pigmentosa. *Invest. Ophthalmol. Vis. Sci.* 34, 3253–3263.

Cideciyan, A. V., and Jacobson, S. G. (1996). An alternative phototransduction model for human rod and cone ERG a-waves: normal parameters and variation with age. *Vision Res.* 36, 2609–2621. doi: 10.1016/0042-6989(95)00327-4

DePristo, M. A., Banks, E., Poplin, R., Garimella, K. V., Maguire, J. R., Hartl, C., et al. (2011). A framework for variation discovery and genotyping using next-generation DNA sequencing data. *Nat. Genet.* 43, 491–498. doi: 10.1038/ng.806

Evans, R. J., Schwarz, N., Nagel-Wolfrum, K., Wolfrum, U., Hardcastle, A. J., and Cheetham, M. E. (2010). The retinitis pigmentosa protein RP2 links pericentriolar vesicle transport between the Golgi and the primary cilium. *Hum. Mol. Genet.* 19, 1358–1367. doi: 10.1093/hmg/ddq012

Fahim, A. T., Daiger, S. P., and Weleber, R. G. (2000). "Nonsyndromic retinitis pigmentosa overview," in *GeneReviews*, eds M. P. Adam, H. H. Ardinger, R. A. Pagon, S. E. Wallace, L. J. H. Bean, G. Mirzaa, et al. (Seattle, WA: University of Washington).

Frederick, J. M., Hanke-Gogokhia, C., Ying, G., and Baehr, W. (2020). Diffuse or hitch a ride: how photoreceptor lipidated proteins get from here to there. *Biol. Chem.* 401, 573–584. doi: 10.1515/hsz-2019-0375

Fu, L., Li, Y., Yao, S., Guo, Q., You, Y., Zhu, X., et al. (2021). Autosomal recessive rod-cone dystrophy associated with compound heterozygous variants in ARL3 gene. *Front. Cell Dev. Biol.* 9:635424. doi: 10.3389/fcell.2021.635424

Garafalo, A. V., Cideciyan, A. V., Héon, E., Sheplock, R., Pearson, A., WeiYang Yu, C., et al. (2020). Progress in treating inherited retinal diseases: early subretinal gene therapy clinical trials and candidates for future initiatives. *Prog. Retin. Eye Res.* 77:100827. doi: 10.1016/j.preteyeres.2019.100827

Gotthardt, K., Lokaj, M., Koerner, C., Falk, N., Gießl, A., and Wittinghofer, A. (2015). A G-protein activation cascade from Arl13B to Arl3 and implications for ciliary targeting of lipidated proteins. *Elife* 4:e11859. doi: 10.7554/eLife.11859

Grayson, C., Bartolini, F., Chapple, J. P., Willison, K. R., Bhamidipati, A., Lewis, S. A., et al. (2002). Localization in the human retina of the X-linked retinitis pigmentosa protein RP2, its homologue cofactor C and the RP2 interacting protein Arl3. *Hum. Mol. Genet.* 11, 3065–3074. doi: 10.1093/hmg/11.24.3065

Hanke-Gogokhia, C., Wu, Z., Gerstner, C. D., Frederick, J. M., Zhang, H., and Baehr, W. (2016). Arf-like protein 3 (ARL3) regulates protein trafficking and ciliogenesis in mouse photoreceptors. *J. Biol. Chem.* 291, 7142–7155. doi: 10.1074/jbc.M115.710954

Hejtmancik, J. F., and Daiger, S. P. (2020). Understanding the genetic architecture of human retinal degenerations. *Proc. Natl. Acad. Sci. U.S.A.* 117, 3904–3906. doi: 10.1073/pnas.1922925117

Holtan, J. P., Teigen, K., Aukrust, I., Bragadóttir, R., and Houge, G. (2019). Dominant ARL3-related retinitis pigmentosa. *Ophthalmic Genet.* 40, 124–128. doi: 10.1080/13816810.2019.1586965

Ismail, S., Chen, Y.-X., Miertzschke, M., Vetter, I. R., Koerner, C., and Wittinghofer, A. (2012). Structural basis for Arl3-specific release of myristoylated ciliary cargo from UNC119. *EMBO J.* 31, 4085–4094. doi: 10.1038/emboj.2012.257

Jacobson, S. G., Cideciyan, A. V., Aleman, T. S., Pianta, M. J., Sumaroka, A., Schwartz, S. B., et al. (2003). Crumbs homolog 1 (CRB1) mutations result in a thick human retina with abnormal lamination. *Hum. Mol. Genet.* 12, 1073–1078. doi: 10.1093/hmg/ddg117

Jacobson, S. G., Voigt, W. J., Parel, J. M., Apáthy, P. P., Nghiem-Phu, L., Myers, S. W., et al. (1986). Automated light- and dark-adapted perimetry for evaluating retinitis pigmentosa. *Ophthalmology* 93, 1604–1611. doi: 10.1016/s0161-6420(86)33522-x

Jacobson, S. G., Yagasaki, K., Feuer, W. J., and Roman, A. J. (1989). Interocular asymmetry of visual function in heterozygotes of X-linked retinitis pigmentosa. *Exp. Eye Res.* 48, 679–691. doi: 10.1016/0014-4835(89)90009-2

Krill, A. E. (1977). *Krill's Hereditary Retinal and Choroidal Diseases*, Vol. 2. Hagerstown, MD: Harper.

Kruczek, K., Qu, Z., Gentry, J., Fadl, B. R., Gieser, L., Hiriyanna, S., et al. (2021). Gene therapy of dominant CRX-Leber congenital amaurosis using patient stem cell-derived retinal organoids. *Stem Cell Rep.* 16, 252–263. doi: 10.1016/j.stemcr.2020.12.018

Kruczek, K., and Swaroop, A. (2020). Pluripotent stem cell-derived retinal organoids for disease modeling and development of therapies. *Stem Cells* 38, 1206–1215. doi: 10.1002/stem.3239

Marmor, M. F., Aguirre, G., Arden, G., Berson, E., Birch, D. G., Boughman, J. A., et al. (1983). Retinitis pigmentosa: a symposium on terminology and methods of examination. *Ophthalmology* 90, 126–131.

Michaelides, M., Chen, L. L., Brantley, M. A. Jr., Andorf, J. L., Isaak, E. M., Jenkins, S. A., et al. (2007). ABCA4 mutations and discordant ABCA4 alleles in patients and siblings with bull's-eye maculopathy. *Br. J. Ophthalmol.* 91, 1650–1655. doi: 10.1136/bjo.2007.118356

O'Sullivan, J., Mullaney, B. G., Bhaskar, S. S., Dickerson, J. E., Hall, G., O'Grady, A., et al. (2012). A paradigm shift in the delivery of services for diagnosis of inherited retinal disease. *J. Med. Genet.* 49, 322–326. doi: 10.1136/jmedgenet-2012-100847

Pagon, R. A. (1988). Retinitis pigmentosa. *Surv. Ophthalmol.* 33, 133–177.

Ratnapriya, R., and Swaroop, A. (2013). Genetic architecture of retinal and macular degenerative diseases: the promise and challenges of next-generation sequencing. *Genome Med.* 5:84.

Retinal Information Network (2021). *RetNet, the Retinal Information Network.* Available online at: https://sph.uth.edu/RetNet/ (Accessed July 1, 2020).

Richards, S., Aziz, N., Bale, S., Bick, D., Das, S., Gastier-Foster, J., et al. (2015). Standards and guidelines for the interpretation of sequence variants: a joint consensus recommendation of the american college of medical genetics and genomics and the association for molecular pathology. *Genet. Med.* 17, 405–424. doi: 10.1038/gim.2015.30

Roberts, L., Ratnapriya, R., du Plessis, M., Chaitankar, V., Ramesar, R. S., and Swaroop, A. (2016). Molecular diagnosis of inherited retinal diseases in indigenous African populations by whole-exome sequencing. *Invest. Ophthalmol. Vis. Sci.* 57, 6374–6381. doi: 10.1167/iovs.16-19785

Rodrigues, C. H. M., Myung, Y., Pires, D. E. V., and Ascher, D. B. (2019). MCSM-PPI2: predicting the effects of mutations on protein-protein interactions. *Nucleic Acids Res.* 47, W338–W344. doi: 10.1093/nar/gkz383

Roman, A. J., Schwartz, S. B., Aleman, T. S., Cideciyan, A. V., Chico, J. D., Windsor, E. A., et al. (2005). Quantifying rod photoreceptor-mediated vision in retinal degenerations: dark-adapted thresholds as outcome measures. *Exp. Eye Res.* 80, 259–272. doi: 10.1016/j.exer.2004.09.00

Sánchez-Bellver, L., Toulis, V., and Marfany, G. (2021). On the wrong track: alterations of ciliary transport in inherited retinal dystrophies. *Front. Cell Dev. Biol.* 9:623734. doi: 10.3389/fcell.2021.623734

Schrick, J. J., Vogel, P., Abuin, A., Hampton, B., and Rice, D. S. (2006). ADP-ribosylation factor-like 3 is involved in kidney and photoreceptor development. *Am. J. Pathol.* 168, 1288–1298. doi: 10.2353/ajpath.2006.050941

Schwarz, N., Hardcastle, A. J., and Cheetham, M. E. (2012). Arl3 and RP2 mediated assembly and traffic of membrane associated cilia proteins. *Vision Res.* 75, 2–4. doi: 10.1016/j.visres.2012.07.016

Sheikh, S. A., Sisk, R. A., Schiavon, C. R., Waryah, Y. M., Usmani, M. A., Steel, D. H., et al. (2019). Homozygous variant in ARL3 causes autosomal recessive cone rod dystrophy. *Invest. Ophthalmol. Vis. Sci.* 60, 4811–4819. doi: 10.1167/iovs.19-27263

Strom, S. P., Clark, M. J., Martinez, A., Garcia, S., Abelazeem, A. A., Matynia, A., et al. (2016). De novo occurrence of a variant in ARL3 and apparent autosomal dominant transmission of retinitis pigmentosa. *PLoS One* 11:e0150944. doi: 10.1371/journal.pone.0150944

Sudharsan, R., and Beltran, W. A. (2019). Progress in gene therapy for rhodopsin autosomal dominant retinitis pigmentosa. *Adv. Exp. Med. Biol.* 1185, 113–118. doi: 10.1007/978-3-030-27378-1_19

Sumaroka, A., Cideciyan, A. V., Charng, J., Wu, V., Powers, C. A., Iyer, B. S., et al. (2019). Autosomal dominant retinitis pigmentosa due to class B *Rhodopsin* mutations: an objective outcome for future treatment trials. *Int. J. Mol. Sci.* 20:5344. doi: 10.3390/ijms20215344

Thiadens, A. A., Phan, T. M., Zekveld-Vroon, R. C., Leroy, B. P., van den Born, L. I., Hoyng, C. B., et al. (2012). Clinical course, genetic etiology, and visual outcome in cone and cone-rod dystrophy. *Ophthalmology* 119, 819–826. doi: 10.1016/j.ophtha.2011.10.011

Veltel, S., Gasper, R., Eisenacher, E., and Wittinghofer, A. (2008). The retinitis pigmentosa 2 gene product is a GTPase-activating protein for arf-like 3. *Nat. Struct. Mol. Biol.* 15, 373–380. doi: 10.1038/nsmb.1396

Verbakel, S. K., van Huet, R., Boon, C., den Hollander, A. I., Collin, R., Klaver, C., et al. (2018). Non-syndromic retinitis pigmentosa. *Prog. Retin. Eye Res.* 66, 157–186. doi: 10.1016/j.preteyeres.2018.03.005

Wang, K., Li, M., and Hakonarson, H. (2010). ANNOVAR: functional annotation of genetic variants from high-throughput sequencing data. *Nucleic Acids Res.* 38:e164. doi: 10.1093/nar/gkq603

Wright, A. F., Chakarova, C. F., Abd El-Aziz, M. M., and Bhattacharya, S. S. (2010). Photoreceptor degeneration: genetic and mechanistic dissection of a complex trait. *Nat. Rev. Genet.* 11, 273–284. doi: 10.1038/nrg2717

Wright, Z. C., Loskutov, Y., Murphy, D., Stoilov, P., Pugacheva, E., Goldberg, A. F. X., et al. (2018). ADP-ribosylation factor-like 2 (ARL2) regulates cilia stability and development of outer segments in rod photoreceptor neurons. *Sci. Rep.* 8:16967.

Wright, Z. C., Singh, R. K., Alpino, R., Goldberg, A. F., Sokolov, M., and Ramamurthy, V. (2016). ARL3 regulates trafficking of prenylated phototransduction proteins to the rod outer segment. *Hum. Mol. Genet.* 25, 2031–2044. doi: 10.1093/hmg/ddw077

Yagasaki, K., and Jacobson, S. G. (1989). Cone-rod dystrophy. phenotypic diversity by retinal function testing. *Arch. Ophthalmol.* 107, 701–708. doi: 10.1001/archopht.1989.01070010719034

13

Variant Profiling of a Large Cohort of 138 Chinese Families With Autosomal Dominant Retinitis Pigmentosa

Ting Xiao†, Yue Xie†, Xin Zhang, Ke Xu, Xiaohui Zhang, Zi-Bing Jin and Yang Li**

Beijing Ophthalmology & Visual Sciences Key Lab, Beijing Tongren Eye Center, Beijing Institute of Ophthalmology, Beijing Tongren Hospital, Capital Medical University, Beijing, China

***Correspondence:**
Zi-Bing Jin
jinzb502@ccmu.edu.cn
Yang Li
yanglibio@aliyun.com

†These authors have contributed equally to this work

Retinitis pigmentosa (RP) is the most common form of inherited retinal dystrophy, and 15–25% of RP is transmitted as an autosomal dominant (ad) trait. The objectives of this study were to establish the variant profile in a large cohort of adRP families and to elucidate the variant spectrum of each adRP gene in Chinese patients. A total of 138 probands clinically diagnosed with RP as a presumed autosomal dominant trait were recruited. All probands underwent ophthalmic examinations by specialists. A combination of molecular screening methods, including targeted next-generation sequencing, Sanger DNA sequencing, and multiplex ligation probe amplification assay, was used to detect variants. We identified heterozygous variants of 11 adRP genes in 73 probands, hemizygous, or heterozygous variants of X-linked RP genes in six patients, compound heterozygous variants of autosomal recessive RP genes in three pseudodominant families, and one heterozygous variant of one ad cone and rod dystrophy gene in one proband. One proband was found carrying both variants in *RPGR* and *FAM161A*. The overall detection rate was 59.4% (82/138). We detected 72 distinct disease-causing variants involving 16 RP genes and one cone-rod dystrophy gene; 33 of these variants have not been reported previously. Disease-causing variants were identified in the adRP genes in 52.9% of the families, followed by 4.3% in the X-linked RP genes, and 2.2% in the autosomal recessive genes. The most frequent mutant genes were *RHO*, *PRPF31*, *RP1*, *SNRNP200*, and *PRPF8*, which explained up to 78.0% of the genetically diagnosed families. Most of the variants identified in adRP genes were missense, and copy number variations were common (7/20) in the *PRPF31* gene. We established the profile of the mutated genes and the variant spectrum of adRP genes in a large cohort of Chinese patients, providing essential information for genetic counseling and future development of therapeutics for retinal dystrophy inherited as a dominant trait.

Keywords: autosomal dominant retinitis pigmentosa, next-generation sequencing, diseasing-causing variant, copy number variation, variant profile

INTRODUCTION

Retinitis pigmentosa (RP) is the most common form of inherited retinal dystrophy (IRD), with a prevalence of about 1 in 4,000 (Ayuso and Millan, 2010). RP is a progressive disorder characterized by initial degeneration of rod photoreceptors, followed by degeneration of cone cells (Ayuso and Millan, 2010). Clinical features include night blindness (usually occurring in adolescence), progressive defects of the peripheral visual field, and ultimately, severe damage to central visual acuity (Ayuso and Millan, 2010; Daiger et al., 2014a). The typical fundus appearance consists of black bone-spicule pigmentation in the midperipheral retina, attenuated retinal arterioles, and a pale optic disc. Electroretinograms (ERGs) present reduced or non-recordable signals (Ayuso and Millan, 2010; Daiger et al., 2014a). Most RP cases (about 70–80%) are non-syndromic, which means that patients display only ocular dysfunction. However, some patients may present highly variable clinical symptoms and progression, even if they come from the same family (Ayuso and Millan, 2010).

RP is a highly genetically heterogeneous disorder and can be transmitted in an autosomal recessive (ar), an autosomal dominant (ad), or an X-linked recessive pattern (xl) (Ayuso and Millan, 2010; Daiger et al., 2014a). Digenic inheritance has been reported in some rare cases (Ayuso and Millan, 2010). Autosomal dominant RP (adRP) accounts for about 15–25% of the total RP cases (Daiger et al., 2014a). At present, 30 causative genes have been identified for adRP (RetNet: https://sph.uth.edu/retnet/home.htm), and more than 1,000 different kinds of variants have been described in those genes (Daiger et al., 2014a; Dias et al., 2018). The most commonly mutated gene is *RHO*, which is responsible for ~20–30% of adRP cases (Daiger et al., 2014a; Dias et al., 2018). Most of the detected variants in the adRP genes are private variants, and a small fraction of the common variants are ethnicity specific; for example, the *RHO* variant p.(P23H) is a founder variant almost exclusively described in Americans of European origin (Sullivan et al., 2013; Daiger et al., 2014a,b; Dias et al., 2018). Copy number variants (CNVs) have also been reported in some adRP genes, and incomplete penetrance has been observed in some specific genes (Sullivan et al., 2013; Daiger et al., 2014a,b; Dias et al., 2018). Taken together, these findings for adRP increase the complexity of its genetic diagnosis, which is very crucial for genetic consulting and gene therapy in patients with this disorder.

In recent years, the application of next-generation sequencing (NGS), mostly as targeted exome sequencing (TES) and whole exome sequencing (WES), has greatly increased the genetic diagnosis rates of different form of IRD (Daiger et al., 2014b; Xu et al., 2014; Costa et al., 2017; Van Cauwenbergh et al., 2017; Martin-Merida et al., 2018; Gao et al., 2019). The profile of mutated genes and the variant spectrum of adRP genes have been established in European and American patients with variant detection rates between 50 and 75% (Daiger et al., 2014b; Costa et al., 2017; Van Cauwenbergh et al., 2017; Martin-Merida et al., 2018). One very recent study that reported genetic analysis using TES in a large cohort of Chinese patients has shown that 72% of the patients could receive a molecular diagnosis (Gao et al., 2019). However, the large cohort included several other IRD cases, such as Bietti crystalline retinopathy, Leber congenital amaurosis, and retinitis punctata albescens, and it did not report the gene profiles for adRP patients (Gao et al., 2019). Several previous studies have reported the gene profiles in the relatively small Chinese adRP cohort (not more than 78 families) (Li et al., 2010; Xu et al., 2014; Huang et al., 2017).

In the current study, we have described the outcomes of a comprehensive molecular analysis of 138 pedigrees with possible adRP by a combination of methods, including TES, Sanger sequencing, and real-time quantitative polymerase chain reaction (q-PCR) analysis or multiplex ligation-dependent probe amplifications (MLPAs).

SUBJECTS AND METHODS

Patients

In total, 138 unrelated families with a clinical diagnosis of RP were enrolled at the Genetics Laboratory of the Beijing Institute of Ophthalmology, Beijing Tongren Ophthalmic Center. Dominant inheritance was presumed when each family had affected members in at least two consecutive generations. This cohort included four previously reported families (Pan et al., 2012; Dong et al., 2013). Patients were diagnosed with RP based on the following criteria: a history of night blindness, progressive visual field defects, fundus displaying bone spicule-like pigment clumping in the midperipheral or peripheral retina and attenuation of retinal vessels, and severe rod-cone dysfunction or non-recordable ERG recording (Ayuso and Millan, 2010). The molecular testing processes were prospectively evaluated and approved by the ethics committee of Beijing Tongren Hospital, and all tests were implemented under the official guidelines of the Beijing Tongren Hospital Joint Committee on Clinical Investigation in compliance with the Declaration of Helsinki. Informed consent was obtained from probands after a detailed explanation of the processes.

Each proband and available family members underwent a regular ophthalmic examination that included best-corrected visual acuity, slit-lamp biomicroscopy, and a fundus examination. Most participants also underwent optical coherence tomography, visual field, and ERG evaluations. Peripheral blood samples were collected from patients and their family members, and genomic DNA was extracted from the leukocytes with a genomic DNA extraction and purification kit (vigorous whole-blood genomic DNA extraction kit; Vigorous Beijing, China), according to the producer's protocol.

PCR-Based Sequencing of the *RHO* Gene

Five exons and flanking splicing sites of the *RHO* gene were first sequenced for all probands diagnosed with adRP, except for the four families that we have previously reported (Pan et al., 2012; Dong et al., 2013). Those four previously reported families were analyzed by linkage mapping following Sanger sequencing (Pan et al., 2012; Dong et al., 2013). The PCR amplifications were performed with regular reaction mixtures, and the purified amplicons were sequenced on an ABI Prism 373A DNA sequencer (Applied Biosystems, Foster City, CA, USA). The sequencing outcomes were matched to the available cDNA sequence of *RHO* (GenBank NM_000539).

TES and Bioinformatics Analysis

We performed TES in 113 patients who did not carry any *RHO* variants using a capture panel developed and evaluated by our group (Sun et al., 2018). This panel comprised 188 known IRD genes, and 26 of them were adRP genes. Details of the procedures, which included the Illumina library preparation, capture experiments, and the enrichment libraries sequencing, have been described previously (Sun et al., 2018). The raw sequencing data processing, calling, and evaluation were carried out as previously reported (Sun et al., 2018). The bioinformatics programs PolyPhen2 (http://genetics.bwh.harvard.edu/pph/), Mutation Taster (http://www.mutationtaster.org/), and SIFT (http://sift.jcvi.org/) were used to predict the pathogenicity of each variant. The programs NetGene2 Server (http://www.cbs.dtu.dk/services/NetGene2/), Human Splice Finder (http://www.umd.be/HSF3/), and Berkeley Drosophila Genome Project (http://www.fruitfly.org/seq_tools/splice.html) were used to analyze any variants involving a splicing effect. We further determined the pathogenicity of each variant by searching the reported pathogenic variants in the HGMD database (http://www.hgmd.cf.ac.uk/ac/index.php) and the LOVD database (https://www.lovd.nl/). We ultimately classified the variants into pathogenic or likely pathogenic variants, variants of uncertain significance (VUS), and benign or likely benign variants according to the standards described by the American College of Medical Genetics and Genomics (ACMG) (Richards et al., 2015). Sanger sequencing was conducted to verify the supposed disease-causing variants and VUS. Segregation analysis was done for the probands and their family members.

CNV Analysis and Validation

We employed the CNV kit software (https://github.com/etal/cnvkit) to identify CNVs from variations in the read depth for the patients who had TES data (Talevich et al., 2016). Real-time q-PCR was then performed to confirm the presence of the presumed CNVs of *PRPF31* in five families and of *FAM161A* in one family, as we previously reported (Dong et al., 2013). MLPA assays were conducted for three probands and their family members using the SALSA MLPA Kit P235 (Amsterdam, the Netherlands), following the producer's protocols.

Supplementary PCR-Based Sequencing

We performed Sanger sequencing of exon 15 [open reading frame 15 (ORF15)] of *RPGR* in all male patients whose disease-causing variants were not found after TES and whose pedigrees could not exclude X-linked transmission.

Statistical Analysis

All statistical analyses were performed using SPSS statistical software (version 25.0, SPSS Inc., Chicago, IL). The Kolmogorov–Smirnov test was used to evaluate whether the onset age of a single group conformed to a normal distribution. The Wilcoxon rank sum test was used to evaluate any difference in the onset age between two groups. $P \leq 0.05$ was considered statistically significant.

RESULTS

Variant Detection Rate and Variant Spectrum

We identified heterozygous autosomal dominant variants that were pathogenic or likely pathogenic in 74 probands, hemizygous, or heterozygous in six probands, and compound heterozygous in three patients, for a general variant detection rate of 59.4% (82/138) (**Table 1**, **Figure 1A**). We found a total of 72 different variants in 17 genes, including 11 adRP genes, two xlRP genes, three arRP genes, and one autosomal dominant cone and rod dystrophy (adCORD) gene (**Figure 1**). Four of the 72 variants were identified three times or more, and the remaining 68 variants were detected either once (88.9%) or twice (5.6%). The most common variants were p.(R135W) and p.(P347L) in *RHO*, with a gene-specific allele frequency of 17.4% (4/23), followed by p.(R677*) in the *RP1* (37.5%, 3/8) and a whole *PRPF31* deletion (15.0%, 3/20) (**Supplementary Table 1**).

Of the 72 putative disease-causing variants, 33 variants were first identified in the current study (**Supplementary Table 1**). These 33 novel variants comprised 16 missense, five frameshift indel, four non-sense, three splicing effect, three CNV, one synonymous, and one stop-codon-lost variant. None of these novel variants were recorded in our in-house and any public databases, such as the Exome Variant Server and 1000 Genomes Database (**Supplementary Table 1**). The 16 novel missense variants were defined as pathogenic or likely pathogenic variants according to the ACMG guidelines and standards (**Supplementary Table 1**). One synonymous variant c.1146G>A, p.(E382E), located in the last base of the exon 11 of *PRPF31*, was predicted to alter the downstream splice effect by NetGene2, HSF, and Mutation Taster. The remaining variants (frameshift small indel, non-sense, splicing effect, and run-on variants) or CNVs were considered to be obviously pathogenic variants. Five variants of *PRPF8* were identified in this cohort, and they all were novel. These five variants contained four missense variants and one frameshift small deletion that escaped non-sense-mediated decay. Three of these variants were located in the C-terminal Jab1 domain, and the other two were in the Linker and RNAseH-like domain (**Figure 2A**). We also detected an unreported missense variant, p.(S216G), which is not located in any domains of PRPF8 (**Figure 2A**). As p.(S216G) was predicted to be benign by both Polyphen2 and SIFT, we defined this variant as a VUS according to the ACMG guidelines and standards.

Variant Profile in the adRP Genes and Related Clinical Features

The 59 putative disease-causing variants of the 11 adRP genes were identified in 73 pedigrees (52.9%, 73/138) and accounted for 89.0% (73/82) of the genetically diagnosed cases in this cohort (**Figure 1B**). Cosegregation analyses were performed in 65 pedigrees of the 73 families (**Supplementary Table 2**). The most frequently mutated gene was *RHO*, identified in 23 of the 138 probands (16.7%), followed by *PRPF31* in 20 unrelated patients (14.5%), *RP1* and *SNRNP200* each in 8 patients (5.8%), and *PRPF8* in 5 patients (3.6%) (**Figure 1A**). Variants in the pre-mRNA splicing factor genes accounted for 24.6% of the families and the variant locations in each gene are displayed in **Figure 2A**. Most of the variants in *RHO*, *SNRNP200*, *PRPF8*, and *IMPDH1* were missense variants, whereas loss-of-function variants, including non-sense, frameshift small indels, and CNVs, were more frequently observed in *PRPF31*, *RP1*, *CRX*, and *TOPORS* (**Table 2**). In the current cohort, CNVs were more

TABLE 1 | Summary of Family Composition and Variant Screening Results in 138 Chinese adRP Families.

	# Family with M to M	%	# Family without M to M	%	#Total	%
adRP gene variant	40	64.5	33	43.4	73	52.9
adCORD gene variant	1	1.6	0	0.0	1	0.7
xlRP gene variant	0	0.0	6*	7.9	6*	4.3
arRP gene variant	2	3.2	1*	1.3	3*	2.2
No variant identified	19	30.7	37	48.7	56	40.6
Total	62		76		138	59.4

*ad, autosomal dominant; ar, autosomal recessive; CORD, cone and rod dystrophy; M to M, male to male transmission; RP, retinitis pigmentosa; xl, x-linked; *one family carrying both variants of RPGR and FAM161A.*

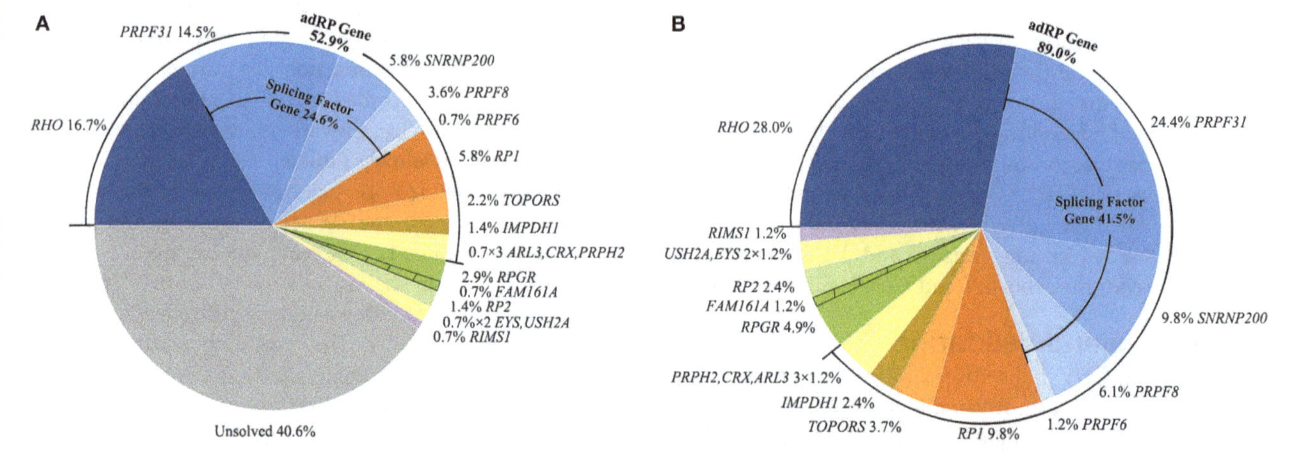

FIGURE 1 | Summary of the proportion of patients in this study with variants in the involved genes. **(A)** Proportion of all probands with variants in each involved gene. **(B)** Proportion in all genetically diagnosed families with variants in each involved gene. The shaded areas indicate a proband carrying both variants of *RPGR* and *FAM161A*.

prevalent in *PRPF31*, with a gene-specific frequency of 35.0% (7/20) (**Figure 2B**).

All probands with the adRP gene variants had typical RP symptoms, and their representative fundus appearances of the patients with variants in the first five common genes are shown in **Figure 3**. The median onset age of all patients with adRP genes was 5 years (range, 1–45 years) (**Table 3**). The median onset age was significantly older for the probands carrying the variants of *RP1* than for all probands with adRP (**Table 3**). Incomplete penetrance was observed in five pedigrees—three carrying variants in *PRPF31*, one in *PRPF8*, and one in *TOPORS*.

Variant Profiles in the xlRP and arRP Genes

Six hemizygous or heterozygous variants of the two xlRP genes were identified in six probands (4.3%, 6/138) and three compound heterozygous variants of three arRP genes in three probands (2.2%) (**Figure 4**). All six families with xlRP gene variants had at least two generations of inheritance; however, none of them showed male-to-male transmission that would exclude X-linked inheritance (**Figure 4**). Proband 0191318 was found to carry one heterozygous variant, p.(Q565Rfs*17), of *RPGR* and a compound heterozygous variant, M1:p.(Q548*) and M2:exon 1-5del, of *FAM161A*. Cosegregation analysis showed that his affected father carried a hemizygous variant of *RPGR* and a heterozygous variant, p.(Q548*), of *FAMI161A*. Pedigree 019207 was a small two-generation family with male-to-male transmission; however, the proband was found to harbor a compound heterozygous variant, p.[(G268R)]; [(P2811T)], of the *USH2A* gene. Cosegregation analysis showed that his affected father only carried a heterozygous variant, p.(G268R). We then conducted TES analysis on his affected father, but we did not detect any other disease-causing variant. Therefore, these two families were considered to be pseudodominant pedigrees (**Figure 4**). Proband 019645 was found to carry a compound heterozygous variant of *EYS*. During his family history review, he stated that his father and sister also had night blindness and visual acuity defects, but his father did not suffer from RP, according to a later ophthalmologic examination.

Variants in Other IRD Genes

Proband 0191323 was found to carry a heterozygous variant, p.(S679T), of *RIMS1*, which is a disease-causing gene for adCORD. Cosegregation analysis showed that his affected mother also harbored this variant. The 51-year-old proband stated that he had experienced night-blindness since the age of 8 years and had developed obvious visual acuity loss and

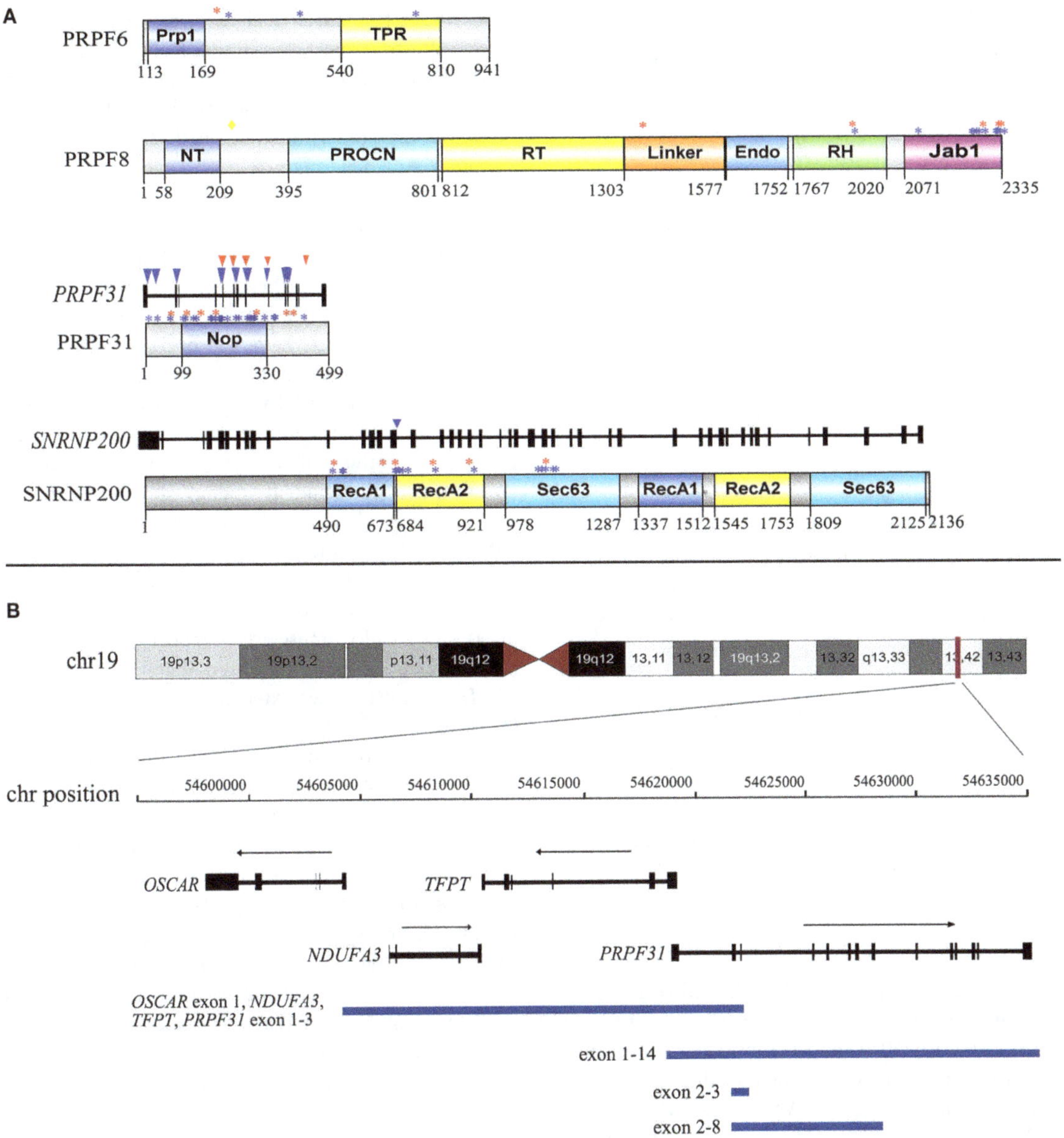

FIGURE 2 | The distribution of 30 distinct variants of *PRPF31*, *SNRNP200*, *PRPF8*, and *PRPF6* identified in our study. **(A)** The distribution of 21 missense variants in the corresponding domain of *PRPF31*, *SNRNP200*, *PRPF8*, and *PRPF6* and the distribution of five splicing effect variants in the exons and introns of *PRPF31* and *SNRNP200*. Numbers under domains indicate amino acid location. Red asterisks indicate missense variants detected in the current cohort. Blue asterisks indicate missense variants reported in HGMD. Yellow diamond indicates the VUS of *PRPF8* detected in the current cohort. Red triangles indicate splicing effect variants detected in the current cohort. Blue triangles indicate splicing effect variants reported in HGMD. Prp1, pre-mRNA processing domain; TPR, tetratricopeptide repeat domain; NT, PRO8NT domain; RT, reverse transcriptase homology domain; Endo, restriction endonuclease homology domain; RH, RNase H homology domain; Jab1, Jun kinase activation binding protein; NOP, nucleolar protein domain; RecA1, repeat helicase ATP-binding domain; RecA2, repeat helicase C-terminal domain; Sec63, secretory-63 domain. **(B)** Lengths and positions of the four gross deletions involving *PRPF31* on chromosome 19q13.42.

photophobia at around age 40 years. His fundus examination showed macular atrophy and black spicule-like pigment in the posterior pole and peripheral retina, and his ERG recording was extinguished. This patient might be in the late stage of CORD, so his fundus examination presented an RP-like appearance.

DISCUSSION

In the current study, we conducted a comprehensive molecular analysis in a large Chinese adRP cohort. We obtained an overall variant detection rate of 59.4% by means of several molecular methods, including linkage mapping, Sanger

TABLE 2 | Prevalence of Disease-Causing Variants in 138 Chinese adRP families and mutation type for each gene.

Gene	No.Families	%	MS	FS	NS	SP	CNV	Others
adRP gene								
ARL3	1	0.7	1	0	0	0	0	0
CRX	1	0.7	0	1	0	0	0	0
IMPDH1	2	1.4	2	0	0	0	0	0
PRPF31	20	14.5	3	1	2	5	7	2
PRPF6	1	0.7	1	0	0	0	0	0
PRPF8	5	3.6	4	1	0	0	0	0
PRPH2	1	0.7	0	1	0	0	0	0
RHO	23	16.7	20	0	3	0	0	0
RP1	8	5.8	1	3	4	0	0	0
SNRNP200	8	5.8	8	0	0	0	0	0
TOPORS	3	2.2	1	2	0	0	0	0
xlRP gene								
RP2	2	1.4	1	0	1	0*	0	0
RPGR	4*	2.9	2	2	0	0	0	0
arRP gene								
EYS	1	0.7	1	0	1	0	0	0
FAM161A	1*	0.7	0	0	1	0	1	0
USH2A	1	0.7	2	0	0	0	0	0
adCORD gene								
RIMS1	1	0.7	1	0	0	0	0	0
Not solved	56	40.6						
Total	138	100						

*ad, autosomal dominant; ar, autosomal recessive; CORD, cone and rod dystrophy; FS, frameshift; MS, missense; NS, non-sense; Other, run-on or synonymous variant; RP, retinitis pigmentosa; SP, splicing effect; *one proband carrying both variants of RPGR and FAM161A.*

sequencing, targeted-exon sequencing, MLPA, and real-time q-PCR analysis. This detection rate is close to the rates recently reported in a large Spanish adRP cohort comprising 258 families (60%), as well as in a previously described small Belgian adRP cohort comprising 86 families (56%) (Van Cauwenbergh et al., 2017; Martin-Merida et al., 2018). However, it is much lower than the rate (70%) described previously in a large American adRP cohort that included 253 families (Daiger et al., 2014b). The variant detection rate is related to the accuracy of the probands' clinical diagnoses. In the current study, the solving rate was much higher for the families with male-to-male transmission (69.3%) than for the families without male-to-male transmission (51.3%). The variant detection rate is also related to molecular screening methods. For the large American adRP cohort, application of next-generation sequencing increased the detection rate from 65% (by only Sanger sequencing) to 70% (Daiger et al., 2014b).

Consistent with several previous studies, *RHO* was the most frequently mutated gene in the current adRP cohort, and its proportion (16.7%) was higher than the proportions reported in Chinese (8.9%) and Japanese (11.5%) adRP cohorts (Xu et al., 2014; Koyanagi et al., 2019) and close to those reported in French (18.3%), Italian (16.0%), and Belgian (14.0%) adRP cohorts (Ziviello et al., 2005; Coussa et al., 2015; Van Cauwenbergh et al., 2017), but much lower than those observed in American (26.9%) adRP cohorts (Daiger et al., 2014a,b). This difference might reflect, in part, the absence of the P23H variant, which is a founder variant and accounts for about 13.2% of the adRP in American families (Daiger et al., 2014a). The second most common mutated gene was *PRPF31*, which showed a 14.5% variant frequency in the current cohort. This frequency was higher than that observed in several adRP cohorts (6.8–10.5%) from Japan, Belgium, America, and Spain (Daiger et al., 2014a; Van Cauwenbergh et al., 2017; Martin-Merida et al., 2018; Koyanagi et al., 2019). The variant frequency of *SNRNP200* was also much higher in the current cohort than in the Spanish and American cohorts (5.8% vs. 2.3 or 1.5%) (Daiger et al., 2014a; Martin-Merida et al., 2018). Therefore, the findings that the variants in the pre-mRNA splicing factor genes were the major cause of the current Chinese adRP cohort and were responsible for 24.6% of the probands were not surprising (**Figure 1B**). By contrast, the variant frequency was much lower for *PRPH2* (0.7%) in our cohort than in the American, Belgian, and Spanish cohorts (7.0, 4.7, and 3.9%, respectively) (Daiger et al., 2014a; Van Cauwenbergh et al., 2017; Martin-Merida et al., 2018). The rate was also lower than the rate previously reported (3.7%, 3/79) in a small Chinese adRP cohort (Xu et al., 2014). Several previous studies have indicated that the variant frequency of *PRPH2* in adRP varies extensively with ethnicity, ranging from 0% (Mexican cohort) up to 10.3% (French cohort) (Sullivan et al., 2006; Matias-Florentino et al., 2009; Manes et al., 2015).

Our cohort showed a greater allelic diversity, and the majority of the observed variants (almost 90%) were private variants responsible for their own respective families. Only four variants in *RHO*, *PRPF31*, and *RP1* were detected three or more times. The most frequent variants, p.(R135W) and p.(P347L) in *RHO*, were variant hotspots that have been reported in several previous studies (Xu et al., 2014; Van Cauwenbergh et al., 2017; Martin-Merida et al., 2018). The common variant p.(R677*) in *RP1* was also a variant hotspot that has been described in many adRP families with different ethnicities (Bowne et al., 1999; Jacobson et al., 2000; Audo et al., 2012; Daiger et al., 2014a,b; Martin-Merida et al., 2018).

The proportion of novel variants identified in the current cohort was relatively high. In the current study, two novel missense variants, p.(R1384W) and p.(T1931M) of *PRPF8*, were not located in the C-terminal Jab1 domain (**Figure 3A**), where almost all reported variants are clustered (RuŽičková and Staněk, 2017). These two variants were situated in highly conserved regions and were predicted to be disease-causing by three *in silico* analysis programs and to cosegregate with their phenotype in the families. They were not found in any public databases, and we defined them as disease-causing variants according to the ACMG guidelines and standards. Additional functional studies are needed to verify their pathogenicity in the future.

Five distinct and large genomic DNA deletions of two genes were identified in eight probands. *PRPF31* showed a high prevalence (5.1%, 7/138) of CNVs in our adRP cohort; this prevalence was much higher than the prevalence of 1.9% recently reported in a large Spanish cohort (Martin-Merida et al., 2018). All five CNVs were in a heterozygous state; therefore, they were

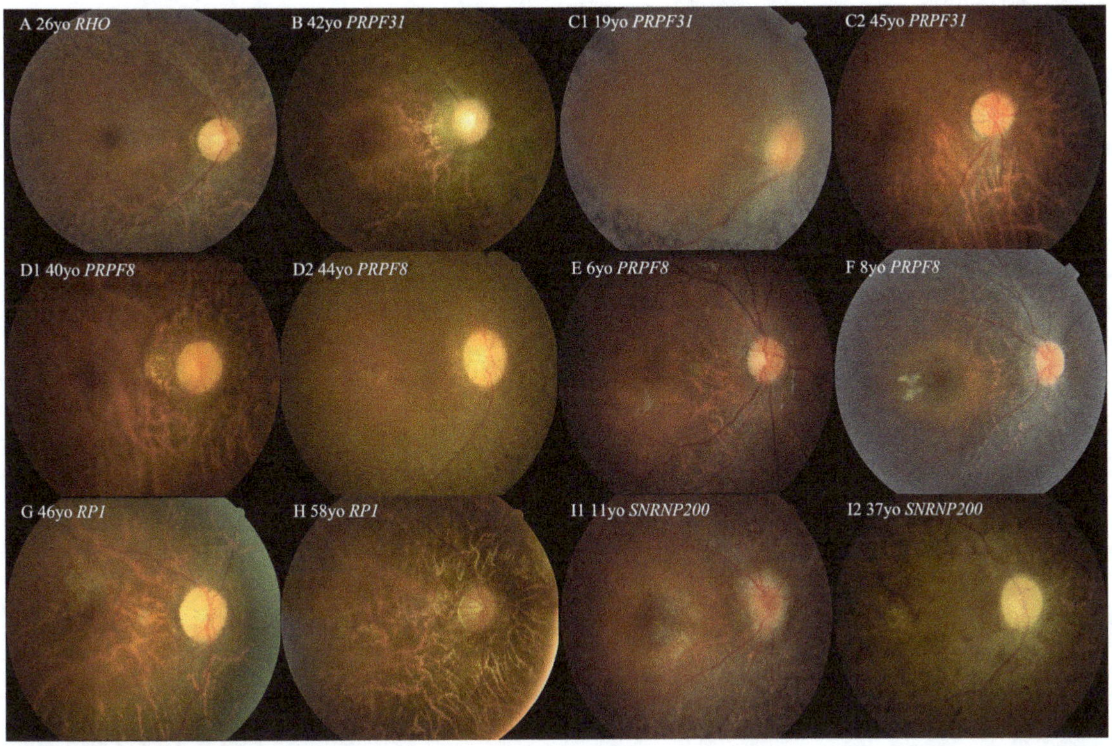

FIGURE 3 | Colored fundus (CF) photographs of patients with variants of *RHO*, *PRPF31*, *SNRNP200*, *RP1*, and *PRPF8*. **(A)** CF image of proband 019875 with the missense variant of *RHO*. **(B)** CF photograph of proband 0191443 with exons 2–3 deletion of *PRPF31*. **(C1,C2)** CF photograph of proband 019417 with the non-sense variant of *PRRF31* shows dense black pigmentation in the midperipheral retina, but CF image of his 45-year-old father with the same variant displaying a normal fundus appearance **(D1,D2)** CF photographs of two affected sisters of pedigree 019917 with the missense variants of *PRPF8* located in the Jab1 domain. **(E,F)** CF photographs of two probands of 010215 and 019444 with the missense variants of *PRPF8* located in the Linker and RH region or domain. **(G,H)** CF photographs of probands 019545 and 0191212 with the variants of *RP1*. **(I1,I2)** CF images of two patients from pedigree 019756 with the missense variant of *SNRNP200*.

undetected by Sanger sequencing. Next-generation sequencing has the capability to detect CNVs, but this capability is related to the coverage depth. A previous study found that CNV analysis could generate ambiguous results in the target regions when the coverage was <250× (Aparisi et al., 2014). In the current cohort, we used comprehensive screening methods, including linkage analysis in the early period, q-PCR, MLPA, and TES read count analysis, to detect the CNVs of *PRPF31*. This comprehensive analysis might be one of the reasons for the high CNV frequency for *PRPF31* observed in the present study.

Six probands (4.3%, 6/138) in the current cohort were found to harbor variants of the xlRP genes (*RPGR* and *RP2*). Four of the six probands were female and did not present a milder phenotype than was observed for the affected individuals in their families. Variant p.(E1031fs*58) (c.3092delA) located in the ORF15 of *RPGR* was identified in the supplementary PCR-based sequencing. The ORF15 where most *RPGR* variants are clustered is poorly covered in the NGS because of its highly repetitive sequence (Huang et al., 2015). Some variants in the ORF15 might be missed by NGS assays; therefore, alternative Sanger sequencing is necessary in patients from any adRP families without male-to-male transmission. A previous study using Sanger sequencing identified variants of *RPGR* and *RP2* in 8.5% (22/258) of adRP families (Churchill et al., 2013).

Obtaining a clear genotype–phenotype correlation is difficult because most probands harbor their own private variants in different genes. In the current cohort, we observed that patients with *RP1* variants had a late onset age and a mild phenotype when compared with patients with other adRP genes variants. This observation was consistent with previous descriptions (Jacobson et al., 2000; Audo et al., 2012). Incomplete penetrance was relatively common in the families with variants of *PRPF31*; however, its prevalence (15%, 3/20) was much lower than the 66.7% observed in Spanish patients (Martin-Merida et al., 2017). Three of our probands carried biallelic variants in three known arRP genes. Cosegregation analysis revealed pseudodominant inheritance in two families, with the remaining family unclear because of an incorrect family history report; this is one of the limitations—we did not perform ophthalmic evaluation in all affected family members of the current study.

Of the 56 probands whose disease-causing genes were not identified, 37 pedigrees did not show male-to-male transmission, and three families presented incomplete penetrance. In addition, 21 of the probands did not undergo ERG recording, which is another limitation of the current study as it means that the probability of a misdiagnosis could not be excluded. Their causal variants might be in areas not covered by

TABLE 3 | Correlations between onset age of patients with different gene variants.

Patients	Number	Onset age, years old		
		Mean ± SD	**Median**	**Range**
Total adRP gene	73	10.7 ± 11.7	5	1–45
With *RHO* variants	23	7.5 ± 9.3	5	1–45
With *PRPF31* variants	20	6.5 ± 5.0	5	1–23
With *RP1* variants	8	33.1 ± 7.8	35†	20–41
With *SNRNP200* variants	8	5.1 ± 3.5	5	1–12
With *PRPF8* variants	5	6.6 ± 7.7	5	1–20
With *TOPORS* variants	3	10.0 ± 8.7	5	5–20
With other adRP gene variants	6	17.7 ± 16.6	9	5–40
With adRP gene variants except for *RP1* gene	65	7.9 ± 8.9	5†	1–45
With splicing factor gene variants (*PRPF31*, *PRPF6*, *PRPF8* and *SNRNP200*)	34	7.1 ± 7.4	5	1–38
Total xlRP	6	5.2 ± 0.4	5	5–6
With *RPGR* variants	4	5.5 ± 0.7	5.5	5–6
With *RP2* variants	2	5.0 ± 0	5	5

†*P* = 0.000.

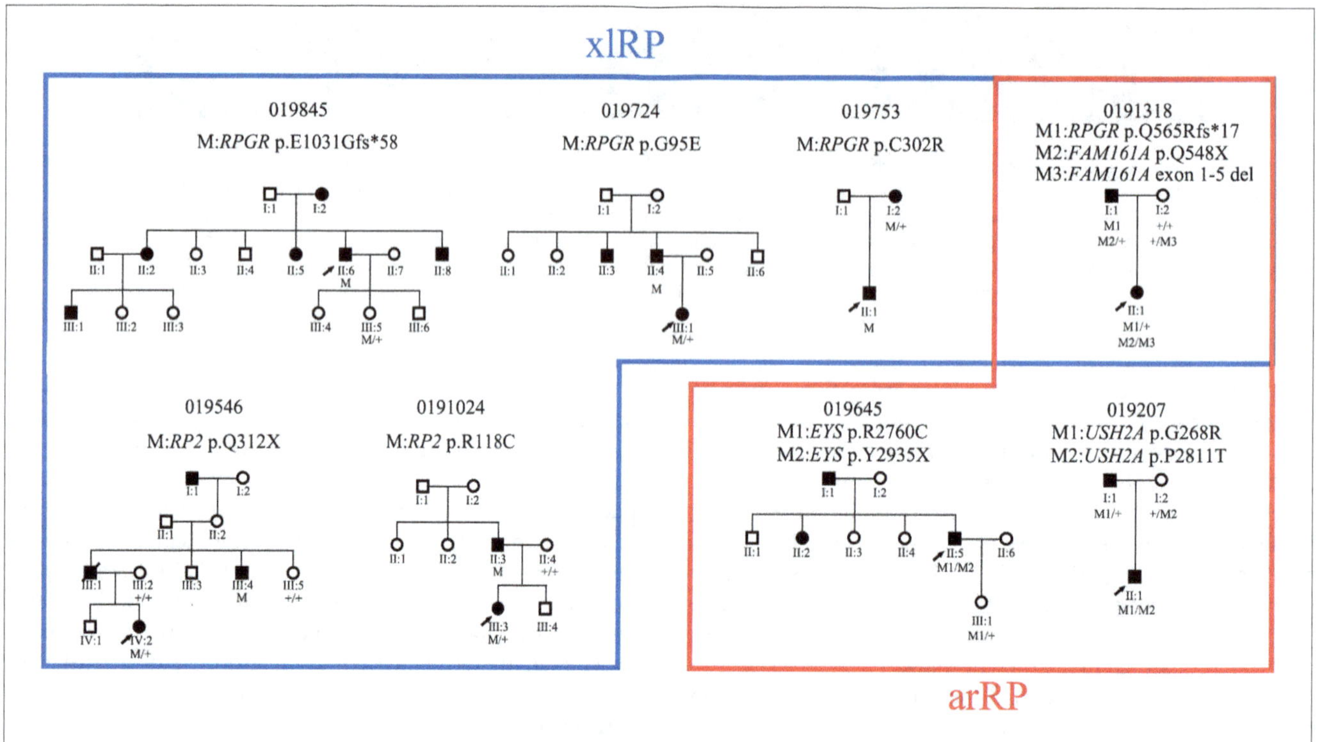

FIGURE 4 | Pedigrees of eight families with xlRP and arRP gene variants and their cosegregation results.

our TES panel, such as the promoter or deep intronic regions of the targeted genes, or they may reside in newly identified genes that were not included in our TES panel. In the future, we will perform WES or WGS analyses for these patients.

In conclusion, we have established the profile of the mutated genes and the variant spectrum of adRP genes in a large cohort of Chinese patients, thereby providing essential information for genetic counseling and future therapeutic development for retinal dystrophy inherited as a dominant trait.

ETHICS STATEMENT

The studies involving human participants were reviewed and approved by Ethics committee of Beijing Tongren Hospital. Written informed consent to participate in this study was provided by the participants' legal guardian/next of kin.

AUTHOR CONTRIBUTIONS

YL and Z-BJ designed and supervised the whole study. TX, YX, XinZ, KX, and XiaZ performed the experiments and interpret the results. TX wrote the manuscript. All authors contributed to the article and approved the submitted version.

REFERENCES

Aparisi, M. J., Aller, E., Fuster-García, C., García-García, G., Rodrigo, R., Vázquez-Manrique, R. P., et al. (2014). Targeted next generation sequencing for molecular diagnosis of usher syndrome. *Orphanet J. Rare Dis.* 9:168. doi: 10.1186/s13023-014-0168-7

Audo, I., Mohand-Saïd, S., Dhaenens, C. M., Germain, A., Orhan, E., Antonio, A., et al. (2012). RP1 and autosomal dominant rod-cone dystrophy: novel variants, a review of published variants, and genotype-phenotype correlation. *Hum. Mutat.* 33, 73–80. doi: 10.1002/humu.21640

Ayuso, C., and Millan, J. M. (2010). Retinitis pigmentosa and allied conditions today: a paradigm of translational research. *Genome Med* 2:34. doi: 10.1186/gm155

Bowne, S. J., Daiger, S. P., Hims, M. M., Sohocki, M. M., Malone, K. A., McKie, A. B., et al. (1999). Variants in the RP1 gene causing autosomal dominant retinitis pigmentosa. *Hum. Mol. Genet.* 8, 2121–2128. doi: 10.1093/hmg/8.11.2121

Churchill, J. D., Bowne, S. J., Sullivan, L. S., Lewis, R. A., Wheaton, D. K., Birch, D. G., et al. (2013). Variants in the X-linked retinitis pigmentosa genes RPGR and RP2 found in 8.5% of families with a provisional diagnosis of autosomal dominant retinitis pigmentosa. *Invest. Ophthalmol. Vis. Sci.* 54, 1411–1416. doi: 10.1167/iovs.12-11541

Costa, K. A., Salles, M. V., Whitebirch, C., Chiang, J., and Sallum, J. M. F. (2017). Gene panel sequencing in Brazilian patients with retinitis pigmentosa. *Int. J. Retina Vitreous* 3:33. doi: 10.1186/s40942-017-0087-6

Coussa, R. G., Chakarova, C., Ajlan, R., Taha, M., Kavalec, C., Gomolin, J., et al. (2015). Genotype and phenotype studies in autosomal dominant retinitis pigmentosa (adRP) of the French Canadian founder population. *Invest. Ophthalmol. Vis. Sci.* 56, 8297–8305. doi: 10.1167/iovs.15-17104

Daiger, S. P., Bowne, S. J., and Sullivan, L. S. (2014a). Genes and variants causing autosomal dominant retinitis pigmentosa. *Cold Spring Harb. Perspect. Med.* 5:a017129. doi: 10.1101/cshperspect.a017129

Daiger, S. P., Bowne, S. J., Sullivan, L. S., Blanton, S. H., Weinstock, G. M., Koboldt, D. C., et al. (2014b). Application of next-generation sequencing to identify genes and variants causing autosomal dominant retinitis pigmentosa (adRP). *Adv. Exp. Med. Biol.* 801, 123–129. doi: 10.1007/978-1-4614-3209-8_16

Dias, M. F., Joo, K., Kemp, J. A., Fialho, S. L., da Silva Cunha, A. Jr., Woo, S. J., et al. (2018). Molecular genetics and emerging therapies for retinitis pigmentosa: basic research and clinical perspectives. *Prog. Retin. Eye Res.* 63, 107–131. doi: 10.1016/j.preteyeres.2017.10.004

Dong, B., Chen, J., Zhang, X., Pan, Z., Bai, F., and Li, Y. (2013). Two novel PRP31 premessenger ribonucleic acid processing factor 31 homolog variants including a complex insertion-deletion identified in Chinese families with retinitis pigmentosa. *Mol. Vis.* 19, 2426–2435.

Gao, F. J., Li, J. K., Chen, H., Hu, F. Y., Zhang, S. H., Qi, Y. H., et al. (2019). Genetic and clinical findings in a large cohort of Chinese patients with suspected retinitis pigmentosa. *Ophthalmology* 126, 1549–1556. doi: 10.1016/j.ophtha.2019.04.038

Huang, L., Zhang, Q., Huang, X., Qu, C., Ma, S., Mao, Y., et al. (2017). Variant screening in genes known to be responsible for retinitis pigmentosa in 98 small han Chinese families. *Sci. Rep.* 7:1948. doi: 10.1038/s41598-017-00963-6

Huang, X. F., Wu, J., Lv, J. N., Zhang, X., and Jin, Z. B. (2015). Identification of false-negative variants missed by next-generation sequencing in retinitis pigmentosa patients: a complementary approach to clinical genetic diagnostic testing. *Genet. Med.* 17, 307–311. doi: 10.1038/gim.2014.193

Jacobson, S. G., Cideciyan, A. V., Iannaccone, A., Weleber, R. G., Fishman, G. A., Maguire, A. M., et al. (2000). Disease expression of RP1 variants causing autosomal dominant retinitis pigmentosa. *Invest. Ophthalmol. Vis. Sci.* 41, 1898–1908.

Koyanagi, Y., Akiyama, M., Nishiguchi, K. M., Momozawa, Y., Kamatani, Y., Takata, S., et al. (2019). Genetic characteristics of retinitis pigmentosa in 1204 Japanese patients. *J. Med. Genet.* 56, 662–670. doi: 10.1136/jmedgenet-2018-105691

Li, S., Xiao, X., Wang, P., Guo, X., and Zhang, Q. (2010). Variant spectrum and frequency of the RHO gene in 248 Chinese families with retinitis pigmentosa. *Biochem. Biophys. Res. Commun.* 401, 42–47. doi: 10.1016/j.bbrc.2010.09.004

Manes, G., Guillaumie, T., Vos, W. L., Devos, A., Audo, I., Zeitz, C., et al. (2015). High prevalence of PRPH2 in autosomal dominant retinitis pigmentosa in france and characterization of biochemical and clinical features. *Am. J. Ophthalmol.* 159, 302–314. doi: 10.1016/j.ajo.2014.10.033

Martin-Merida, I., Aguilera-Garcia, D., Fernandez-San Jose, P., Blanco-Kelly, F., Zurita, O., Almoguera, B., et al. (2018). Toward the variantal landscape of autosomal dominant retinitis pigmentosa: a comprehensive analysis of 258 Spanish families. *Invest. Ophthalmol. Vis. Sci.*59, 2345–2354. doi: 10.1167/iovs.18-23854

Martin-Merida, I., Sanchez-Alcudia, R., Fernandez-San Jose, P., Blanco-Kelly, F., Perez-Carro, R., Rodriguez-Jacy da Silva, L., et al. (2017). Analysis of the PRPF31 gene in Spanish autosomal dominant retinitis pigmentosa patients: a novel genomic rearrangement. *Invest. Ophthalmol. Vis. Sci.* 58, 1045–1053. doi: 10.1167/iovs.16-20515

Matias-Florentino, M., Ayala-Ramirez, R., Graue-Wiechers, F., and Zenteno, J. C. (2009). Molecular screening of rhodopsin and peripherin/RDS genes in Mexican families with autosomal dominant retinitis pigmentosa. *Curr. Eye Res.* 34, 1050–1056. doi: 10.3109/02713680903283169

Pan, Z., Lu, T., Zhang, X., Dai, H., Yan, W., Bai, F., et al. (2012). Identification of two variants of the RHO gene in two Chinese families with retinitis pigmentosa: correlation between genotype and phenotype. *Mol. Vis.* 18, 3013–3020.

Richards, S., Aziz, N., Bale, S., Bick, D., Das, S., Gastier-Foster, J., et al. (2015). Standards and guidelines for the interpretation of sequence variants: a joint consensus recommendation of the American college of medical genetics and genomics and the association for molecular pathology. *Genet. Med.* 17, 405–424. doi: 10.1038/gim.2015.30

RuŽičková, Š., and Staněk, D. (2017). Variants in spliceosomal proteins and retina degeneration. *RNA Biol.* 14, 544–552. doi: 10.1080/15476286.2016.1191735

Sullivan, L. S., Bowne, S. J., Birch, D. G., Hughbanks-Wheaton, D., Heckenlively, J. R., Lewis, R. A., et al. (2006). Prevalence of disease-causing variants in families with autosomal dominant retinitis pigmentosa: a screen of known genes in 200 families. *Invest. Ophthalmol. Vis. Sci.* 47, 3052–3064. doi: 10.1167/iovs.05-1443

Sullivan, L. S., Bowne, S. J., Reeves, M. J., Blain, D., Goetz, K., Ndifor, V., et al. (2013). Prevalence of variants in eyeGENE probands with a diagnosis of autosomal dominant retinitis pigmentosa. *Invest. Ophthalmol. Vis. Sci.* 54, 6255–6261. doi: 10.1167/iovs.13-12605

Sun, T., Xu, K., Ren, Y., Xie, Y., Zhang, X., Tian, L., et al. (2018). Comprehensive molecular screening in Chinese usher syndrome patients. *Invest. Ophthalmol. Vis. Sci.* 59, 1229–1237. doi: 10.1167/iovs.17-23312

Talevich, E., Shain, A. H., Botton, T., and Bastian, B. C. (2016). CNVkit: genome-wide copy number detection and visualization from targeted DNA sequencing. *PLoS Comput. Biol.* 12:e1004873. doi: 10.1371/journal.pcbi.1004873

Van Cauwenbergh, C., Coppieters, F., Roels, D., De Jaegere, S., Flipts, H., De Zaeytijd, J., et al. (2017). Variants in splicing factor genes are a major cause of autosomal dominant retinitis pigmentosa in belgian families. *PLoS ONE* 12:e0170038. doi: 10.1371/journal.pone.0170038

Xu, Y., Guan, L., Shen, T., Zhang, J., Xiao, X., Jiang, H., et al. (2014). Variants of 60 known causative genes in 157 families with retinitis pigmentosa based on exome sequencing. *Hum. Genet.* 133, 1255–1271. doi: 10.1007/s00439-014-1460-2

Ziviello, C., Simonelli, F., Testa, F., Anastasi, M., Marzoli, S. B., Falsini, B., et al. (2005). Molecular genetics of autosomal dominant retinitis pigmentosa (ADRP): a comprehensive study of 43 Italian families. *J. Med. Genet.* 42:e47. doi: 10.1136/jmg.2005.031682

14

Long-Read Sequencing to Unravel Complex Structural Variants of *CEP78* Leading to Cone-Rod Dystrophy and Hearing Loss

*Giulia Ascari[1,2], Nanna D. Rendtorff[3], Marieke De Bruyne[1,2], Julie De Zaeytijd[4], Michel Van Lint[5], Miriam Bauwens[1,2], Mattias Van Heetvelde[1,2], Gavin Arno[6,7,8], Julie Jacob[9], David Creytens[10,11], Jo Van Dorpe[10,11], Thalia Van Laethem[1,2], Toon Rosseel[1,2], Tim De Pooter[12,13], Peter De Rijk[12,13], Wouter De Coster[14,15], Björn Menten[1,2], Alfredo Dueñas Rey[1,2], Mojca Strazisar[12,13], Mette Bertelsen[3,16], Lisbeth Tranebjaerg[3,17] and Elfride De Baere[1,2]**

[1] Center for Medical Genetics Ghent, Ghent University Hospital, Ghent, Belgium, [2] Department of Biomolecular Medicine, Ghent University, Ghent, Belgium, [3] The Kennedy Center, Department of Clinical Genetics, Rigshospitalet, Copenhagen University Hospital, Copenhagen, Denmark, [4] Department of Ophthalmology, Ghent University Hospital, Ghent, Belgium, [5] Department of Ophthalmology, Antwerp University Hospital, Antwerp, Belgium, [6] Great Ormond Street Hospital, London, United Kingdom, [7] Moorfields Eye Hospital, London, United Kingdom, [8] UCL Institute of Ophthalmology, London, United Kingdom, [9] Department of Ophthalmology, University Hospitals Leuven, Leuven, Belgium, [10] Department of Pathology, Ghent University Hospital, Ghent, Belgium, [11] Department of Diagnostic Sciences, Ghent University, Ghent, Belgium, [12] Neuromics Support Facility, VIB Center for Molecular Neurology, VIB, Antwerp, Belgium, [13] Neuromics Support Facility, Department of Biomedical Sciences, University of Antwerp, Antwerp, Belgium, [14] Applied and Translational Neurogenomics Group, VIB Center for Molecular Neurology, VIB, Antwerp, Belgium, [15] Applied and Translational Neurogenomics Group, Department of Biomedical Sciences, University of Antwerp, Antwerp, Belgium, [16] Department of Ophthalmology, Rigshospitalet-Glostrup, University of Copenhagen, Glostrup, Denmark, [17] Institute of Clinical Medicine, University of Copenhagen, Copenhagen, Denmark

***Correspondence:**
Elfride De Baere
Elfride.DeBaere@UGent.be

Inactivating variants as well as a missense variant in the centrosomal *CEP78* gene have been identified in autosomal recessive cone-rod dystrophy with hearing loss (CRDHL), a rare syndromic inherited retinal disease distinct from Usher syndrome. Apart from this, a complex structural variant (SV) implicating *CEP78* has been reported in CRDHL. Here we aimed to expand the genetic architecture of typical CRDHL by the identification of complex SVs of the *CEP78* region and characterization of their underlying mechanisms. Approaches used for the identification of the SVs are shallow whole-genome sequencing (sWGS) combined with quantitative polymerase chain reaction (PCR) and long-range PCR, or ExomeDepth analysis on whole-exome sequencing (WES) data. Targeted or whole-genome nanopore long-read sequencing (LRS) was used to delineate breakpoint junctions at the nucleotide level. For all SVs cases, the effect of the SVs on *CEP78* expression was assessed using quantitative PCR on patient-derived RNA. Apart from two novel canonical *CEP78* splice variants and a frameshifting single-nucleotide variant (SNV), two SVs affecting *CEP78* were identified in three unrelated individuals with CRDHL: a heterozygous total gene deletion of 235 kb and a partial gene deletion of 15 kb in a heterozygous and homozygous state, respectively. Assessment of the molecular consequences of the SVs on patient's materials displayed a loss-of-function effect. Delineation and characterization of the

15-kb deletion using targeted LRS revealed the previously described complex *CEP78* SV, suggestive of a recurrent genomic rearrangement. A founder haplotype was demonstrated for the latter SV in cases of Belgian and British origin, respectively. The novel 235-kb deletion was delineated using whole-genome LRS. Breakpoint analysis showed microhomology and pointed to a replication-based underlying mechanism. Moreover, data mining of bulk and single-cell human and mouse transcriptional datasets, together with CEP78 immunostaining on human retina, linked the CEP78 expression domain with its phenotypic manifestations. Overall, this study supports that the *CEP78* locus is prone to distinct SVs and that SV analysis should be considered in a genetic workup of CRDHL. Finally, it demonstrated the power of sWGS and both targeted and whole-genome LRS in identifying and characterizing complex SVs in patients with ocular diseases.

Keywords: CEP78, inherited retinal disease, cone-rod dystrophy with hearing loss, long-read sequencing, structural variants, single-cell gene expression analysis

INTRODUCTION

During the last years, next-generation sequencing (NGS) techniques mostly relying on short-read sequencing (SRS) have accelerated molecular diagnoses in individuals with inherited retinal diseases (IRDs) (Jespersgaard et al., 2019). IRD is characterized by a tremendous genetic heterogeneity with variants identified in more than 270 genes [RetNet (Retinal Information Network)[1]]. Different types of variants can give rise to IRD, both single-nucleotide variants (SNVs) as well as structural variants (SVs), of which copy number variants (CNVs) have been most frequently reported (Khateb et al., 2016; Ellingford et al., 2018; Van Schil et al., 2018; Daiger et al., 2019; Zampaglione et al., 2020). The latter are estimated to contribute to at least 7%–10% of pathogenic alleles in IRD (Khateb et al., 2016; Ellingford et al., 2018; Daiger et al., 2019; Zampaglione et al., 2020). Interestingly, genomic features such as gene size have been shown to correlate with CNV occurrence in IRD genes (Van Schil et al., 2018).

Structural variant detection based on standard molecular karyotyping and on sequencing depth algorithms is capable of detecting only large CNVs, such as deletions and duplications greater than 50 kb in size, whereas cryptic SVs, such as smaller CNVs, copy neutral, and complex rearrangements, may be missed (Lindstrand et al., 2019). Nowadays, it is possible to detect approximately 27,000 SVs (>50 bp) per human genome only using a combination of technologies, where the majority of these SVs is located in the non-coding part of the genome and missed using exome-based approaches (Belkadi et al., 2015; Chaisson et al., 2019; Mahmoud et al., 2019). Whole-genome sequencing (WGS) proved to be particularly powerful to detect SVs, variants in GC-rich regions, and variants in non-coding regulatory regions (Nishiguchi et al., 2013; Ellingford et al., 2016; Carss et al., 2017; de Bruijn et al., 2020). While predictions are indicating that at least 48% of deletions and 83% of insertions are routinely missed by short-read-calling algorithms (Eichler, 2019), long-read sequencing (LRS) is particularly valuable for detecting SVs, as the long reads provide the necessary context to call and resolve SVs, regardless of their sequence composition (De Coster and Van Broeckhoven, 2019).

One of the more recently identified disease genes that contribute to the genetic heterogeneity of IRD is the centrosomal gene *CEP78* (MIM# 617110), in which several types of variants, inactivating sequence variants as well as a unique missense variant have been found in autosomal recessive cone-rod dystrophy with hearing loss (CRDHL; MIM# 617236), a recognizable phenotype distinct from Usher syndrome (Fu et al., 2016; Namburi et al., 2016; Nikopoulos et al., 2016; Ascari et al., 2020). Apart from CRDHL, sperm abnormalities causing infertility have been reported in two unrelated affected males (Ascari et al., 2020). Functional studies pointed to a loss-of-function effect with decreased amounts of protein, normal subcellular localization, and elongated primary cilia in patients' cells (Namburi et al., 2016; Nikopoulos et al., 2016; Ascari et al., 2020). Interestingly, a complex SV implicating *CEP78* has been reported in one individual with CRDHL, being a homozygous deletion–inversion–deletion overlapping *CEP78* (Sanchis-Juan et al., 2018). CEP78 localizes to the mature centrioles (Brunk et al., 2016), which are the main components of the centrosomes, key microtubule-organizing hubs in eukaryotic cells, with the mother centriole acting as the basal body during cilia formation (Gönczy and Hatzopoulos, 2019). Centrioles duplicate once per cell cycle, and irregularities in their structure, or number, are associated with several diseases including cancer or ciliopathies (Nigg and Raff, 2009; Gönczy, 2015).

Here, we report *CEP78* SVs and SNVs in four unrelated CRDHL families of Belgian, Danish, and Turkish origin. Interestingly, two distinct SVs were identified in three of the four CRDHL families using a combination of NGS technologies. Targeted or whole-genome nanopore LRS was used to delineate breakpoint junctions at the nucleotide level. For the smallest SV, a founder effect was shown. Overall, this study supports that the *CEP78* locus is prone to distinct SVs and emphasizes the importance of SV analysis in the genetic workup of CRDHL,

[1] https://sph.uth.edu/retnet

leveraging the power of shallow whole-genome sequencing (sWGS) and both targeted and whole-genome LRS. Furthermore, data mining of bulk and single-cell (sc) transcriptional datasets, in combination with CEP78 immunostaining, displayed a CEP78 expression domain in agreement with the phenotypic manifestations of CRDHL.

MATERIALS AND METHODS

Ethics Statement

This study followed the tenets of the Declaration of Helsinki, and ethical approval was given by the local ethics committee (Ghent University Hospital, EC UZG 2017/1540). All individuals involved gave their informed consent prior to inclusion in this study.

Phenotypic Evaluation

Affected individuals were subjected to ophthalmologic evaluation including best-corrected visual acuity measurement, funduscopy, visual field assessment, infrared and blue light reflectance and autofluorescence imaging, spectral-domain optical coherence tomography, and electroretinography, when possible. In addition, an audiological assessment was performed before or after the molecular diagnosis.

Whole-Exome Sequencing and Variant Validation

Genomic DNA (gDNA) was extracted from leukocytes according the manufacturer's guidelines. Whole-exome sequencing (WES) was performed using SureSelectXT Human All Exon V6 enrichment (Agilent Technologies) and HiSeq 3000 sequencing (Illumina) (F1 and F4), or SureSelectXT Low Input Human All Exon V7 kit (Agilent Technologies) and NovaSeq 6000 sequencing (Illumina) (F3). Reads were aligned to the human hg38 reference genome with BWA (v0.7.15) (Li and Durbin, 2009). SNVs and small insertions and deletions were detected with the GATK HaplotypeCaller (v3.8[2]). The VCF (variant call format) files were annotated with the Ensembl Variant Effect Predictor (release 95) and the dbNSFP (v3.4a) and dbscSNV (v1.1) databases. Variants were scored heterozygous or homozygous and were assessed with our in-house variant filtering and visualization tool. A selection of 272 and 275 RetNet genes was assessed, respectively (versions 3 and 4 of the RetNet panel). Nucleotide numbering was done following HGVS guidelines[3] with nucleotide "A" of the ATG as "c.1." Classification of variants was based on the ACMG and ACGS guidelines with adaptations (Richards et al., 2015; Nykamp et al., 2017; Abou Tayoun et al., 2018; Ellard et al., 2019). CNVs were assessed using ExomeDepth (Plagnol et al., 2012) (v1.1.10) and Pindel (Ye et al., 2009). Pathogenic (likely) variants were confirmed *via* Sanger sequencing. Sanger sequencing was performed using an ABI 3730xl DNA Analyzer (Applied Biosystems) with the BigDye Terminator Cycle Sequencing Kit (Applied Biosystems).

For F2, II:1 gene panel sequencing of 13 genes [*ABHD12*, *ADGRV1* (*GPR98*), *CDH23*, *CIB2*, *CLRN1*, *DFNB31* (*WHRN*), *HARS1*, *MYO7A*, *PCDH15*, *PDZD7*, *USH1C*, *USH1G*, and *USH2A*] associated with Usher syndrome was performed using a HaloPlex custom design created by use of Agilent SureDesign and included exons and 50 bp of the intron at each intron–exon boundary. The enrichment library from patient DNA was sequenced on a MiSeq sequencer (Illumina). FASTQ files were analyzed using SureCall v.3.0.1.4 (Agilent Technologies) using default settings. Whole-exome trio sequencing was performed for F2, II:1 and her parents. Library preparation was done using the Ion AmpliSeq exome kit (Thermo Fisher), and libraries were sequenced using the IonProton system (Thermo Fisher). Base calling, read alignment, and variant calling were performed using the Torrent Suite including the Torrent Variant Caller (Thermo Fisher). VarSeq (GoldenHelix) was used for annotation and filtering of the variants. Confirmation of the identified *CEP78* variant was performed *via* Sanger sequencing using NM_001098802.2 as reference sequence.

Shallow WGS

Shallow whole-genome sequencing was performed using the Hiseq3000 (Illumina), starting from 200 ng of gDNA. For library construction the NEXTflex Rapid DNA Sequencing kit (Bio Scientific) was used. Pipetting steps were automated using a Hamilton Star robot (Hamilton). Library concentrations were measured by the Qubit High-Sensitivity kit (Thermo Fisher Scientific), and equimolar concentrations were pooled before sequencing. The minimal number of mapped reads was set at 50 million. Copy number analysis was performed with WisecondorX and further visualized with the ViVar platform (Sante et al., 2014; Raman et al., 2019).

Quantitative and Long-Range Polymerase Chain Reaction for Deletion Confirmation and Delineation

Copy number variants were confirmed by quantitative polymerase chain reaction (qPCR), and primers were designed in coding exons or intronic regions as previously described (D'haene et al., 2010). Assays were prepared using SsoAdvanced Universal SYBR Green Supermix (Bio-Rad Laboratories) and run on LightCycler 480 System (Roche). Data were analyzed with qbase + software (Biogazelle). *ZNF80* and *GPR15* were used as reference genes. Subsequent to iterative qPCRs (long-range), PCR was performed to obtain junction deletion products using Phusion High-Fidelity PCR kit (New England Biolabs) and visualized on 1% UltraPure Agarose (Thermo Fisher Scientific) gels. Primer design was done using Primer3Plus. Primers sequences are listed in **Supplementary Table 1**.

Targeted LRS

Amplified (long-range) PCR product was quality checked using DropSense (Trinean), Qubit (ThermoFisher), and Fragment

[2]https://www.biorxiv.org/content/10.1101/201178v3
[3]http://www.hgvs.org

Analyzer (Agilent), using DNF-492 Large Fragment analysis kit (Agilent). A library was constructed according to the Ligation sequencing protocol (SQK-LSK109, Oxford Nanopore Technologies, ONT; GDE_9063_v109_revU_14Aug2019) with minor adaptations. DNA repair and end-prep using ONT consumables (SQK-LSK109) and NEBNext FFPE DNA repair mix and NEBNext Ultra II End repair/dA tailing Module (M6630, E7546 both from New England Biolabs) started with 100 fmol of the PCR amplicon, with extended enzymatic incubation times, 30 min at 20°C and 30 min at 65°C. Repaired and end-prepped amplicon was Ampure XP (Beckman Coulter) cleaned up for increased adaptor ligation efficiency, using a ratio of 1:1 (vol/vol) and extended incubation (10 min on Hulamixer). After bead cleanup, the pellet was eluted in 32 μL Nuclease Free Water, of which 30 μL was used for adapter ligation. Adapter ligation using SQK-LSK109, ONT, and NEBNext Quick Ligation Module (E6056, New England Biolabs) was performed according to the protocol with extension of the ligation incubation to 30 min at room temperature. The ligation reaction was cleaned up using Ampure XP (Beckman Coulter) in vol/vol ratio of 0.4 with extended incubation (10 min on Hulamixer). A purified pellet was eluted in 10 μL of MilliQ water with the final yield of library calculated using concentration and size information (F1, II:1 yield = 508.2 ng/72.6 fmol and F3, II:1 yield = 462 ng/61 fmol). Ten fmol (64 ng for F1, II:1) and 20 fmol (151.5 ng for F3, II:1) amount of the library was loaded and sequenced on MinION using Flongle Flowcell (both Oxford Nanopore Technologies) with, respectively, 85 (F1, II:1) and 47 (F3, II:1) number of pores sequencing after loading of the library. Sequencing was complete in 24 h and generated in total 1.08 Gb (F1, II:1) and 827.9 Mb (F3, II:1) of data, equaling 172.75 K (F1, II:1) and 140.99 K (F3, II:1) reads with an estimated N50 of 10.55 kb (F1, II:1) and 10.7 kb (F3, II:1).

Whole-Genome LRS

Extracted DNA was checked for concentration, purity, and integrity using DropSense (Trinean), Qubit (ThermoFisher), and Fragment Analyzer (Agilent), using 464 High Sensitivity Large Fragment 50-Kb kit (Agilent). The sample was sheared using Mega3 (Diagenode) to the final average size of the peak 21,015 bp (smear analysis 25,230 bp). Short fragments were eliminated using SRE XS (Circulomics). Sheared and size-selected DNA sample was used in library prep following the protocol gDNA by Ligation (SQK-LSK109, GDE_9063_v109_revU_14Aug2019, Oxford Nanopore Technologies) with minor adaptations. DNA repair and end-prep using ONT consumables (SQK-LSK109) and NEBNext FFPE DNA repair mix and NEBNext Ultra II End repair/dA tailing Module (M6630, E7546 both New England Biolabs) started with 182 fmol of the PCR amplicon, with extended enzymatic incubation times, 30 min at 20°C and 30 min at 65°C. Repaired and end-prepped amplicon was Ampure XP (Beckman Coulter) cleaned up for increased adaptor ligation efficiency, using a ratio of 1:1 (vol/vol) and extended incubation (10 min on Hulamixer). After bead cleanup, the pellet was eluted in 63 μL nuclease-free water, of which 60 μL was used for adapter ligation. Adapter ligation using SQK-LSK109, ONT, and NEBNext Quick Ligation Module (E6056, New England Biolabs) was performed according to the protocol with extension of the ligation incubation to 30 min at room temperature. The ligation reaction was cleaned up using Ampure XP (Beckman Coulter) in vol/vol ratio of 0.4 with extended incubation (10 min on Hulamixer). A purified pellet was eluted in 40 μL of MilliQ water with final yield of library calculated using concentration and size information (yield = 1,627.4 ng/105.6 fmol). Thirty femtomoles of the final library prep was loaded onto PromethION Flow cells (Oxford Nanopore Technologies). In order to generate enough data, the sample was loaded on three flow cells (FCs). Runs started with 6,844 (FC1), 5,835 (FC2), and 6,314 (FC3) sequenceable pores and ran for 72 h, generating in total 32.55 Gb (FC1), 36.18 Gb (FC2), and 40.99 Gb (FC3) of data, equaling 2.12 M (FC1), 2.39 M (FC2), and 2.68 M (FC3) reads with an estimated N50 of 27.86 kb (FC1), 28.76 kb (FC2), and 28.96 kb (FC3).

Data Analysis LRS

Base calling of the Nanopore data was performed using the Guppy base caller (v4.0.9 + 92ae093). Further analysis was performed using a pipeline integrated in GenomeComb (0.101.0) (Reumers et al., 2012). Reads were aligned to the hg38 genome reference (Schneider et al., 2017) using minimap2 (2.17-r941) (Li, 2018), and the resulting SAM file sorted and converted to BAM using Samtools (1.10) (Li et al., 2009). SVs were called using Sniffles (1.0.11) (Sedlazeck et al., 2018). The region of interest was filtered out and scanned for well-supported SVs using GenomeComb (Reumers et al., 2012).

Expression Analysis on Patient's Material and Splicing Assessment

For quantitative reverse transcription–PCR (RT-PCR), total RNA was extracted from short-term cultured lymphocytes or fibroblasts using MagCore according the manufacturer's guidelines. cDNA was synthesized with the iScript cDNA Synthesis Kit (Bio-Rad Laboratories). For each cDNA sample, assays were prepared using SsoAdvanced Universal SYBR Green Supermix (Bio-Rad Laboratories) and run on LightCycler 480 System (Roche). Data were analyzed with qbase + and normalized to the *YWHAZ* and *HMBS* or *SDHA* genes. Primers were designed using Primer3plus, and sequences are listed in **Supplementary Table 1**. For non-quantitative RT-PCR, cDNA was synthesized using SuperScript IV Reverse Transcriptase kit (Thermo Fisher) and underwent standard PCR, loaded on 2% UltraPure Agarose gel, and Sanger sequenced.

Haplotype Analysis

In total, 18 single-nucleotide polymorphisms (SNPs) (dbSNP, build 151) were selected for haplotype reconstruction in the upstream and downstream areas flanking *CEP78*. SNPs were Sanger sequenced according to the standard procedures (see above). PCR primers were designed with Primer3Plus, and sequences can be found in **Supplementary Table 2**.

CEP78 Expression in Mouse and Human Retina and Inner Ear

Data Mining in Single-Cell Retinal and Cochlear Transcriptional Datasets

Human adult retinal and murine P1 cochlear sc transcriptional datasets were mined for evaluating *CEP78* expression at the sc level. Expression matrices derived from pooling three donor neural retinal (Cowan et al., 2020) and four cochlear samples (Kolla et al., 2020) were retrieved and processed separately using SCANPY (v1.4.6) (Wolf et al., 2018). Preprocessing and quality control were conducted to remove outlier cells. Briefly, we considered only genes with counts of at least three cells and filtered out cells that had unique feature counts <200 or >2,500 and/or that expressed >5% mitochondrial counts. The data were then total-count normalized, logarithmized, filtered for highly variable features, and scaled to unit variance. After quality control preprocessing, a total of 19,768 retinal and 11,332 cochlear cells were kept for subsequent dimensionality reduction, embedding, and clustering. Markers associated with major neural retina and cochlear cell populations were used to assess *CEP78* expression at the sc level.

Data Mining in Bulk Retinal and Cochlear Transcriptional Datasets

Retina| Expression levels by transcripts per million (TPMs) were retrieved from postmortem retina samples characterized in Ratnapriya et al. (2019). From 453 samples that passed quality control, we only considered donor retinas that showed no age-related macular degeneration progression (n = 102) to avoid confounding variables in downstream analyses. To remove potential noise, 20% of genes with the lowest mean expression across all samples were filtered out. TPM values were then filtered for a set of candidate genes, which included all genes reported to cause IRD (RetNet) and ciliary genes (SCGSv1) (van Dam et al., 2013). A total of 519 genes were eventually considered. Before evaluating correlations in the expression of the candidate genes, the set was subjected to a variance-stabilizing transformation to correct for mean-variance dependency (Zwiener et al., 2014). We then examined the expression of *CEP78* and several ciliary genes listed in the top 10 of the Human Gene Connectome (HGC) (Itan et al., 2013) (*SCLT1*, *MKS1*, *CEP57*, *CEP76*, *CEP135*, *CEP152*, *CEP63*, *CEP164*, *OFD1*, and *CEP250*). Spearman correlations were computed along with pairwise p values adjusted for multiple comparisons (Holm method). A correlogram was then generated for visualization.

Cochlea| We retrieved paired-end FASTQ files (GSE111348) derived from adult (P28-P32) mouse inner (IHC) and outer (OHC) cochlear hair cells (~1,000 cells per sample; n = 4 and 6 for IHC and OHC, respectively) (Li et al., 2018). Transcripts were quantified through pseudoalignment by Kallisto (v.0.46.1), for which default parameters were used for both index build and transcript quantification (Bray et al., 2016). Additionally, data generated by Schrauwen et al. (2016) were used to retrieve expression values of *CEP78* in adult human cochlea and components of the vestibular labyrinth.

CEP78 Immunostaining on Human Retina

Human retina used for immunohistochemistry was fixed in 10% neutral buffered formaldehyde and embedded in paraffin. Staining for CEP78 was performed on 3-μm-thick sections using an automatic immunostainer (BenchMark Ultra, Ventana Medical Systems, Tucson, AZ, United States). The rabbit polyclonal antibody anti-CEP78 (1:100; LN2004459, LabNed) was used, and visualization was achieved with the OptiView Amplification Kit (Ventana Medical Systems). Heat-induced epitope retrieval was performed using Cell Conditioning 2 (Ventana Medical Systems).

RESULTS

The CRDHL families included in this study are of Belgian (F1 and F3), Danish (F2), and Turkish origin (F4). Consanguinity was reported for F4. Pedigrees are represented in **Figure 1**.

CNV Analysis on WES Data, sWGS, Long-Range PCR, and Targeted LRS in F1

For F1, II:1 CNV analysis on WES data using ExomeDepth revealed a potential homozygous deletion overlapping *CEP78* [initial coordinates (hg38) chr9: g.78236351–78243636]. Subsequent sWGS confirmed the homozygous deletion spanning exons 1–5 of *CEP78* [new coordinates (hg38) chr9:g.78230001–78245000], covering a region of 15–20 kb. The sWGS output is available in **Supplementary Table 3**. The deletion could be refined up to ~12 kb using iterative qPCRs, and a junction product could be obtained *via* long-range PCR (**Supplementary Figure 1**). Targeted LRS on the long-range PCR amplicon allowed final delineation, identifying a complex deletion–inversion–deletion (**Figure 2**). The left breakpoint is located at (hg38) chr9:78228782, whereas the right breakpoint at chr9:78244762. The inverted segment spans chr9:78234546–78234844 [nearby an L1ME3Cz repetitive element (chr9:78234521–78234902)]. The SV overlaps with the one previously described in a British patient by Sanchis-Juan et al. (2018), delineated using microarray and Sanger sequencing (Sanchis-Juan et al., 2018). A smaller deletion, overlapping exons 2 and 3 in *CEP78*, is reported in gnomAD SV (DEL_9_103019; gnomAD SVs v2.1). Segregation analysis was performed *via* qPCR and confirmed both parents as heterozygous carriers of the deletion. Expression analysis of *CEP78* mRNA on available lymphocytes (F1, II:1) and three controls showed complete loss of *CEP78* expression due to the homozygous deletion (**Supplementary Figure 2**).

Segregation Analysis, sWGS, and Whole-Genome LRS in F2

For F2, II:1, initial targeted gene panel sequencing was negative, as it was carried out before the *CEP78* gene had been associated with CRDHL. Thus, trio WES was performed for the proband

A

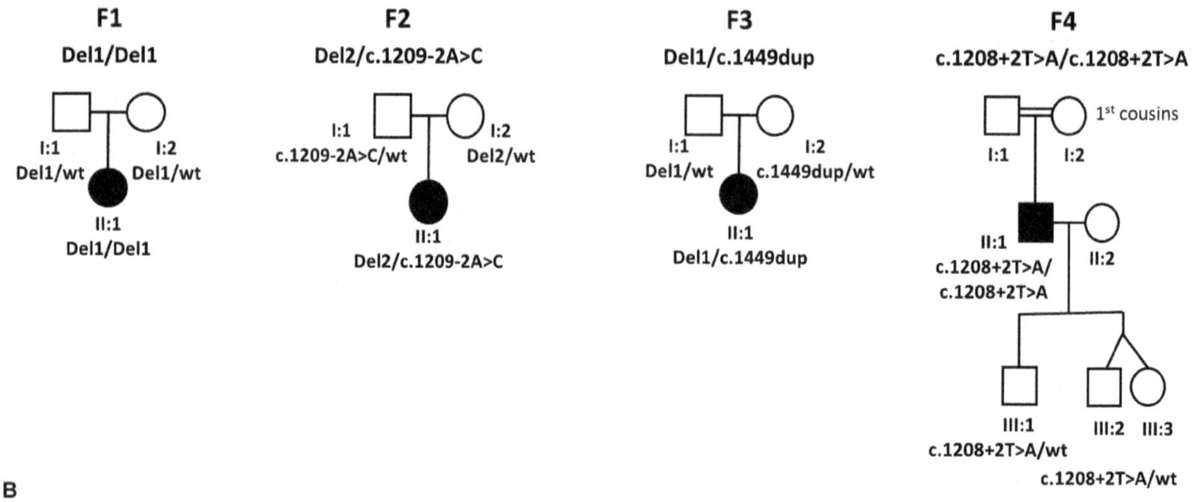

B

Marker	F1, II:1	F3, II:1	F3, I:2	F3, I:1	SV Sanchis-Juan *et al.*
rs10156442	GG	GA	GG	AA	AA
rs1953019	AA	AC	CC	AA	CC
rs2026000	GG	GG	GA	GG	GG
rs4877499	NA	GG	CG	CC	NA
CEP78	Del1/Del1	Del1/c.1449dup	c.1449dup/wt	Del1/wt	Del1/Del1
rs2521904	GG	GG	GA	GG	GG
rs7869495	GG	GC	CG	GC	GG
rs11792810	TT	TT	TC	TT	TT
rs10780305	GG	GG	GA	GG	GG
rs946806	AA	AG	GG	AG	AA
rs7039267	AA	AG	GG	AG	AA
rs7041989	TT	TG	TT	TG	TT

FIGURE 1 | Pedigrees segregating the *CEP78* structural and sequence variants and haplotype reconstruction for the shared SV. **(A)** F1, II:1 is homozygous for a complex deletion–inversion–deletion involving exons 1–5 of *CEP78*. F2, II:1 is compound heterozygous for a deletion of 235 kb overlapping *CEP78* and *PSAT1* and for splice site variant c.1209-2A>C. F3, II:1 is compound heterozygous for the same deletion–inversion–deletion of F1, II:1 and the c.1449dup variant in *CEP78*. F4, II:1 is homozygous for splice site variant c.1208+2T>A. Extended F4 pedigree available in **Supplementary Clinical Data 2**. **(B)** Genotyping of 18 flanking single-nucleotide polymorphisms (SNPs) revealed a common haplotype of 1.9 Mb, between the individuals carrying the deletion–inversion–deletion [F1, F3 and the case originally described by Sanchis-Juan et al. (2018)]. Extended version available in **Supplementary Table 5**. Abbreviations: Del, deletion (or deletion–inversion–deletion); wt, wild type.

and revealed a novel heterozygous splice variant c.1209-2A>C p.(?) (NM_001098802.2) in *CEP78*. The c.1209-2A>C variant in *CEP78* was confirmed *via* Sanger sequencing, where the proband appeared homozygous, the father heterozygous and the mother wild-type (**Supplementary Figure 3**). No additional family members have been tested. The splice variant is located in the acceptor splice site of intron 9, reported in dbSNP (rs778035330) with a frequency of 0.00002628 (gnomAD), and predictions suggest a skip of exon 10. It is predicted to disrupt the consensus splice site and likely results in an absent or disrupted protein product and loss of function. Subsequent RT-PCR confirmed the skip of exon 10 (**Supplementary Figure 3**). Population frequencies and *in silico* predictions of the *CEP78* splice variant are listed in **Supplementary Table 4** and **Supplementary Figure 4**. To our knowledge, this variant has not been reported in literature, but is reported as likely pathogenic in one case in ClinVar (ID 851351). Segregation analysis suggested a heterozygous genomic deletion of the *CEP78* region in F2, II:1, *in trans* with the splice variant. The heterozygous deletion was confirmed by sWGS, showing an interval of 225–240 kb spanning the entire *CEP78* and *PSAT1* genes (chr9: g.78105001–78330000). The sWGS output is available in **Supplementary Table 3**. The final delineation was obtained *via* whole-genome LRS allowing the identification of a heterozygous (13 reference sequence reads, 21 deletion reads) deletion spanning the region chr9:78096930–78331887 and covering 235 kb (**Figure 2**). Breakpoint junction

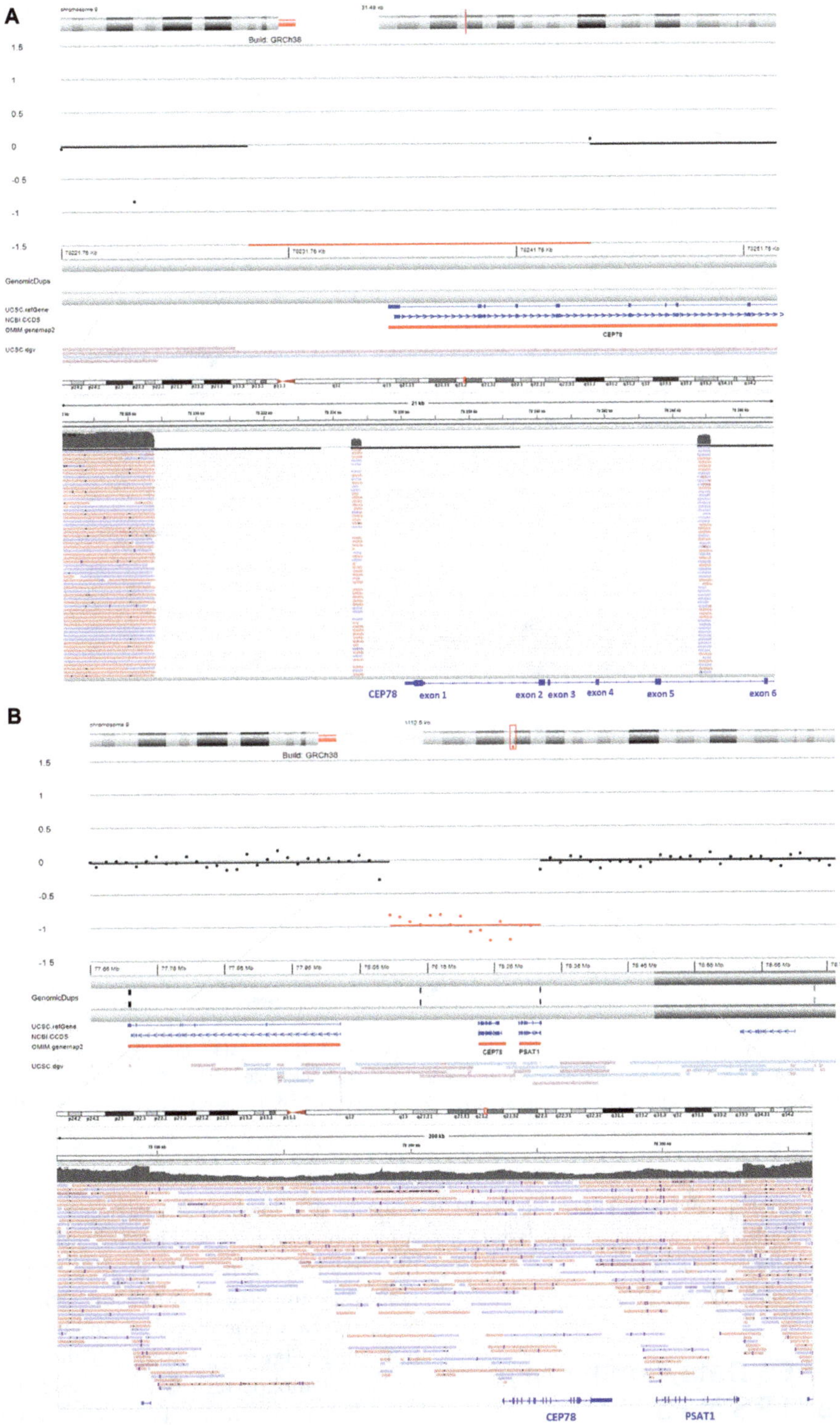

FIGURE 2 | sWGS output and integrative genomics viewer (IGV) view of the structural variants (SVs) detected *via* long-read sequencing (LRS) in F1 and F2. **(A)** sWGS in F1, II:1 revealed a homozygous deletion of the region spanning exons 1–5 of *CEP78* (top). Subsequent delineation of the SV *via* targeted LRS of the junction product identified a complex deletion–inversion–deletion (bottom). The left breakpoint is located at (hg38) chr9:78228782, whereas the right breakpoint is located at chr9:78244762. The inverted segment spans chr9:78234546–78234844 [nearby an L1ME3Cz repetitive element (chr9:78234521–78234902)]. The SV overlaps with a previously described SV affecting *CEP78* (Sanchis-Juan et al., 2018). **(B)** sWGS in F2, II:1 identified a heterozygous deletion spanning the entire *CEP78* and *PSAT1* genes (top). Final delineation was obtained *via* whole-genome LRS, coordinates are crossing chr9: 78096930–78331887 and cover 235 kb (bottom).

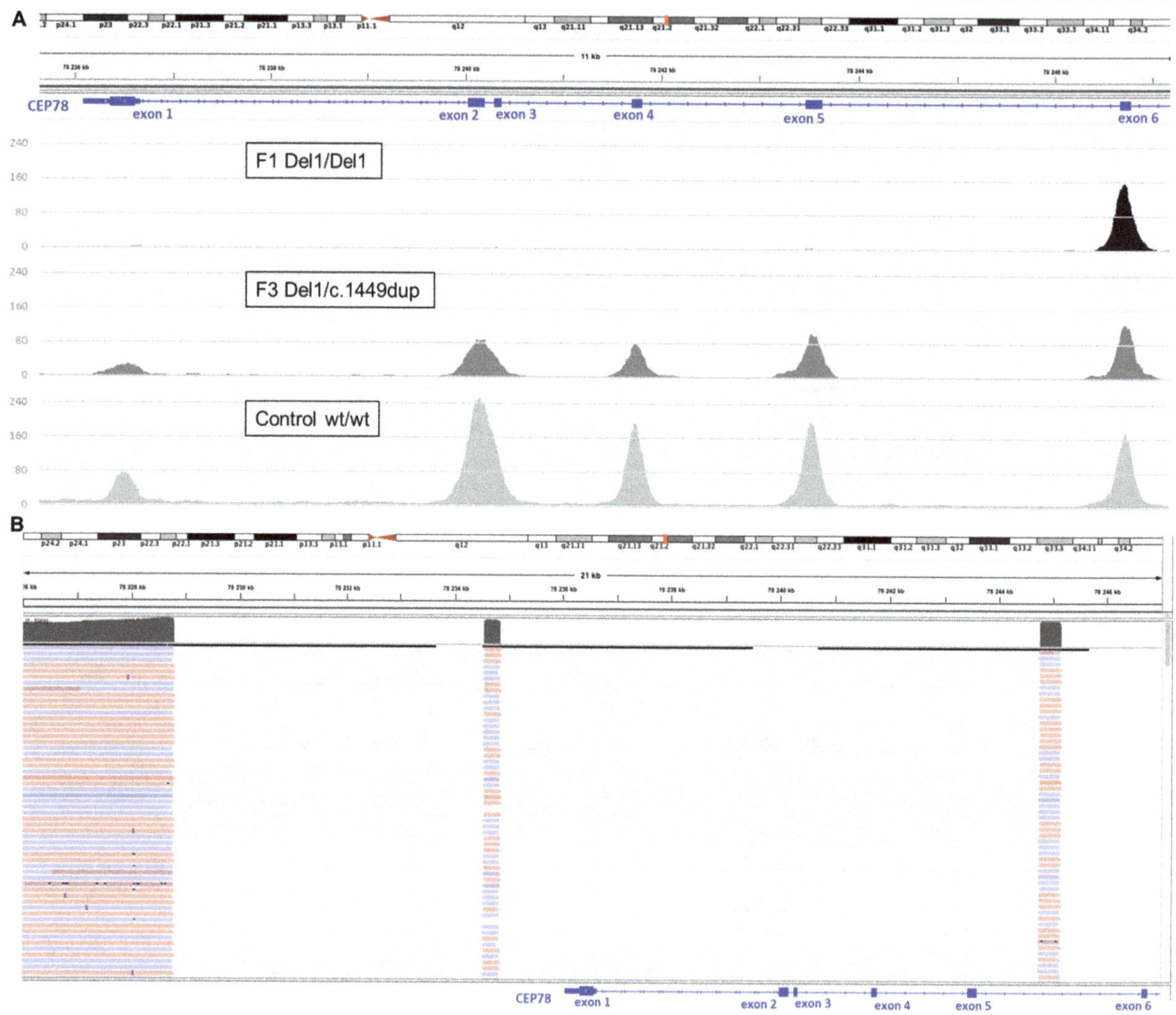

FIGURE 3 | Deletion coverage plots and IGV view of the complex SV detected *via* targeted LRS in F3, II:1. **(A)** ExomeDepth coverage plots for homozygous deletion (F1, II:1, top) and heterozygous deletion (F3, II:1, middle) compared to control (bottom). Coverage suggested for F3, II:1 the same deletion described for F1, II:1 but in heterozygous state. **(B)** Delineation of the SV *via* targeted LRS of the junction product obtained in F3, II:1 identified the same complex deletion–inversion–deletion found previously in F1, II:1.

analysis highlighted microhomology (**Supplementary Figure 5**). Expression analysis of *CEP78* mRNA on available fibroblasts (F2, II:1) and two controls showed loss of *CEP78* expression due to the *CEP78* genotype (**Supplementary Figure 2**).

CNV Analysis on WES Data, Long-Range PCR, and Targeted LRS in F3

For F3, II:1 CNV analysis on WES data using ExomeDepth revealed a heterozygous deletion overlapping *CEP78* with the same coordinates of the deletion in F1, II:1 (**Figure 3**) in combination with c.1449dup [p.(Arg484Thrfs*4)]. The latter is a novel 1-bp duplication in exon 12, creating a frameshift starting at codon Arg484. The new reading frame ends in a stop codon at position 4 (**Supplementary Table 4**). Segregation analysis confirmed the presence of c.1449dup on the maternal allele, while the deletion has paternal origin (**Supplementary Figure 6**). A junction product could be obtained *via* long-range PCR using the same primers used for F1, II:1. Targeted LRS on the long-range PCR amplicon allowed a final delineation, identifying once more the same complex deletion–inversion–deletion as found in F1, II:1 (**Figure 3**). Expression analysis of *CEP78* mRNA on available lymphocytes (F3 I:1, I:2, and II:1) and three controls showed extremely reduced *CEP78* expression due to the variants in the index case (**Supplementary Figure 2**).

Haplotype Reconstruction for Recurrent Deletion–Inversion–Deletion of *CEP78* Identified in F1 and F3

The same deletion–inversion–deletion, originally described by Sanchis-Juan et al. (2018), has been identified here in F1

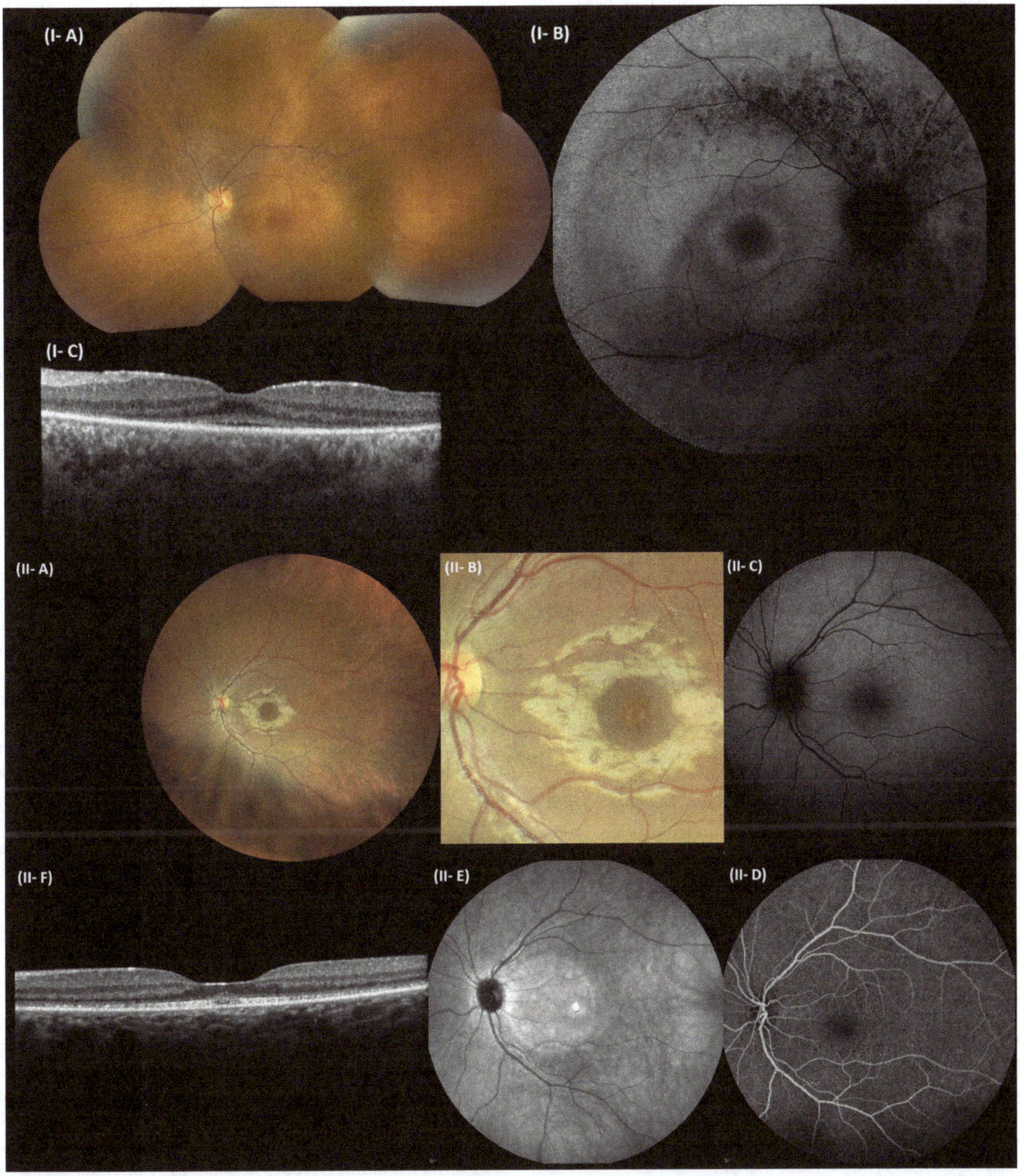

FIGURE 4 | Representative ophthalmological pictures of individuals from F1 and F3 carrying *CEP78* structural variants. **(I)** F1, II:1. **(I-A)** Color fundus photograph of LE with normal optic disk, minimal narrowing of retinal arterioles, RPE mottling around the temporal vascular arcades, no bone spiculae. **(I-B)** BAF of the RE with hyperautofluorescent ring surrounding the fovea and granular hypo-autofluorescence around the temporal vascular arcades. **(I-C)** Spectral-domain OCT of the LE depicting loss of perifoveal photoreceptor layer and better foveal quality with loss, however, of integrity of photoreceptor outer segments. **(II)** F3, II:1. **(II-A)** Eye fundus of the left eye with perifoveal fine, granular, yellowish material upon close inspection. Normal aspect of optic disk, peripheral retina, and retinal vessels. **(II-B)** Close-up of the macular area, demonstrating the fine, granular, yellowish material encircling the fovea. **(II-C)** BAF of the LE without obvious abnormalities. **(II-D)** Fluorescein angiography of the LE with normal fluorescence. **(II-E)** Near-infrared imaging of the LE (hyperintense circular area is an artifact). **(II-F)** Spectral-domain OCT of the LE, revealing a mottled aspect of the ellipsoid zone and subfoveal collection of fluffy material. Enlarged and flat foveal depression. BAF, blue-light autofluorescence imaging; OCT, spectral-domain optical coherence tomography; RE, right eye; LE, left eye; RPE, retinal pigment epithelium.

(homozygous) and F3 (heterozygous, with paternal inheritance); therefore, haplotype reconstruction using genotyping of 18 SNPs was performed in the proband of F1 (II:1) and in the proband and parents of F3 (II:1, I:1, and I:2). In addition, the haplotype of the homozygous *CEP78* SV reported by Sanchis-Juan et al. (2018), was reconstructed here on the basis of available WGS data. A common shared haplotype of at least 1.9 Mb was identified (**Supplementary Table 5**).

Phenotypic Expression of *CEP78* Disease Caused by SVs and SNVs

In F4, II:1 WES filtering revealed a novel homozygous splice variant c.1208+2T>A [p.(?)] (NM_001098802.2), located in the donor splice site of intron 9 and predicted to cause skipping of exon 9. The variant involves the same intron as the one affected by c.1209-2A>C in F2, II:1 and is not reported in gnomAD. Segregation analysis in two of the obligate carrier children confirmed they are heterozygous carriers. Population frequencies, *in silico* predictions, and variant classification according to ACMG and ACGS criteria are listed in **Supplementary Table 4** and **Supplementary Figure 4**. All patients included received an initial (F1, F2, and F3) or *post hoc*, genotype-driven (F4) clinical diagnosis compatible with CRDHL. In agreement with previous studies, the IRD phenotype displays a more pronounced cone dysfunction at the onset. The age at onset of the IRD ranged from the second to third decade and, of the hearing loss, from congenital to the first decade of life. More detailed clinical features are provided in **Figure 4**, **Table 1**, and **Supplementary Clinical Data 1, 2**. Affected individuals from F1 to F3 are females, whereas the affected individual from F4 is a male, without signs of subfertility/infertility. Apart from CRDHL, no additional clinical features were reported except for a balance disorder in F1. Overall, no genotype–phenotype correlation could be observed for the IRD phenotype in probands with biallelic *CEP78* SVs, SNVs, or a combination of both.

CEP78 Expression in Human and Mouse Tissues Affected in CRDHL

In line with the main systems affected in CRDHL, i.e., neural retina and the inner ear, we examined *CEP78* expression in sc transcriptional datasets of human neural retina together with mouse and human cochlear or inner ear cells. This showed that *CEP78* is predominantly expressed in cone photoreceptor and in hair cell clusters, respectively (**Figure 5** and **Supplementary Figures 7, 8**). Next, the expression patterns of *CEP78* and other ciliary genes listed in the top 10 of the HGC (Itan et al., 2013), *SCLT1*, *MKS1*, *CEP57*, *CEP76*, *CEP135*, *CEP152*, *CEP63*, *CEP164*, *OFD1*, and *CEP250*, in human adult bulk retinal transcriptional datasets were assessed for coordinated correlation, reasoning that this could offer insight into possible regulatory interactions. Interestingly, a matrix correlation plot (**Supplementary Figure 9**) showed *CEP78* expression to be correlated with *SCLT1* ($\rho = 0.63$, $p < 0.001$) and to be anticorrelated with *CEP250* ($\rho = -0.53$, $p = 0.0007$), both of them already associated with IRD (Khateb et al., 2014; Tonda et al., 2016; Kubota et al., 2018). Immunohistochemistry analysis of human retina shows predominant cytoplasmic expression of CEP78 in both cones and rods, with strong staining at the base of the inner segments, concordant with previous findings (**Figure 5**; Namburi et al., 2016; Nikopoulos et al., 2016).

DISCUSSION

In this study, we focused on *CEP78*-associated IRD, of which several studies have linked *CEP78* variants with a presumed loss-of-function effect to CRDHL. Interestingly, a homozygous complex SV affecting *CEP78*, i.e., a deletion–inversion–deletion, was recently described in a case of CRDHL (Sanchis-Juan et al., 2018). We assessed the role of SVs in CRDHL cases and found two distinct SVs affecting the *CEP78* region, emphasizing their role in *CEP78* disease. We showed the efficacy of CNV analysis of WES data to identify subtle CNVs; more specifically, we identified a deletion spanning exons 1–5 of *CEP78*, in both homozygous and heterozygous states, leading to loss of function. Furthermore, we showed the power of combined sWGS, qPCR, and targeted or whole-genome LRS to delineate and characterize SVs at the nucleotide level. This approach revealed a complex 15-kb deletion–inversion–deletion, which proved to be the same as the previously reported *CEP78* SV that was found and characterized by combined molecular karyotyping and Sanger sequencing. As this deletion was identified in the two families of Belgian origin and in a previously published case of a British patient, haplotype reconstruction was performed and suggested a founder effect. Apart from this, a distinct larger SV, being a 235-kb heterozygous deletion, was identified using molecular karyotyping and characterized using whole-genome LRS. This deletion encompasses the *CEP78* and *PSAT1* (MIM #610936) genes, the latter of which has so far only been implicated in recessive phosphoserine aminotransferase deficiency (MIM # 610992) and Neu-Laxova syndrome 2 (MIM # 616038) (Hart et al., 2007; Acuna-Hidalgo et al., 2014). Overall, for all cases with *CEP78* SVs identified by us, loss of *CEP78* expression was confirmed on patient-derived material. The latter is in line with the molecular effects of the previously reported *CEP78* sequence variants.

Sanchis-Juan et al. (2018) reported that the sequences surrounding all the breakpoints of the described SV in *CEP78* present high similarity to long interspersed nuclear elements (LINEs). It was hypothesized that repetitive elements enable replication-based SV formation, providing the necessary microhomology islands or increasing the vulnerability of the region to the formation of secondary DNA structures, which can lead to replication fork collapse (Sanchis-Juan et al., 2018). We performed a similar extensive *in silico* analysis of all breakpoints and junctions of the SVs identified in this study (**Supplementary Figures 5, 10** and **Supplementary Tables 6, 7**). Interestingly, all breakpoint junctions, including the 235-kb *CEP78-PSAT1* deletion, showed microhomology, supporting repetitive element-mediated replication-based SV formation underlying *CEP78* SVs/complex SVs. Our findings underscore that SVs contribute to the genetic diversity of the human genome and are of high relevance for the molecular pathogenesis of rare diseases. Very

TABLE 1 | Overview of clinical findings in *CEP78*-associated CRDHL.

	Age/sex	Origin	Age at onset	BCVA (RE/LE)	Goldmann visual fields	Fundus imaging	BAF	OCT	ERG	Hearing impairment	Other findings reported
F1 II:1	45 y/F	Belgian	22 y	0.1/0.1	Small central island of less than 5°, surrounded by large absolute (mid)peripheral scotoma (100° horizontal, 70° vertical) and normal peripheral limits	Normal optic disk, normal veins, narrowing of the arteries, perimacular grayish mottling around the vascular arcades and midperiphery, absence of bone spiculae	Mottled hypofluo rescence around the large vascular arcades, perifoveal hyperfluo rescent ring	Loss of outer retinal layers with sparing of subfoveal region with foveal swelling and blending	Maximum tendency toward electronegativity, scotopic function flat, cone function: both 30-Hz flicker and single flash present but delayed and reduced	Present since the age of 12 y, hearing aids	No fertility problems, balance disorder
F2 II:1	52 y/F	Danish	30 y	0.25/0.2 (49 y)	Paracentral scotomas, normal outer borders (49 y)	Normal optic disk, attenuated vessels, absence of hyperpigme ntations (49 y)	Mottled appearance midperiphery (49 y)	Attenuation of outer retinal layers (49 y)	Reduced cone and rod responses (39 y)	Congenital progressive hearing loss, hearing aids	None
F3 II:1	25 y/F	Belgian	24 y	0.3/0.2	Pericentral concentric scotoma	Discrete macular mottling	Unremarkable	Wide foveal depression	Lowered cone and rod responses, but worse for cones	High frequencies	Subtle mottling in central macula on infrared
F4 II:1	57 y/M	Turkish	NA	0.08/0.08	Small central island less than 5°, currently stable	Pale optic disk, narrow blood vessels, grayish discoloration, some bone spiculae in midperiphery	Mottled hypoautoflu orescence around the large vascular arcades and nasally, perifoveal hyperflu orescent ring	Attenuation of outer retina	Extinguished responses of cones and rods	Present since childhood, not progressive	None

BAF, blue-light autofluorescence imaging; BCVA, best-corrected visual acuity; CF, counting fingers; ERG, full-field flash electroretinography; F, female; HM, hand movements; M, male; NA, not available; OCT, spectral-domain optical coherence tomography; RE, right eye; LE, left eye.

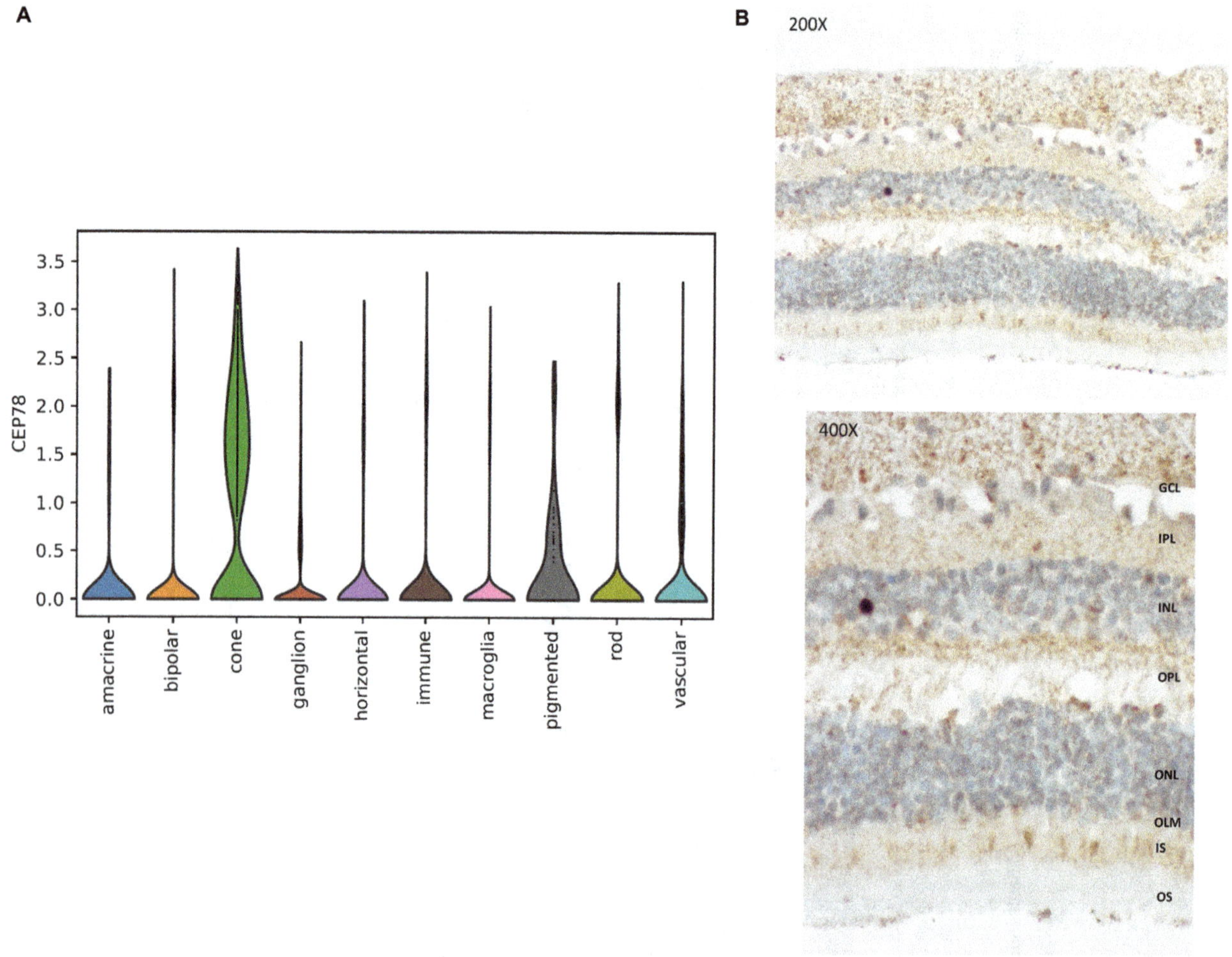

FIGURE 5 | Single-cell transcriptional data in human retina and immunohistochemistry of CEP78 in adult human retina. **(A)** Violin plot for visualization of scaled and corrected expression of *CEP78* in 19,768 human neural retinal cells. Cells belonging to the cone cell population exhibit the highest expression. **(B)** Immunostaining of the CEP78 protein is visible in light brown. Light microscopy at 200 × (top) and 400 × (bottom). Predominant cytoplasmic expression of CEP78 can be seen in both cone and rod photoreceptors with strong staining at the base of the inner segments. Antibody: LN2004459 (1:100, rabbit, LabNed). GCL, ganglion cell layer; IPL, inner plexiform layer; INL, inner nuclear layer; OPL, outer plexiform layer; ONL, outer nuclear layer; OLM, outer limiting membrane; IS, inner segments; OS, outer segments.

recently, SVs were mapped and characterized in 17,795 deeply sequenced human genomes (Abel et al., 2020). It is estimated that SVs account for 17.2% of rare alleles genome-wide and that approximately 90% of such SVs are non-coding deletions. The number of complex SVs as a cause of genetic diseases is emerging. This is illustrated by *de novo* interspersed repeat insertions found in 124 cases with a genetic disease, 76 of which are caused by *Alu* short interspersed elements (SINEs), and 30 can be attributed to LINE-1 insertions (Payer et al., 2017). Two remarkable examples of complex SVs as a cause of IRD are SVA retrotransposon insertions in *MFSD8*- and *BBS1*-associated disease, of which the first SV served as a target for antisense oligonucleotide treatment, and the second appears to be a frequent cause of Bardet–Biedl syndrome (Kim et al., 2019; Delvallée et al., 2020). Another recent example is the identification of 33 pathogenic SVs in a cohort of 722 patients with autosomal dominant retinitis pigmentosa (adRP). Indeed, eight distinct complex non-coding SVs were found as the underlying mechanism of RP17-linked adRP in 22 affected families with >300 affected individuals, clearly emphasizing the importance of the non-coding genome as target for SVs in IRD (de Bruijn et al., 2020).

Given a high contribution of CNVs to ~7%–10% of the pathogenic alleles in IRD, the fact that the majority of the SVs in our genome are non-coding and the emerging number of non-coding or complex SVs causing IRD (Abel et al., 2020; Zampaglione et al., 2020), it can be expected that SVs represent an important part of missing heritability of IRD. Hence, there is a need to assess the impact and frequency of SVs in IRD cohorts more systematically. Here, we showed how CNV calling on WES data, sWGS, and targeted or whole-genome LRS led to a confirmed molecular diagnosis in *CEP78*-associated IRD cases. CNV assessment using NGS-based algorithms has been already described as a reliable method to enhance the diagnostic rate of IRD (Khateb et al., 2016; Ellingford et al., 2018). Furthermore, this study supports the superiority of LRS for fast characterization of complex SVs. Massively parallel sequencing is currently dominated by second-generation sequencing technology, mainly relying on SRS, having its limitations for the identification of cryptic SVs, sequencing repetitive regions, phasing of alleles, and distinguishing highly homologous genomic regions, mainly due to its short-read lengths. Third-generation or LRS technologies offer improvements in the characterization of genetic variation and regions that are difficult to assess with the current SRS approaches. The main advantage of LRS compared to SRS technologies comes from the use of long reads (>10 kb on average), originating from single-DNA molecules. Apart from this, the sequencing occurs in real time without the need of PCR amplification, therefore being mostly free from PCR-related bias. The power of LRS approaches to overcome specific limitations of second generation–based analyses will further become clear when LRS will be implemented in routine genetic testing workflows.

Apart from the *CEP78* SVs, the two novel splice variants found here expand the spectrum of *CEP78* (likely) pathogenic SNVs: a novel canonical acceptor and donor splice variant of intron 9, respectively, c.1209-2A>C (p.?), predicted to lead to an exon 10 skip, and c.1208 + 2T > A (p.?), predicted to cause an exon 9 skip. Interestingly, skipping of the 46-bp exon 10 was previously reported for c.1254 + 5G>A (*CEP78*, NM_032171) (Fu et al., 2016). When comparing the phenotypes found in CRDHL cases with SNV and SVs, no apparent genotype–phenotype correlation could be demonstrated that would allow discriminating between the two classes of variants, emphasizing the need for a systematic SV assessment in the genetic workup of CRDHL cases, in which a *CEP78* genotype is suspected or in "atypical" Usher syndrome cases.

Using data mining of bulk or sc transcriptional datasets from human retina, mouse cochlea, and human inner ear, we showed expression in cone photoreceptors and in hair cell clusters. These expression domains are in agreement with the main systems affected in CRDHL, i.e., neural retina and the inner ear. Apart from this, a correlation study of *CEP78* expression strengthened the importance of CEP78 in the ciliary machinery.

To conclude, this study supports that the *CEP78* locus is prone to microhomology-mediated, replication-based SV formation and that (complex) SV analysis should be included in molecular genetic testing of CRDHL or "atypical" Usher syndrome. Finally, it demonstrates the power of WES-based CNV assessment, sWGS, and whole or targeted LRS in identifying and characterizing suspected complex SVs in patients with *CEP78*-associated IRD. Systematic SV assessment in IRD will certainly close a diagnostic gap and will contribute to precision medicine in IRD.

ETHICS STATEMENT

The studies involving human participants were reviewed and approved by Ethics Committee Ghent University Hospital, Ghent University Hospital, Ghent. Written informed consent to participate in this study was provided by the participants' legal guardian/next of kin. Written informed consent was obtained from the individual(s), and minor(s)' legal guardian/next of kin, for the publication of any potentially identifiable images or data included in this article.

AUTHOR CONTRIBUTIONS

GAs and EDB designed the study and wrote the overall manuscript. GAs, NR, MDB, MVH, DC, JVD, TVL, TDP, AR, and EDB performed the research. JDZ, MVL, JJ, MBe, and LT clinically evaluated and described the families included in the study. GAs, NR, MDB, MBa, MVH, GAr, DC, JVD, TR, TDP, PDR, WDC, BM, AR, MS, and EDB analyzed and described the data. All authors reviewed the manuscript.

ACKNOWLEDGMENTS

Lone Sandbjerg Hindbaek is thanked for excellent technical help with RT-PCR studies. Sarah De Jaegere and Valerie Baumont are thanked for their assistance. We are also grateful to the families for their participation in the study.

REFERENCES

Abel, H. J., Larson, D. E., Regier, A. A., Chiang, C., Das, I., Kanchi, K. L., et al. (2020). Mapping and characterization of structural variation in 17,795 human genomes. *Nature* 583, 83–89. doi: 10.1038/s41586-020-2371-0

Abou Tayoun, A. N., Pesaran, T., DiStefano, M. T., Oza, A., Rehm, H. L., Biesecker, L. G., et al. (2018). Recommendations for interpreting the loss of function PVS1 ACMG/AMP variant criterion. *Hum. Mutat.* 39, 1517–1524. doi: 10.1002/humu.23626

Acuna-Hidalgo, R., Schanze, D., Kariminejad, A., Nordgren, A., Kariminejad, M. H., Conner, P., et al. (2014). Neu-laxova syndrome is a heterogeneous metabolic disorder caused by defects in enzymes of the l-serine biosynthesis pathway. *Am. J. Hum. Genet.* 95, 285–93. doi: 10.1016/j.ajhg.2014.07.012

Ascari, G., Peelman, F., Farinelli, P., Rosseel, T., Lambrechts, N., Wunderlich, K. A., et al. (2020). Functional characterization of the first missense variant in CEP78, a founder allele associated with cone-rod dystrophy, hearing loss and reduced male fertility. *Hum. Mutat.* 41, 998–1011. doi: 10.1002/humu.23993

Belkadi, A., Bolze, A., Itan, Y., Cobat, A., Vincent, Q. B., Antipenko, A., et al. (2015). Whole-genome sequencing is more powerful than whole-exome sequencing for detecting exome variants. *Proc. Natl. Acad. Sci. U.S.A.* 112, 5473–5478. doi: 10.1073/pnas.1418631112

Bray, N. L., Pimentel, H., Melsted, P., and Pachter, L. (2016). Near-optimal probabilistic RNA-seq quantification. *Nat. Biotechnol.* 34, 525–527. doi: 10.1038/nbt.3519

Brunk, K., Zhu, M., Bärenz, F., Kratz, A., Haselmann-Weiss, U., Antony, C., et al. (2016). Cep78 is a new centriolar protein involved in Plk4-induced centriole overduplication. *J. Cell Sci.* 129, 2713–2718. doi: 10.1242/jcs.184093

Carss, K., Arno, G., Erwood, M., Stephens, J., Sanchis-Juan, A., Hull, S., et al. (2017). Comprehensive rare variant analysis via whole-genome sequencing to determine the molecular pathology of inherited retinal disease. *Am. J. Hum. Genet.* 100, 75–90. doi: 10.1016/j.ajhg.2016.12.003

Chaisson, M. J. P., Sanders, A. D., Zhao, X., Malhotra, A., Porubsky, D., Rausch, T., et al. (2019). Multi-platform discovery of haplotype-resolved structural variation in human genomes. *Nat. Commun.* 10:1784. doi: 10.1038/s41467-018-08148-z

Cowan, C. S., Renner, M., De Gennaro, M., Gross-Scherf, B., Goldblum, D., Hou, Y., et al. (2020). Cell types of the human retina and its organoids at single-cell resolution. *Cell* 182, 1623–1640.e34. doi: 10.1016/j.cell.2020.08.013

D'haene, B., Vandesompele, J., and Hellemans, J. (2010). Accurate and objective copy number profiling using real-time quantitative PCR. *Methods* 50, 262–270. doi: 10.1016/j.ymeth.2009.12.007

Daiger, S. P., Sullivan, L. S., Bowne, S. J., Cadena, E. D., Koboldt, D., Bujakowska, K. M., et al. (2019). Detection of large structural variants causing inherited retinal diseases. *Adv. Exp. Med. Biol.* 1185, 197–202. doi: 10.1007/978-3-030-27378-1_32

de Bruijn, S. E., Fiorentino, A., Ottaviani, D., Fanucchi, S., Melo, U. S., Corral-Serrano, J. C., et al. (2020). Structural variants create new topological-associated domains and ectopic retinal enhancer-gene contact in dominant retinitis pigmentosa. *Am. J. Hum. Genet.* 107, 802–814. doi: 10.1016/j.ajhg.2020.09.002

De Coster, W., and Van Broeckhoven, C. (2019). Newest methods for detecting structural variations. *Trends Biotechnol.* 37, 973–982. doi: 10.1016/j.tibtech.2019.02.003

Delvallée, C., Nicaise, S., Antin, M., Leuvrey, A., Nourisson, E., Leitch, C. C., et al. (2020). A BBS1 SVA F retrotransposon insertion is a frequent cause of Bardet-Biedl syndrome. *Clin. Genet.* 99, 318–324. doi: 10.1111/cge.13878

Eichler, E. E. (2019). Genetic variation, comparative genomics, and the diagnosis of disease. *N. Engl. J. Med.* 381, 64–74. doi: 10.1056/nejmra1809315

Ellard, S., Baple, E. L., Berry, I., Forrester, N., Turnbull, C., Owens, M., et al. (2019). ACGS best practice guidelines for variant classification 2019. *Assoc. Clin. Genet. Sci.* 1–32.

Ellingford, J. M., Barton, S., Bhaskar, S., Williams, S. G., Sergouniotis, P. I., O'Sullivan, J., et al. (2016). Whole genome sequencing increases molecular diagnostic yield compared with current diagnostic testing for inherited retinal disease. *Ophthalmology* 123, 1143–1150. doi: 10.1016/j.ophtha.2016.01.009

Ellingford, J. M., Horn, B., Campbell, C., Arno, G., Barton, S., Tate, C., et al. (2018). Assessment of the incorporation of CNV surveillance into gene panel next-generation sequencing testing for inherited retinal diseases. *J. Med. Genet.* 55, 114–121. doi: 10.1136/jmedgenet-2017-104791

Fu, Q., Xu, M., Chen, X., Sheng, X., Yuan, Z., Liu, Y., et al. (2016). CEP78 is mutated in a distinct type of Usher syndrome. *J. Med. Genet.* 54, 190–195. doi: 10.1136/jmedgenet-2016-104166

Gönczy, P. (2015). Centrosomes and cancer: revisiting a long-standing relationship. *Nat. Rev. Cancer* 15, 639–652. doi: 10.1038/nrc3995

Gönczy, P., and Hatzopoulos, G. N. (2019). Centriole assembly at a glance. *J. Cell Sci.* 132:jcs228833. doi: 10.1242/jcs.228833

Hart, C. E., Race, V., Achouri, Y., Wiame, E., Sharrard, M., Olpin, S. E., et al. (2007). Phosphoserine aminotransferase deficiency: a novel disorder of the serine biosynthesis pathway. *Am. J. Hum. Genet.* 80, 931–937. doi: 10.1086/517888

Itan, Y., Zhang, S.-Y., Vogt, G., Abhyankar, A., Herman, M., Nitschke, P., et al. (2013). The human gene connectome as a map of short cuts for morbid allele discovery. *Proc. Natl. Acad. Sci. U.S.A.* 110, 5558–5563. doi: 10.1073/pnas.1218167110

Jespersgaard, C., Fang, M., Bertelsen, M., Dang, X., Jensen, H., Chen, Y., et al. (2019). Molecular genetic analysis using targeted NGS analysis of 677 individuals with retinal dystrophy. *Sci. Rep.* 9:1219. doi: 10.1038/s41598-018-38007-2

Khateb, S., Hanany, M., Khalaileh, A., Beryozkin, A., Meyer, S., Abu-Diab, A., et al. (2016). Identification of genomic deletions causing inherited retinal degenerations by coverage analysis of whole exome sequencing data. *J. Med. Genet.* 53, 600–607. doi: 10.1136/jmedgenet-2016-103825

Khateb, S., Zelinger, L., Mizrahi-Meissonnier, L., Ayuso, C., Koenekoop, R. K., Laxer, U., et al. (2014). A homozygous nonsense CEP250 mutation combined with a heterozygous nonsense C2orf71 mutation is associated with atypical Usher syndrome. *J. Med. Genet.* 51, 460–469. doi: 10.1136/jmedgenet-2014-102287

Kim, J., Hu, C., Moufawad El Achkar, C., Black, L. E., Douville, J., Larson, A., et al. (2019). Patient-customized oligonucleotide therapy for a rare genetic disease. *N. Engl. J. Med.* 381, 1644–1652. doi: 10.1056/nejmoa1813279

Kolla, L., Kelly, M. C., Mann, Z. F., Anaya-Rocha, A., Ellis, K., Lemons, A., et al. (2020). Characterization of the development of the mouse cochlear epithelium at the single cell level. *Nat. Commun.* 11:2389. doi: 10.1038/s41467-020-1113-y

Kubota, D., Gocho, K., Kikuchi, S., Akeo, K., Miura, M., Yamaki, K., et al. (2018). CEP250 mutations associated with mild cone-rod dystrophy and sensorineural hearing loss in a Japanese family. *Ophthalmic Genet.* 39, 500–507. doi: 10.1080/13816810.2018.1466338

Li, H. (2018). Minimap2: pairwise alignment for nucleotide sequences. *Bioinformatics* 34, 3094–3100. doi: 10.1093/bioinformatics/bty191

Li, H., and Durbin, R. (2009). Fast and accurate short read alignment with Burrows-Wheeler transform. *Bioinformatics* 25, 1754–1760. doi: 10.1093/bioinformatics/btp324

Li, H., Handsaker, B., Wysoker, A., Fennell, T., Ruan, J., Homer, N., et al. (2009). The sequence alignment / map (SAM) Format and SAMtools 1000 Genome project data processing subgroup. *Bioinformatics* 25, 2078–2079.

Li, Y., Liu, H., Giffen, K. P., Chen, L., Beisel, K. W., and He, D. Z. Z. (2018). Transcriptomes of cochlear inner and outer hair cells from adult mice. *Sci. Data* 5:180199. doi: 10.1038/sdata.2018.199

Lindstrand, A., Eisfeldt, J., Pettersson, M., Carvalho, C. M. B., Kvarnung, M., Grigelioniene, G., et al. (2019). From cytogenetics to cytogenomics: whole-genome sequencing as a first-line test comprehensively captures the diverse spectrum of disease-causing genetic variation underlying intellectual disability. *Genome Med.* 11:68. doi: 10.1186/s13073-019-0675-1

Mahmoud, M., Gobet, N., Cruz-Dávalos, D. I., Mounier, N., Dessimoz, C., and Sedlazeck, F. J. (2019). Structural variant calling: the long and the short of it. *Genome Biol.* 20:246. doi: 10.1186/s13059-019-1828-7

Namburi, P., Ratnapriya, R., Khateb, S., Lazar, C. H., Kinarty, Y., Obolensky, A., et al. (2016). Bi-allelic truncating mutations in CEP78, encoding centrosomal protein 78, cause cone-rod degeneration with sensorineural hearing loss. *Am. J. Hum. Genet.* 99, 777–784. doi: 10.1016/j.ajhg.2016.07.010

Nigg, E. A., and Raff, J. W. (2009). Centrioles, centrosomes, and cilia in health and disease. *Cell* 139, 663–678. doi: 10.1016/j.cell.2009.10.036

Nikopoulos, K., Farinelli, P., Giangreco, B., Tsika, C., Royer-Bertrand, B., Mbefo, M. K., et al. (2016). Mutations in CEP78 cause cone-rod dystrophy and hearing loss associated with primary-cilia defects. *Am. J. Hum. Genet.* 99, 770–776. doi: 10.1016/j.ajhg.2016.07.009

Nishiguchi, K. M., Tearle, R. G., Liu, Y. P., Oh, E. C., Miyake, N., Benaglio, P., et al. (2013). Whole genome sequencing in patients with retinitis pigmentosa reveals pathogenic DNA structural changes and NEK2 as a new disease gene. *Proc. Natl. Acad. Sci. U.S.A.* 110, 16139–16144. doi: 10.1073/pnas.1308243110

Nykamp, K., Anderson, M., Powers, M., Garcia, J., Herrera, B., Ho, Y. Y., et al. (2017). Sherloc: a comprehensive refinement of the ACMG-AMP variant classification criteria. *Genet. Med.* 19, 1105–1117. doi: 10.1038/gim.2017.37

Payer, L. M., Steranka, J. P., Yang, W. R., Kryatova, M., Medabalimi, S., Ardeljan, D., et al. (2017). Structural variants caused by Alu insertions are associated with risks for many human diseases. *Proc. Natl. Acad. Sci. U.S.A.* 114, E3984–E3992. doi: 10.1073/pnas.1704117114

Plagnol, V., Curtis, J., Epstein, M., Mok, K. Y., Stebbings, E., Grigoriadou, S., et al. (2012). A robust model for read count data in exome sequencing experiments and implications for copy number variant calling. *Bioinformatics* 28, 2747–2754. doi: 10.1093/bioinformatics/bts526

Raman, L., Dheedene, A., De Smet, M., Van Dorpe, J., and Menten, B. (2019). WisecondorX: improved copy number detection for routine shallow whole-genome sequencing. *Nucleic Acids Res.* 47, 1605–1614. doi: 10.1093/nar/gky1263

Ratnapriya, R., Sosina, O. A., Starostik, M. R., Kwicklis, M., Kapphahn, R. J., Fritsche, L. G., et al. (2019). Retinal transcriptome and eQTL analyses identify genes associated with age-related macular degeneration. *Nat. Genet.* 51, 606–610. doi: 10.1038/s41588-019-0351-9

Reumers, J., De Rijk, P., Zhao, H., Liekens, A., Smeets, D., Cleary, J., et al. (2012). Optimized filtering reduces the error rate in detecting genomic variants by short-read sequencing. *Nat. Biotechnol.* 30, 61–68. doi: 10.1038/nbt.2053

Richards, S., Aziz, N., Bale, S., Bick, D., Das, S., Gastier-Foster, J., et al. (2015). Standards and guidelines for the interpretation of sequence variants: a joint consensus recommendation of the American college of medical genetics and genomics and the association for molecular pathology. *Genet. Med.* 17, 405–424. doi: 10.1038/gim.2015.30

Sanchis-Juan, A., Stephens, J., French, C. E., Gleadall, N., Mégy, K., Penkett, C., et al. (2018). Complex structural variants in mendelian disorders: identification and breakpoint resolution using short- and long-read genome sequencing. *Genome Med.* 10:95. doi: 10.1186/s13073-018-0606-6

Sante, T., Vergult, S., Volders, P. J., Kloosterman, W. P., Trooskens, G., De Preter, K., et al. (2014). ViVar: a comprehensive platform for the analysis and visualization of structural genomic variation. *PLoS One* 9:e113800. doi: 10.1371/journal.pone.0113800

Schneider, V. A., Graves-Lindsay, T., Howe, K., Bouk, N., Chen, H. C., Kitts, P. A., et al. (2017). Evaluation of GRCh38 and de novo haploid genome assemblies demonstrates the enduring quality of the reference assembly. *Genome Res.* 27, 849-864. doi: 10.1101/gr.213611.116

Schrauwen, I., Hasin-Brumshtein, Y., Corneveaux, J. J., Ohmen, J., White, C., Allen, A. N., et al. (2016). A comprehensive catalogue of the coding and non-coding transcripts of the human inner ear. *Hear. Res.* 333, 266–274. doi: 10.1016/j.heares.2015.08.013

Sedlazeck, F. J., Rescheneder, P., Smolka, M., Fang, H., Nattestad, M., Von Haeseler, A., et al. (2018). Accurate detection of complex structural variations using single-molecule sequencing. *Nat. Methods* 15, 461–468. doi: 10.1038/s41592-018-0001-7

Tonda, R., Escudero-ferruz, P., Andre, R., Castro-miro, M., De Ciccioli, M., Hidalgo, D. A., et al. (2016). Novel candidate genes and a wide spectrum of structural and point mutations responsible for inherited retinal dystrophies revealed by exome sequencing. *PLoS One* 11:e0168966. doi: 10.1371/journal.pone.0168966

van Dam, T. J., Wheway, G., Slaats, G. G., Huynen, M. A., and Giles, R. H. (2013). The SYSCILIA gold standard (SCGSv1) of known ciliary components and its applications within a systems biology consortium. *Cilia* 2:7. doi: 10.1186/2046-2530-2-7

Van Schil, K., Naessens, S., Van de Sompele, S., Carron, M., Aslanidis, A., Van Cauwenbergh, C., et al. (2018). Mapping the genomic landscape of inherited retinal disease genes prioritizes genes prone to coding and noncoding copy-number variations. *Genet. Med.* 20, 202–213. doi: 10.1038/gim.2017.97

Wolf, F. A., Angerer, P., and Theis, F. J. (2018). SCANPY: large-scale single-cell gene expression data analysis. *Genome Biol.* 19:15. doi: 10.1186/s13059-017-1382-0

Ye, K., Schulz, M. H., Long, Q., Apweiler, R., and Ning, Z. (2009). Pindel: a pattern growth approach to detect break points of large deletions and medium sized insertions from paired-end short reads. *Bioinformatics* 25, 2865–2871. doi: 10.1093/bioinformatics/btp394

Zampaglione, E., Kinde, B., Place, E. M., Navarro-Gomez, D., Maher, M., Jamshidi, F., et al. (2020). Copy-number variation contributes 9% of pathogenicity in the inherited retinal degenerations. *Genet. Med.* 22, 1079–1087. doi: 10.1038/s41436-020-0759-8

Zwiener, I., Frisch, B., and Binder, H. (2014). Transforming RNA-Seq data to improve the performance of prognostic gene signatures. *PLoS One* 9:e85150. doi: 10.1371/journal.pone.0085150

15

Dominant RP in the Middle While Recessive in Both the N- and C-Terminals Due to *RP1* Truncations: Confirmation, Refinement and Questions

Junwen Wang, Xueshan Xiao, Shiqiang Li, Panfeng Wang, Wenmin Sun* and Qingjiong Zhang*

State Key Laboratory of Ophthalmology, Zhongshan Ophthalmic Center, Sun Yat-sen University, Guangzhou, China

***Correspondence:**
Wenmin Sun
sunwenmin@gzzoc.com
Qingjiong Zhang
zhangqji@mail.sysu.edu.cn;
zhangqingjiong@gzzoc.com

RP1 truncation variants, including frameshift, nonsense, and splicing, are a common cause of retinitis pigmentosa (RP). *RP1* is a unique gene where truncations cause either autosomal dominant RP (adRP) or autosomal recessive RP (arRP) depending on the location of the variants. This study aims to clarify the boundaries between adRP and arRP caused by *RP1* truncation variants based on a systemic analysis of 165 *RP1* variants from our in-house exome-sequencing data of 7,092 individuals as well as a thorough review of 185 *RP1* variants from published literature. In our cohort, potential pathogenic variants were detected in 16 families, including 11 new and five previously described families. Of the 16, seven families with adRP had heterozygous truncations in the middle portion, while nine families with either arRP (eight) or macular degeneration had biallelic variants in the N- and C-terminals, involving 10 known and seven novel variants. In the literature, 147 truncations in *RP1* were reported to be responsible for either arRP (85) or adRP (58) or both (four). An overall evaluation of *RP1* causative variants suggested three separate regions, i.e., the N-terminal from c.1 (p.1) to c.1837 (p.613), the middle portion from c.1981 (p.661) to c.2749 (p.917), and the C-terminal from c.2816 (p.939) to c.6471 (p.2157), where truncations in the middle portion were associated with adRP, while those in the N- and C-terminals were responsible for arRP. Heterozygous truncations alone in the N- and C- terminals were unlikely pathogenic. However, conflict reports with reverse situation were present for 13 variants, suggesting a complicated pathogenicity awaiting to be further elucidated. In addition, pathogenicity for homozygous truncations around c.5797 and thereafter might also need to be further clarified, so as for missense variants and for truncations located in the two gaps. Our data not only confirmed and refined the boundaries between dominant and recessive *RP1* truncations but also revealed unsolved questions valuable for further investigation. These findings remind us that great care is needed in interpreting the results of *RP1* variants in clinical gene testing as well as similar features may also be present in some other genes.

Keywords: *RP1*, retinitis pigmentosa, exome sequencing, variants, inheritance pattern

INTRODUCTION

RP1 (OMIM 603937), mapped to chromosome 8q11.2–12.1, is an axonemal microtubule-associated gene with four exons, where the protein-coding region is in the last three (Blanton et al., 1991; Pierce et al., 1999; Méndez-Vidal et al., 2014). It encodes a 2,156-amino acid protein that is specifically expressed in photoreceptor connecting cilia (Liu et al., 2002, 2003), participating in protein transport between the inner and outer segments of the photoreceptors via two domains: the doublecortin (DCX) domain and the bifocal (BIF) domain (Pierce et al., 1999; Liu et al., 2002; Siemiatkowska et al., 2012; Méndez-Vidal et al., 2014).

Variants in *RP1* were initially identified to be responsible for autosomal dominant retinitis pigmentosa (adRP) and later for autosomal recessive retinitis pigmentosa (arRP) (OMIM 180100) (Pierce et al., 1999; Sullivan et al., 1999; Khaliq et al., 2005). *RP1* is listed as the top seventh of the most frequently implicated genes in inherited retinal disease based on a large cohort (Pontikos et al., 2020). To date, a large number of potential pathogenic variants in *RP1* have been reported, demonstrating a unique correlation between mutation location and pattern of inheritance. Usually, heterozygous truncation variants in the middle portion contributed to adRP, while biallelic truncation variants in the N- and C- terminals were associated with arRP. The boundaries between dominant and recessive variants have been suggested in previous studies but conflict reports were also present (Chen et al., 2010; Al-Rashed et al., 2012; Siemiatkowska et al., 2012; Eisenberger et al., 2013; El Shamieh et al., 2015; Kabir et al., 2016; Nanda et al., 2019; Riera et al., 2020). It is expected to confirm and refine the boundaries as well as the genotype–phenotype correlation of *RP1* variants based on a large dataset, especially at the era of widespread application of clinical genetic testing.

In this study, *RP1* variants were selected and analyzed based on our in-house exome-sequencing data from 7,092 individuals with different forms of eye conditions. *RP1* variants in published literature were systematically reviewed. These data further confirmed and refined the boundaries of *RP1* truncation variants, in which adRP associated with heterozygous variants in the middle portion, while arRP associated with biallelic variants in the N- and C- terminals. Besides, conflict reports in a reverse situation may call attention and be studied further. In clinical gene testing, pathogenicity of individual truncation variants in *RP1* might be complicated and should be explained with great care, especially for novel variants as well as those variants with conflict consequence.

MATERIALS AND METHODS

Subjects

Individuals with various forms of eye conditions were collected by our team based on our ongoing program on genetic study of inherited eye diseases. Prior to their participation, written informed consent adhering to the tenets of the Declaration of Helsinki was obtained from participants or their guardians. Clinical data and peripheral venous blood samples were collected from these individuals and their available family members. Genomic DNA was extracted from the leukocytes of peripheral blood based on procedures as described in our previously study (Wang et al., 2010). This study was approved by the institutional review board of the Zhongshan Ophthalmic Center.

RP1 Variant Identification From Our In-House Data

Exome sequencing was performed on genomic DNA samples from the 7,092 individuals, including whole-exome sequencing (WES) on 5,307 and targeting exome sequencing (TES) on 1,785. The procedures used to perform WES and TES were described in detail in our previous studies (Li et al., 2015; Wang et al., 2019).

RP1 variants were collected from exome-sequencing data of 7,092 individuals with various forms of eye conditions, including 1,019 with RP, 1,217 with glaucoma, 1,299 with high myopia, 492 normal controls, and 3,065 with other eye conditions. *RP1* variants were initially filtered following the procedures described in our previous studies (Jiang et al., 2014; Li et al., 2015). The candidate variants in *RP1* were then annotated as the following steps: (1) the allelic frequency of each variant was annotated according to the gnomAD database[1]; (2) missense variants were predicted using five *in silico* online tools, including REVEL[2], CADD[3], SIFT[4], PolyPhen2[5], and PROVEAN[6]; (3) the splicing effect of variants in the intronic region as well as synonymous variants were predicted using the Berkeley Drosophila Genome Project (BDGP[7]); (4) genotype–phenotype correlation was used to identify potential pathogenic variants. Sanger sequencing was used to validate potential pathogenic variants and segregation analysis in available family members was carried out to further validate the pathogenicity. The primers used herein were designed using the Primer3 online tool[8].

Literature Review of *RP1* Variants

The "RP1" was used as the keyword to search PubMed[9], Google Scholar[10], and The Human Gene Mutation Database (HGMD[11]) on September 1, 2020. The *RP1* variants were collected from these resources and annotated as noted in the above section. The phenotypes associated with these *RP1* variants are summarized.

Statistical Analysis

All statistical analyses were performed by using SPSS software version 25.0 (Armonk, NY: IBM Corp). The difference of proportion of macular abnormalities between the two groups

[1] https://gnomad.broadinstitute.org/
[2] https://sites.google.com/site/revelgenomics/
[3] https://cadd.gs.washington.edu/
[4] http://sift.jcvi.org/www/SIFT_enst_submit.html
[5] http://genetics.bwh.harvard.edu/pph2/index.shtml
[6] http://provean.jcvi.org
[7] http://www.fruitfly.org/
[8] http://primer3.ut.ee/
[9] https://www.ncbi.nlm.nih.gov/pubmed/
[10] http://so.hiqq.com.cn/
[11] http://www.hgmd.cf.ac.uk/ac/index.php

of patients with adRP and arRP was analyzed using the Chi-square test. The difference of the frequency of truncation variants between in-house exome sequencing data and gnomAD database was tested via the Chi-square test. A Mann–Whitney *U*-test was used to determine the phenotypic differences between the two groups of patients because the data were not distributed normally. A *P*-value of less than 0.05 was considered statistically significant.

RESULTS

RP1 Variants Detected in Our In-House Data

Totally, 165 variants were detected based on our exome sequencing data, including 143 missense variants, 20 truncation variants (10 nonsense, nine frameshift, and one splicing change variants), and two inframe variants. Potential pathogenic variants were detected in 16 families, including 11 new families and five previously described families (Xu et al., 2014; Wang et al., 2019). Of the 16 families, seven families with adRP had heterozygous truncation variants in the middle portion, while eight families with arRP and one family with macular degeneration (MD) had biallelic variants in the N- and C-terminals, involving 17 variants (**Table 1** and **Supplementary Table S1**). Of the 17 variants, seven were novel, i.e., c.256C > A (p.Pro86Thr), c.1987A > T (p.Lys663*), c.2062G > T (p.Gly688*), c.2399_2400del (p.Lys800Serfs*6), c.2700dup (p.Pro901Thrfs*2), c.5017del (p.Tyr1673Metfs*37), and c.6341_6343del (p.Ser2114del). These variants were confirmed by Sanger sequencing and co-segregated with the disease in families with available family members (**Supplementary Figure S1**). Biallelic missense variants were detected in five probands, in which one was with adRP, while the other four were with other conditions (**Supplementary Table S2**).

In addition, 12 single heterozygous truncation variants were identified in 44 individuals from our cohort. Of the 12 variants, 11 located at the N- and C- terminals were identified in 43 unrelated individuals and were considered non-pathogenic. Of the 43 individuals, seven were affected with RP and the remaining 36 with various conditions other than RP (**Supplementary Table S3**). Five different truncations involved in the seven patients with RP were unlikely pathogenic based on the following evidence: (1) the c.257dup (p.Arg87Serfs*48) was detected in three patients with RP and four individuals with unrelated conditions; (2) the c.1826C > G (p.Ser609*) was detected in one patient with RP who had biallelic pathogenic variants in *EYS*; (3) the c.4690del (p.Val1564*) was detected in a patient with X-linked RP and a patient with other condition; (4) the c.5017del (p.Tyr1673Metfs*37) was detected in one patient with isolated RP and four patients with other conditions; and (5) the c.5797C > T (p.Arg1933*) was detected in one patient with RP and 19 unrelated individuals with other conditions. These heterozygous variants were not enriched in patients with RP, and their frequency in our cohort is comparable with that in the East Asian population in gnomAD database ($P = 0.94$), suggesting that these 11 variants were unlikely pathogenic for retinal degeneration in heterozygous status. Apart from the 11, the remaining heterozygous c.2391_2392del (p.Asp799*) variant was located in the middle portion of *RP1* and was detected in a college student with late-onset high myopia without any sign of RP. The p.Asp799* is a known variant associated with cone-rod dystrophy (CRD) in homozygous status in a previous study (El Shamieh et al., 2015). Besides, none of the heterozygous missense variants predicted to be damaging were associated with adRP in our cohort.

RP1 Variants Reported in the Literature

A total of 185 *RP1* variants have been reported in the literature, including 147 truncation variants (51 nonsense, 95 frameshift, and one splicing) (**Supplementary Table S4**) and 38 missense variants (**Supplementary Table S5**). Of the 147 truncation variants, 85 were reported to cause recessive diseases, 58 were reported to lead to dominant diseases, and four were identified in patients with both dominant and recessive diseases. Of the 38 missense variants, 22 were reported to be recessive, 15 were reported to be dominant, and one was reported to be both dominant and recessive (**Supplementary Table S5**). The diseases associated with the 185 variants of *RP1* included RP, CRD, Leber congenital amaurosis (LCA), MD, and unclassified inherited retinal dystrophy (IRD) (**Supplementary Tables S4, S5**).

The Location of *RP1* Truncation Variants

In our cohort, the six *RP1* heterozygous truncation variants associated with adRP in seven families were located in the region from c.1987 (p.663) to c.2700 (p.901), which was immediately downstream of the BIF domain (**Table 1** and **Figure 1**). For the nine families with biallelic variants, five had homozygous truncation variants located in the C-terminal region, including c.4690del (p.Val1564*) in three families, c.5017del (p.Tyr1673Metfs*37) in one, and c.5797C > T (p.Arg1933*) in one; one had compound heterozygous truncations, c.257dup (p.Arg87Serfs*48) and c.4804C > T (p.Gln1602*); two had compound heterozygous variants, one truncation and one missense; the remaining one had compound heterozygous variants, one inframe and one missense (**Table 1** and **Supplementary Table S1**). In addition, 11 likely benign single heterozygous truncation variants were located at N- and C- terminals (**Supplementary Table S3**).

From the literature, 58 heterozygous truncation variants of *RP1* were reported to be associated with dominant diseases. Of the 58, 55 from 152 families were located in a region from c.1981 (p.661) to c.2749 (p.917) (**Figure 1**). Of the 85 biallelic variants from the literature, 79 from 117 families were located in the N- and C-terminal regions, namely, c.1 (p.1)–c.1837 (p.613) and c.2816 (p.939)–c.6471 (p.2157) (**Figure 1**). Combining our in-house data and the data from the literature, three regions in *RP1* were suggested, N-terminal from c.1 (p.1) to c.1837 (p.613), middle portion from c.1981 (p.661) to c.2749 (p.917), and C-terminal from c.2816 (p.939) to c. 6471 (p.2157) (**Figure 1**). A common feature could be identified as follows: truncations in the middle portion are associated with adRP, while those in the N- and C- terminals are responsible for arRP, which was supported by most truncation variants (91.9%, 147/160).

TABLE 1 | Potential pathogenic variants associated with retinitis pigmentosa (RP) in our cohort.

Position	Exon	Nucleotide change (NM_006269.1)	Effect	Status	Family number New + Reported#	Family ID (Reported#)	Allele in gnomAD	HGMD	References
1. Single heterozygous variants									
5,5538,429	4	c.1987A > T	p.Lys663*	Het	1 + 0	20,455	/	/	Novel
5,5538,471	4	c.2029C > T	p.Arg677*	Het	2 + 0	7,948, 18,926	/	DM	Guillonneau et al., 1999; Pierce et al., 1999; Martin-Merida et al., 2018
5,5538,504	4	c.2062G > T	p.Gly688*	Het	1 + 0	9,053	/	/	Novel
5,5538,558	4	c.2117del	p.Gly706Valfs*7	Het	0 + 1	(4,293)	/	DM	Xu et al., 2014
5,5538,841	4	c.2399_2400del	p.Lys800Serfs*6	Het	1 + 0	12,426	/	/	Novel
5,5539,142	4	c.2700dup	p.Pro901Thrfs*2	Het	1 + 0	18,611	/	/	Novel
2. Biallelic variants									
5,5533,782	2	c.256C > A	p.Pro86Thr	ComHet	1 + 0	12,349	22/282,760	/	Novel
5,5533,779	2	c.257dup	p.Arg87Serfs*48	ComHet	0 + 1	(14,948)	DM	/	Huang et al., 2015; Wang et al., 2019
5,5533,952	2	c.426dup	p.Ala143Serfs*86	ComHet	0 + 1	(6,170)	/	DM	Xu et al., 2014
5,5534,133	2	c.607G > C	p.Gly203Arg	ComHet	0 + 1	(6,170)	/	DM	Xu et al., 2014
5,5538,558	4	c.2116G > C	p.Gly706Arg	ComHet	0 + 1	(13,159)	89/282,438	DM	Wang et al., 2019
5,5540,748	4	c.4306del	p.Ser1436Profs*16	ComHet	0 + 1	(13,159)	/	DM	Wang et al., 2019
5,5541,132	4	c.4690del	p.Val1564*	Hom	3 + 0	6,609, 21,210, 21,311	/	DM	Wang et al., 2019
5,5541,246	4	c.4804C > T	p.Gln1602*	ComHet	0 + 1	(14,948)	3/251,080	DM	Avila-Fernandez et al., 2012; Ezquerra-Inchausti et al., 2018; Wang et al., 2019
5,5541,459	4	c.5017del	p.Tyr1673Metfs*37	Hom	1 + 0	8,089	/	/	Novel
5,5542,239	4	c.5797C > T	p.Arg1933*	Hom	0 + 1	(13,685)	49/281,934	DM?	Yeung et al., 2001; Fujinami et al., 2016; Li et al., 2018; Wang et al., 2019
5,5542,783	4	c.6341_6343del	p.Ser2114del	ComHet	1 + 0	12,349	10/280,914	/	Novel

#Families that have been reported by us previously. The genome build for these chromosomal positions was UCSC GRCh37/hg19. RP, retinitis pigmentosa; Het, heterozygous; Hom, homozygous; ComHet, compound heterozygous; DM, disease-causing mutations.

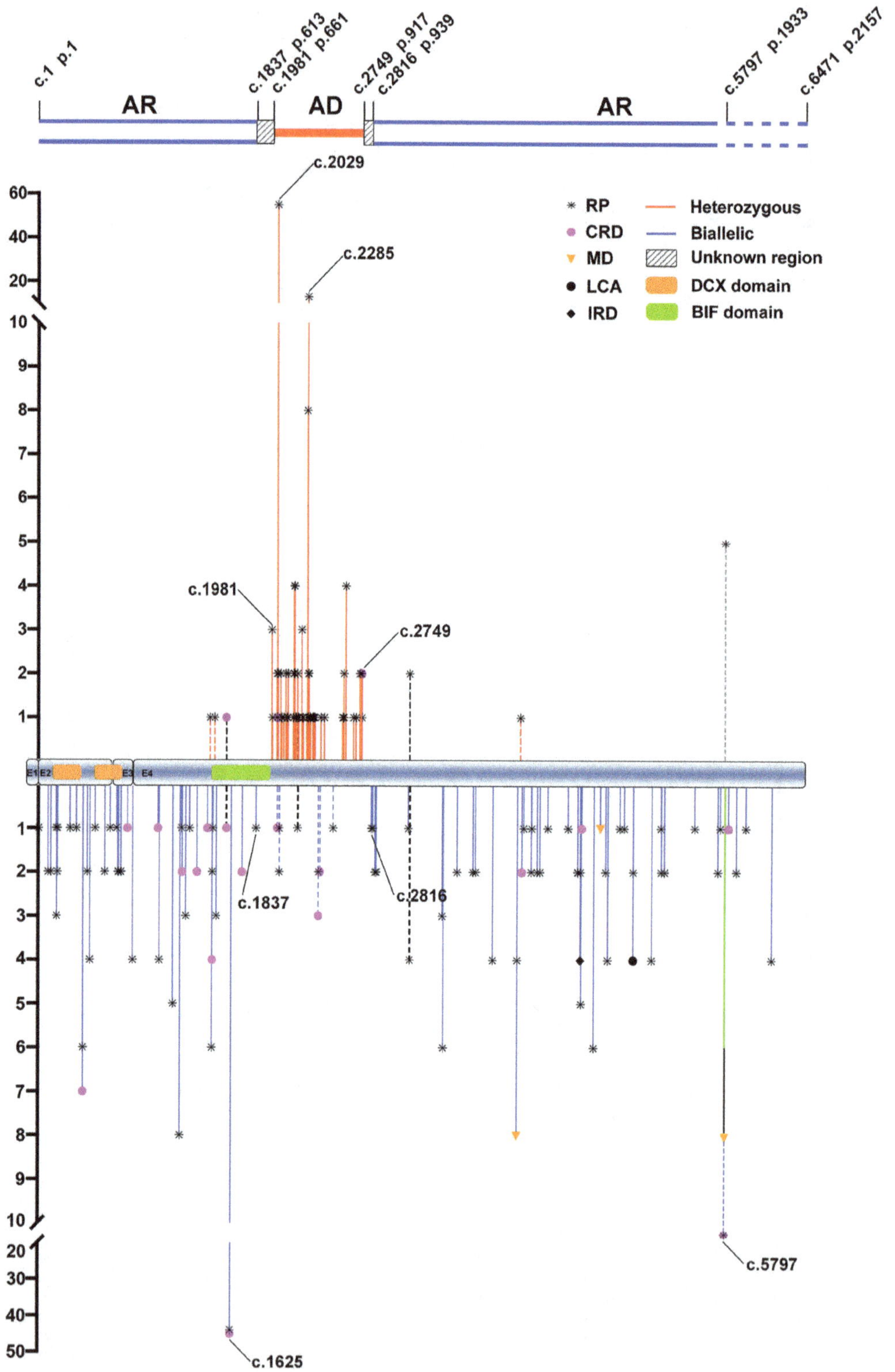

FIGURE 1 | The distribution and frequency of the potential pathogenic truncation variants in *RP1* identified in the present and previous studies. AR, autosomal recessive; AD, autosomal dominant; RP, retinitis pigmentosa; CRD, cone-rod dystrophy; MD, macular degeneration; LCA, Leber congenital amaurosis; IRD, inherited retinal disease. The positions and allele counts of the heterozygous *RP1* variants are displayed above, while those of the biallelic *RP1* variants are displayed below. The two blue lines above represent the autosomal recessive retinitis pigmentosa (arRP) region, the single red line represents the autosomal dominant retinitis pigmentosa (adRP) region, and the diagonal line between them represents the unknown regions. The two blue dashed lines are used to indicate the pathogenicity of homozygous truncations around the c.5797, and thereafter, need to be further clarified. DCX domain: c.106–354 (p.36–188) and c.460-699 (p.154–233). BIF domain: c.1456–1959 (p.486–653).

However, conflict results were reported for at least 13 truncation variants in *RP1* (Jacobson et al., 2000; Payne et al., 2000; Baum et al., 2001; Xiaoli et al., 2002; Kawamura et al., 2004; Eisenberger et al., 2013; Sullivan et al., 2013; El Shamieh et al., 2015; Yoon et al., 2015; Carrigan et al., 2016; Ellingford et al., 2016; Huang et al., 2017; Van Cauwenbergh et al., 2017; Li et al., 2018; Martin-Merida et al., 2019; Nikopoulos et al., 2019; Verbakel et al., 2019; Huckfeldt et al., 2020; **Supplementary Table S6**). Of the 13 variants, seven located in the middle portion were reported to be responsible for arRP rather than adRP, while six located in the N- and C-terminals caused adRP rather than arRP. Surprisingly, four of the 13 were involved in both adRP and arRP (**Supplementary Table S6**). In addition, the c.2391_2392del (p.Asp799*) located in the middle portion was reported to cause arCRD in homozygous status, which was supported by our study where a heterozygous carrier did not have any sign of RP. These raise questions on how to explain the common feature vs. the rare conflict results.

The Missense Variants in *RP1*

For the 38 missense variants from the literature, 22 variants involved in recessive retinal degeneration, and all of them were located at the N- and C-terminals (**Supplementary Figure S2**). The c.606C > A (p.Asp202Glu) variant was the most common and was detected in 17 families in homozygous status, including 13 families with arMD (Huckfeldt et al., 2020; Riera et al., 2020), three families with arRP (Aldahmesh et al., 2009; Huckfeldt et al., 2020), and one family with arCRD (Huckfeldt et al., 2020). This variant was absent from the gnomAD database. In contrast, 15 missense variants were reported to cause adRP and distributed scattered across the whole coding region of *RP1*, but segregation information was not described for 13 of the 15 variants. The remaining one, c.1118C > T (p.Thr373Ile), with a frequency of 3434/282692 in gnomAD database, was reported in patients with either dominant or recessive retinal degeneration, which is apparently a non-pathogenic variant. No heterozygous missense variant predicted to be damaging was identified to be responsible for adRP in our cohort.

Genotype–Phenotype Correlation of *RP1* Variants in our In-House Data and the Literature

From our in-house data, a total of 21 individuals from 16 families were detected with potential pathogenic truncation variants in *RP1*. Clinical data were available in 17 of the 21 individuals. These individuals complained of a variety of initial clinical manifestation, including night blindness, decreased visual acuity, or narrowing of visual field. The age at onset of these individuals ranged from childhood to 52 years old. The age at examination ranged from 9 to 57 years with visual acuity varying from no light perception to 0.5 (Snellen equivalent). Sixteen of the 17 individuals with potential pathogenic variants showed typical RP fundus changes including waxy pale optic disc, attenuated vessels, and periphery degeneration with bone spicule pigmentation with or without obvious macula involvement (**Figure 2**). Electroretinogram recordings of four patients showed severely decreased to distinguished responses for both of the rods and cones at the ages of 10, 34, 37, and 53 years old, respectively. The remaining one of the 17, a 53 year-old patient with a homozygous c.5797C > T (p.Arg1933*) had macular degeneration rather than RP (**Figure 2C**). Combined with our in-house data and the data obtained from the literature review (**Figure 3**), patients with arRP due to biallelic *RP1* variants had a significantly earlier age at onset (**Figure 3B**, $Z = -6.66$, $P = 2.76*10^{-11}$), worse visual acuity (**Figure 3C**, $Z = -3.75$, $P = 1.75*10^{-4}$), and seemingly more likely to have degeneration involving both of the macular and mid-peripheral retina (**Figures 2**, **3D**, $P = 0.061$) (compared to adRP due to heterozygous *RP1* variants, in which mid-peripheral retina was mainly affected).

DISCUSSION

In this study, results from a systemic analysis of *RP1* variants from our in-house data as well as those from published literature demonstrate some common features of pathogenic variants in this gene, including: (1) about 80% of pathogenic variants are truncation variants; (2) truncation variants in the middle portion (c.1981 to c.2749) are associated with adRP, while those in the N-terminal (c.1 to c.1837) and C-terminal (c.2816 to c.6471) are responsible for arRP, supported by 91.9% of truncations; and (3) heterozygous truncation variants alone in the N- and C-terminals are unlikely pathogenic. Several questions remain to be clarified in future studies regarding the pathogenicity of the following *RP1* variants: (1) truncation variants located in the two gaps between the N-terminal and middle portion as well as between the middle portion and C-terminal; (2) homozygous truncation variants around the c.5797 and thereafter; (3) missense variants, especially those with adRP; (4) the mechanism for the common features of *RP1* truncation variants; and (5) the possible reasons for 8.1% of truncation variants with phenotypes contrary to the common feature. Awareness of these common features and unsolved questions is important in this era of widespread application of clinical gene testing.

The pathogenicity of truncation variants of *RP1* has been previously reported to be related to the location of the gene. Chen et al. (2010) first defined four classes of truncation variants in *RP1*: Class I, from p.1 to p.263, does not cause RP; Class II, from p.500 to p.1053, causes adRP; Class III, from p.263 to p.500 and from p.1053 to p.1751, causes arRP; Class IV, from p.1816 to p.2156, does not cause RP. However, variants in the non-pathogenic Class I and Class IV regions have subsequently been identified in patients with arRP (Avila-Fernandez et al., 2012; Eisenberger et al., 2013; Xu et al., 2014; Bravo-Gil et al., 2016; Kabir et al., 2016; Perez-Carro et al., 2016; Verbakel et al., 2019; Riera et al., 2020; Silva et al., 2020). In addition, some variants in the Class II region, associated with adRP, have been reported to cause arRP in homozygous or compound heterozygous status (Avila-Fernandez et al., 2012; Corton et al., 2013; Bravo-Gil et al., 2017; Ezquerra-Inchausti et al., 2018; Li et al., 2018; Martin-Merida et al., 2019; Silva et al., 2020). Therefore, several studies reported that the *RP1* variants at N-terminal and C-terminal

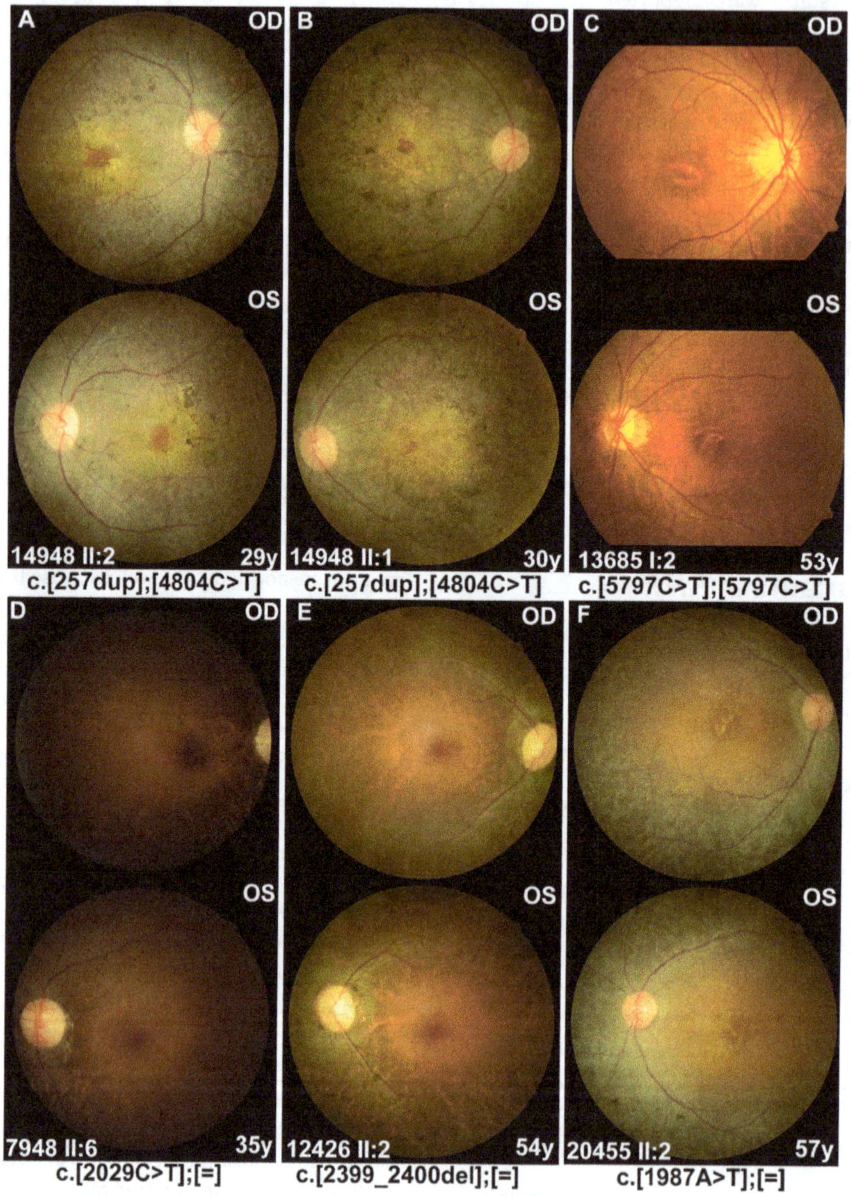

FIGURE 2 | Fundus photographs of the affected individuals with *RP1* variants. **(A,B)** Severe phenotypes were shown in patients with biallelic *RP1* variants, including waxy pale optic disc, attenuated vessels, and periphery degeneration with bone spicule pigmentation and involving macular region. **(C)** A 53 year-old patient diagnosed with macular degeneration rather than RP, who carried homozygous variant c.5797C > T (p.Arg1933*) in our cohort. **(D–F)** Patients with heterozygous *RP1* variants were characterized by peripheral pigment disorders and scattered distribution of bone spicule pigmentation, both of which were often absent in the macular region.

regions were associated with arRP and those at the middle region resulted in adRP (Kabir et al., 2016; Nanda et al., 2019), and Nanda et al. (2019) suggested that the boundary of the region associated with adRP was located between p.677 and p.917. In our cohort, the c.257dup (p.Arg87Serfs*48) variant, located in the Class I region, was identified in two siblings from one family with typical RP changes in trans with the c.4804C > T (p.Gln1602*) (**Figures 2A,B**). Furthermore, the boundaries of these three regions were refined based on a systemic analysis of our in-house exome-sequencing data and the literature review, namely, the arRP region, from c.1 (p.1) to c.1837 (p.613) in the N-terminal and from c.2816 (p.939) to c.6471 (p.2157) in the C-terminal, and the adRP region, from c.1981 (p.661) to c.2749 (p.917) in the middle portion. The difference of the middle portion for adRP between this study and the previous studies is the extension of this region between p.677 and p.917 to p.661–p.917. The c.1981G > T (p.Glu661*) variant is defined as the upstream boundary of the middle portion because it has been identified in three independent families with adRP and cosegregated with adRP in one family (Fernandez-San Jose et al., 2015; Martin-Merida et al., 2018; Riera et al., 2020). Although the boundaries among different regions have been well outlined

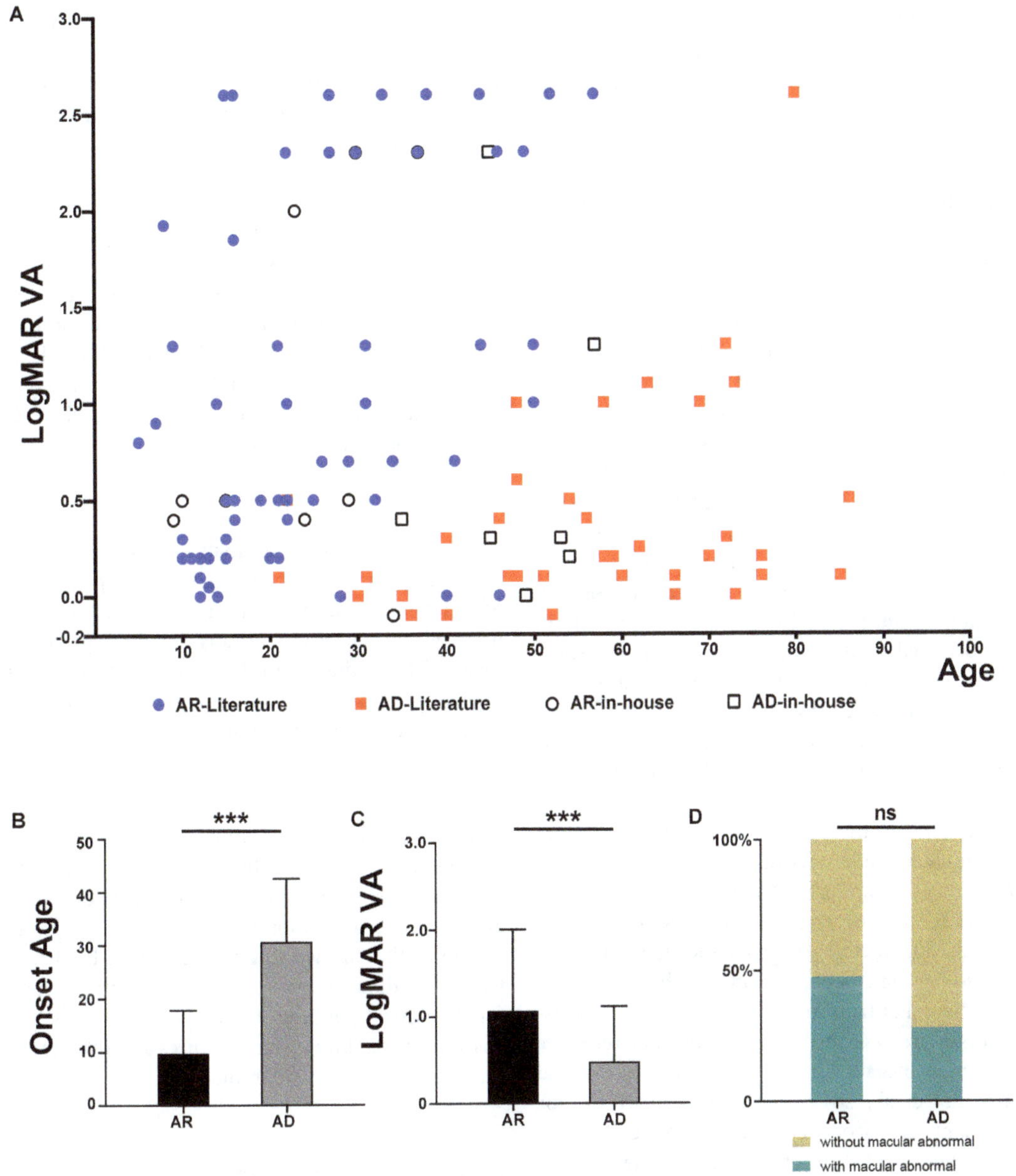

FIGURE 3 | Comparison of phenotypes in patients with an inheritance pattern for arRP and adRP. **(A)** Scatter plots of the LogMAR visual acuity of patients with AR and AD inheritance from our in-house data and the previously published literature. **(B)** Comparison of the onset ages of patients with AR and AD inheritance from our in-house data and the previously published literature. ***$P = 2.76*10^{-11}$. **(C)** Comparison of the LogMAR visual acuity of patients with AR and AD inheritance from our in-house data and the previously published literature. ***$P = 1.75*10^{-4}$. **(D)** Comparison of the macular abnormalities, including macular degeneration or macular atrophy, of patients with AR and AD inheritance from our in-house data and the previously published literature. ns mean not significant ($P = 0.061$).

based on our data and data from at least 291 families, there are still two gaps in between without enough information. As for the 13 truncation variants contrary to the common feature, some might be problematic while the others may represent a variable expression of phenotypes. For example, four truncation variants were initially reported to cause dominant retinal degeneration and then were reported to cause recessive diseases in trans with the other allele in subsequent studies. Clinically variable expression from hardly identifiable to typical phenotypes have been observed in RP patients from the same family with the same mutation in other gene like *RHO* (Luo et al., 2020), and such phenomenon could not be excluded for *RP1* variants. In addition, age-dependent expression of the diseases might also be considered. In these cases, wide-field examination of fundus such as scanning laser ophthalmoscope and electroretinogram may be of help in identifying mild or early signs of RP, especially in those carriers of individuals with variants associated with both dominant and recessive retinal degeneration. Co-segregation of those variants as well as well-defined phenotypes in family members may provide additional information in clarifying these conflict results. Moreover, a few variants with conflict result may represent a unique point-dependent rather than region-dependent pathogenicity of dominant or recessive nature. For example, the c.2391_2392del (p.Asp799*), located in the middle portion and supposed to be causative for adRP, has been reported to cause arCRD with firm evidence in previous study (El Shamieh et al., 2015) and is identified in an adult without any sign of RP in heterozygous status in our cohort.

Besides, the c.5797C > T (p.Arg1933*) variant located at the C-terminal has been reported to be non-pathogenic either in heterozygous or in homozygous status (Baum et al., 2001; Xiaoli et al., 2002; Nikopoulos et al., 2019). However, it can cause recessive diseases in trans with another truncation variant of *RP1* located upstream (Li et al., 2018; Nikopoulos et al., 2019; Verbakel et al., 2019). It has been suggested that the effect of the c.5797C > T (p.Arg1933*) variant might be between monogenic and complex diseases (Baum et al., 2001; Xiaoli et al., 2002; Nikopoulos et al., 2019). In our cohort, this variant in homozygosis was identified in a 53 year-old singleton case with macular degeneration (**Figure 2C**). No pathogenic variants in other genes were detected in this patient based on the whole exome sequencing. Unfortunately, further clinical examination of the patients is unavailable except for fundus photographs. This raises questions on whether the c.5797C > T variant as well as other truncations downstream are pathogenic or not in homozygous status.

So far, it is unclear for the molecular mechanism about dominant in the middle while recessive in the N- and C-terminals for *RP1* truncation variants. Mutations in several other genes such as *GUCY2D* (Sharon et al., 2018), *RHO* (Luo et al., 2020), *CRX* (Yi et al., 2019), etc., are also associated with both dominant and recessive retinal degeneration, but the situation is a little different for them. For truncations in *CRX* and *RHO*, loss-of-function mutations are responsible for autosomal recessive diseases while dominant-negative mutations lead to autosomal dominant diseases (Yi et al., 2019; Luo et al., 2020). As for *GUCY2D*, most variants are associated with autosomal recessive LCA but the heterozygous substitution of the arginine at p.838 could cause autosomal dominant CRD (Sharon et al., 2018). The arginine at p.838 is the most sensitive position of GUCY2D protein. The mutants at arginine 838 shift the Ca^{2+}-sensitivity in the guanylate cyclase-activating proteins mediated activation. This shift can be overactive and in some reported cases the activity level does not return to the basal level. The abnormal higher activity from the heterozygous 838 mutations leads to CRD, while the loss of partial or total function is tolerable in heterozygous status but is causative and leads LCA in biallelic status (Sharon et al., 2018). For *RP1* truncation variants, some studies have excluded haploinsufficiency and gain-of-function as the causative mechanism of *RP1* variants (Liu et al., 2012; Nanda et al., 2019). The variants involving the BIF domain, which is crucial for the photoreceptor (Bahri et al., 1997; Pierce et al., 1999), will lead to haploinsufficiency of *RP1* either by triggering nonsense-mediated decay or by producing a loss-of-function protein. Therefore, heterozygous variants located within or upstream of the BIF domain will not cause diseases. For the variants associated with adRP, the truncated production will preserve the BIF domain and may cause disease via a dominant-negative effect (Chen et al., 2010; Nanda et al., 2019). However, the variants at the C-terminal recessive region, which can also produce a protein with the BIF domain, would not cause diseases in heterozygous status. It has been assumed that an unrecognized domain is present downstream of the BIF domain (Baum et al., 2001). The unknown domain may be important for the interaction of *RP1* with other proteins by cooperating with the BIF domain. It implies that the heterozygous variants will be non-pathogenic either loss of both the BIF domain and the unrecognized domain or preserve with both domains, while the heterozygous variants will cause retinal degeneration with preserved BIF domain but loss of the unrecognized domain. Functional studies are expected to disclose the exact mechanism of the unique feature associated with *RP1* variants.

Genotype–phenotype analysis revealed that patients with biallelic variants showed more severe phenotypes than those with heterozygous variants, including an earlier age at onset, worse visual acuity, and fundus changes especially in the macular region. The limitation of this study is not knowing the exact age at onset because of the nature of a retrospective study and lack of supporting evidence from functional studies.

In conclusion, in this study, a pooled analysis of our exome-sequencing data and the literature review confirmed and refined the common features and the boundaries between dominant and recessive truncation variants in *RP1*. It also raises unsolved problems that are worth investigating in the future. The unique features and questions identified in *RP1* may not only be valuable for its clinical application and further studies but also reminds us of the possibility of such features and questions in other genes that are awaited to be identified.

ETHICS STATEMENT

The studies involving human participants were reviewed and approved by the institutional review board of the Zhongshan Ophthalmic Center. Written informed consent to participate in this study was provided by the participants' legal guardian/next of kin.

AUTHOR CONTRIBUTIONS

XX, SL, and QZ recruited the individuals diagnosed with different forms of eye conditions. XX, JW, and QZ collected the clinical records. XX, SL, PW, and QZ performed the whole-exome analysis and targeted-exome sequencing. JW, WS, and QZ performed the bioinformatic analysis and designed the study and discussed the results and wrote the manuscript. JW and WS confirmed the variants by Sanger sequencing and did the statistical analysis of clinical data. JW, WS, and QZ discussed the results and wrote the manuscript. All authors reviewed and approved the manuscript.

ACKNOWLEDGMENTS

We thank the patients and their family members for their participation.

SUPPLEMENTARY MATERIAL

Supplementary Figure 1 | Pedigrees and Sanger sequencing chromatography of unrelated families with identified *RP1* variants in this study. For each family, the pedigree is shown in the left column and the sequence changes are shown in the right column. Mx, mutant allele; +, wild-type allele.

Supplementary Figure 2 | The distributions and frequencies of the missense variants in *RP1*. The positions and allele counts of the heterozygous *RP1* variants are displayed above, while those of the biallelic *RP1* variants are displayed below. RP, retinitis pigmentosa; CRD, cone-rod dystrophy; MD, macular degeneration; IRD, inherited retinal disease; LCA, Leber congenital amaurosis; STGD, Stargardt disease. **DCX domain:** c.106–354 (p.36–188) and c.460–699 (p.154–233). BIF domain: c.1456-1959 (p.486-653). **(A)** Distributions and frequencies of the missense variants in the gnomAD database. **(B)** Distributions and frequencies of the missense variants in the published literature. **(C)** Distributions and frequencies of the missense variants in this study.

Supplementary Table 1 | Clinical information of probands with *RP1* variants in our cohort.

Supplementary Table 2 | Biallelic variants in *RP1* not associated with RP.

Supplementary Table 3 | Single heterozygous truncation variants in *RP1* that were not associated with RP in our cohort.

Supplementary Table 4 | Truncation *RP1* variants in published literature.

Supplementary Table 5 | All missense *RP1* variants in published literature.

Supplementary Table 6 | Truncation variants in *RP1* reported in patients with conflict pattern of inheritance.

REFERENCES

Aldahmesh, M. A., Safieh, L. A., Alkuraya, H., Al-Rajhi, A., Shamseldin, H., Hashem, M., et al. (2009). Molecular characterization of retinitis pigmentosa in Saudi Arabia. *Mol. Vis.* 15, 2464–2469.

Al-Rashed, M., Abu Safieh, L., Alkuraya, H., Aldahmesh, M. A., Alzahrani, J., Diya, M., et al. (2012). RP1 and retinitis pigmentosa: report of novel mutations and insight into mutational mechanism. *Br. J. Ophthalmol.* 96, 1018–1022. doi: 10.1136/bjophthalmol-2011-301134

Avila-Fernandez, A., Corton, M., Nishiguchi, K. M., Muñoz-Sanz, N., Benavides-Mori, B., Blanco-Kelly, F., et al. (2012). Identification of an RP1 prevalent founder mutation and related phenotype in Spanish patients with early-onset autosomal recessive retinitis. *Ophthalmology* 119, 2616–2621. doi: 10.1016/j.ophtha.2012.06.033

Bahri, S. M., Yang, X., and Chia, W. (1997). The *Drosophila bifocal* gene encodes a novel protein which colocalizes with actin and is necessary for photoreceptor morphogenesis. *Mol. Cell Biol.* 17, 5521–5529. doi: 10.1128/mcb.17.9.5521

Baum, L., Chan, W. M., Yeung, K. Y., Lam, D. S., Kwok, A. K., and Pang, C. P. (2001). RP1 in Chinese: eight novel variants and evidence that truncation of the extreme C-terminal does not cause retinitis pigmentosa. *Hum. Mutat.* 17:436. doi: 10.1002/humu.1127

Blanton, S. H., Heckenlively, J. R., Cottingham, A. W., Friedman, J., Sadler, L. A., Wagner, M., et al. (1991). Linkage mapping of autosomal dominant retinitis pigmentosa (RP1) to the pericentric region of human chromosome 8. *Genomics* 11, 857–869. doi: 10.1016/0888-7543(91)90008-3

Bravo-Gil, N., González-Del Pozo, M., Martín-Sánchez, M., Méndez-Vidal, C., Rodríguez-De La Rúa, E., Borrego, S., et al. (2017). Unravelling the genetic basis of simplex Retinitis Pigmentosa cases. *Sci. Rep.* 7:41937.

Bravo-Gil, N., Méndez-Vidal, C., Romero-Pérez, L., González-Del Pozo, M., Rodríguez-De La Rúa, E., Dopazo, J., et al. (2016). Improving the management of Inherited Retinal Dystrophies by targeted sequencing of a population-specific gene panel. *Sci. Rep.* 6:23910.

Carrigan, M., Duignan, E., Malone, C. P., Stephenson, K., Saad, T., Mcdermott, C., et al. (2016). Panel-based population next-generation sequencing for inherited retinal degenerations. *Sci. Rep.* 6:33248.

Chen, L. J., Lai, T. Y., Tam, P. O., Chiang, S. W., Zhang, X., Lam, S., et al. (2010). Compound heterozygosity of two novel truncation mutations in RP1 causing autosomal recessive retinitis pigmentosa. *Invest. Ophthalmol. Vis. Sci.* 51, 2236–2242. doi: 10.1167/iovs.09-4437

Corton, M., Nishiguchi, K. M., Avila-Fernández, A., Nikopoulos, K., Riveiro-Alvarez, R., Tatu, S. D., et al. (2013). Exome sequencing of index patients with retinal dystrophies as a tool for molecular diagnosis. *PLoS One* 8:e65574. doi: 10.1371/journal.pone.0065574

Eisenberger, T., Neuhaus, C., Khan, A. O., Decker, C., Preising, M. N., Friedburg, C., et al. (2013). Increasing the yield in targeted next-generation sequencing by implicating CNV analysis, non-coding exons and the overall variant load: the example of retinal dystrophies. *PLoS One* 8:e78496. doi: 10.1371/journal.pone.0078496

El Shamieh, S., Boulanger-Scemama, E., Lancelot, M. E., Antonio, A., Démontant, V., Condroyer, C., et al. (2015). Targeted next generation sequencing identifies novel mutations in RP1 as a relatively common cause of autosomal recessive rod-cone dystrophy. *Biomed. Res. Int.* 2015:485624.

Ellingford, J. M., Barton, S., Bhaskar, S., O'sullivan, J., Williams, S. G., Lamb, J. A., et al. (2016). Molecular findings from 537 individuals with inherited retinal disease. *J. Med. Genet.* 53, 761–767. doi: 10.1136/jmedgenet-2016-103837

Ezquerra-Inchausti, M., Anasagasti, A., Barandika, O., Garay-Aramburu, G., Galdós, M., López De Munain, A., et al. (2018). A new approach based on targeted pooled DNA sequencing identifies novel mutations in patients with Inherited Retinal Dystrophies. *Sci. Rep.* 8:15457.

Fernandez-San Jose, P., Corton, M., Blanco-Kelly, F., Avila-Fernandez, A., Lopez-Martinez, M. A., Sanchez-Navarro, I., et al. (2015). Targeted next-generation sequencing improves the diagnosis of autosomal dominant retinitis Pigmentosa in Spanish patients. *Invest. Ophthalmol. Vis. Sci.* 56, 2173–2182. doi: 10.1167/iovs.14-16178

Fujinami, K., Kameya, S., Kikuchi, S., Ueno, S., Kondo, M., Hayashi, T., et al. (2016). Novel *RP1L1* variants and genotype-photoreceptor microstructural phenotype associations in cohort of Japanese patients with occult macular dystrophy. *Invest Ophthalmol. Vis. Sci.* 57, 4837–4846. doi: 10.1167/iovs.16-19670

Guillonneau, X., Piriev, N. I., Danciger, M., Kozak, C. A., Cideciyan, A. V., Jacobson, S. G., et al. (1999). A nonsense mutation in a novel gene is associated with retinitis pigmentosa in a family linked to the RP1 locus. *Hum. Mol. Genet.* 8, 1541–1546. doi: 10.1093/hmg/8.8.1541

Huang, X. F., Huang, F., Wu, K. C., Wu, J., Chen, J., Pang, C. P., et al. (2015). Genotype-phenotype correlation and mutation spectrum in a large cohort of patients with inherited retinal dystrophy revealed by next-generation sequencing. *Genet. Med.* 17, 271–278. doi: 10.1038/gim.2014.138

Huang, L., Zhang, Q., Huang, X., Qu, C., Ma, S., Mao, Y., et al. (2017). Mutation screening in genes known to be responsible for Retinitis Pigmentosa in 98 small Han Chinese families. *Sci. Rep.* 7:1948.

Huckfeldt, R. M., Grigorian, F., Place, E., Comander, J. I., Vavvas, D., Young, L. H., et al. (2020). Biallelic RP1-associated retinal dystrophies: Expanding the mutational and clinical spectrum. *Mol. Vis.* 26, 423–433.

Jacobson, S. G., Cideciyan, A. V., Iannaccone, A., Weleber, R. G., Fishman, G. A., Maguire, A. M., et al. (2000). Disease expression of RP1 mutations causing autosomal dominant retinitis pigmentosa. *Invest. Ophthalmol. Vis. Sci.* 41, 1898–1908.

Jiang, D., Li, J., Xiao, X., Li, S., Jia, X., Sun, W., et al. (2014). Detection of mutations in LRPAP1, CTSH, LEPREL1, ZNF644, SLC39A5, and SCO2 in 298 families with early-onset high myopia by exome sequencing. *Invest. Ophthalmol. Vis. Sci.* 56, 339–345. doi: 10.1167/iovs.14-14850

Kabir, F., Ullah, I., Ali, S., Gottsch, A. D., Naeem, M. A., Assir, M. Z., et al. (2016). Loss of function mutations in RP1 are responsible for retinitis pigmentosa in consanguineous familial cases. *Mol. Vis.* 22, 610–625.

Kawamura, M., Wada, Y., Noda, Y., Itabashi, T., Ogawa, S., Sato, H., et al. (2004). Novel 2336-2337delCT mutation in RP1 gene in a Japanese family with autosomal dominant retinitis pigmentosa. *Am. J. Ophthalmol.* 137, 1137–1139. doi: 10.1016/j.ajo.2003.12.037

Khaliq, S., Abid, A., Ismail, M., Hameed, A., Mohyuddin, A., Lall, P., et al. (2005). Novel association of RP1 gene mutations with autosomal recessive retinitis pigmentosa. *J. Med. Genet.* 42, 436–438. doi: 10.1136/jmg.2004.024281

Li, J., Jiang, D., Xiao, X., Li, S., Jia, X., Sun, W., et al. (2015). Evaluation of 12 myopia-associated genes in Chinese patients with high myopia. *Invest. Ophthalmol. Vis. Sci.* 56, 722–729. doi: 10.1167/iovs.14-14880

Li, S., Yang, M., Liu, W., Liu, Y., Zhang, L., Yang, Y., et al. (2018). Targeted next-generation sequencing reveals novel RP1 mutations in autosomal recessive retinitis pigmentosa. *Genet. Test. Mol. Biomarkers* 22, 109–114. doi: 10.1089/gtmb.2017.0223

Liu, Q., Collin, R. W., Cremers, F. P., Den Hollander, A. I., Van Den Born, L. I., and Pierce, E. A. (2012). Expression of wild-type Rp1 protein in Rp1 knock-in mice rescues the retinal degeneration phenotype. *PLoS One* 7:e43251. doi: 10.1371/journal.pone.0043251

Liu, Q., Lyubarsky, A., Skalet, J. H., Pugh, E. N. Jr., and Pierce, E. A. (2003). RP1 is required for the correct stacking of outer segment discs. *Invest. Ophthalmol. Vis. Sci.* 44, 4171–4183. doi: 10.1167/iovs.03-0410

Liu, Q., Zhou, J., Daiger, S. P., Farber, D. B., Heckenlively, J. R., Smith, J. E., et al. (2002). Identification and subcellular localization of the RP1 protein in human and mouse photoreceptors. *Invest. Ophthalmol. Vis. Sci.* 43, 22–32.

Luo, H., Xiao, X., Li, S., Sun, W., Yi, Z., Wang, P., et al. (2020). Spectrum-frequency and genotype-phenotype analysis of rhodopsin variants. *Exp. Eye Res.* 203:108405. doi: 10.1016/j.exer.2020.108405

Martin-Merida, I., Aguilera-Garcia, D., Fernandez-San Jose, P., Blanco-Kelly, F., Zurita, O., Almoguera, B., et al. (2018). Toward the mutational landscape of autosomal dominant retinitis Pigmentosa: a comprehensive analysis of 258 Spanish families. *Invest. Ophthalmol. Vis. Sci.* 59, 2345–2354. doi: 10.1167/iovs.18-23854

Martin-Merida, I., Avila-Fernandez, A., Del Pozo-Valero, M., Blanco-Kelly, F., Zurita, O., Perez-Carro, R., et al. (2019). Genomic landscape of sporadic retinitis Pigmentosa: findings from 877 Spanish cases. *Ophthalmology* 126, 1181–1188. doi: 10.1016/j.ophtha.2019.03.018

Méndez-Vidal, C., Bravo-Gil, N., González-Del Pozo, M., Vela-Boza, A., Dopazo, J., Borrego, S., et al. (2014). Novel RP1 mutations and a recurrent BBS1 variant explain the co-existence of two distinct retinal phenotypes in the same pedigree. *BMC Genet.* 15:143. doi: 10.1186/s12863-014-0143-2

Nanda, A., Mcclements, M. E., Clouston, P., Shanks, M. E., and Maclaren, R. E. (2019). The location of exon 4 mutations in RP1 raises challenges for genetic counseling and gene therapy. *Am. J. Ophthalmol.* 202, 23–29. doi: 10.1016/j.ajo.2019.01.027

Nikopoulos, K., Cisarova, K., Quinodoz, M., Koskiniemi-Kuendig, H., Miyake, N., Farinelli, P., et al. (2019). A frequent variant in the Japanese population determines quasi-Mendelian inheritance of rare retinal ciliopathy. *Nat. Commun.* 10:2884.

Payne, A., Vithana, E., Khaliq, S., Hameed, A., Deller, J., Abu-Safieh, L., et al. (2000). RP1 protein truncating mutations predominate at the RP1 adRP locus. *Invest. Ophthalmol. Vis. Sci.* 41, 4069–4073.

Perez-Carro, R., Corton, M., Sánchez-Navarro, I., Zurita, O., Sanchez-Bolivar, N., Sánchez-Alcudia, R., et al. (2016). Panel-based NGS reveals novel pathogenic mutations in autosomal recessive retinitis Pigmentosa. *Sci. Rep.* 6:19531.

Pierce, E. A., Quinn, T., Meehan, T., Mcgee, T. L., Berson, E. L., and Dryja, T. P. (1999). Mutations in a gene encoding a new oxygen-regulated photoreceptor protein cause dominant retinitis pigmentosa. *Nat. Genet.* 22, 248–254. doi: 10.1038/10305

Pontikos, N., Arno, G., Jurkute, N., Schiff, E., Ba-Abbad, R., Malka, S., et al. (2020). Genetic basis of inherited retinal disease in a molecularly characterized cohort of more than 3000 families from the United Kingdom. *Ophthalmology* 127, 1384–1394. doi: 10.1016/j.ophtha.2020.04.008

Riera, M., Abad-Morales, V., Navarro, R., Ruiz-Nogales, S., Méndez-Vendrell, P., Corcostegui, B., et al. (2020). Expanding the retinal phenotype of RP1: from retinitis pigmentosa to a novel and singular macular dystrophy. *Br. J. Ophthalmol.* 104, 173–181. doi: 10.1136/bjophthalmol-2018-313672

Sharon, D., Wimberg, H., Kinarty, Y., and Koch, K. W. (2018). Genotype-functional-phenotype correlations in photoreceptor guanylate cyclase (GC-E) encoded by GUCY2D. *Prog. Retin. Eye Res.* 63, 69–91. doi: 10.1016/j.preteyeres.2017.10.003

Siemiatkowska, A. M., Astuti, G. D., Arimadyo, K., Den Hollander, A. I., Faradz, S. M., Cremers, F. P., et al. (2012). Identification of a novel nonsense mutation in RP1 that causes autosomal recessive retinitis pigmentosa in an Indonesian family. *Mol. Vis.* 18, 2411–2419.

Silva, R. S., Salles, M. V., Motta, F. L., and Sallum, J. M. F. (2020). Retinitis *Pigmentosa* due to Rp1 biallelic variants. *Sci. Rep.* 10:1603.

Sullivan, L. S., Bowne, S. J., Reeves, M. J., Blain, D., Goetz, K., Ndifor, V., et al. (2013). Prevalence of mutations in eyeGENE probands with a diagnosis of autosomal dominant retinitis pigmentosa. *Invest. Ophthalmol. Vis. Sci.* 54, 6255–6261. doi: 10.1167/iovs.13-12605

Sullivan, L. S., Heckenlively, J. R., Bowne, S. J., Zuo, J., Hide, W. A., Gal, A., et al. (1999). Mutations in a novel retina-specific gene cause autosomal dominant retinitis pigmentosa. *Nat. Genet.* 22, 255–259. doi: 10.1038/10314

Van Cauwenbergh, C., Coppieters, F., Roels, D., De Jaegere, S., Flipts, H., De Zaeytijd, J., et al. (2017). Mutations in splicing factor genes are a major cause of autosomal dominant retinitis pigmentosa in belgian families. *PLoS One* 12:e0170038. doi: 10.1371/journal.pone.0170038

Verbakel, S. K., Van Huet, R. A. C., Den Hollander, A. I., Geerlings, M. J., Kersten, E., Klevering, B. J., et al. (2019). Macular dystrophy and cone-rod dystrophy caused by mutations in the RP1 gene: extending the RP1 disease spectrum. *Invest. Ophthalmol. Vis. Sci.* 60, 1192–1203.

Wang, P., Li, S., Sun, W., Xiao, X., Jia, X., Liu, M., et al. (2019). An ophthalmic targeted exome sequencing panel as a powerful tool to identify causative mutations in patients suspected of hereditary eye diseases. *Transl. Vis. Sci. Technol.* 8:21. doi: 10.1167/tvst.8.2.21

Wang, Q., Wang, P., Li, S., Xiao, X., Jia, X., Guo, X., et al. (2010). Mitochondrial DNA haplogroup distribution in Chaoshanese with and without myopia. *Mol. Vis.* 16, 303–309.

Xiaoli, Z., Weiling, F., Pang, C. P., and Yeung, K. Y. (2002). Screening for mutations in a novel retinal-specific gene among Chinese patients with retinitis pigmentosa. *Chin. Med. Sci. J.* 17, 225–230.

Xu, Y., Guan, L., Shen, T., Zhang, J., Xiao, X., Jiang, H., et al. (2014). Mutations of 60 known causative genes in 157 families with retinitis pigmentosa based on exome sequencing. *Hum. Genet.* 133, 1255–1271. doi: 10.1007/s00439-014-1460-2

Yeung, K. Y., Baum, L., Chan, W. M., Lam, D. S., Kwok, A. K., and Pang, C. P. (2001). Molecular diagnostics for retinitis pigmentosa. *Clin. Chim. Acta* 313, 209–215. doi: 10.1016/s0009-8981(01)00674-x

Yi, Z., Xiao, X., Li, S., Sun, W., and Zhang, Q. (2019). Pathogenicity discrimination and genetic test reference for CRX variants based on genotype-phenotype analysis. *Exp. Eye Res.* 189:107846. doi: 10.1016/j.exer.2019.107846

Yoon, C. K., Kim, N. K., Joung, J. G., Shin, J. Y., Park, J. H., Eum, H. H., et al. (2015). The diagnostic application of targeted re-sequencing in Korean patients with retinitis *Pigmentosa*. *BMC Genomics* 16:515. doi: 10.1186/s12864-015-1723-x

16

CircRNA is a Rising Star in Researches of Ocular Diseases

Chengshou Zhang[1], *Jianghua Hu*[1,2] *and Yibo Yu*[1]*

[1] *Eye Center of the Second Affiliated Hospital, School of Medicine, Zhejiang University, Hangzhou, China,* [2] *Department of Ophthalmology, Jiande Branch, The Second Affiliated Hospital, School of Medicine, Zhejiang University, Hangzhou, China*

Correspondence:
Yibo Yu
yuyibo@zju.edu.cn

A newly rediscovered subclass of noncoding RNAs, circular RNAs (circRNAs), is produced by a back-splicing mechanism with a covalently closed loop structure. They not only serve as the sponge for microRNAs (miRNAs) and proteins but also regulate gene expression and epigenetic modification, translate into peptides, and generate pseudogenes. Dysregulation of circRNA expression has opened a new chapter in the etiology of various human disorders, including cancer and cardiovascular, neurodegenerative, and ocular diseases. Recent studies recognized the vital roles that circRNAs played in the pathogenesis of various eye diseases, highlighting circRNAs as promising biomarkers for diagnosis and assessment of progression and prognosis. Interventions targeting circRNAs provide insights for developing novel treatments for these ocular diseases. This review summarizes our current perception of the properties, biogenesis, and functions of circRNAs and the development of circRNA researches related to ophthalmologic diseases, including diabetic retinopathy, age-related macular degeneration, retinopathy of prematurity, glaucoma, corneal neovascularization, cataract, pterygium, proliferative vitreoretinopathy, retinoblastoma, and ocular melanoma.

Keywords: circular RNA, noncoding RNA, microRNA sponge, ocular diseases, ophthalmology

---

Abbreviations: ADAR1, adenosine deaminase acting on RNA 1; Ago, argonaute; AMD, age-related macular degeneration; ARCs, age-related cataracts; BAMBI, BMP and activin membrane bound inhibitor; CBS, cystathionine-β-synthase; CDK2, cyclin-dependent kinase 2; circRNA, circular RNA; ciRNAs, intronic circRNAs; CM, conjunctival melanoma; CNV, choroidal neovascularization; CRYAA, crystallin alpha A; CSPG4, chondroitin sulfate proteoglycan 4; DM, diabetes mellitus; DMNT3B, DNA (cytosine-5-)-methyltransferase 3 beta; DR, diabetic retinopathy; dsRNA, double-stranded RNA; E2F3, E2F transcription factor 3; ecircRNAs, exonic circRNAs; ECs, endothelial cells; EIciRNAs, exon-intron circRNAs; EMT, epithelial-mesenchymal transition; ERMs, epiretinal membranes; FVM, fibrovascular membranes; FVMs, fibrovascular membranes; FZD4, frizzled-4; HCEKs, corneal epithelial keratinocytes; Hcy, homocysteine; HG, high glucose; HHcy, hyperhomocysteinemia; HIPK3, homeodomain interacting protein kinase 3; HNRNPK, heterogeneous nuclear ribonucleoprotein K; HRMECs, human retinal microvascular endothelial cells; HRVECs, human retinal vascular endothelial cells; HuR, human antigen R; HUVECs, human umbilical vein endothelial cells; IOP, intraocular pressure; IRES, internal ribosome entry site; KIFAP3, kinesin-associated protein 3; lncRNAs, long noncoding RNAs; LOXL2, lysyl oxidase homolog 2; MBL, muscleblind; MEF2A, myocyte-specific enhancer factor 2A; METRN, meteorin; miRNAs, micro RNAs; MMP-2, matrix metallopeptidase 2; MREs, miRNA recognition elements; MTUS1, microtubule-associated scaffold protein 1; nAMD, neovascular age-related macular degeneration; ncRNAs, noncoding RNAs; NR3C1, nuclear receptor subfamily 3 group C member 1; nt, nucleotide; OIR, oxygen-induced retinopathy; PTEN, phosphatase and tensin homolog on chromosome ten; PVR, proliferative vitreoretinopathy; PWWP2A, PWWP domain containing 2A; QKI, quaking; RB, retinoblastoma; RBPs, RNA-binding proteins; RCMs, reverse complementary matches; RD, retinal detachment; RGCs, retinal ganglion cells; RISC, RNA-induced silencing complex; RNase R, ribonuclease R; ROP, retinopathy of prematurity; RPE, retinal pigment epithelium; RUNX2, runt-related transcription factor 2; SIRT1, sirtuin 1; SP1, specificity protein 1; ss, splice sites; STAT3, signal transducer and activator of transcription 3; UM, uveal melanoma; UTRs, untranslated regions; UV, ultraviolet radiation; VCAM1, vascular cell adhesion molecule 1; VEGF, vascular endothelial growth factor; WNT2, Wnt family member 2; XIAP, X-linked inhibitor of apoptosis; ZBTB44, zinc finger and BTB domain containing 44; ZNF, zinc finger protein; ZRANB1, zinc finger RAN-binding domain containing 1.

INTRODUCTION

Noncoding RNAs (ncRNAs), containing microRNAs (miRNAs) and long noncoding RNAs (lncRNAs) comparatively studied extensively, are identified to have vital functions in the regulation of gene expression and development of many human diseases (Esteller, 2011). A rising star in studies of endogenous ncRNAs is circular RNA (circRNA), which has a single-stranded covalently closed structure without 5′ caps and 3′ poly-A tails (Lasda and Parker, 2014) and has attracted interest from many researchers. Although circRNAs were initially discovered in plant viroids four decades ago (Sanger et al., 1976) and then sporadically in hepatitis delta virus and transcripts of the DCC gene, SRY gene and cytochrome P450 2C24 gene (Patop et al., 2019), these molecules were not well understood and treated as by-products of aberrant RNA splicing because they appeared in low abundance and had unknown biological functions (Cocquerelle et al., 1993). However, due to advances in bioinformatics tools and RNA high-throughput sequencing technology, circRNAs have been confirmed to exist in high abundance and be highly diverse and conserved. It has also been confirmed that they are widely expressed in eukaryotes with a cell/tissue- and developmental stage-specific manner (Salzman et al., 2012, 2013; Jeck et al., 2013; Memczak et al., 2013). Since the circRNA called CDR1as/ciRS-7 has been first reported to function as the sponge for miR-7, circRNAs are becoming the focus of biomedical studies (Hansen et al., 2013a; Memczak et al., 2013). Their unique properties and mysterious functions are being uncovered gradually. For instance, it has been found that, in addition to acting as miRNA sponges, circRNAs can interact with RNA-binding proteins (RBPs) (Ashwal-Fluss et al., 2014; Westholm et al., 2014; Conn et al., 2015; Ivanov et al., 2015), regulate RNA splicing or transcription (Ashwal-Fluss et al., 2014; Li Z. et al., 2015), and translate into peptides or proteins (Legnini et al., 2017; Pamudurti et al., 2017; Yang et al., 2017). CircRNAs are also implicated in various biological processes, such as cell differentiation, proliferation, migration and death, carcinogenesis, angiogenesis, neuronal genesis, and innate immune responses (Guo et al., 2014; Lasda and Parker, 2014; Li X. et al., 2018). Furthermore, emerging studies have revealed that circRNAs play a vital role in the pathogenesis of various diseases, including cancer (Su et al., 2019), cardiovascular disease (Aufiero et al., 2019), neurodegenerative diseases (Kumar et al., 2017), and ocular diseases (Guo et al., 2019). Thus, circRNAs can serve as novel biomarkers and therapeutic targets for many diseases.

In recent years, circRNA studies have begun to shed light on studies in the ophthalmology area. Dysregulated circRNAs exert a significant influence on the development of eye tissue and the pathogenesis of ocular diseases (George et al., 2019; Guo et al., 2019). However, to fully reveal the importance of circRNAs, greater knowledge is required, which can be obtained through further researches. Here, we present an overview of the characteristics, biogenesis, and functions of circRNAs (**Figure 1**) and their current recognition of and development for regulating ocular diseases (**Table 1**).

PROPERTIES OF CIRCULAR RNA

Abundance

At first, most discoveries of circular isoforms in the genes of live beings were perceived as mis-splicing occurrences (Cocquerelle et al., 1993). A sea change occurred in 2012 when Salzman et al. (2012) applied RNA-sequencing and computation analysis to identify the global expression of circRNAs in diverse human cell lines. Since then, circRNAs have been found to be abundant and widespread not only in metazoans including mice, *Drosophila*, and zebrafish but also in protists, fungi, and plants (Li X. et al., 2018). Although circRNAs generally have a low expression level (Jeck et al., 2013; Memczak et al., 2013; Salzman et al., 2013; Guo et al., 2014), in some cases, their abundance can exceed that of cognate linear mRNAs due to higher expression or spatiotemporal accumulation (Ashwal-Fluss et al., 2014; Westholm et al., 2014; Conn et al., 2015; Rybak-Wolf et al., 2015; Szabo et al., 2015; Venø et al., 2015; You et al., 2015).

Specificity

The expression patterns of circRNAs are very diverse in different cell and tissue types, as well as developmental stages (Han et al., 2018). As well known, the SRY gene in adult mouse testes produces a circular isoform exclusively instead of linear mRNA (Capel et al., 1993), and the expression of circRNAs is generally induced in the embryonic development stage (Westholm et al., 2014; Szabo et al., 2015). In humans, pigs, and mice, circRNAs are much more abundant in the brains, where the circRNA modulation is correlated with neuronal development and differentiation, homeostatic neuronal activity, and synaptogenesis (Rybak-Wolf et al., 2015; Szabo et al., 2015; Venø et al., 2015; You et al., 2015). Furthermore, the transcription of circRNAs is also dynamic during different biological processes, such as epithelial-mesenchymal transition (EMT) (Conn et al., 2015).

Conservation

Wang et al. (2014) argued that the gene expression of circRNAs was either highly conserved or the result of repeated convergent evolution. Orthologous genes in mice and humans were estimated to produce approximately 5–30% of conserved circRNAs (Jeck et al., 2013; Memczak et al., 2013; Guo et al., 2014; Rybak-Wolf et al., 2015). In addition, nearly 20% of porcine splice sites (ss) correlated with circRNA production were functionally conserved between mice and humans (Venø et al., 2015). Moreover, mechanisms of circRNA biogenesis and similar structural features of circRNA were also judged to be conserved (Jeck et al., 2013; Ashwal-Fluss et al., 2014; Liang and Wilusz, 2014; Zhang et al., 2014). It is worth noting that circular exons were better conserved than flanking exons, which were more likely to be flanked by introns with reverse complementary matches (RCMs) (Rybak-Wolf et al., 2015).

Stability

Ribonuclease R (RNase R) is a 3′ to 5′ exoribonuclease and is capable of catalyzing the degradation of linear RNA, so the

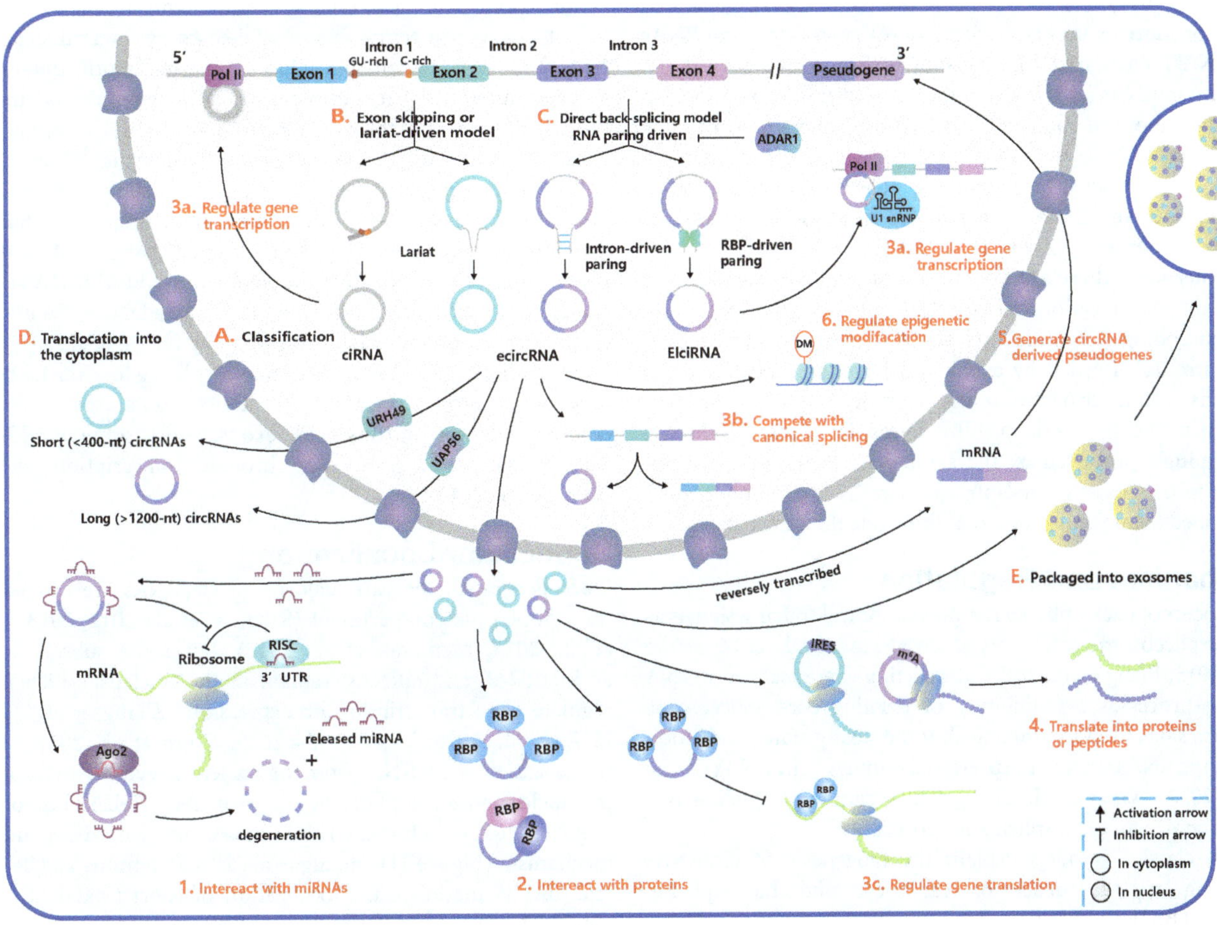

FIGURE 1 | The basic acknowledgment of circular RNA (circRNA). **(A)** CircRNA classification. CircRNAs can be classified into intronic circRNA (ciRNA), exonic circRNA (ecircRNA), and exon-intron circRNA (ElciRNA). **(B)** Exon skipping or lariat-driven mechanism of circRNA biogenesis. Lariats contained skipping exons and introns, can produce ecircRNAs and ElciRNAs. And ciRNAs are produced from a lariat intron with special GU-rich element at 5′ splice sites (ss) and C-rich element at 3′ branchpoint site. **(C)** Direct back-splicing or RNA pairing-driven mechanism of circRNA biogenesis. Special elements in introns like inverted repetitive Alu elements and reverse complementary matches (RCMs) and special RNA-binding proteins (RBPs) like NF90/110, quaking (QKI), and muscleblind (MBL) can facilitate the RNA-pairing. But adenosine deaminase acting on RNA 1 (ADAR1) can inhibit the RNA-pairing and reduce circRNA expression. **(D)** The translocation of circRNAs from the nucleus into the cytoplasm. Short (<400 nt) and long (>1,200 nt) circRNAs were transported into the cytoplasm based on the URH49 and UAP56, respectively. **(E)** Packaged into exosomes. CircRNAs can execute the regulatory function by exporting exosomes. **(1–6)** The function of circRNAs. **(1)** Interact with miRNAs. CircRNAs can work as miRNA sponges and promote the translation of miRNA-targeted genes. But some miRNAs can trigger the circRNA degeneration in the Ago2-slicer-dependent manner, which leads to the release of binding miRNAs. **(2)** Interact with proteins. CircRNAs can serve as transporters, decoys, or scaffolds for proteins and regulate their activities. **(3a–c)** Regulate gene transcription, splicing, and translation. **(3a)** CircRNAs can inhibit gene translation by competing for special RBPs. **(3b)** CiRNA and EcliRNA can promote parent gene transcription by interacting with Pol II. **(3c)** CircRNA biogenesis competes with canonical splicing and circRNAs like circMbl can regulate gene splicing. **(4)** Translate into proteins or peptides. CircRNAs like circZNF609 have internal ribosome entry site (IRES) within their sequences and can be translated. CircRNA translation also can be driven by N^6-methyladenosine (m^6A) modification in a cap-independent manner. **(5)** Generate pseudogenes. **(6)** Regulate epigenetic alterations. CircRNAs can adjust epigenetic modifications, such as DNA or histone methylation.

absence of 3′ and 5′ terminals in circRNAs allows them to resist RNase R degradation (Suzuki, 2006). Jeck et al. (2013) found circRNAs had half-lives exceeding 48 h, while linear transcripts occurred for less than 20 h. Thus, circRNAs are much more stable in cells, tissues, blood, saliva, urine, exosomes, etc., than their linear counterparts due to their covalently closed loop structure. In the aging process of the brain, stable circRNAs can accumulate and exist in richer abundance in quiescent and postmitotic cells (Westholm et al., 2014; Rybak-Wolf et al., 2015).

These characteristics make circRNA production another special feature of genomes rather than transcriptional noise. Besides, circRNAs are delicately regulated, play a vital role in living organisms, and serve as potential biomarkers in bodily fluid for disease diagnosis.

BIOGENESIS OF THE CIRCULAR RNA

Classification

According to recent studies, most of the circRNAs in eukaryotes can be divided into three subtypes depending on their components (**Figure 1A**; Lasda and Parker, 2014;

Liu J. et al., 2017): (1) exonic circRNAs (ecircRNAs): generated by one or more exons circularization; (2) exon-intron circRNAs (EIciRNAs): circularized from exons with introns reserved; (3) intronic circRNAs (ciRNAs): composed only of introns. Different from the canonical splicing, circRNAs are generally formed by the joining of an upstream 3′ acceptor and a downstream 5′ donor, which is called "back-splicing" (Lasda and Parker, 2014). The sequence of ciRNAs is assembled head-to-tail by a 2′, 5′ phosphodiester bond (Zhang et al., 2013).

Furthermore, there are five subsets of circRNA classification based on the location relationship between circRNAs and adjacent coding RNA (Liu J. et al., 2017): (1) and (2) "exonic" and "intronic": formed by exons and introns, respectively; (3) "antisense": transcribed into the opposite strand from their gene locus being overlapped by linear isoforms; (4) "sense overlapping": produced by the same gene locus but does not belong to the "exonic" or "intronic" circRNA; (5) "intergenic": transcribed from the location that is outside the gene loci.

Mechanism and Regulation

The process of back-splicing requires canonical splicing signals as well as spliceosome machinery (Ashwal-Fluss et al., 2014; Starke et al., 2015; Liang et al., 2017). Restricting canonical pre-mRNA splicing processes by inhibiting or deleting core spliceosome complexes has been reported to shift the steady-state production of linear mRNAs toward the preferred output of circRNAs (Liang et al., 2017; Wang et al., 2019). Thus, canonical splicing is a default choice for gene splicing in most cases.

Two classical models explain the biogenesis of circRNAs according to the order of canonical and back-splicing (**Figures 1B,C**):

(1) The "direct back-splicing" model or RNA pairing model (Chen and Yang, 2015; Li X. et al., 2018; Han et al., 2018): Back-splicing occurs first, then a circular structure with intermediate exons and introns are generated directly and are processed into the final product. In this model, RNA pairing across flanking introns brings back-splicing sites into closer proximity and promotes efficient biogenesis of circRNAs. RNA pairing can be driven by repetitive flanking intron sequences, such as inverted repetitive Alu elements, or RCMs (Liang and Wilusz, 2014; Zhang et al., 2014; Ivanov et al., 2015; Kramer et al., 2015). In addition, some double-stranded RBPs, such as immune factors NF90/110, can facilitate RNA pairing formation and some RBPs without dsRNA binding domains, such as muscleblind (MBL) and quaking (QKI), can bind to specific targets in introns (Ashwal-Fluss et al., 2014; Conn et al., 2015; Li et al., 2017; Liu J. et al., 2017). The QKI dimerization at binding sites in the flanking introns can increase the production of many circRNAs (Conn et al., 2015). However, adenosine deaminase acting on RNA 1 (ADAR1) can recognize and diminish the double-stranded RNA (dsRNA) pairing structure through A-to-I editing in dsRNA regions, exerting opposite influence on the biogenesis of circRNAs (Ivanov et al., 2015; Rybak-Wolf et al., 2015).

(2) The "exon skipping" or "lariat-driven" model (Barrett et al., 2015; Chen and Yang, 2015; Li X. et al., 2018; Han et al., 2018): In this model, canonical splicing occurs first, then a lariat structure is generated with skipping exons and introns. Following introns being dislodged, retained components are ligated head-to-tail to produce ecircRNAs or EIciRNAs by internal splicing. Note that a lariat intron, which has a consistent motif containing a seven-nucleotide (nt) Adjacent bases of guanine and uracil (GU)-rich element at the 5′ ss and an 11-nt C-rich element at the 3′ branchpoint site, can be generated and can avoid debranching and degradation (Zhang et al., 2013). Then stable ciRNAs are produced from the lariat intron after removing the 3′ tail in the downstream of the branchpoint site (Zhang et al., 2013). Interestingly, a circRNA from the *Arabidopsis* SEPALLATA3 gene can bind to the cognate DNA locus and form a DNA:RNA hybrid (R-loop), promoting further exon skipping (Conn et al., 2017).

In a single gene locus, alternative splicing occurs in both models to produce various circRNAs containing different combinations of introns and exons. And some circRNAs can be generated from readthrough transcription events (Liang et al., 2017).

Subcellular Localization

Once generated, the vast majority of circRNAs are located in the cytoplasmic compartment (Salzman et al., 2012, 2013; Jeck et al., 2013; Memczak et al., 2013), but some subsets, such as EIciRNAS and ciRNAs, remain in the nucleus, which may regulate gene transcription or expression (Zhang et al., 2013; Li Z. et al., 2015; Venø et al., 2015; Conn et al., 2017). The translocation of circRNAs from the nucleus to cytoplasm through the nuclear pore complex relies on proteins – Hel25E homologs (UAP56/URH49 in humans) and is based on a length-dependent mechanism (**Figure 1D**; Huang et al., 2018). In humans, URH49 and UAP56 modulate the localization of short (<400 nt) and long (>1,200 nt) circRNAs, respectively (Huang et al., 2018). However, the localization of circRNAs is not stationary. You et al. (2015) showed circZEB1 was transited from the cytoplasm and perinuclear sites at E60 to the nucleus at E80, and many circRNAs were enriched in synapses. Moreover, circRNAs can be exported through exosomes and execute their functions (**Figure 1E**). And more than 1,000 circRNAs have been found enriched in human serum exosomes (Li Y. et al., 2015).

Adjustable expression levels and subcellular localization of circRNAs are indicated to be tightly correlated with their function manipulation. While mechanisms that modulate the biogenesis and translocation of many circRNAs have been discovered, molecular details are still poorly understood.

FUNCTIONS OF CIRCULAR RNA

MicroRNA Sponges or Reservoirs

The miRNA, a type of short single-stranded ncRNA, is capable of binding to the 3′ untranslated regions (UTRs) of protein-coding mRNAs and inhibiting their translation by forming an RNA-induced silencing complex (RISC) with the argonaute 2 (Ago2) (Baek et al., 2008). CircRNAs contain miRNA recognition elements (MREs) and rescue mRNAs from miRNA combination through competitive binding. CDR1as/ciRS-7, containing more than 70 MREs of miR-7, was the first circRNA to be identified as a miRNA sponge (**Figure 1.1**; Hansen et al., 2013a;

Memczak et al., 2013). However, the cleavage of ciRS-7, triggered by miR-671 in an Ago2-slicer-dependent manner (Hansen et al., 2011), could lead to immediate spatiotemporal activation of miR-7 and repression of mRNA targets (Hansen et al., 2013b). Thus, ciRS-7 may function as the reservoir or storage of miR-7 and transport it to the specific subcellular location (Hansen et al., 2013b; Memczak et al., 2013).

Interaction With Proteins

The interaction between proteins and circRNAs is much intricate, and circRNAs can serve as transporters, decoys, or scaffolds for proteins (**Figure 1.2**; Patop et al., 2019). CircFoxo3, for example, can have a high binding affinity to some transcription factors and inhibit their nuclear translocation and anti-tress function during cardiac stress (Du et al., 2017b). Another study found circFoxo3 facilitated the inhibition of CDK2 by p21 by generating a ternary complex with p21 and CDK2 (Du et al., 2016). It is first to show that circRNAs can act as a scaffold to form the protein-protein complex and modulate protein interactions (Du et al., 2016). And it has been determined that dynamic tertiary structures of circRNAs enable them to interact with various proteins (Du et al., 2017a,c). Many circRNAs are likely to create a molecular reservoir for antiviral proteins NF90/110 before a viral infection occurs. This behavior supports the hypothesis that circRNAs may regulate activities of proteins *via* cooperative actions (Li et al., 2017).

Regulation of Transcription, Splicing, and Translation

Some circRNAs, such as EIciRNAs and ciRNAs, are positioned in the nucleus and regulate gene transcription and splicing (**Figures 1.3a,b**). For example, based on a specific RNA-RNA interaction, EIciRNAs-U1 snRNP complexes combine with RNA Pol II to promote cognate gene transcription (Li Z. et al., 2015). In addition, ciRNAs can perform cis-regulation by interacting with Pol II, and the depletion of ciRNAs can lead to a significant downregulation of parent gene transcription (Zhang et al., 2013). CircMBL, on the other hand, can strongly bind to MBL and promote back-splicing to produce more circMBL instead of MBL mRNA, which forms a negative-feedback regulation loop (Ashwal-Fluss et al., 2014). CircRNAs can also regulate mRNA translation (**Figure 1.3c**). For instance, circPABPN1 can reduce the expression of PABPN1 by competing with its cognate linear mRNA for human antigen R (HuR, an RBP) (Abdelmohsen et al., 2017).

Translation Into Peptides or Proteins

Synthetic circRNAs implanted with an internal ribosome entry site (IRES) have already been proven to be translated *in vivo* and *in vitro* (Chen and Sarnow, 1995; Wang and Wang, 2015). CircZNF609 was the first natural circRNA discovered to translate to protein through the splicing-dependent and cap-independent mechanisms (Legnini et al., 2017). It was also discovered that circMBL from fly heads encodes a protein (Pamudurti et al., 2017). Both translatable circRNAs have IRES embedded within their sequences. The translation of circRNAs also can be driven by N^6-methyladenosine (m^6A) modification in a cap-independent manner (**Figure 1.4**), which requires initiation factor eIF4G2 and m^6A reader YTHDF3 (Yang et al., 2017).

Generation of CircRNA-Derived Pseudogenes

Pseudogenes are important regulators at the DNA, RNA, or protein level in diverse physiological and pathological processes (Xiao-Jie et al., 2015). Similar to mRNAs, circRNAs have the potential to be reverse transcribed and integrated into their host genomes to generate pseudogenes (**Figure 1.5**). Dong et al. (2016) determined that circRNA-derived pseudogenes may reshape genome architecture by providing additional CCCTC binding factor-binding sites. However, the mysterious generation mechanism and functions of circRNA-derived pseudogenes are still unknown.

Regulate Epigenetic Alterations

A few circRNAs have been found to affect epigenetic modifications by acting on DNA or histone methylation (**Figure 1.6**; Chen et al., 2018; Su et al., 2019). For instance, circFECR1 can bind to the promoter of FLI1 in cis and lead to DNA hypomethylation by recruiting a demethylase TET1 (Chen et al., 2018). It can also bind to and downregulate trans DNMT1, a methyltransferase that is essential for maintaining DNA methylation (Chen et al., 2018). Through epigenetic modification, circFECR1 positively activates the FLI1 and underlines the deep mechanism of tumor growth and metastasis (Chen et al., 2018, 1). Several circRNAs can indirectly regulate histone methylation by sponging miRNAs that inhibit the expression of an N-methyltransferase enzyme called EZH2 (Su et al., 2019).

Although most of the identified functional circRNAs act as miRNA sponges, they have varied biological functions that support our recognition of the importance of circRNAs in parental cell activities. Additionally, exosomal circRNAs may regulate biological processes in distant cells and tissues (Li Y. et al., 2015; Shi et al., 2020).

INVOLVEMENT OF CIRCULAR RNA RESEARCH IN OCULAR DISEASES

Recently, in a study conducted by Sun et al. (2019), retinal circRNA repertoires showed conservation and variation across six vertebrate species, and the expression pattern of circRNAs had specific signatures in different stages of retinal development and degeneration (Chen X.-J. et al., 2020). The deficiency of circTulp4 in mice caused the mouse retinas to have abnormal structures and defective functions (Chen X.-J. et al., 2020). These studies further convince us to highlight the potential key biological functions of circRNAs in regulating eye development as well as ocular diseases. In this part, we focus on accumulative evidence that has identified that circRNAs play a crucial role in the pathogenesis and progression of some ocular diseases (**Table 1**). CircRNAs can serve as potentially diagnostic, progressive, and prognostic

TABLE 1 | Verified circRNAs involved in various ocular diseases.

Ocular diseases	circRNAs	Expression	Functions	Related networks	References
DR	circ_0005015	Upregulated in the plasma, vitreous samples, and FVMs of DR patients.	Promote the angiogenic function of HRVECs *in vitro*.	miR-519d-3p-MMP-2/STAT3/XIAP	Zhang S.-J. et al., 2017
	circHIPK3	Upregulated in HRVECs under HG conditions, DR models, the plasma, vitreous samples, and FVMs of DR patients.	Promote the angiogenic function of HRVECs under HG conditions *in vitro*. Aggravate the DM-induced retinal vascular dysfunction *in vivo*.	c-myb, miR-30a-3p/ VEGFC/FZD4/WNT2	Shan et al., 2017
	circZNF609	Upregulated in HUVECs under HG conditions, DR models, the plasma, and FVMs of DR patients.	Promote the angiogenic function of HUVECs under HG conditions *in vitro*. Aggravate the DM-induced retinal vascular dysfunction *in vivo*.	miR-615-5p-MEF2A	Liu C. et al., 2017
	circDMNT3B	Downregulated in HRMECs under HG conditions and the FVMs of DR patients.	Suppress the angiogenic function of HRMECs under HG conditions *in vitro*. Ameliorate DM-induced retinal vascular dysfunction and visual damage *in vivo*.	miR-20b-5p-BAMBI	Zhu et al., 2019
	circPWWP2A	Upregulated in retinal pericytes under DM related stresses instead of HRVECs, DR models, and the FVMs of DR patients.	Promote the viability, proliferation, antiapoptosis, recruitment toward HRVECs of pericytes under DM-related stresses *in vitro* but affect HRVECs indirectly *via* exosomes. Ameliorate DM-induced retinal vascular dysfunction and pericyte dysfunction *in vivo*.	miR-579-angiopoietin1/ occludin/SIRT1	Liu et al., 2019
	circZNF532	Upregulated in retinal pericytes following DM-related stresses, DR models, and the vitreous samples of DR patients.	Promote the viability, proliferation, antiapoptosis, recruitment toward HRVECs of pericytes under DM-related stresses *in vitro*. Ameliorate DM-induced retinal vascular dysfunction and pericyte dysfunction *in vivo*.	SP1, miR-29a-3p-CSPG4/LOXL2/CDK2	Jiang et al., 2020
ROP	circZNF609	Upregulated at the neovascularization stage of OIR models.	Aggravate the oxygen-induced retinal vascular dysfunction *in vivo*.	miR-615-5p-MEF2A	Liu C. et al., 2017
Exudative AMD	circZBTB44	Upregulated in chorioretinal ECs under hypoxic conditions, CNV models, the aqueous humor of nAMD patients.	Promote the angiogenic function of chorioretinal vascular ECs under hypoxic conditions *in vitro*. Aggravate the CNV development *in vivo*.	miR-578-VEGFA/VCAM1	Zhou et al., 2020
Atrophic AMD	circNR3C1	Downregulated in RPE cells under oxidative stress and the blood serum of AMD patients.	Maintain the RPE phenotypes and functions *in vitro* and *in vivo* to prevent AMD progression.	miR-382-5p-PTEN-AKT/mTOR	Chen X. et al., 2020
Glaucoma	circZRANB1	Upregulated in glaucoma model and the aqueous humor of glaucoma patients.	Promote the viability, proliferation, and activation of Müller cells directly, but indirectly inhibit RGC function *in vitro*. Promote the retinal reactive gliosis and glia cell activation (glaucomatous retinal neuropathy) *in vivo*.	miR-217-RUNX2	Wang et al., 2018b
	circZNF609	Upregulated in glaucoma model and the aqueous humor of glaucoma patients.	Promote the viability, proliferation, and activation of Müller cells directly, but indirectly inhibit RGC function *in vitro*. Promote the retinal reactive gliosis and glia cell activation (glaucomatous retinal neuropathy), but inhibit RGC survival *in vivo*.	miR-615-METRN	Wang et al., 2018a
ARC	circHIPK3	Downregulated in lens capsules of patients with various types of ARC.	Promote the viability, proliferation, EMT and antiapoptosis upon oxidative stress of HLECs *in vitro*.	miR-193a-3p-CRYAA	Liu et al., 2018, 3
Corneal neovascularization	circZNF609	Upregulated in the corneal epithelium of corneal neovascularization models.	Promote the angiogenic function of HCEKs *in vivo*. Aggravate the corneal angiogenesis *in vivo*.	miR-184-AKT/β-catenin/VEGF	Wu et al., 2020
	circKIFAP3	Downregulated in alkali burn-induced neovascularization corneal models and patients' vascularized corneas.	Suppress the angiogenic function of HUVECs *in vitro*.		Zhou Y.-F. et al., 2019
Pterygium	circ_0085020	Upregulated in pterygium tissues	Promote the viability, proliferation, migration, and antiapoptosis under UV exposure of pterygium fibroblasts and epithelial cells *in vitro*.		Li X.-M. et al., 2018

(Continued)

TABLE 1 | Continued

Ocular diseases	circRNAs	Expression	Functions	Related networks	References
PVR	circ_0043144	Upregulated in serum ERMs of PVR patient.	Promote the proliferation, migration, and secretion ability of RPE cells *in vitro*.		Yao et al., 2019
Retinoblastoma	circ_0001649	Downregulated in RB cell lines and RB tissues of patients.	Suppress the proliferation and antiapoptosis of RB cells *in vitro*. Suppress the xenograft tumor growth of RB *in vivo*.	AKT/mTOR	Xing et al., 2018
	circ–0075804	Upregulated in RB cell lines and RB tissues of patients.	Promote the proliferation and antiapoptosis of RB cells *in vitro*. Promote the xenograft tumor growth of RB *in vivo*.	E2F3, HNRNPK	Zhao et al., 2020
Conjunctival melanoma	circMTUS1	Upregulated in CM tissues.	Promote the proliferation of CM cell lines *in vitro*. Promote the xenograft tumor growth of CM *in vivo*.		Shang et al., 2019

DR, Diabetic retinopathy; FVM, fibrovascular membrane; HRVECs, human retinal vascular ECs; MMP-2, matrix metallopeptidase 2; STAT3, signal transducer and activator of transcription 3; XIAP, x-linked inhibitor Of apoptosis; HIPK3, homeodomain interacting protein kinase 3; HG, high glucose; DM, diabetes mellitus; VEGF, vascular endothelial growth factor; FZD4, frizzled-4; WNT2, Wnt family member 2; ZNF, zinc finger protein; HUVECs, human umbilical vein endothelial cells; MEF2A, myocyte-specific enhancer factor 2A; DMNT3B, DNA (cytosine-5-)-methyltransferase 3 beta; ECs, endothelial cells; HRMECs, human retinal microvascular ECs; BAMBI, BMP and activin membrane bound inhibitor; PWWP2A, PWWP domain containing 2A; SIRT1, sirtuin 1; SP1, specificity protein 1; CSPG4, chondroitin sulfate proteoglycan 4; LOXL2, lysyl oxidase homolog 2; CDK2, cyclin-dependent kinase 2; ROP, Retinopathy of prematurity; OIR, oxygen?induced retinopathy; AMD, Age-related macular degeneration; ZBTB44, zinc finger and BTB domain containing 44; VCAM1, vascular cell adhesion protein 1; nAMD, neovascular AMD; CNV, choroidal neovascularization; NR3C1, nuclear receptor subfamily 3 group C member 1; RPE, retinal pigment epithelium; PTEN, phosphatase and tensin homolog on chromosome ten; mTOR, mammalian target of rapamycin; ZRANB1, zinc finger RAN-binding domain containing 1; RGCs, retinal ganglion cells; RUNX2, runt-related transcription factor 2; METRN, meteorin; ARC, age-related cataracts; EMT, epithelial-mesenchymal transition; HLECs, human lens epithelial cells; CRYAA, crystallin alpha A; HCEKs, corneal epithelial keratinocytes; KIFAP3, kinesin-associated protein 3; UV, ultraviolet radiation; PVR, proliferative vitreoretinopathy; ERMs, epiretinal membranes; RB, retinoblastoma; E2F3, E2F transcription factor 3; HNRNPK, heterogeneous nuclear ribonucleoprotein K; MTUS1, microtubule-associated scaffold protein 1; CM, conjunctival melanoma.

biomarkers for these diseases, and it is promising to treat them by intervening circRNA expression.

Retinal Diseases

Diabetic Retinopathy

Diabetic retinopathy (DR) is a common microvascular complication among people with diabetes mellitus (DM) and is one of the main causes of visual damage and blindness for them (Yau et al., 2012). In DM, diabetes-related stresses can cause retinal vasculatures to undergo early and prevalent damage, and disequilibrium of endothelial cells (ECs) can increase vascular exudation and macula edema and promote retinal angiogenesis (Duh et al., 2017). The combination of abnormal vascular endothelial growth factor (VEGF) expression and other factors, such as advanced glycation end products, oxidative stress, activated protein kinase C, and Phosphatidylinositol 3-kinase (PI3K)/Akt signaling pathways, has also been identified to underlie vascular dysfunction in DR (Schalkwijk and Stehouwer, 2005; Potenza et al., 2009).

Circ_0005015 has been identified as a putative circRNA biomarker in DR, which is significantly increased in the plasma, vitreous samples, and preretinal fibrovascular membranes (FVMs) of people with DR (Zhang S.-J. et al., 2017). In addition, circ_0005015 can promote the retinal endothelial angiogenesis by working as the miR-519d-3p sponge, which regulates the expression of matrix metallopeptidase (MMP)-2, signal transducer and activator of transcription (STAT)3, and X-linked inhibitor of apoptosis protein (XIAP) (**Figure 2**; Zhang S.-J. et al., 2017). Similar to circ_005015, overexpressed circHIPK3 promotes cell viability, proliferation, migration, and tube formation in human retinal vascular ECs (HRVECs) and aggravates diabetic retinal vascular dysfunction by increasing vascular leakage and the number of the acellular capillary (Shan et al., 2017). The transcription factor c-myb is responsible for the upregulation of circHIPK3 under diabetes-related stresses, and then the regulatory network of circHIPK3-miR-30a-3p-VEGFC/FZD4/WNT2 is activated (**Figure 2**; Shan et al., 2017). cZNF609 is another highly expressed circRNA in patients with DR, and its defect suppresses pathological angiogenesis in the DR model (**Figure 2**; Liu C. et al., 2017). Conversely, circDNMT3B has a decreased concentration in FVMs and human retinal microvascular ECs (HRMECs) under the high-glucose (HG) treatment. MiR-20b-5p, targeted by circDNMT3B, has been found to positively regulate endothelial angiogenesis through modulating the expression of BAMBI (**Figure 2**; Zhu et al., 2019). Earlier works have shown that BAMBI is involved in capillary growth regulation and angiogenesis (Guillot et al., 2012).

The dysfunction of pericytes is a leading pathologic feature of inchoate DR and the unbalanced pericyte-EC crosstalk induces the dysfunction of the retinal microvasculature system in DR (Hammes et al., 2002; Armulik et al., 2005). Researchers have verified cPWWP2A and cZNF532 are attractive targets for alternative therapies of pericyte degeneration and DR (Liu et al., 2019; Jiang et al., 2020). Upregulated expressions of cPWWP2A and cZNF532 were found in pericytes under DM-related stresses and in clinical samples from people with DR, but not in

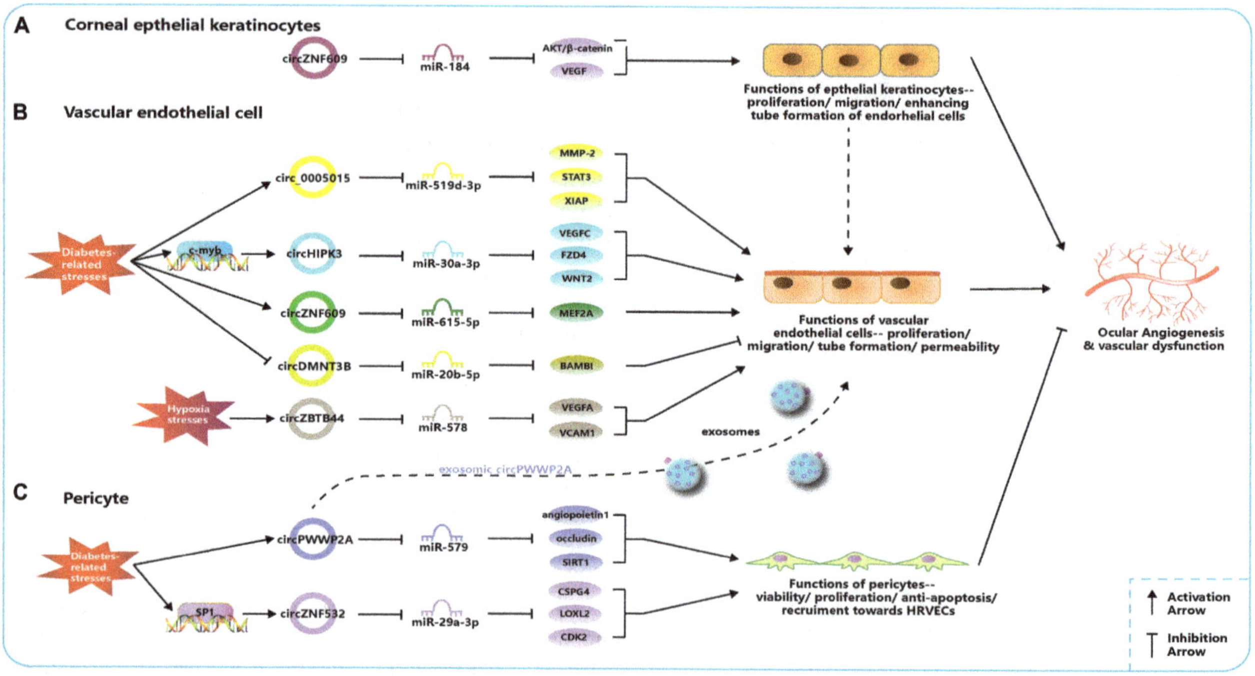

FIGURE 2 | Related circular RNAs (circRNAs) in the pathogenesis of ocular neovascular diseases. **(A)** In corneal epithelial keratinocytes, circZNF609 regulates the function of epithelial cells and promote the ocular angiogenesis through miR-184-AKT/β-catenin/vascular endothelial growth factor (VEGF) network. **(B)** In vascular endothelial cells, networks of circ_0005015-miR-519d-3p-matrix metallopeptidase (MMP)-2/STAT3/X-linked inhibitor of apoptosis protein (XIAP), circHIPK3-miR-30a-3p-VEGFC/FZD4/WNT2, circZNF609-miR-615-5p-MEF2A, circDMNT3B-miR-20b-5p-BMP, and activin membrane bound inhibitor (BAMBI), and circZBTB44-miR-578-VEGFA/vascular cell adhesion molecule (VCAM)1 regulate the function of endothelial cells and the ocular angiogenesis. Circ_0005015, circHIPK3, and circZNF609 can promote angiogenesis and be upregulated under diabetes-related stresses, which is opposite to circDMNT3B. CircZBTB44 can promote angiogenesis and be upregulated under diabetes-related stresses. **(C)** In pericytes, networks of circPWWP2A-miR-579-angiopoietin1/occludin/sirtuin (SIRT)1 and circZNF532-miR-29a-3p-CSPG4/LOXL2/CDK2 regulate the function of pericytes and the ocular angiogenesis. CircPWWP2A and circZNF532 can inhibit the angiogenesis and maintain the normal vascular structure. CircPWWP2A is also packaged into exosomes and transported from pericytes to the endothelial cells.

ECs, which were verified to antagonize the diabetes-induced disruption to vascular homeostasis (Liu et al., 2019; Jiang et al., 2020). And the severity of DR was also correlated to rising levels of cZNF532 in the vitreous (Jiang et al., 2020). The SP1, a transcription factor activated in diabetic condition, could bind to the promoter of cZNF532 and take charge of increasing cZNF532 expression (Jiang et al., 2020). In pericytes, cZNF532 can promote the expression of CSPG4, LOXL2, and CDK2 by sequestering the miR-29a-3p binding sites, which results in increased cell viability, proliferation, and recruitment toward HRVECs, ameliorated diabetic stress-induced cell apoptosis, and decreased the macromolecular permeability (**Figure 2**; Jiang et al., 2020). However, manipulating the cZNF532 expression had almost no effect on HRVECs (Jiang et al., 2020). cPWWP2A had similar effects to those of cZNF532 on the regulation of pericyte functions *via* a different network—cPWWP2A-miR-579-angiopoietin1/occludin/SIRT1, but, unlike cZNF532, it was able to indirectly modulate HRVEC angiogenic activities and pericyte-EC crosstalk through a paracrine approach in exosomes from pericytes (**Figure 2**; Liu et al., 2019). In conclusion, the overexpression of cZNF532 and cPWWP2A or the silencing of miR-29a-3p and miR-579 was found to alleviate the diabetes-related damage to pericyte functions *in vitro* and retinal vasculatures *in vivo*, as it resulted in an increase in pericyte coverage and a reduction of vascular leakage, the acellular vascular area, and the amount of microaneurysm (Liu et al., 2019; Jiang et al., 2020).

Another two studies identified altered expression profiles of circRNAs in serum samples and the vitreous humor of people with DR, which could serve as a foundation for future studies on the role of circRNAs in DR (Gu et al., 2017a; He et al., 2020).

Retinopathy of Prematurity

Retinopathy of prematurity (ROP), a retinal vasoproliferative disease, primarily occurs in premature infants and may cause blindness (Chen and Smith, 2007; Chan-Ling et al., 2018). The pathogenesis of ROP is known to have two phases: Phase 1 is hyperoxia-induced incomplete retinal vessel growth after premature birth, and Phase 2 is hypoxia-driven pathological vessel proliferation (Chen and Smith, 2007; Chan-Ling et al., 2018). Current ablation treatments, the injection of anti-VEGF agents, and other relatively effective treatments contribute to reduced blindness and improved long-term prognosis for people with ROP (Chan-Ling et al., 2018).

The oxygen-induced retinopathy (OIR) newborn mouse model is widely used for mimicking the development of ROP and studying the pathogenesis of retinal neovascularization (Scott and Fruttiger, 2010). Using the OIR model, it was found that cZNF609 was downregulated at the vaso-obliteration stage (Postnatal Days 7–12), but it was upregulated at the neovascularization stage (P12–17) (Liu C. et al., 2017). The reduction in cZNF609 dramatically shrunk the avascular area and suppressed pathologic angiogenesis *in vivo* at P12 and P17 (Liu C. et al., 2017). Decreased cZNF609 also positively regulated human umbilical vein endothelial cell (HUVEC) functions by targeting miR-615-5p-MEF2A network (**Figure 2**). Therefore, MEF2A silencing can have a mimicking effect on HUVECs as cZNF609 (Liu C. et al., 2017). Two more pieces of research contain a microarray analysis of circRNAs based on the OIR model, providing further research targets for ROP pathogenesis (Cao et al., 2019; Zhou H. et al., 2019).

Age-Related Macular Degeneration

Exudative age-related macular degeneration

Age-related macular degeneration (AMD) is one of the leading causes of irreversible blindness in the elderly. AMD is classified into two subtypes–exudative AMD and atrophic AMD–according to whether choroidal vessels disruptively invade the retina (Lim et al., 2012). Exudative AMD, also called neovascular AMD (nAMD) or wet AMD, is characterized by choroidal neovascularization (CNV) leading to retinal pigment epithelium (RPE) rupture, leaking lipids and blood, and fibrous scarring (Lim et al., 2012). Intraocular injection of anti-VEGF agents is the current main treatment for nAMD (Bloch et al., 2012). Whether dysregulated circRNA contributes to developing nAMD is being studied recently.

Liu et al. (2020) investigated circRNA expression profiles using the laser-induced CNV mouse model and constructed circRNA-miRNA-mRNA networks potentially regulating the CNV development. Zhou et al. (2020) identified that cZBTB44 could regulate the pathogenesis of CNV. They also found that cZBTB44, as well as VEGFA and vascular cell adhesion molecule (VCAM)1, was significantly upregulated not only in chorioretinal vascular ECs under hypoxic conditions and CNV lesions from mouse models but also in the aqueous humor of patients with nAMD (Zhou et al., 2020). Moreover, the silencing of cZBTB44 led to the reduction of the CNV lesion area *in vivo* and reduced the size of the choroidal capillary area and the sprouting area in choroidal sprouting assay *ex vivo* (Zhou et al., 2020). cZBTB44 can promote endothelial angiogenic effect by sponging the miR-578 and then modulating the level of VEGFA/VCAM1 indirectly in choroid-retinal ECs (**Figure 2**; Zhou et al., 2020).

Atrophic age-related macular degeneration

Atrophic AMD, also called dry AMD, is characterized by persistent atrophy of the RPE, choriocapillaris, and photoreceptors (Lim et al., 2012). RPE cells can maintain retinal functions through vital activities, such as light absorption, nutrient or metabolic waste transportation, and growth factor secretion (Strauss, 2005; Chen X. et al., 2020). RPE abnormalities, like dedifferentiation and degeneration, underlines the pathogenesis of early atrophic AMD, and the strategies for RPE protection will be a promising therapy in the future (Strauss, 2005; Lim et al., 2012).

A recent study revealed that the expression of circNR3C1 was downregulated in serum samples of people with atrophic AMD patients and RPE cells under oxidative stress (Chen X. et al., 2020). CircNR3C1 was found to protect RPE functions *via* regulating the miR-382-5p-phosphatase and tension homolog on chromosome ten (PTEN)-AKT/mammalian target of rapamycin (mTOR) networks (Chen X. et al., 2020). More specifically, insufficient endogenous circNR3C1 expression could disturb RPE ultrastructure, reduce RPE markers, interrupt phagocytosis, and promote RPE proliferation (Chen X. et al., 2020). PTEN, an inhibitor of the AKT/mTOR signaling pathway, enables RPE cells to function normally, but the activation of the AKT/mTOR pathway triggers RPE dedifferentiation and retinal degeneration (Kim et al., 2008; Lee et al., 2011; Zhao et al., 2011; Jiang et al., 2016).

Glaucoma

As circRNAs are abundant, well conserved, and dynamically expressed in the central nervous system (Rybak-Wolf et al., 2015; You et al., 2015), they play a vital role in the modulation of neurodegeneration disorders (Kumar et al., 2017). Glaucoma is an irreversible and progressive retinal neurodegenerative disease and is the second leading cause of blindness worldwide (Kingman, 2004). It is caused by the progressive loss of retinal ganglion cells (RGCs) (Weinreb et al., 2014). The only method to delay or halt the progression of glaucoma and help RGC survival is to reduce intraocular pressure through surgery and medication (Weinreb et al., 2014).

Although the pathogenesis of glaucoma is highly complex and still unclear, two recent studies have revealed that circRNAs played an important role in glaucoma (Wang et al., 2018a,b). Wang et al. determined that the expression levels of Wang et al. (2018a) and Wang et al. (2018b) were upregulated by elevating the intraocular pressure (IOP) in the rat microbead injection-induced glaucoma model, which was consistent with the detection results in aqueous humor from people with glaucoma. *In vivo*, knockdown of cZNF609 and cZRANB1 inhibited the reaction of retinal gliosis and facilitated the survival of RGCs, but it did not affect the amacrine cells, photoreceptors, or bipolar cells. *In vitro*, silencing cZNF609 or cZRANB1 suppressed the viability, proliferation, and activation of Müller cells. However, the silencing indirectly regulated RGC function by reducing the proapoptotic effects of Müller cells on RGCs under oxidative stress and glutamate toxicity stress. cZNF609 was validated to function as the sponge for miR-615, targeting METRN. In addition, the cZRANB1-miR-217-RUNX2 network was uncovered in Müller cells. Moreover, circRNAs showed abnormal expression patterns in a much earlier stage, before the onset of retinal degeneration diseases, in *in vivo* models (Chen X.-J. et al., 2020). The RUNX2 is involved in mammalian neural development, and METRN influences glial cell differentiation and axonal network formation (Nishino et al., 2004; Zagami et al., 2009). A therapy targeting cZNF609 and cZRANB1 that would indirectly regulate these target genes may be promising as a glaucoma treatment.

Cataract

Age-Related Cataract

Cataract is characterized by the loss of transparency of the human lens. Severe opacification leads to visual impairment or blindness at last. Cataracts can be categorized based on the etiology: age-related cataracts (ARCs), congenital cataracts, and secondary cataracts (cataracts caused by other factors, such as diabetic cataracts) (Liu Y.-C. et al., 2017). The etiopathogenesis of ARC can include the accumulation of insoluble crystallin and dysregulated biological activities of human lens epithelial cells (HLECs), such as abnormal cell growth, cell death, and differentiation (Michael and Bron, 2011). Although cataract surgery is an efficient way to manage cataracts, the rapidly increasing demand for cataract surgery poses a great economic burden on society (Rao et al., 2011; Liu Y.-C. et al., 2017). A more precise molecule mechanism is being studied to find promising alternative pharmacological means for ARC treatment.

Liu et al. (2018) found a general decrease in the expression of circHIPK3 in all three subtypes of ARC (cortical, nuclear, and posterior subcapsular ARC). CircHIPK3 is an abundant and highly conserved circRNA that is involved in a series of physiological or pathological activities (Xie et al., 2020). Silencing circHIPK3 led to the suppression of various cell activities in primary cultured HLECs, such as cell viability, proliferation, EMT, and anti-apoptosis under oxidative stress (Liu et al., 2018). The function of circHIPK3 was manipulated through the circHIPK3-miR-193a-3p-CRYAA axis in HLECs. The CRYAA encodes the αA-crystallin, which is necessary for the maintenance of lens transparency and lens epithelium survival (Andley, 2009).

Diabetic Cataract

Cataract often occurs at an earlier age and keeps progressing faster in people with DM (Harding et al., 1993). The proliferation, apoptosis, and autophagy of HLECs are often induced by the hyperglycemic and hyperosmotic microenvironment combined with impaired antioxidant systems (Pollreisz and Schmidt-Erfurth, 2010; Zhang L. et al., 2017). Cataract surgery for patients with DM should be carried out more cautiously and has higher complication rates (Pollreisz and Schmidt-Erfurth, 2010). Interventions that target the pathogenic mechanism of diabetic cataract to delay or confine its onset and progression remain not well understand.

Fan et al. (2019) identified the expression profiling of circRNAs in people with DR first. They detected that circKMT2E was significantly upregulated in circRNAs of the anterior capsular tissues of the lens in those patients, which was the opposite of the results for the promising miRNA target—miR-204-5p, which is related to cell autophagy (Cost and Czyzyk-Krzeska, 2015; Zhang L. et al., 2017; Fan et al., 2019). The autophagy-related circKMT2E/miRNA/mRNA interaction network was only putatively depicted in this study, which may affect the pathogenesis of diabetic cataract (Fan et al., 2019). Thus, the function of circKMT2E in cataract is still imprecise.

Corneal Diseases

The cornea is a transparent and avascular part of the eye when it is healthy, while the corneal limbus has many blood vessels to support the survival of stem cells (Chang et al., 2001). However, in people with immunologic, traumatic, or infectious disorders on the ocular surface, corneal neovascularization results from newborn blood vessels from the limbus invading the cornea (Casey and Li, 1997; Chang et al., 2001). Corneal neovascularization often leads to profound vision loss and increases the risk of graft failure and rejection after corneal transplantation (Chang et al., 2001; Bachmann et al., 2010).

The expressions of cZFP609 (cZNF609 in humans) and cKifap3 are the most upregulated and downregulated circRNAs, respectively, in the alkali burn-induced corneal neovascularization model, with results consistent with those of patients' vascularized corneas (Zhou Y.-F. et al., 2019). The phenomenon of persistent upregulated cZNF609 and downregulated miR-184 was also discovered in the rat cornea after corneal suture surgery (Wu et al., 2020). *In vitro*, cKifap3 knockdown improved the angiogenic function of HUVECs (Zhou Y.-F. et al., 2019). In addition, cZNF609 was found to promote angiogenesis by acting as a sponge for miR-184 and activating downstream AKT/β-catenin/VEGF in human corneal epithelial keratinocytes (HCEKs) (**Figure 2**). This circRNA was revealed to increase the proliferation and migration of HCEKs and enhance the tube formation of ECs (Wu et al., 2020). Thus, topical administration to upregulate the miR-184 or attenuate the cZNF609 was effective in decreasing corneal neovascularization in corneal sutured rats (Wu et al., 2020).

As mentioned above, enhanced expressions of circ_0005015, cZNF609, circHIPK3, and cZBTB44 or decreased expressions of circDMNT3B can promote the angiogenic function of vascular endothelial cells. The overexpression of cZNF609 can strengthen the angiogenesis effect in corneal epithelial keratinocytes, and the overexpression of cPWWP2A or cZNF532 can regulate pericyte functions and alleviate retinal vascular dysfunction *in vivo*. These dysregulated circRNAs, together with their regulatory networks, disrupt the balance of angiogenic and angiostatic factors and modulate the cell activities of endothelial cells, epithelial keratinocytes, and pericytes (**Figure 2**). These findings provide new insights into the pathogenesis of vascular eye diseases.

Ocular Surface Diseases

Pterygium, a common ocular surface disorder, is characterized by benign noncancerous overgrowth of conjunctiva over the sclera (Liu et al., 2013). Visual function is significantly affected if the hyperplastic fibrovascular tissue invades the cornea or causes inflammation (Liu et al., 2013). Genetic factors (e.g., DNA repair, cell proliferation and migration, and angiogenesis) and environmental factors [e.g., human papillomavirus infection and chronic ultraviolet radiation (UV) exposure] underlie the pathogenesis of pterygium (Liu et al., 2013). However, the precise molecular mechanism of pterygium formation is not clear, and pterygium has a relatively high recurrence ratio with the current treatments (Hacıoğlu and Erdöl, 2017).

In a recent study, 669 circRNAs were found to be abnormally expressed in pterygium tissues (Li X.-M. et al., 2018). Further analysis revealed that the most enriched biological process and regulatory network of dysregulated circRNAs are the extracellular matrix organization and focal adhesion signaling pathways, respectively, which are highly correlated with the pathogenesis of pterygium (Li X.-M. et al., 2018). The researchers focused on significantly upregulated circ_0085020 (circLAPTM4B) and found that its silencing weakened cellular viability, proliferation, and migration of pterygium fibroblasts and pterygium epithelial cells but increased UV-induced apoptosis (Li X.-M. et al., 2018). More researches are required to more thoroughly understand the regulatory network of circ_0085020.

Vitreous Diseases

Proliferative vitreoretinopathy (PVR) commonly occurs after retinal detachment (RD) surgery or other intraocular surgeries due to the genesis of membranes on the surface between the detached retina and the posterior hyaloid (Pastor et al., 2016). The migration and proliferation of RPE and glial cells have been considered essential elements of the pathogenesis of PVR (Pastor et al., 2016). Proliferating membranes may lead to further tractional RD, and current surgical treatments carry the risk of retina re-detachment (Charteris et al., 2002), so it is important to prevent the development of PVR.

Yao et al. (2019) screened 91 circRNAs that were dysregulated in the epiretinal membranes (ERMs) of people with rhegmatogenous RD who were diagnosed with PVR. Among the 91 circRNAs was circ_0043144, which has a dynamic expression consistent with established PVR markers, and its circulating molecular concentration in serum samples positively increased in a PVR severity assessment, but there was no difference after the surgery for PVR (Yao et al., 2019). In *in vitro* studies, the silence of circ_0043144 induced the dysfunction of RPE cells, such as suppressed proliferation and migration and attenuated secretion of cytokines and growth factors that may prevent the formation of ERMs (Yao et al., 2019). Circ_0043144 may be able to perform as an indicator for the diagnosis and aggravation of PVR, as well as a potential therapeutic target.

Hyperhomocysteinemia-Induced Ocular Diseases

Hyperhomocysteinemia (HHcy) is a type of metabolic disease in which there is an abnormally high level of homocysteine (Hcy) in the patient's plasma caused by a deficiency of cystathionine-β-synthase (CBS), methionine synthase, and other factors involved in the metabolism, such as vitamins B6 and B12 (Ajith and Ranimenon, 2015). Many pieces of evidence have supported that HHcy can induce various ocular pathological changes correlated with glaucoma, cataract, retinopathy, optic neuropathy, retinal vascular diseases, and many other eye disorders (Ajith and Ranimenon, 2015).

A profile of differentially expressed circRNAs was identified in the eyes of the CBS-deficient murine model with HHcy (Singh et al., 2018). On the other hand, Singh et al. (2019) found 54 dysregulated circRNAs in the RPE cells exposed to high levels of Hcy. In the future, more functional circRNAs should be verified to help us better understand the role of circRNAs in HHcy-induced ocular diseases.

Ocular Malignancies

Retinoblastoma

Retinoblastoma (RB) is a progressive intraocular cancer that occurs most commonly in young children (Dimaras et al., 2012). This has an approximate mortality ratio of 70% in pediatric patients with RB in underdeveloped countries (Dimaras et al., 2012). The genetic etiology or pathogenesis of RB is suspected to be what is known as the Knudson's "two-hit" hypothesis. According to this hypothesis, there is first a mutation of the RB1 gene and then the second hit occurs in the RB1 alleles (Knudson, 1971). However, more research has revealed a more complex landscape of genetics and epigenetics in which other biological molecules and events affect the origin and prognosis of RB, including DNA methylation, miRNA, and circRNAs (Reis et al., 2012).

Has_circ_0001649, transcribed from an antioncogene SHPRH, is a novel cancer-associated circRNA found in several cancers, such as cholangiocarcinoma (Xing et al., 2018; Xu et al., 2018). The downregulation of circ_0001649 was found in RB tissues and human RB cell lines, and it was correlated with a larger bulk of tumors, more severe retinoblastoma, and reduced 5-year survival rate after surgeries (Xing et al., 2018). Furthermore, overexpressed circ_0001649 was shown to inhibit the proliferative ability of RB cells by modulating the signaling pathway of AKT/mTOR and slow down the xenograft growth of RB in the mouse model (Xing et al., 2018). In another study, circ_0075804 and its homologous mRNA derived from gene E2F3 were highly expressed in RB cells (Zhao et al., 2020). Interestingly, circ_0075804 was found to enhance the stability of E2F3 mRNA with the help of HNRNPK (a type of RBP) (Zhao et al., 2020). Thus, the level of E2F3 mRNA and coding protein was upregulated by circ_0075804, but E2F3 had no impact on circ_0075804 (Zhao et al., 2020). The silencing of circ_0075804 can lead to downregulated E2F3 and then inhibit its proliferation, promote apoptosis of RB cells, and slow down RB progression (Zhao et al., 2020).

Lyu et al. (2019) found that there was a correlation between the parental genes of dysregulated circRNAs in RB samples and the function of chromatin modification, which is an important part of the pathogenesis of RB. A potential regulatory axis of has_circ_0093996-miR-183-PDCD4 is predicted to play a role in RB pathogenesis (Lyu et al., 2019).

Ocular Melanoma

Malignant melanoma, a type of highly invasive tumor made up of melanocytes, often occurs in sun-exposed skin. Ocular melanoma occurs most commonly in the uvea, and uveal melanoma (UM) usually leads to unfavorable clinical outcomes and early metastasis (Shields, 2010; Krantz et al., 2017). Conjunctival melanoma (CM) is much rarer but also has a high degree of malignancy (Shields, 2000, 2010). The mortality rate following the initial diagnosis of UM is ~30% at 5 years, but only 8% of people with UM survived 2 years with tumor metastasis (Shields, 2010; Krantz et al., 2017). The rate of survival for CM is ~7% at 5 years (Shields, 2000). Due to the limitations in the treatment of these malignant tumors, there is an urgent need for a greater understanding of the role of circular molecules in melanoma especially in UM and CM.

In a study on CM, researchers screened out circMTUS1 (has_circ_0083444) from the highly expressed circRNAs in CM tissues compared with those of adjacent normal tissues (Shang et al., 2019). The host gene MTUS1 of circMTUS1 has been recognized as an antioncogene in multiple types of cancer, such as lung cancer (Gu et al., 2017b). In addition, it was found that circMTUS1 knockdown inhibited melanoma cell proliferation *in vitro* and suppressed tumor growth and the final weight of xenograft tumors in the mouse model (Shang et al., 2019). Furthermore, the bioinformatic analyses suggested that circMTUS1 may participate in CM progression through the ErbB, mitogen-activated protein kinase (MAPK), and Wnt signaling pathways and by targeting miR-1208 and miR-622 (Shang et al., 2019). The miR-622 is a proven tumor suppressor in cutaneous melanoma (Dietrich et al., 2018).

Yang et al. (2018) investigated dysregulated circRNA profiles in UM. Of studied circRNAs, upregulated circ_0128533 was predicted to work as a tumor promoter and protect UM cells from apoptosis by binding miR-145 whose overexpression could produce reverse effects (Li et al., 2014). Future studies should verify the function of these promising circRNAs.

In recent years, more and more circRNAs have been revealed to be involved in special characteristics of cancer, including resistance to cell death, limitless replication, sustained angiogenesis, tissue invasion, and metastasis (Su et al., 2019). Here, except for normal sponging miRNAs, circRNAs such as circ_0075804 can also perform oncogenesis regulation in cells by interacting with RBPs (Zhao et al., 2020). Listed studies reveal a novel scale of the role of circRNAs in ocular malignancy pathogenesis. Circ_0001649 and circ_0075804 may serve as diagnostic biomarkers, prognostic indicators for RB in the clinical works in the future as well as circMTUS1 for CM. These promising findings suggest that new treatment targeting these functional circRNAs may cure or suppress the formation of tumors in the eyes.

CONCLUSION

In summary, through greater recognition of circular RNAs and powerful high-throughput sequencing combined with bioinformatic tools, more circRNAs are attracting the interest of researchers. CircRNAs play a vital role in regulating different molecules, signaling pathways, pathophysiological activities, and diseases. Herein, we depict the current landscape of the properties, biogenesis, and functions of circRNAs based on our understanding, and we introduce up-to-date advancements of circRNA studies in the scope of ocular diseases to help us focus on this rising star in research. The main finding is that dysregulation of specific circRNAs can act as potential biomarkers and make promising candidates for therapeutic intervention. However, except for circRNAs listed in **Table 1**, there are still many unknown circRNAs that can affect the development of eyes and the pathogenesis of ocular diseases (more than diseases that we discussed in this review), so more researches are urgently needed.

AUTHOR CONTRIBUTIONS

CZ and YY collected the information and drafted and revised the manuscript. JH contributed to collecting information and editing the manuscript. YY directed the work and finalized the manuscript. All authors read and approved the final manuscript.

REFERENCES

Abdelmohsen, K., Panda, A. C., Munk, R., Grammatikakis, I., Dudekula, D. B., De, S., et al. (2017). Identification of HuR target circular RNAs uncovers suppression of PABPN1 translation by CircPABPN1. *RNA Biol.* 14, 361–369. doi: 10.1080/15476286.2017.1279788

Ajith, T. A., and Ranimenon. (2015). Homocysteine in ocular diseases. *Clin. Chim. Acta* 450, 316–321. doi: 10.1016/j.cca.2015.09.007

Andley, U. (2009). Effects of α-crystallin on lens cell function and cataract pathology. *Curr. Mol. Med.* 9, 887–892. doi: 10.2174/156652409789105598

Armulik, A., Abramsson, A., and Betsholtz, C. (2005). Endothelial/pericyte interactions. *Circ. Res.* 97, 512–523. doi: 10.1161/01.RES.0000182903.16652.d7

Ashwal-Fluss, R., Meyer, M., Pamudurti, N. R., Ivanov, A., Bartok, O., Hanan, M., et al. (2014). circRNA biogenesis competes with Pre-mRNA splicing. *Mol. Cell* 56, 55–66. doi: 10.1016/j.molcel.2014.08.019

Aufiero, S., Reckman, Y. J., Pinto, Y. M., and Creemers, E. E. (2019). Circular RNAs open a new chapter in cardiovascular biology. *Nat. Rev. Cardiol.* 16, 503–514. doi: 10.1038/s41569-019-0185-2

Bachmann, B., Taylor, R. S., and Cursiefen, C. (2010). Corneal Neovascularization as a risk factor for graft failure and rejection after keratoplasty: an evidence-based meta-analysis. *Ophthalmology* 117, 1300–1305.e7. doi: 10.1016/j.ophtha.2010.01.039

Baek, D., Villén, J., Shin, C., Camargo, F. D., Gygi, S. P., and Bartel, D. P. (2008). The impact of microRNAs on protein output. *Nature* 455, 64–71. doi: 10.1038/nature07242

Barrett, S. P., Wang, P. L., and Salzman, J. (2015). Circular RNA biogenesis can proceed through an exon-containing lariat precursor. *eLife* 4:e07540. doi: 10.7554/eLife.07540

Bloch, S. B., Larsen, M., and Munch, I. C. (2012). Incidence of legal blindness from age-related macular degeneration in denmark: year 2000 to 2010. *Am. J. Ophthalmol.* 153, 209–213.e2. doi: 10.1016/j.ajo.2011.10.016

Cao, M., Zhang, L., Wang, J.-H., Zeng, H., Peng, Y., Zou, J., et al. (2019). Identifying circRNA-associated-ceRNA networks in retinal neovascularization in mice. *Int. J. Med. Sci.* 16, 1356–1365. doi: 10.7150/ijms.35149

Capel, B., Swain, A., Nicolis, S., Hacker, A., Walter, M., Koopman, P., et al. (1993). Circular transcripts of the testis-determining gene Sry in adult mouse testis. *Cell* 73, 1019–1030. doi: 10.1016/0092-8674(93)90279-Y

Casey, R., and Li, W. W. (1997). Factors controlling ocular angiogenesis. *Am. J. Ophthalmol.* 124, 521–529. doi: 10.1016/S0002-9394(14)70868-2

Chang, J. H., Gabison, E. E., Kato, T., and Azar, D. T. (2001). Corneal neovascularization. *Curr. Opin. Ophthalmol.* 12, 242–249. doi: 10.1097/00055735-200108000-00002

Chan-Ling, T., Gole, G. A., Quinn, G. E., Adamson, S. J., and Darlow, B. A. (2018). Pathophysiology, screening and treatment of ROP: a multi-disciplinary perspective. *Prog. Retin. Eye Res.* 62, 77–119. doi: 10.1016/j.preteyeres.2017.09.002

Charteris, D. G., Sethi, C. S., Lewis, G. P., and Fisher, S. K. (2002). Proliferative vitreoretinopathy—developments in adjunctive treatment and retinal pathology. *Eye* 16, 369–374. doi: 10.1038/sj.eye.6700194

Chen, C., and Sarnow, P. (1995). Initiation of protein synthesis by the eukaryotic translational apparatus on circular RNAs. *Science* 268, 415–417. doi: 10.1126/science.7536344

Chen, J., and Smith, L. E. H. (2007). Retinopathy of prematurity. *Angiogenesis* 10, 133–140. doi: 10.1007/s10456-007-9066-0

Chen, L.-L., and Yang, L. (2015). Regulation of circRNA biogenesis. *RNA Biol.* 12, 381–388. doi: 10.1080/15476286.2015.1020271

Chen, N., Zhao, G., Yan, X., Lv, Z., Yin, H., Zhang, S., et al. (2018). A novel FLI1 exonic circular RNA promotes metastasis in breast cancer by coordinately regulating TET1 and DNMT1. *Genome Biol.* 19:218. doi: 10.1186/s13059-018-1594-y

Chen, X., Jiang, C., Sun, R., Yang, D., and Liu, Q. (2020). Circular Noncoding RNA NR3C1 Acts as a miR-382-5p Sponge to Protect RPE Functions via Regulating PTEN/AKT/mTOR Signaling Pathway. *Mol. Ther.* 28, 929–945. doi: 10.1016/j.ymthe.2020.01.010

Chen, X.-J., Zhang, Z.-C., Wang, X.-Y., Zhao, H.-Q., Li, M.-L., Ma, Y., et al. (2020). The Circular RNome of developmental retina in mice. *Mol. Ther. Nucleic Acids* 19, 339–349. doi: 10.1016/j.omtn.2019.11.016

Cocquerelle, C., Mascrez, B., Hétuin, D., and Bailleul, B. (1993). Mis-splicing yields circular RNA molecules. *FASEB J.* 7, 155–160. doi: 10.1096/fasebj.7.1.7678559

Conn, S. J., Pillman, K. A., Toubia, J., Conn, V. M., Salmanidis, M., Phillips, C. A., et al. (2015). The RNA binding protein quaking regulates formation of circRNAs. *Cell* 160, 1125–1134. doi: 10.1016/j.cell.2015.02.014

Conn, V. M., Hugouvieux, V., Nayak, A., Conos, S. A., Capovilla, G., Cildir, G., et al. (2017). A circRNA from SEPALLATA3 regulates splicing of its cognate mRNA through R-loop formation. *Nat. Plants* 3:17053. doi: 10.1038/nplants.2017.53

Cost, N. G., and Czyzyk-Krzeska, M. F. (2015). Regulation of autophagy by two products of one gene: TRPM3 and miR-204. *Mol. Cell. Oncol.* 2:e1002712. doi: 10.1080/23723556.2014.1002712

Dietrich, P., Kuphal, S., Spruss, T., Hellerbrand, C., and Bosserhoff, A. K. (2018). MicroRNA-622 is a novel mediator of tumorigenicity in melanoma by targeting Kirsten rat sarcoma. *Pigment Cell Melanoma Res.* 31, 614–629. doi: 10.1111/pcmr.12698

Dimaras, H., Kimani, K., Dimba, E. A., Gronsdahl, P., White, A., Chan, H. S., et al. (2012). Retinoblastoma. *Lancet* 379, 1436–1446. doi: 10.1016/S0140-6736(11)61137-9

Dong, R., Zhang, X.-O., Zhang, Y., Ma, X.-K., Chen, L.-L., and Yang, L. (2016). CircRNA-derived pseudogenes. *Cell Res.* 26, 747–750. doi: 10.1038/cr.2016.42

Du, W. W., Fang, L., Yang, W., Wu, N., Awan, F. M., Yang, Z., et al. (2017a). Induction of tumor apoptosis through a circular RNA enhancing Foxo3 activity. *Cell Death Differ.* 24, 357–370. doi: 10.1038/cdd.2016.133

Du, W. W., Yang, W., Chen, Y., Wu, Z.-K., Foster, F. S., Yang, Z., et al. (2017b). Foxo3 circular RNA promotes cardiac senescence by modulating multiple factors associated with stress and senescence responses. *Eur. Heart J.* 38, 1402–1412. doi: 10.1093/eurheartj/ehw001

Du, W. W., Yang, W., Liu, E., Yang, Z., Dhaliwal, P., and Yang, B. B. (2016). Foxo3 circular RNA retards cell cycle progression via forming ternary complexes with p21 and CDK2. *Nucleic Acids Res.* 44, 2846–2858. doi: 10.1093/nar/gkw027

Du, W. W., Zhang, C., Yang, W., Yong, T., Awan, F. M., and Yang, B. B. (2017c). Identifying and characterizing circRNA-Protein interaction. *Theranostics* 7, 4183–4191. doi: 10.7150/thno.21299

Duh, E. J., Sun, J. K., and Stitt, A. W. (2017). Diabetic retinopathy: current understanding, mechanisms, and treatment strategies. *JCI Insight* 2:e93751. doi: 10.1172/jci.insight.93751

Esteller, M. (2011). Non-coding RNAs in human disease. *Nat. Rev. Genet.* 12, 861–874. doi: 10.1038/nrg3074

Fan, C., Liu, X., Li, W., Wang, H., Teng, Y., Ren, J., et al. (2019). Circular RNA circ KMT2E is up-regulated in diabetic cataract lenses and is associated with miR-204-5p sponge function. *Gene* 710, 170–177. doi: 10.1016/j.gene.2019.05.054

George, A. K., Master, K., Majumder, A., Homme, R. P., Laha, A., Sandhu, H. S., et al. (2019). Circular RNAs constitute an inherent gene regulatory axis in the mammalian eye and brain 1. *Can. J. Physiol. Pharmacol.* 97, 463–472. doi: 10.1139/cjpp-2018-0505

Gu, Y., Ke, G., Wang, L., Zhou, E., Zhu, K., and Wei, Y. (2017a). Altered Expression Profile of Circular RNAs in the serum of patients with diabetic retinopathy revealed by microarray. *Ophthalmic Res.* 58, 176–184. doi: 10.1159/000479156

Gu, Y., Liu, S., Zhang, X., Chen, G., Liang, H., Yu, M., et al. (2017b). Oncogenic miR-19a and miR-19b co-regulate tumor suppressor MTUS1 to promote cell proliferation and migration in lung cancer. *Protein Cell* 8, 455–466. doi: 10.1007/s13238-017-0393-7

Guillot, N., Kollins, D., Gilbert, V., Xavier, S., Chen, J., Gentle, M., et al. (2012). BAMBI regulates angiogenesis and endothelial homeostasis through modulation of alternative TGFβ Signaling. *PLoS One* 7:e39406. doi: 10.1371/journal.pone.0039406

Guo, J. U., Agarwal, V., Guo, H., and Bartel, D. P. (2014). Expanded identification and characterization of mammalian circular RNAs. *Genome Biol.* 15:409. doi: 10.1186/s13059-014-0409-z

Guo, N., Liu, X., Pant, O. P., Zhou, D.-D., Hao, J., and Lu, C. (2019). Circular RNAs: novel promising biomarkers in ocular diseases. *Int. J. Med. Sci.* 16, 513–518. doi: 10.7150/ijms.29750

Hacıoğlu, D., and Erdöl, H. (2017). Developments and current approaches in the treatment of pterygium. *Int. Ophthalmol.* 37, 1073–1081. doi: 10.1007/s10792-016-0358-5

Hammes, H.-P., Lin, J., Renner, O., Shani, M., Lundqvist, A., Betsholtz, C., et al. (2002). Pericytes and the pathogenesis of diabetic retinopathy. *Diabetes* 51, 3107–3112. doi: 10.2337/diabetes.51.10.3107

Han, B., Chao, J., and Yao, H. (2018). Circular RNA and its mechanisms in disease: from the bench to the clinic. *Pharmacol. Ther.* 187, 31–44. doi: 10.1016/j.pharmthera.2018.01.010

Hansen, T. B., Jensen, T. I., Clausen, B. H., Bramsen, J. B., Finsen, B., Damgaard, C. K., et al. (2013a). Natural RNA circles function as efficient microRNA sponges. *Nature* 495, 384–388. doi: 10.1038/nature11993

Hansen, T. B., Kjems, J., and Damgaard, C. K. (2013b). Circular RNA and miR-7 in Cancer. *Cancer Res.* 73, 5609–5612. doi: 10.1158/0008-5472.CAN-13-1568

Hansen, T. B., Wiklund, E. D., Bramsen, J. B., Villadsen, S. B., Statham, A. L., Clark, S. J., et al. (2011). miRNA-dependent gene silencing involving Ago2-mediated cleavage of a circular antisense RNA: miRNA mediated cleavage of circular antisense RNA. *EMBO J.* 30, 4414–4422. doi: 10.1038/emboj.2011.359

Harding, J. J., Egerton, M., van Heyningen, R., and Harding, R. S. (1993). Diabetes, glaucoma, sex, and cataract: analysis of combined data from two case control studies. *Br. J. Ophthalmol.* 77, 2–6.

He, M., Wang, W., Yu, H., Wang, D., Cao, D., Zeng, Y., et al. (2020). Comparison of expression profiling of circular RNAs in vitreous humour between diabetic retinopathy and non-diabetes mellitus patients. *Acta Diabetol.* 57, 479–489. doi: 10.1007/s00592-019-01448-w

Huang, C., Liang, D., Tatomer, D. C., and Wilusz, J. E. (2018). A length-dependent evolutionarily conserved pathway controls nuclear export of circular RNAs. *Genes Dev.* 32, 639–644. doi: 10.1101/gad.314856.118

Ivanov, A., Memczak, S., Wyler, E., Torti, F., Porath, H. T., Orejuela, M. R., et al. (2015). Analysis of Intron sequences reveals hallmarks of circular RNA biogenesis in animals. *Cell Rep.* 10, 170–177. doi: 10.1016/j.celrep.2014.12.019

Jeck, W. R., Sorrentino, J. A., Wang, K., Slevin, M. K., Burd, C. E., Liu, J., et al. (2013). Circular RNAs are abundant, conserved, and associated with ALU repeats. *RNA* 19, 141–157. doi: 10.1261/rna.035667.112

Jiang, C., Qin, B., Liu, G., Sun, X., Shi, H., Ding, S., et al. (2016). MicroRNA-184 promotes differentiation of the retinal pigment epithelium by targeting the AKT2/mTOR signaling pathway. *Oncotarget* 7, 52340–52353. doi: 10.18632/oncotarget.10566

Jiang, Q., Liu, C., Li, C., Xu, S., Yao, M., Ge, H., et al. (2020). Circular RNA-ZNF532 regulates diabetes-induced retinal pericyte degeneration and vascular dysfunction. *J. Clin. Invest.* 130, 3833–3847. doi: 10.1172/JCI123353

Kim, J. W., Kang, K. H., Burrola, P., Mak, T. W., and Lemke, G. (2008). Retinal degeneration triggered by inactivation of PTEN in the retinal pigment epithelium. *Genes Dev.* 22, 3147–3157. doi: 10.1101/gad.1700108

Kingman, S. (2004). Glaucoma is second leading cause of blindness globally. *Bull. World Health Organ.* 82, 887–888.

Knudson, A. G. (1971). Mutation and cancer: statistical study of retinoblastoma. *Proc. Natl. Acad. Sci. U.S.A.* 68, 820–823. doi: 10.1073/pnas.68.4.820

Kramer, M. C., Liang, D., Tatomer, D. C., Gold, B., March, Z. M., Cherry, S., et al. (2015). Combinatorial control of Drosophilai circular RNA expression by intronic repeats, hnRNPs, and SR proteins. *Genes Dev.* 29, 2168–2182. doi: 10.1101/gad.270421.115

Krantz, B. A., Dave, N., Komatsubara, K. M., Marr, B. P., and Carvajal, R. D. (2017). Uveal melanoma: epidemiology, etiology, and treatment of primary disease. *Clin. Ophthalmol.* 11, 279–289. doi: 10.2147/OPTH.S89591

Kumar, L., Shamsuzzama, Haque, R., Baghel, T., and Nazir, A. (2017). Circular RNAs: the emerging class of non-coding RNAs and their potential role in human neurodegenerative diseases. *Mol. Neurobiol.* 54, 7224–7234. doi: 10.1007/s12035-016-0213-8

Lasda, E., and Parker, R. (2014). Circular RNAs: diversity of form and function. *RNA* 20, 1829–1842. doi: 10.1261/rna.047126.114

Lee, E. J., Kim, N., Kang, K. H., and Kim, J. W. (2011). Phosphorylation/inactivation of PTEN by Akt-independent PI3K signaling in retinal pigment epithelium. *Biochem. Biophys. Res. Commun.* 414, 384–389. doi: 10.1016/j.bbrc.2011.09.083

Legnini, I., Di Timoteo, G., Rossi, F., Morlando, M., Briganti, F., Sthandier, O., et al. (2017). Circ-ZNF609 is a circular RNA that can be translated and functions in myogenesis. *Mol. Cell* 66, 22–37.e9. doi: 10.1016/j.molcel.2017.02.017

Li, X., Liu, C.-X., Xue, W., Zhang, Y., Jiang, S., Yin, Q.-F., et al. (2017). Coordinated circRNA biogenesis and function with NF90/NF110 in viral infection. *Mol. Cell* 67, 214–227.e7. doi: 10.1016/j.molcel.2017.05.023

Li, X., Yang, L., and Chen, L.-L. (2018). The biogenesis, functions, and challenges of circular RNAs. *Mol. Cell* 71, 428–442. doi: 10.1016/j.molcel.2018.06.034

Li, X.-M., Ge, H.-M., Yao, J., Zhou, Y.-F., Yao, M.-D., Liu, C., et al. (2018). Genome-wide identification of circular RNAs as a novel class of putative biomarkers for an ocular surface disease. *Cell. Physiol. Biochem.* 47, 1630–1642. doi: 10.1159/000490982

Li, Y., Huang, Q., Shi, X., Jin, X., Shen, L., Xu, X., et al. (2014). MicroRNA 145 may play an important role in uveal melanoma cell growth by potentially targeting insulin receptor substrate-1. *Chin. Med. J.* 127, 1410–1416.

Li, Y., Zheng, Q., Bao, C., Li, S., Guo, W., Zhao, J., et al. (2015). Circular RNA is enriched and stable in exosomes: a promising biomarker for cancer diagnosis. *Cell Res.* 25, 981–984. doi: 10.1038/cr.2015.82

Li, Z., Huang, C., Bao, C., Chen, L., Lin, M., Wang, X., et al. (2015). Exon-intron circular RNAs regulate transcription in the nucleus. *Nat. Struct. Mol. Biol.* 22, 256–264. doi: 10.1038/nsmb.2959

Liang, D., Tatomer, D. C., Luo, Z., Wu, H., Yang, L., Chen, L.-L., et al. (2017). The output of protein-coding genes shifts to circular RNAs When the Pre-mRNA processing machinery is limiting. *Mol. Cell* 68, 940–954.e3. doi: 10.1016/j.molcel.2017.10.034

Liang, D., and Wilusz, J. E. (2014). Short intronic repeat sequences facilitate circular RNA production. *Genes Dev.* 28, 2233–2247. doi: 10.1101/gad.251926.114

Lim, L. S., Mitchell, P., Seddon, J. M., Holz, F. G., and Wong, T. Y. (2012). Age-related macular degeneration. *Lancet* 379, 1728–1738. doi: 10.1016/S0140-6736(12)60282-7

Liu, C., Ge, H.-M., Liu, B.-H., Dong, R., Shan, K., Chen, X., et al. (2019). Targeting pericyte–endothelial cell crosstalk by circular RNA-cPWWP2A inhibition aggravates diabetes-induced microvascular dysfunction. *Proc. Natl. Acad. Sci. U.S.A.* 116, 7455–7464. doi: 10.1073/pnas.1814874116

Liu, C., Yao, M.-D., Li, C.-P., Shan, K., Yang, H., Wang, J.-J., et al. (2017). Silencing Of Circular RNA-ZNF609 ameliorates vascular endothelial dysfunction. *Theranostics* 7, 2863–2877. doi: 10.7150/thno.19353

Liu, J., Liu, T., Wang, X., and He, A. (2017). Circles reshaping the RNA world: from waste to treasure. *Mol. Cancer* 16:58. doi: 10.1186/s12943-017-0630-y

Liu, T., Liu, Y., Xie, L., He, X., and Bai, J. (2013). Progress in the Pathogenesis of Pterygium. *Curr. Eye Res.* 38, 1191–1197. doi: 10.3109/02713683.2013.823212

Liu, X., Liu, B., Zhou, M., Fan, F., Yu, M., Gao, C., et al. (2018). Circular RNA HIPK3 regulates human lens epithelial cells proliferation and apoptosis by targeting the miR-193a/CRYAA axis. *Biochem. Biophys. Res. Commun.* 503, 2277–2285. doi: 10.1016/j.bbrc.2018.06.149

Liu, X., Zhang, L., Wang, J.-H., Zeng, H., Zou, J., Tan, W., et al. (2020). Investigation of circRNA expression profiles and analysis of circRNA-miRNA-mRNA networks in an animal (Mouse) model of age-related macular degeneration. *Curr. Eye Res.* 45, 1173–1180. doi: 10.1080/02713683.2020.1722179

Liu, Y.-C., Wilkins, M., Kim, T., Malyugin, B., and Mehta, J. S. (2017). Cataracts. *Lancet* 390, 600–612. doi: 10.1016/S0140-6736(17)30544-5

Lyu, J., Wang, Y., Zheng, Q., Hua, P., Zhu, X., Li, J., et al. (2019). Reduction of circular RNA expression associated with human retinoblastoma. *Exp. Eye Res.* 184, 278–285. doi: 10.1016/j.exer.2019.03.017

Memczak, S., Jens, M., Elefsinioti, A., Torti, F., Krueger, J., Rybak, A., et al. (2013). Circular RNAs are a large class of animal RNAs with regulatory potency. *Nature* 495, 333–338. doi: 10.1038/nature11928

Michael, R., and Bron, A. J. (2011). The ageing lens and cataract: a model of normal and pathological ageing. *Philos. Trans. R. Soc. Lond. B. Biol. Sci.* 366, 1278–1292. doi: 10.1098/rstb.2010.0300

Nishino, J., Yamashita, K., Hashiguchi, H., Fujii, H., Shimazaki, T., and Hamada, H. (2004). Meteorin: a secreted protein that regulates glial cell differentiation and promotes axonal extension. *EMBO J.* 23, 1998–2008. doi: 10.1038/sj.emboj.7600202

Pamudurti, N. R., Bartok, O., Jens, M., Ashwal-Fluss, R., Stottmeister, C., Ruhe, L., et al. (2017). Translation of CircRNAs. *Mol. Cell* 66, 9–21.e7. doi: 10.1016/j.molcel.2017.02.021

Pastor, J. C., Rojas, J., Pastor-Idoate, S., Di Lauro, S., Gonzalez-Buendia, L., and Delgado-Tirado, S. (2016). Proliferative vitreoretinopathy: a new concept of disease pathogenesis and practical consequences. *Prog. Retin. Eye Res.* 51, 125–155. doi: 10.1016/j.preteyeres.2015.07.005

Patop, I. L., Wüst, S., and Kadener, S. (2019). Past, present, and future of circRNAs. *EMBO J.* 38:e100836. doi: 10.15252/embj.2018100836

Pollreisz, A., and Schmidt-Erfurth, U. (2010). Diabetic Cataract—Pathogenesis, Epidemiology and Treatment. *J. Ophthalmol.* 2010:608751. doi: 10.1155/2010/608751

Potenza, M., Gagliardi, S., Nacci, C., Carratu, M., and Montagnani, M. (2009). Endothelial dysfunction in diabetes: from mechanisms to therapeutic targets. *Curr. Med. Chem.* 16, 94–112. doi: 10.2174/092986709787002853

Rao, G. N., Khanna, R., and Payal, A. (2011). The global burden of cataract. *Curr. Opin. Ophthalmol.* 22, 4–9. doi: 10.1097/ICU.0b013e3283414fc8

Reis, A. H. O., Vargas, F. R., and Lemos, B. (2012). More epigenetic hits than meets the eye: microRNAs and genes associated with the tumorigenesis of retinoblastoma. *Front. Genet.* 3:284. doi: 10.3389/fgene.2012.00284

Rybak-Wolf, A., Stottmeister, C., Glažar, P., Jens, M., Pino, N., Giusti, S., et al. (2015). Circular RNAs in the mammalian brain are highly abundant. Conserved, and Dynamically Expressed. *Mol. Cell* 58, 870–885. doi: 10.1016/j.molcel.2015.03.027

Salzman, J., Chen, R. E., Olsen, M. N., Wang, P. L., and Brown, P. O. (2013). Cell-type specific features of circular RNA expression. *PLoS Genet.* 9:e1003777. doi: 10.1371/journal.pgen.1003777

Salzman, J., Gawad, C., Wang, P. L., Lacayo, N., and Brown, P. O. (2012). Circular RNAs are the predominant transcript isoform from hundreds of human genes in diverse cell types. *PLoS One* 7:e30733. doi: 10.1371/journal.pone.0030733

Sanger, H. L., Klotz, G., Riesner, D., Gross, H. J., and Kleinschmidt, A. K. (1976). Viroids are single-stranded covalently closed circular RNA molecules existing as highly base-paired rod-like structures. *Proc. Natl. Acad. Sci. U.S.A.* 73, 3852–3856. doi: 10.1073/pnas.73.11.3852

Schalkwijk, C. G., and Stehouwer, C. D. A. (2005). Vascular complications in diabetes mellitus: the role of endothelial dysfunction. *Clin. Sci.* 109, 143–159. doi: 10.1042/CS20050025

Scott, A., and Fruttiger, M. (2010). Oxygen-induced retinopathy: a model for vascular pathology in the retina. *Eye* 24, 416–421. doi: 10.1038/eye.2009.306

Shan, K., Liu, C., Liu, B.-H., Chen, X., Dong, R., Liu, X., et al. (2017). Circular noncoding RNA HIPK3 mediates retinal vascular dysfunction in diabetes mellitus. *Circulation* 136, 1629–1642. doi: 10.1161/CIRCULATIONAHA.117.029004

Shang, Q., Li, Y., Wang, H., Ge, S., and Jia, R. (2019). Altered expression profile of circular RNAs in conjunctival melanoma. *Epigenomics* 11, 787–804. doi: 10.2217/epi-2019-0029

Shi, X., Wang, B., Feng, X., Xu, Y., Lu, K., and Sun, M. (2020). circRNAs and exosomes: a mysterious frontier for human cancer. *Mol. Ther. Nucleic Acids* 19, 384–392. doi: 10.1016/j.omtn.2019.11.023

Shields, C. L. (2000). Conjunctival melanomarisk factors for recurrence, exenteration, metastasis, and death in 150 consecutive patients. *Arch. Ophthalmol.* 118, 1497–1507. doi: 10.1001/archopht.118.11.1497

Shields, C. L. (2010). Ocular melanoma: relatively rare but requiring respect. *Yearb. Ophthalmol.* 2010:221. doi: 10.1016/S0084-392X(10)79224-8

Singh, M., George, A. K., Homme, R. P., Majumder, A., Laha, A., Sandhu, H. S., et al. (2018). Circular RNAs profiling in the cystathionine-β-synthase mutant mouse reveals novel gene targets for hyperhomocysteinemia induced ocular disorders. *Exp. Eye Res.* 174, 80–92. doi: 10.1016/j.exer.2018.05.026

Singh, M., George, A. K., Homme, R. P., Majumder, A., Laha, A., Sandhu, H. S., et al. (2019). Expression analysis of the circular RNA molecules in the human retinal cells treated with homocysteine. *Curr. Eye Res.* 44, 287–293. doi: 10.1080/02713683.2018.1542005

Starke, S., Jost, I., Rossbach, O., Schneider, T., Schreiner, S., Hung, L.-H., et al. (2015). Exon circularization requires canonical splice signals. *Cell Rep.* 10, 103–111. doi: 10.1016/j.celrep.2014.12.002

Strauss, O. (2005). The retinal pigment epithelium in visual function. *Physiol. Rev.* 85, 845–881. doi: 10.1152/physrev.00021.2004

Su, M., Xiao, Y., Ma, J., Tang, Y., Tian, B., Hang, Y., et al. (2019). Circular RNAs in Cancer: emerging functions in hallmarks, stemness, resistance and roles as potential biomarkers. *Mol. Cancer* 18:90. doi: 10.1186/s12943-019-1002-6

Sun, L.-F., Zhang, B., Chen, X.-J., Wang, X.-Y., Zhang, B.-W., Ji, Y.-Y., et al. (2019). Circular RNAs in human and vertebrate neural retinas. *RNA Biol.* 16, 821–829. doi: 10.1080/15476286.2019.1591034

Suzuki, H. (2006). Characterization of RNase R-digested cellular RNA source that consists of lariat and circular RNAs from pre-mRNA splicing. *Nucleic Acids Res.* 34:e63. doi: 10.1093/nar/gkl151

Szabo, L., Morey, R., Palpant, N. J., Wang, P. L., Afari, N., Jiang, C., et al. (2015). Statistically based splicing detection reveals neural enrichment and tissue-specific induction of circular RNA during human fetal development. *Genome Biol.* 16:126. doi: 10.1186/s13059-015-0690-5

Venø, M. T., Hansen, T. B., Venø, S. T., Clausen, B. H., Grebing, M., Finsen, B., et al. (2015). Spatio-temporal regulation of circular RNA expression during porcine embryonic brain development. *Genome Biol.* 16:245. doi: 10.1186/s13059-015-0801-3

Wang, J.-J., Liu, C., Shan, K., Liu, B.-H., Li, X.-M., Zhang, S.-J., et al. (2018a). Circular RNA-ZNF609 regulates retinal neurodegeneration by acting as miR-615 sponge. *Theranostics* 8, 3408–3415. doi: 10.7150/thno.25156

Wang, J.-J., Shan, K., Liu, B.-H., Liu, C., Zhou, R.-M., Li, X.-M., et al. (2018b). Targeting circular RNA-ZRANB1 for therapeutic intervention in retinal neurodegeneration. *Cell Death Dis.* 9:540. doi: 10.1038/s41419-018-0597-7

Wang, M., Hou, J., Müller-McNicoll, M., Chen, W., and Schuman, E. M. (2019). Long and repeat-rich intronic sequences favor circular RNA formation under conditions of reduced spliceosome activity. *iScience* 20, 237–247. doi: 10.1016/j.isci.2019.08.058

Wang, P. L., Bao, Y., Yee, M.-C., Barrett, S. P., Hogan, G. J., Olsen, M. N., et al. (2014). Circular RNA is expressed across the eukaryotic tree of life. *PLoS One* 9:e90859. doi: 10.1371/journal.pone.0090859

Wang, Y., and Wang, Z. (2015). Efficient backsplicing produces translatable circular mRNAs. *RNA* 21, 172–179. doi: 10.1261/rna.048272.114

Weinreb, R. N., Aung, T., and Medeiros, F. A. (2014). The pathophysiology and treatment of glaucoma: a review. *JAMA* 311, 1901–1911. doi: 10.1001/jama.2014.3192

Westholm, J. O., Miura, P., Olson, S., Shenker, S., Joseph, B., Sanfilippo, P., et al. (2014). Genome-wide analysis of drosophila circular rnas reveals their structural and sequence properties and age-dependent neural accumulation. *Cell Rep.* 9, 1966–1980. doi: 10.1016/j.celrep.2014.10.062

Wu, P., Zhang, D., Geng, Y., Li, R., and Zhang, Y. (2020). Circular RNA-ZNF609 regulates corneal neovascularization by acting as a sponge of miR-184. *Exp. Eye Res.* 192:107937. doi: 10.1016/j.exer.2020.107937

Xiao-Jie, L., Ai-Mei, G., Li-Juan, J., and Jiang, X. (2015). Pseudogene in cancer: real functions and promising signature. *J. Med. Genet.* 52, 17–24. doi: 10.1136/jmedgenet-2014-102785

Xie, Y., Yuan, X., Zhou, W., Kosiba, A. A., Shi, H., Gu, J., et al. (2020). The circular RNA HIPK3 (circHIPK3) and its regulation in cancer progression: review. *Life Sci.* 254:117252. doi: 10.1016/j.lfs.2019.117252

Xing, L., Zhang, L., Feng, Y., Cui, Z., and Ding, L. (2018). Downregulation of circular RNA hsa_circ_0001649 indicates poor prognosis for retinoblastoma and regulates cell proliferation and apoptosis via AKT/mTOR signaling pathway. *Biomed. Pharmacother.* 105, 326–333. doi: 10.1016/j.biopha.2018.05.141

Xu, Y., Yao, Y., Zhong, X., Leng, K., Qin, W., Qu, L., et al. (2018). Downregulated circular RNA hsa_circ_0001649 regulates proliferation, migration and invasion in cholangiocarcinoma cells. *Biochem. Biophys. Res. Commun.* 496, 455–461. doi: 10.1016/j.bbrc.2018.01.077

Yang, X., Li, Y., Liu, Y., Xu, X., Wang, Y., Yan, Y., et al. (2018). Novel circular RNA expression profile of uveal melanoma revealed by microarray. *Chin. J. Cancer Res.* 30, 656–668. doi: 10.21147/j.issn.1000-9604.2018.06.10

Yang, Y., Fan, X., Mao, M., Song, X., Wu, P., Zhang, Y., et al. (2017). Extensive translation of circular RNAs driven by N6-methyladenosine. *Cell Res.* 27, 626–641. doi: 10.1038/cr.2017.31

Yao, J., Hu, L.-L., Li, X.-M., Shan, K., Zhou, R.-M., Ge, H.-M., et al. (2019). Comprehensive circular RNA profiling of proliferative vitreoretinopathy and its clinical significance. *Biomed. Pharmacother.* 111, 548–554. doi: 10.1016/j.biopha.2018.12.044

Yau, J. W. Y., Rogers, S. L., Kawasaki, R., Lamoureux, E. L., Kowalski, J. W., Bek, T., et al. (2012). Global prevalence and major risk factors of diabetic retinopathy. *Diabetes Care* 35, 556–564. doi: 10.2337/dc11-1909

You, X., Vlatkovic, I., Babic, A., Will, T., Epstein, I., Tushev, G., et al. (2015). Neural circular RNAs are derived from synaptic genes and regulated by development and plasticity. *Nat. Neurosci.* 18, 603–610. doi: 10.1038/nn.3975

Zagami, C. J., Zusso, M., and Stifani, S. (2009). Runx transcription factors: lineage-specific regulators of neuronal precursor cell proliferation and post-mitotic neuron subtype development. *J. Cell. Biochem.* 107, 1063–1072. doi: 10.1002/jcb.22221

Zhang, L., Cheng, R., and Huang, Y. (2017). MiR-30a inhibits BECN1-mediated autophagy in diabetic cataract. *Oncotarget* 8, 77360–77368. doi: 10.18632/oncotarget.20483

Zhang, S.-J., Chen, X., Li, C.-P., Li, X.-M., Liu, C., Liu, B.-H., et al. (2017). Identification and characterization of circular RNAs as a new class of putative biomarkers in diabetes retinopathy. *Investig. Opthalmology Vis. Sci.* 58, 6500–6509. doi: 10.1167/iovs.17-22698

Zhang, X.-O., Wang, H.-B., Zhang, Y., Lu, X., Chen, L.-L., and Yang, L. (2014). Complementary sequence-mediated exon circularization. *Cell* 159, 134–147. doi: 10.1016/j.cell.2014.09.001

Zhang, Y., Zhang, X.-O., Chen, T., Xiang, J.-F., Yin, Q.-F., Xing, Y.-H., et al. (2013). Circular intronic long noncoding RNAs. *Mol. Cell* 51, 792–806. doi: 10.1016/j.molcel.2013.08.017

Zhao, C., Yasumura, D., Li, X., Matthes, M., Lloyd, M., Nielsen, G., et al. (2011). mTOR-mediated dedifferentiation of the retinal pigment epithelium initiates photoreceptor degeneration in mice. *J. Clin. Invest.* 121, 369–383. doi: 10.1172/JCI44303

Zhao, W., Wang, S., Qin, T., and Wang, W. (2020). Circular RNA (circ-0075804) promotes the proliferation of retinoblastoma via combining heterogeneous nuclear ribonucleoprotein K (HNRNPK) to improve the stability of E2F transcription factor 3 E2F3. *J. Cell. Biochem.* 121, 3516–3525. doi: 10.1002/jcb.29631

Zhou, H., Song, H., Wu, Y., Liu, X., Li, J., Zhao, H., et al. (2019). Oxygen-induced circRNA profiles and coregulatory networks in a retinopathy of prematurity mouse model. *Exp. Ther. Med.* 18, 2037–2050. doi: 10.3892/etm.2019.7819

Zhou, R., Shi, L., Shan, K., Sun, Y., Wang, S., Zhang, S., et al. (2020). Circular RNA-ZBTB44 regulates the development of choroidal neovascularization. *Theranostics* 10, 3293–3307. doi: 10.7150/thno.39488

Zhou, Y.-F., Shi, L.-J., Yao, J., Sun, Y.-N., Shan, K., Jiang, Q., et al. (2019). Microarray analysis of circRNA expression pattern in corneal neovascularization. *Cornea* 38, 1443–1449. doi: 10.1097/ICO.0000000000002089

Zhu, K., Hu, X., Chen, H., Li, F., Yin, N., Liu, A. L., et al. (2019). Downregulation of circRNA DMNT3B contributes to diabetic retinal vascular dysfunction through targeting miR-20b-5p and BAMBI. *EBioMedicine* 49, 341–353. doi: 10.1016/j.ebiom.2019.10.004

17

Whole-Exome Sequencing in a Cohort of High Myopia Patients in Northwest China

Yang Liu[1†], Jin-Jin Zhang[2†], Shun-Yu Piao[3], Ren-Juan Shen[4], Ya Ma[4], Zhong-Qi Xue[5], Wen Zhang[3], Juan Liu[1], Zi-Bing Jin[4*] and Wen-Juan Zhuang[3*]*

[1] School of Basic Medical Sciences, Third Clinical Medical College of Ningxia Medical University (People's Hospital of Ningxia Hui Autonomous Region), Yinchuan, China, [2] Clinical Medical College, Ningxia Medical University, Yinchuan, China, [3] Ningxia Eye Hospital, People's Hospital of Ningxia Hui Autonomous Region, Third Clinical Medical College of Ningxia Medical University, Yinchuan, China, [4] Beijing Institute of Ophthalmology, Beijing Tongren Eye Center, Beijing Tongren Hospital, Capital Medical University, Beijing Ophthalmology and Visual Science Key Laboratory, Beijing, China, [5] Department of Ophthalmology, Affiliated Hospital of Qingdao Binhai University, Qingdao, China

***Correspondence:**
Juan Liu
ryuken0518@163.com
Zi-Bing Jin
jinzibing@foxmail.com
Wen-Juan Zhuang
zh_wenj@163.com*

† These authors have contributed equally to this work

High myopia (HM) is one of the leading causes of visual impairment worldwide. In order to expand the myopia gene spectrum in the Chinese population, we investigated genetic mutations in a cohort of 27 families with HM from Northwest China by using whole-exome sequencing (WES). Genetic variations were filtered using bioinformatics tools and cosegregation analysis. A total of 201 candidate mutations were detected, and 139 were cosegregated with the disease in the families. Multistep analysis revealed four missense variants in four unrelated families, including c.904C>T (p.R302C) in *CSMD1*, c.860G>A (p.R287H) in *PARP8*, c.G848A (p.G283D) in *ADAMTSL1*, and c.686A>G (p.H229R) in *FNDC3B*. These mutations were rare or absent in the Exome Aggregation Consortium (ExAC), 1000 Genomes Project, and Genome Aggregation Database (gnomAD), indicating that they are new candidate disease-causing genes. Our findings not only expand the myopia gene spectrum but also provide reference information for further genetic study of heritable HM.

Keywords: high myopia, cohort, mutation, gene, Northwest China

INTRODUCTION

Myopia, also known as shortsightedness, is globally increasing in prevalence. Approximately 108 million people are currently affected, and myopia is expected to become the leading cause of blindness across the globe (Bourne et al., 2013). In East Asian countries, the prevalence of myopia has been reported to be twice as high as in western countries (Pan et al., 2015).

High myopia (HM), which is the extreme form of myopia, is diagnosed in cases with refractive error worse than or equal to −6 diopters (D) and/or ocular axial length (AL) > 26.00 mm (Percival, 1987; Young et al., 2007). Recently meta-analyses have estimated that the prevalence of myopia will rise to 49.8% in 2050 and that the prevalence of HM will increase to 9.8% (Holden et al., 2016). The complications associated with HM, such as cataract, glaucoma, retinal detachment, chorioretinal degeneration, and choroidal neovascularization, may lead to severe visual impairment and blindness (Morgan et al., 2012; Tham et al., 2018).

Both environmental and genetic factors are known to contribute to HM (Morgan et al., 2012).

Familial aggregation and twin studies have demonstrated that genetic factors play critical roles in the development of HM (Katz et al., 1997; Hammond et al., 2001). To date, 25 loci (MYP1–MYP3, MYP5–MYP26) associated with HM have been discovered *via* genome-wide association studies (GWAS), family-based linkage analyses, and whole-exome sequencing (WES) and documented in the Online Mendelian Inheritance in Man (OMIM) (Zhang, 2015; Fan et al., 2016; Cai et al., 2019a). However, only a limited number of causative genes have been identified (Cai et al., 2019a). WES has identified several genes responsible for HM, including two X-linked genes, *OPN1LW* (Li et al., 2015) and *ARR3* (Xiao et al., 2016); six autosomal dominant genes, *ZNF644* (Shi et al., 2011a), *SCO2* (Tran-Viet et al., 2013), *SLC39A5* (Guo et al., 2014), *P4HA2* (Guo et al., 2015), *BSG* (Jin et al., 2017), and *CCDC111* (Zhao et al., 2013); and three autosomal recessive genes, *LEPREL1* (Mordechai et al., 2011), *LRPAP1* (Aldahmesh et al., 2013), and *CTSH* (Jiang et al., 2015). Nevertheless, these genes explain the pathogenesis of HM in a limited number of patients (Kloss et al., 2017). Therefore, numerous HM-related genes surely remain to be discovered. In this study, we identified candidate mutations and genes in 27 non-syndromic families with HM from Northwest China.

MATERIALS AND METHODS

Patient Subjects

Twenty-seven families with HM were recruited in this study. The study was performed in accordance with the tenets of the Declaration of Helsinki. Written informed consent was obtained from the participants or their statutory guardians, with approval from the institutional review board of the People's Hospital of Ningxia Hui Autonomous Region, Third Clinical Medical College of Ningxia Medical University. Refractive error and AL of the patients in each family were concisely recorded in **Table 1**, a collection of the upper and lower limits of clinical data of all patients in each of the 27 families. The pedigree and clinical information of the 27 families were integrated in **Supplementary Figure 1**. Genomic DNAs were extracted from peripheral blood samples.

All 27 families included in this study were from Ningxia Hui Autonomous Region.

Patients were recruited according to the following inclusion criteria: (1) refractive error worse than or equal to −6 D and/or AL >26.00 mm; and (2) no other known ocular diseases or systemic disorders.

Whole-Exome Sequencing

Whole-exome sequencing was performed as previously described with the Exome Enrichment V5 Kit (Agilent Technologies, United States) (Jin et al., 2018; Cai et al., 2019b; Zhou et al., 2020). DNA fragments were sequenced on Illumina HiSeq 2000 Analyzers (90 cycles per read). The Illumina libraries were prepared and generated using a sequencing platform (Hiseq2000; Illumina, Inc.), according to the manufacturer's instructions. Local realignments, quality control text, and variant calling were assembled using the Genome Analysis Toolkit (GATK). All sequencing reads were mapped against a human reference genome (hg19/GRCH37) with BWA-MEM software as described (Kumar et al., 2009). WES yielded a mean read depth of ~30×. Median coverage of the targeted regions was >95%.

Variant Filtering

We focused on rare variants in ocular diseases and HM; the ocular disease genes were assembled from the databases: genes associated with the myopia phenotype term (HP:0000545) in Human Phenotype Ontology (HPO[1]) or ocular disease genes from RetNet database[2] and OMIM[3]. The complete list of genes associated with myopia and ocular disease was shown in **Supplementary Table 1**.

The WES results from patients with HM were filtered as follows: (1) variants outside of the exonic splicing site predicted by the Berkeley Drosophila Genome Project[4] were excluded; (2) synonymous variants were excluded without altering splice-site regions; (3) variants with minor allele frequencies (MAFs)

[1] http://human-phenotype-ontology.github.io
[2] http://www.sph.uth.tmc.edu/retnet/
[3] https://www.omim.org/
[4] http://www.fruitfly.org/

TABLE 1 | Clinical data from 27 families with high myopia.

Family	Proband age	Affected individuals	SE range	SE median	AL range	AL median
85	57	2	−19.50/−23.75	−20.25	29.61/31.72	30.85
89	19	1	−9.75/−10.11	−9.93	27.80/27.90	27.85
90	19	1	−7.75/−8.25	−8.01	28.17/28.35	28.26
91	19	2	−8.50/−16.50	−11.88	27.52/28.67	27.81
92	23	1	−7.75/−8.75	−8.25	26.85/26.87	26.86
93	21	2	−10.00/−11.75	−10.81	24.75/27.22	25.85
94	22	2	−8.00/−9.25	−8.50	27.01/27.53	27.32
95	21	1	−6.75/−7.25	−7.00	26.45/26.75	26.60
96	18	1	−6.75/−7.00	−6.86	26.65/26.71	26.68
97	23	2	−6.25/−14.00	−11.25	26.58/29.86	28.03
99	19	1	−8.75/−9.00	−8.88	27.97/28.18	28.08
100	22	2	−6.00/−7.00	−6.50	24.98/26.27	25.60
101	20	1	−8.50/−8.75	−8.63	27.32/27.37	27.35
102	17	1	−7.50/−7.50	−7.50	27.46/27.50	27.48
103	18	1	−8.00/−8.75	−8.38	26.96/27.28	27.12
104	15	2	−5.75/−10.50	−6.71	26.12/26.91	26.28
105	33	1	−8.25/−9.25	−8.75	27.43/27.63	27.53
106	27	2	−5.50/−11.50	−8.56	26.05/27.33	26.62
107	20	3	−6.50/−13.00	−9.63	25.10/27.33	25.85
109	19	1	−7.25/−8.25	−7.75	27.14/27.75	27.45
110	24	1	−7.75/−9.25	−8.50	26.51/26.79	26.65
111	18	1	−6.00/−6.00	−6.00	26.65/26.76	26.71
112	23	1	−10.00/−10.50	−10.25	27.35/27.36	27.36
113	21	2	−12.75/−14.50	−9.31	26.64/26.91	26.42
114	18	1	−7.75/−9.00	−8.38	26.85/27.16	27.01
115	22	2	−6.00/−9.75	−8.28	26.60/28.55	27.62
116	20	1	−10.00/−10.50	−10.25	27.96/28.17	28.07

SE, refractive error; AL, axial length.

greater than or equal to 0.01 in any of the three public population databases [Exome Aggregation Consortium (ExAC), 1000 Genomes Project (1000G), and Genome Aggregation Database (gnomAD)] were excluded; (4) variants that were not heterozygous in all AD families were excluded, as the variants that were not homozygous in all AR families. Meanwhile, *de novo* variants were also excluded, and these *de novo* variants were displayed in **Supplementary Table 2**. After these filtering steps, cosegregation analysis was performed for all family members. Finally, variant scores corresponding to the quality of biological and statistical evidence were assigned. Strong candidates were validated by Sanger sequencing (**Figure 1**).

All identified variants were assessed with the following tools and databases. The pathogenicity of gene mutations was predicted with 10 bioinformatics tools:

SIFT (Adzhubei et al., 2010)[5], PolyPhen-2-HDIV, PolyPhen-2-HVAR (Schwarz et al., 2010)[6], Mutation Taster (Desmet et al., 2009)[7], LRT, Mutation Assessor, FATHMM, Radial SVM, LR, and DANN. Splicing mutations were analyzed with Human Splicing Finder software (Huang et al., 2015)[8]. Mutations with a MAF were evaluated with the ExAC[9], 1000G (Bahcall, 2015) (1000G[10]), and gnomAD[11]. The RaptorX structure prediction web server[12] was used to simulate the wild-type and mutant protein three-dimensional (3D) models. Changes in protein folding and crystal structure were visualized with PyMol software (version 1.5).

RESULTS

Strong Candidate Genetic Causes Yielded by Computational Assessments and Cosegregation Analysis

A total of 201 potential variants were identified in 27 families: 139 were well cosegregated with the disease in 15 families. Sixty-two variants not cosegregated were excluded (**Figure 2**). Each variant was reported at a frequency of less than 1 in 100 alleles in the ExAC, 1000G, and gnomAD. For the 139 genes that cosegregated, none of the variants were identified in unaffected family members (refractive error less than 2.00 D). Fifty-eight of the 139 variants were novel changes that were unreported in public databases (**Supplementary Table 3**). Eighty-one of the 139 variants were rare changes (less than 1 in 1,000 alleles in any population) (**Supplementary Table 4**). Among 139 variants, 59 had been presented in 10 pathogenicity prediction tools with biological relevance (**Supplementary Figure 2**).

The 20 variants with the highest scores are shown (**Figure 3**). Four missense variants in the *CSMD1*, *PARP8*, *ADAMTSL1*, and *FNDC3B* genes in four unrelated families achieved the highest scores, including c.904C>T (p.R302C) in *CSMD1*, c.860G>A (p.R287H) in *PARP8*, c.G848A (p.G283D) in *ADAMTSL1*, and c.686A>G (p.H229R) in *FNDC3B*. These variants were well cosegregated with the disease. Further analysis was performed according to the guidelines of the American College of Medical Genetics and Genomics (Bahcall, 2015). After these multistep systematic analyses, these genetic variants were estimated as potentially pathogenic and were rare or absent from the ExAC, 1000G, and gnomAD. The scores of DANN in *CSMD1*, *PARP8*, *ADAMTSL1*, and *FNDC3B* were 0.999, 0.915, 0.998, and 0.98, respectively.

Candidate Genes Identified

The p.R302C substitution (c.904C>T) in *CSMD1* was detected in a 22-year-old man and his father (**Figure 4A**). The individual and his father had refractive error less than −8.50 D in both eyes, with AL >27 mm, without oculopathy or systemic diseases. Interestingly, proband and their affected family member both had HM before school age according to their self-report. Electroretinogram (ERG) and optical coherence tomography (OCT) examinations revealed the normal retinal appearance of proband and his father (**Figure 5** and **Supplementary Figure 3**), as did his mother in family 94 (**Supplementary Figure 4**). This mutation was predicted to be pathogenic by eight pathogenicity prediction tools (SIFT, Polyphen-2, Mutation Taster, Mutation Assessor, FATHMM, RadialSVM, LR, and DANN) and listed as novel in the ExAC, 1000G, and gnomAD. The substitution p.R302C occurred at a highly conserved region in multiple orthologous sequence alignments, which demonstrates that the associated protein plays an important role (**Figure 6A**), and this site may have an important effect on protein function. Three-dimensional modeling demonstrated the absence of a bond between the mutated cysteine at residue 302 and the arginine at residue 301 (**Figure 7A**).

A heterozygous mutation in *PARP8* was detected in a 25-year-old woman and her mother (**Figure 4B**), both of whom had extreme myopia, with average spherical equivalent refractive error greater than −20 D and AL >29 mm. This mutation was also detected in the proband's younger brother, who had AL of 25.06 mm in the right eye and 25.14 mm in the left eye. But there were no other symptoms of oculopathy or systemic diseases. The c.860G>A mutation is a rare single-nucleotide polymorphism (SNP) (rs142224685) located in exon 11. The pathogenicity of the p.R287H mutation in *PARP8* (c.860G>A) was verified by SIFT, Mutation Taster, and PolyPhen-2. Furthermore, the p.R287H variant was detected as an SNP with a MAF of 0.0014 in ExAC. This amino acid mutation is evolutionarily conserved among species (**Figure 6B**). Three-dimensional protein modeling demonstrated the absence of a bond between mutated residue 287 and residues 285 and 291 (**Figure 7B**).

The c.848G>A, p.G283D variant in *ADAMTSL1* was identified in a 21-year-old female (**Figure 4C**), whose spherical equivalent refractive error was −15.25 D in the right eye, with an AL of 26.64 mm and −13.50 D in the left eye with AL 26.91 mm. This mutation in *ADAMTSL1* was a novel conservative mutation (**Figure 6C**) that was predicted to be disease-causing by SIFT, Polphen-2, and Mutation Taster. Three-dimensional structural

---

[5] http://sift.jcvi.org/

[6] http://genetics.bwh.harvard.edu/pph2/index.shtml

[7] http://www.mutationtaster.org/

[8] http://www.umd.be/HSF/

[9] http://ExAC.broadinstitute.org/

[10] ftp://1000genomes.ebi.ac.uk/vol1/ftp

[11] https://gnomad.broadinstitute.org/

[12] http://raptorx.uchicago.edu/

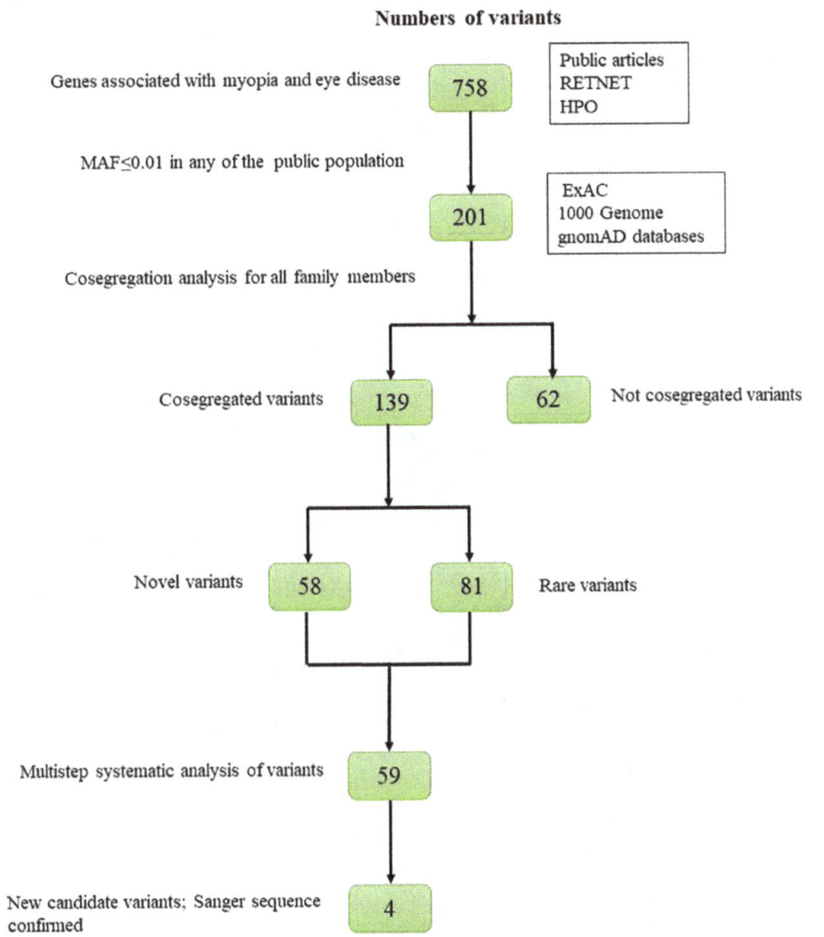

FIGURE 1 | Overview of the variant filtering strategy.

modeling revealed a newly formed bond between residue 283 and residues 282 and 284 (**Figure 7C**), and this mutation is absent in the ExAC, 1000G, and gnomAD, indicating its disease causality.

A heterozygous mutation (c.686A>G; p.H229R) in *FNDC3B* was found in a proband from Family 104 and her mother (**Figure 4D**). The proband, a 15-year-old female, presented with concomitant severe anisometropia. Her spherical equivalent refractive error was −6.25 D in the right eye and −10.50 D in the left eye. According to the results of the corneal topography, the thickness of the thinnest point is 504 μm, and ^{K}m is 56.2 D for her left eye (**Supplementary Figure 5**). The p.H229R mutation in *FNDC3B* (c.686A>G) was predicted to be pathogenic by six *in silico* tools (SIFT, Polphen-2, Mutation Taster, LRT, Mutation Assessor, and DANN). The mutation was in a region extremely conserved across eight homologous species (**Figure 6D**), in line with the changes of 3D protein folding (**Figure 7D**).

Mutations in Known Genes Responsible for High Myopia

The screening of 11 known HM genes revealed four variants to be highly pathogenic, including c.518A>T (p.D173V) in *SCO2*, c.3266A>G (p.Y1089C) in *ZNF644*, c.758C>A (p. A253E) in *SLC39A5* (Family 89), and c.577G>A (p. D193N) in *SLC39A5* (Family 95). Notably, Families 89 and 95 exhibited an AR mode of inheritance. We detected the same mutation in the mother of the proband from Family 89 and the father of the proband from Family 95. The c.758C>A mutation in *SLC39A5*, which was predicted to be deleterious by eight of the 10 computational tools, was absent from the 1000G, ExAC, and gnomAD East Asian databases. The c.577G>A mutation in *SLC39A5*, which was predicted to be deleterious by Polyphen2_HDIV and MutationTaster, was extremely rare in healthy populations. The 1000G and ExAC databases listed MAF as 0.001 and 0.00007462 and MAF in gnomAD is 0.00008761, well below the Popmax Filtering AF 0.0001781 in the East Asian population.

SCO2, located at MYP6, was identified as an AD gene. The c.518A>T (p.D173V) mutation in *SCO2* was detected in Family 111, with a recessive mode of inheritance.

This variant was listed as novel in 1000G and gnomAD, associated with (MAF) 0.0000269 in the ExAC database. The SIFT and FATHMM predicted that this mutation would be deleterious. The MAF of c.3266A>G (p.Y1089C) in *ZNF644*, identified in the proband and his father of Family 115, was 0.001in 1000G,

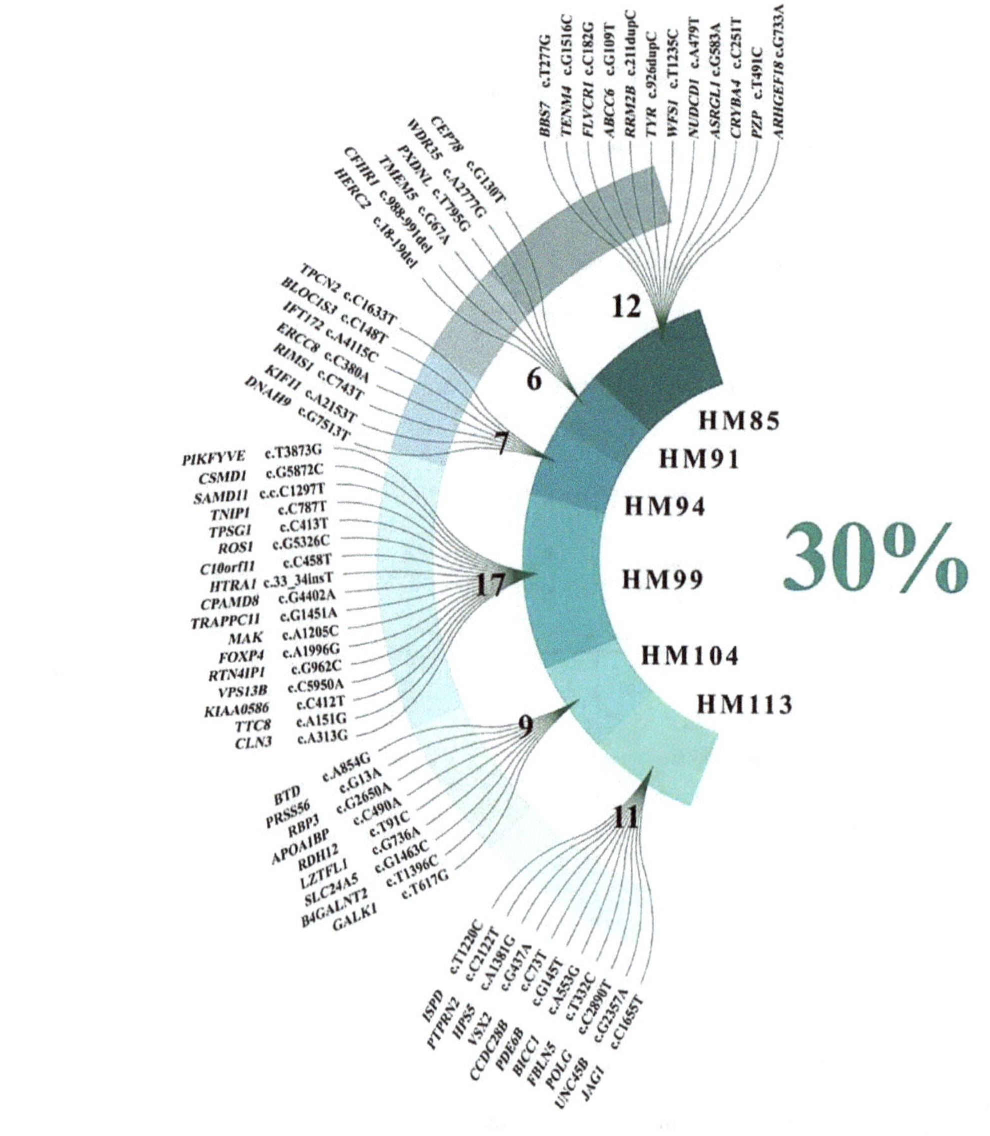

FIGURE 2 | Sixty-two variants related to high myopia and ocular disease that were not cosegregated with high myopia.

0.0003 in the ExAC, and 0.002456 in gnomAD. This mutation was predicted to be deleterious by five of 10 computational tools.

DISCUSSION

Up to now, only a few genes responsible for non-syndromic myopia have been discovered. In our previous study of large-scale screening of eight causative genes in 731 patients with HM, we merely identified mutations in 6.16% cases (Cai et al., 2019c). In this study, we identified four new candidate genes associated with HM. All mutations in these genes affect the function of the coding region according to the 3D structure model, and *CSMD1*, *ADAMTSL1*, and *FNDC3B* were absent in three examined databases (ExAC, 1000G, gnomAD). SIFT, PolyPhen-2-HDIV, PolyPhen-2-HVAR, Mutation Taster, LRT, Mutation Assessor, FATHMM, RadialSVM, and LR were employed to assess the mutation changes in protein function and mutation changes in protein spatial conformation, which further cause harmful changes in physiological functions (Mahfuz and Khan, 2020).

CSMD1, located on MYP10 and mapped to chromosome 8p23.2, was highly expressed in the central nervous system and epithelial tissues. Furthermore, Wan et al. (2018) found that the *CSMD1* gene is expressed at extremely high levels in peripheral retina and the area surrounding the macula. It seems that *CSMD1* plays a critical role in the growth of cones, including signal transduction and matrix adhesion (Kraus et al., 2006). The *de novo* mutations of *CSMD1* have been reported in a Chinese family with early-onset high myopia (EOHM) (Jin et al., 2017). We hypothesize *CSMD1* is also a candidate gene for HM in addition to neurological effects. In our study, a heterozygous missense mutation (c.904C>T) in

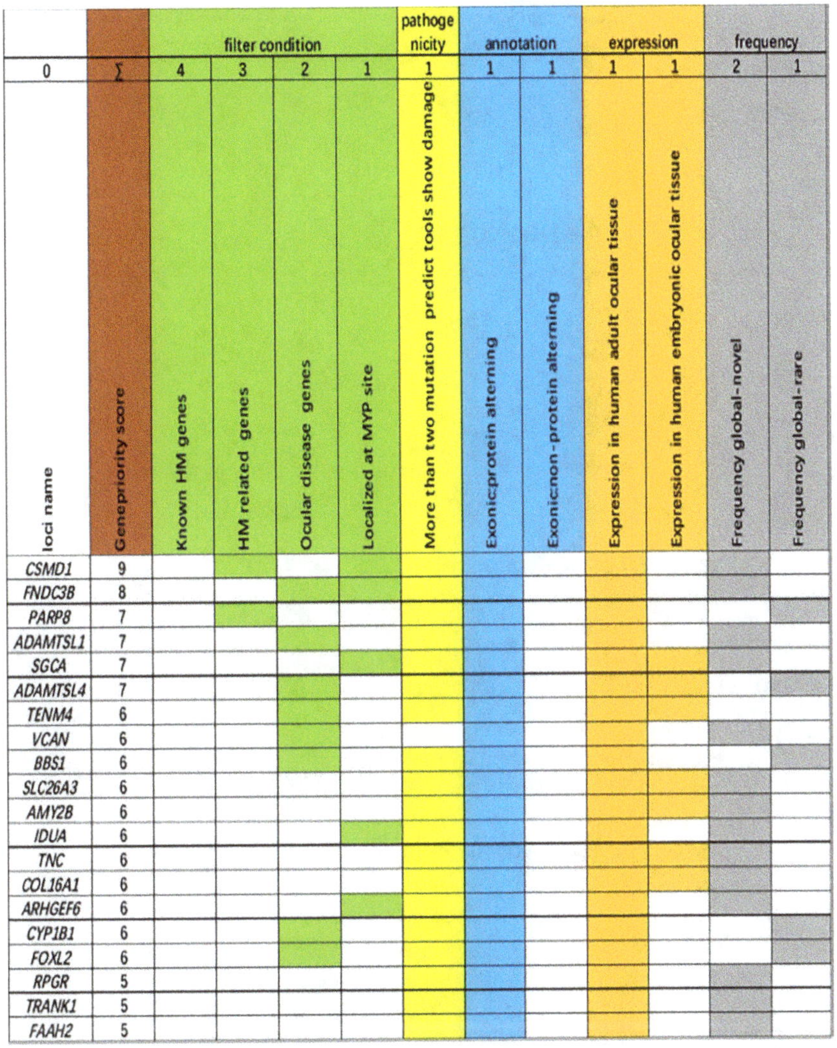

FIGURE 3 | Genes ranked according to biological and statistical evidence. Genes were ranked based on 11 categories that can be divided into five categories: filter condition [green: genes are related to known high myopia (HM) genes, HM-related genes, ocular disease genes, or localized at the MYP site], pathogenicity (light yellow: more than two mutation predict tools show damage), annotation (light blue: genetic variant harboring an exonic protein altering variant or non-protein-altering variant), expression (dark yellow: expression in adult human ocular tissue, expression in human embryonic ocular tissue), and frequency [light dark: frequency global in Exome Aggregation Consortium (ExAC) database, novel; frequency global in ExAC database, rare].

CSMD1 was found in two patients of Family 94, which shows the characteristics of dominant inheritance and is consistent with family cosegregation. However, there were no significant retina changes from the OCT and ERG results of the proband and his father. Further molecular mechanism study about how *CSMD1* plays a role in the development of HM is needed. Meanwhile, our results provide more genetic evidence for the hypothesis that *CSMD1* is the causative gene for HM.

PARP8 is a critical regulator of eukaryotic physiology, localized to the nuclear envelope, and resulted in cell morphology defects that showed potential functions for *PARPs* in the assembly or maintenance of membranous organelles (Vyas et al., 2013). As reported, *PARP* is the major risk factor associated with age-related cataract in central India (Ughade et al., 1998). Fan et al. (2012) first investigated the SNPs rs282544, rs2404958, rs32396, rs12055210, and rs11954386 on *PARP8*, which is closely related to the AL with p-values $< 1 \times 10^{-5}$.

Dongyan (2019) subsequently identified SNPs in *PARP8* gene including rs1195438, rs2404958, rs282544, and rs32396, which are significantly associated with HM in the Han southwest Chinese population. In this study, we also found a rare SNP (rs142224685) as a heterozygous missense mutation c.860G>A in *PARP8*. The research on the association between SNP on *PARP8* and HM needs to be further explored.

A recent study reported a heterozygous c.124T>C (p. Trp42Arg) mutation in the first thrombospondin type 1 (TSR) motif of *ADAMTSL1*, which is responsible for a complex disorder with features including developmental glaucoma, myopia, and/or retinal defects (Hendee et al., 2017). Moreover, *ADAMTSL1* caused the dislocation of microspherophakic lens

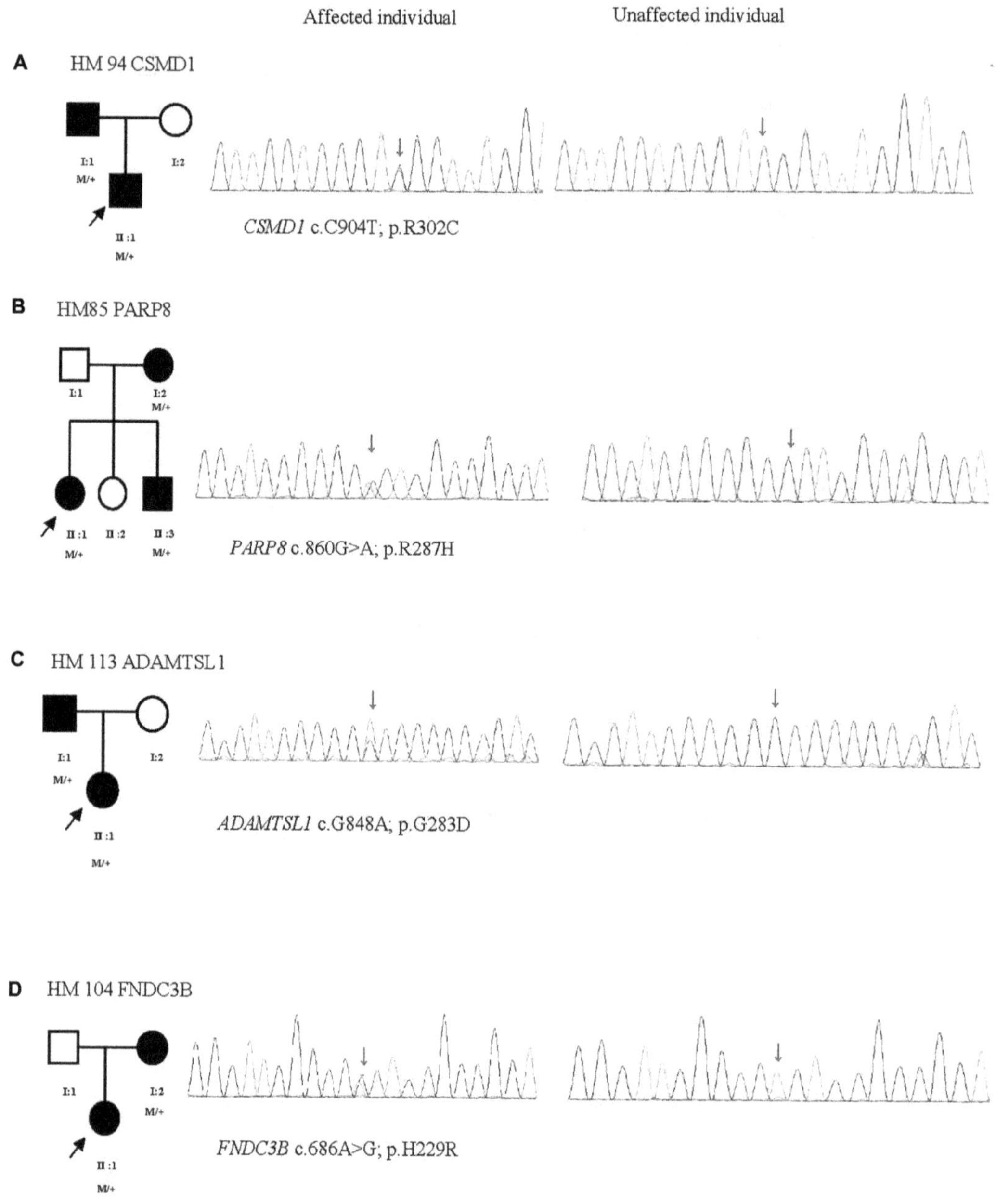

FIGURE 4 | Four potentially pathogenic variants detected in this study. The black arrow represents the patient. +, wild-type; M, mutation. From left to right: pedigree plots of mutations, sequences from affected individual with identified mutation, sequences from unaffected control **(A–D)**.

that causes severe myopia, glaucoma, or cataract. Two modes of inheritance have been reported: autosomal dominant and autosomal recessive (Delhon et al., 2016).

The c.848G>A (p.G283D) variant in *ADAMTSL1*, identified in the proband and her father in Family 113 accompanied by extremely HM, shows a dominant inheritance model. This result is consistent with the previous study in that *ADAMTSL1* accounts for the myopia, especially for severe HM (Hendee et al., 2017).

FNDC3B, located on MYP8, which maps to chromosome 3q26.31, plays an important role in central corneal thickness (CCT), intraocular pressure, and anterior chamber angle depth (Rong et al., 2017). As we know, previous studies mainly focused on the association of *FNDC3B* with glaucoma and keratoconus (Shi et al., 2011b). CCT as one of the most heritable human traits was related to many eye diseases, especially for myopia (Pedersen et al., 2005). CCT reduction related to myopia was also reported (Hao et al., 2015; Rong et al., 2017). In our study, we identified a heterozygous mutation (c.686A>G; p.H229R) in *FNDC3B* from Family 104, and the left eye of the proband with higher refractive error showed typical keratoconus symptoms (−6.25 D/−10.50 D). Based on our findings, we speculate that the clinical phenotype of mutations in *FNDC3B* may be HM for

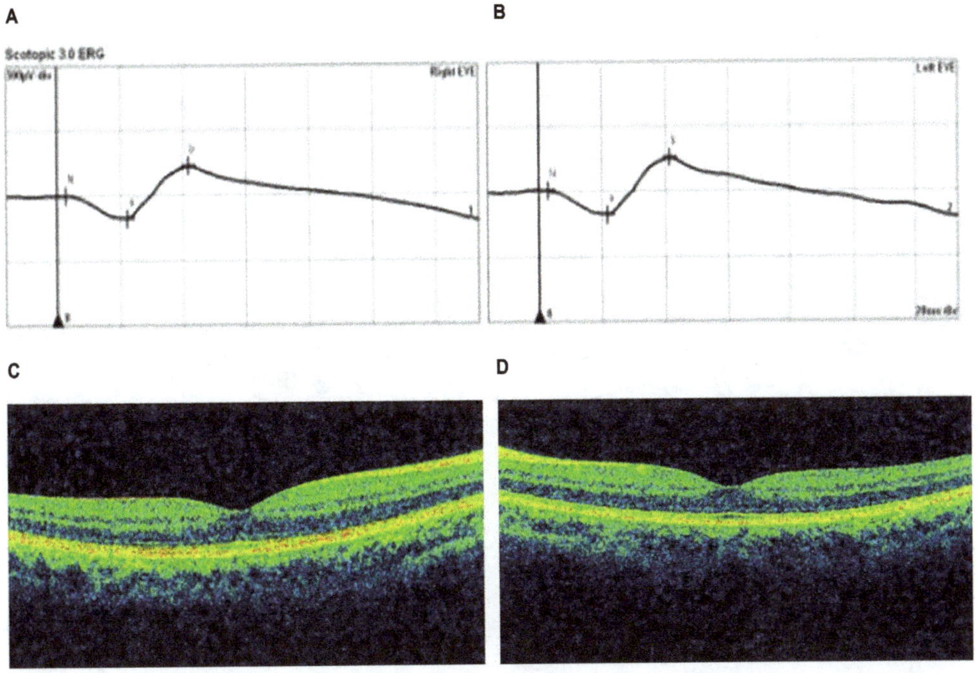

FIGURE 5 | Optical coherence tomography (OCT) and electroretinogram (ERG) results of proband in Family 94. **(A,B)** Standard scotopic response of full-field ERG of the right and left eye showing normal b-wave amplitude. **(C,D)** OCT images of the right and left eye reveal the normal retinal appearance.

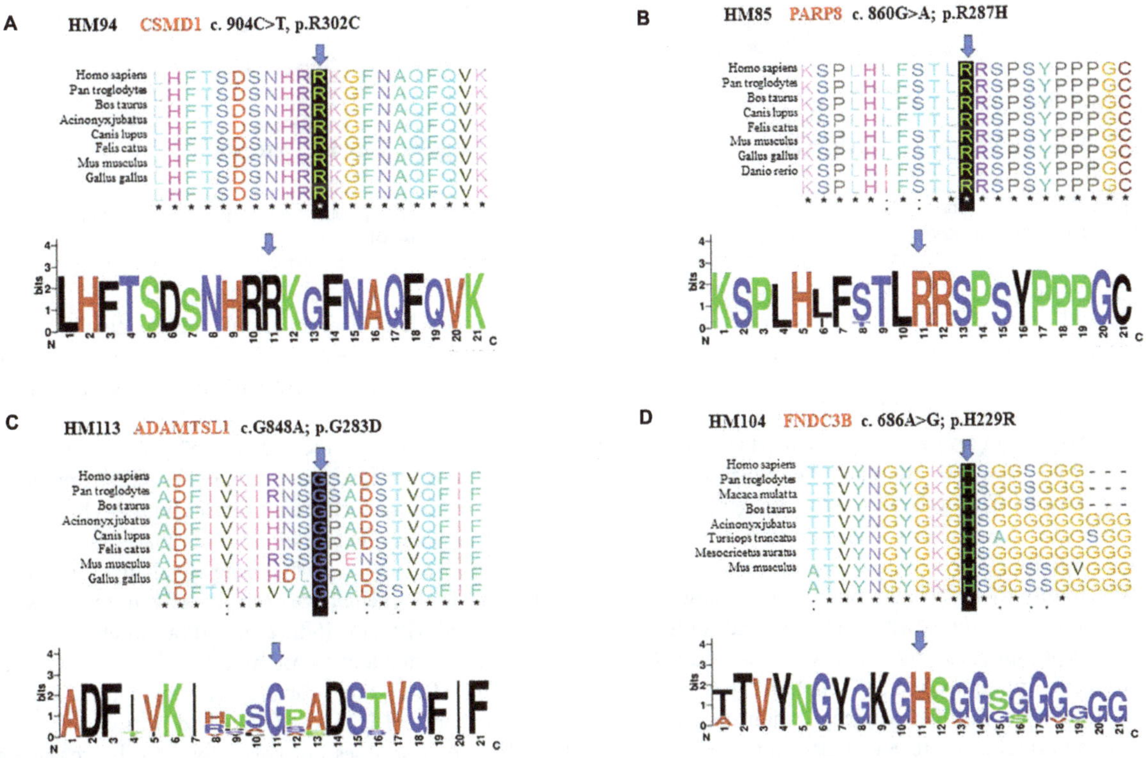

FIGURE 6 | Conservation analysis revealed evolutionary conservation of the mutation. It shows multiple alignments of the amino acids from different species. The arrow indicates the location of the mutation **(A–D)**.

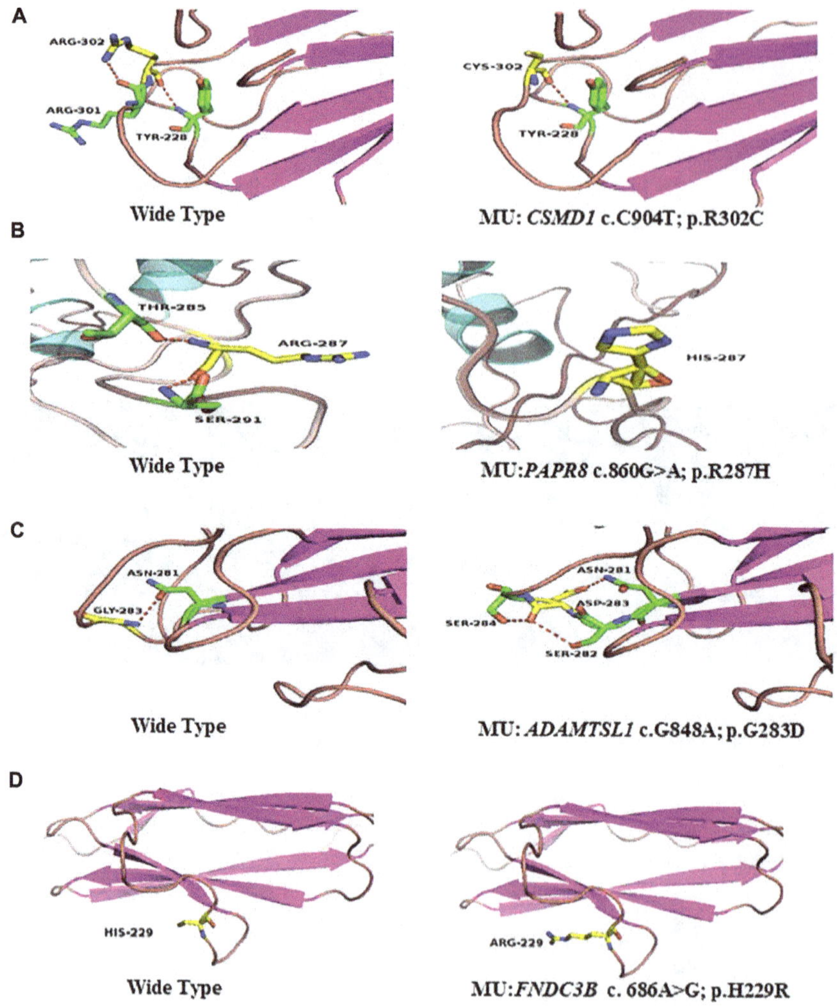

FIGURE 7 | Predicted three-dimensional (3D) structure of proteins. Predicted crystal structures of wild-type (left) and mutant (right) proteins. Yellow shows residue of wild-type and mutant; green represents residues interact with wild-type (left), and mutant residue (right) **(A–D)**.

some people, and it may also be keratoconus for other people, so whether it is an HM candidate disease-causing gene remains to be further evaluated.

The association of known HM genes with HM has been previously investigated in several studies (Jiang et al., 2015; Rong et al., 2017). For this study, we examined the associations within our own HM cohort. The screening of 11 known HM genes revealed four variants in *SCO2*, *ZNF644*, and *SLC39A5* to be highly potentially pathogenic.

SCO2 was found to be related to HM in a large three-generation family in Europe, with nine affected individuals with HM (average spherical refractive error of −22.00 D). Four heterozygous mutations, p.G53*, p.A114H, p.G140L, and p.A259V, in *SCO2* were identified; these mutations may truncate or destabilize the protein structure and lead to retinal neuronal thinning (Tran-Viet et al., 2013). Moreover, R120W, R112W, and A97V were reported in subsequent studies (Jiang et al., 2015; Wakazono et al., 2016).Tran-Viet et al. (2013) observed Sco2 protein localization in the retina, retinal pigment epithelium (RPE), and scleral wall in mouse ocular tissues. We further identified mutations A201P and I221V in *SCO2* in 2019 (Cai et al., 2019c). Here, a new variant c.518A>T (p.D173V) in *SCO2* is detected.

ZNF644, which is located at 1p22.2, can inhibit histone methyltransferase complex through G9a/GLP, functioning as a regulator of histone methyltransferase complex (Bian et al., 2015). *ZNF644* is widely expressed in eye, placenta, and liver and is assumed to play a pivotal role in changes in ocular wall. Mutations in this gene have been reported in previous studies to be associated with HM (Shi et al., 2011a; Jin et al., 2017). In this study, we detected a missense mutation c.3266A>G (p.Y1089C) in *ZNF644* from the proband and his father. Interestingly, while the son had HM, the father had normal vision. It seems that this situation does not correspond to the cosegregation of the clinical phenotype. Further functional studies are needed to elucidate this.

SLC39A5, located at 12q13.3, encodes zinc transporter (Xia et al., 2020). A heterozygous truncation mutation in the *SLC39A5* gene p.Y47* was first reported in 2014 (Guo et al., 2014). Subsequently, the missense mutation p.M304T was detected in the same family; p.G413A (Jiang et al., 2015), p.A84T, p.P87L, p.A319T, and p.A243fs*140 were found to be responsible for HM (Feng et al., 2017; Liu et al., 2020). Other studies have shown that the bone morphogenetic protein (BMP)/transforming growth factor-beta (TGF-β) pathway is related to myopia, and c.141C>G, p.Y47* mutation may cause the loss of function (Jobling et al., 2009; Guo et al., 2014). It has been demonstrated that destruction of BMP/TGF-β pathway may lead to refractive errors (Wu et al., 2018). In the present study, two missense mutations, c.758C>A (p. A253E) and c.577G>A (p.D193N), in *SLC39A5* were detected in two unrelated families. The relationship between these mutations and functions needs to be further studied.

In our study, 62 variants that were highly potentially pathogenic and related to ocular disease or HM were incompatible with cosegregation; they may be used as references for subsequent research. Notably, our technology failed to detect variants in 12 families. On one hand, we set stringent screening criteria, which may have reduced the number of genes for selection. On the other hand, most published articles on HM genetics are focused on families with dominant patterns of inheritance, which means that families with dominant genetic patterns of inheritance may be easier to screen for genes associated with HM. In our study, 18 of 27 families had a recessively inherited clinical phenotype. HM is a very clinically heterogeneous disease, even between patients in the same family. Refractive status and AL are different between patients. This point was also verified in our investigation of the four families in the sibships (Families 85, 99, 100, and 107). In Family 85, the 14-year-old brother of the patient showed the eye AL above 25 mm, and his diopter was less than 3.00 D; with the increase in age, the patient's brother was very likely to develop into HM characterized by excessive AL. The younger brother of the proband in Family 99 is now 13 years old with refractive error −1.75 D in the right eye and −2.25 D in the left eye. On the other hand, the AL of his eyes is about 25 mm. There is also a risk of developing axial HM. Interestingly, the situation of Family 107 is opposite to that of Families 85 and 99. The three sisters are patients, and all showed HM with high diopter and low AL.

Especially the two sisters of the proband showed the diopter was greater than −6.00 D with the AL less than 26 mm. The two patients in Family 100 are of similar age; the older sister is 22 years old and the younger brother is 21 years old. The refractive error and AL of their eyes are relatively similar, in addition to the common genetic factors. The consistency of their living background may also play an important role in the development of their myopia for HM is a disease in which environmental and genetic factors work together. Different life backgrounds, dietary habits, and near-work habits may all contribute to the development of HM.

This study had some limitations. Because environmental and genetic factors determine the manifestation of HM, environmental factors may be an important influencing factor that causes inconsistency between the genotype and the clinical phenotype. This study did not focus on the impact of environmental factors, which may explain our observations of non-cosegregated genes, and we did not carry out functional verification tests. However, analysis of the pathogenicity of gene mutations based on the interpretation standards and guidelines of gene mutations developed by the American College of Medical Genetics and Genomics (ACMG) showed that four new candidate genes met the evidence criteria for possibly pathogenic mutations. The mechanisms underlying the effects of these genetic variants in the context of HM require further elucidation through additional studies. In addition, we have not investigated the impact of copy number variation (Huang et al., 2017) and somatic mosaicism (Jin et al., 2007) in these patients. Finally, targeted exome sequencing including a panel of disease-causing genes, likewise the strategy of inherited retinal dystrophy (Huang et al., 2013, 2015; Xing et al., 2014; Chen et al., 2020), might be more appropriate for future genetic diagnosis of genetic HM.

CONCLUSION

In conclusion, we identified 201 genetic variants related to the development of HM by WES and bioinformatics analysis. To our knowledge, this is the first study of WES in patients with HM from Northwest China. The findings presented four new candidate genes associated with HM, providing additional evidence of heritable HM in Chinese patients. These findings expand the mutation spectrum of myopia genes and provide clues for further genetic study of HM.

ETHICS STATEMENT

The studies involving human participants were reviewed and approved by the Institutional Review Board of People's Hospital of Ningxia Hui Autonomous Region, Third Clinical Medical College of Ningxia Medical University. Written informed consent to participate in this study was provided by the participants' legal guardian/next of kin.

AUTHOR CONTRIBUTIONS

W-JZ, Z-BJ, and JL designed and supervised the whole study. YL, J-JZ, and S-YP performed the experiments. YL, R-JS, YM, Z-QX, and WZ interpreted the results. YL drafted the manuscript. Z-BJ and W-JZ revised the manuscript. All authors contributed to the article and approved the submitted version.

Science Foundation (Z200014 to Z-BJ). This work was supported by the Ningxia Natural Science Foundation (2021AAC03301).

REFERENCES

Adzhubei, I. A., Schmidt, S., Peshkin, L., Ramensky, V. E., Gerasimova, A., Bork, P., et al. (2010). A method and server for predicting damaging missense mutations. *Nat. Methods* 7, 248–249. doi: 10.1038/nmeth0410-248

Aldahmesh, M. A., Khan, A. O., Alkuraya, H., Adly, N., Anazi, S., Al-Saleh, A. A., et al. (2013). Mutations in LRPAP1 are associated with severe myopia in humans. *Am. J. Hum. Genet.* 93, 313–320. doi: 10.1016/j.ajhg.2013.06.002

Bahcall, O. G. (2015). Genetic testing. ACMG guides on the interpretation of sequence variants. *Nat. Rev. Genet.* 16, 256–257.

Bian, C., Chen, Q., and Yu, X. (2015). The zinc finger proteins ZNF644 and WIZ regulate the G9a/GLP complex for gene repression. *Elife* 4:e05606.

Bourne, R. R., Stevens, G. A., White, R. A., Smith, J. L., Flaxman, S. R., and Price, H. (2013). Causes of vision loss worldwide, 1990–2010: a systematic analysis. *Lancet Glob. Health* 1, e339–e349.

Cai, X. B., Shen, S. R., Chen, D. F., Zhang, Q., and Jin, Z. B. (2019a). An overview of myopiagenetics. *Exp. Eye Res.* 188:107778.

Cai, X. B., Wu, K. C., Zhang, X., Lv, J. N., Jin, G. H., Xiang, L., et al. (2019b). Whole-exome sequencing identified ARL2 as a novel candidate genefor MRCS (microcornea, rod-cone dystrophy, cataract, and posterior staphyloma) syndrome. *Clin. Genet.* 96, 61–71.

Cai, X. B., Zheng, Y. H., Chen, D. F., Zhou, F. Y., Xia, L. Q., Wen, X. R., et al. (2019c). Expanding the phenotypic and genotypic landscape of nonsyndromic high myopia: a cross-sectional study in 731 Chinese patients. *Invest. Ophthalmol. Vis. Sci.* 60, 4052–4062.

Chen, Z. J., Lin, K. H., Lee, S. H., Shen, R. J., Feng, Z. K., Wang, X. F., et al. (2020). Mutation spectrum and genotype-phenotype correlation of inherited retinal dystrophy in Taiwan. *Clin. Exp. Ophthalmol.* 48, 486–499. doi: 10.1111/ceo.13708

Delhon, L., Cormier-Daire, V., and Le Goff, C. (2016). Metalloproteinases and their inhibitors in the pathophysiology of heritable connective tissue disorders: current evidence. *Metalloproteinases Med.* 3, 1–9. doi: 10.2147/mnm.s63634

Desmet, F.-O., Hamroun, D., Lalande, M., Collod-Béroud, G., Claustres, M., and Béroud, C. (2009). Human splicing finder: an online bioinformatics tool to predict splicing signals. *Nucleic Acids Res.* 37:e67. doi: 10.1093/nar/gkp215

Dongyan, L. (2019). "Association of PARP8 gene Polymorphisms as genetic risk factors with High Myopia in a Chinese population," in *Proceedings of the 2nd China Conference on Clinical Molecular Diagnosis*, (Chengdu, China).

Fan, Q., Barathi, V. A., Cheng, C. Y., Zhou, X., Meguro, A., Nakata, I., et al. (2012). Genetic variants on chromosome 1q41 influence ocular axial length and high myopia. *PLoS Genet.* 8:e1002753. doi: 10.1371/journal.pgen.1002753

Fan, Q., Guo, X., Tideman, J. W., Williams, K. M., Yazar, S., Hosseini, S. M., et al. (2016). Childhood gene-environment interactions and age-dependent effects ofgenetic variants associated with refractive error and myopia: the CREAM consortium. *Sci. Rep.* 6:25853.

Feng, C. Y., Huang, X. Q., Cheng, X. W., Wu, R. H., Lu, F., and Jin, Z. B. (2017). Mutational screening of SLC39A5, LEPREL1 and LRPAP1 in a cohort of 187 high myopia patients. *Sci. Rep.* 7:1120.

Guo, H., Jin, X., Zhu, T., Wang, T., Tong, P., Tian, L., et al. (2014). SLC39A5 mutations interfering with the BMP/TGF-β pathway in non-syndromic high myopia. *J. Med. Genet.* 51, 518–525. doi: 10.1136/jmedgenet-2014-102351

Guo, H., Tong, P., Liu, Y., Xia, L., Wang, T., Tian, Q., et al. (2015). Mutations of P4HA2 encoding prolyl 4-hydroxylase 2 are associated with nonsyndromic high myopia. *Genet. Med.* 17, 300–306. doi: 10.1038/gim.2015.28

Hammond, C. J., Snieder, H., Gilbert, C. E., and Spector, T. D. (2001). Genes and environment in refractive error: the twin eye study. *Invest. Ophthalmol. Vis. Sci.* 42, 1232–1236.

Hao, X. D., Chen, P., Chen, Z. L., Li, S. X., and Wang, Y. (2015). Evaluating the association between keratoconus and reported genetic loci in a Han Chinese population. *Ophthalmic Genet.* 36, 132–136. doi: 10.3109/13816810.2015.1005317

Hendee, K., Wang, L. W., Reis, L. M., Rice, G. M., Apte, S. S., and Semina, E. V. (2017). Identification and functional analysis of an ADAMTSL1 variant associated with a complex phenotype including congenital glaucoma, craniofacial, and other systemic features in a three-generation human pedigree. *Hum. Mut.* 38, 1485–1490. doi: 10.1002/humu.23299

Holden, B. A., Fricke, T. R., Wilson, D. A., Jong, M., Naidoo, K. S., Sankaridurg, P., et al. (2016). Global prevalence of myopia and high myopia and temporal trendsfrom 2000 through 2050. *Ophthalmology* 123, 1036–1042. doi: 10.1016/j.ophtha.2016.01.006

Huang, X.-F., Huang, F., Wu, K. C., Wu, J., Chen, J., Pang, C. P., et al. (2015). Genotype–phenotype correlation and mutation spectrum in a large cohort of patients with inherited retinal dystrophy revealed by next-generation sequencing. *Genet. Med.* 17, 271–278. doi: 10.1038/gim.2014.138

Huang, X. F., Mao, J. Y., Huang, Z. Q., Rao, F. Q., Cheng, F. F., Li, F. F., et al. (2017). Genome-wide detection of copy number variations in unsolved inherited retinal disease. *Invest. Ophthalmol. Vis. Sci.* 58, 424–429. doi: 10.1167/iovs.16-20705

Huang, X. F., Xiang, P., Chen, J., Xing, D. J., Huang, N., Min, Q., et al. (2013). Targeted exome sequencing identified novel USH2A mutations in Usher syndrome families. *PLoS One* 8:e63832. doi: 10.1371/journal.pone.0063832

Jiang, D., Li, J., Xiao, X., Li, S., Jia, X., Sun, W., et al. (2015). Detection of mutations in LRPAP1, CTSH, LEPREL1, ZNF644, SLC39A5, and SCO2 in 298 families with early-onset high myopia by exome sequencing. *Invest. Ophthalmol. Vis. Sci.* 56, 339–345. doi: 10.1167/iovs.14-14850

Jin, Z. B., Gu, F., Matsuda, H., Yukawa, N., Ma, X., and Nao-i, N. (2007). Somatic and gonadal mosaicism in X-linked retinitis pigmentosa. *Am. J. Med. Genet. A* 143A, 2544–2548. doi: 10.1002/ajmg.a.31984

Jin, Z. B., Li, Z., Liu, Z., Jiang, Y., Cai, X. B., and Wu, J. (2018). Identification of de novo germline mutations and causal genes for sporadic diseases using trio-based whole-exome/genome sequencing. *Biol. Rev.* 93, 1014–1031. doi: 10.1111/brv.12383

Jin, Z.-B., Wu, J., Huang, X. F., Feng, C. Y., Cai, X. B., Mao, J. Y., et al. (2017). Trio-based exome sequencing arrests de novo mutations in early-onset high myopia. *Proc. Natl. Acad. Sci. U.S.A.* 114, 4219–4224. doi: 10.1073/pnas.1615970114

Jobling, A. I., Wan, R., Gentle, A., Bui, B. V., and McBrien, N. A. (2009). Retinal and choroidal TGF-β in the tree shrew model of myopia: isoform expression, activation and effects on function. *Exp. Eye Res.* 88, 458–466.

Katz, J., Tielsch, J. M., and Sommer, A. (1997). Prevalence and risk factors for refractive errors in an adult inner city population. *Invest. Ophthalmol. Vis. Sci.* 38, 334–340.

Kloss, B. A., Tompson, S. W., Whisenhunt, K. N., Quow, K. L., Huang, S. J., Pavelec, D. M., et al. (2017). Exome sequence analysis of 14 families with high myopia. *Invest. Ophthalmol. Vis. Sci.* 58, 1982–1990. doi: 10.1167/iovs.16-20883

Kraus, D. M., Elliott, G. S., Chute, H., Horan, T., Pfenninger, K. H., Sanford, S. D., et al. (2006). CSMD1 is a novel multiple domain complement-regulatory protein highly expressed in the central nervous system and epithelial tissues. *J. Immunol.* 176, 4419–4430. doi: 10.4049/jimmunol.176.7.4419

Kumar, P., Henikoff, S., and Ng, P. C. (2009). Predicting the effects of coding non-synonymous variants on protein function using the SIFT algorithm. *Nat. Protoc.* 4:1073. doi: 10.1038/nprot.2009.86

Li, J., Gao, B., Guan, L., Xiao, X., Zhang, J., Li, S., et al. (2015). Unique variants in OPN1LW cause both syndromic and nonsyndromic X-linked high myopia mapped to MYP1. *Invest. Ophthalmol. Vis. Sci.* 56, 4150–4155. doi: 10.1167/iovs.14-16356

Liu, F., Wang, J., Xing, Y., and Li, T. (2020). Mutation screening of 17 candidate genes in a cohort of 67 probands with early—onset high myopia. *Ophthalmic Physiol. Opt.* 40, 271–280. doi: 10.1111/opo.12683

Mahfuz, A., and Khan, M. A. (2020). Identification of deleterious single nucleotide polymorphism (SNP) s in the human TBX5 gene & prediction of their structural & functional consequences: an in silico approach. *bioRxiv* [Preprint] doi: 10.1101/2020.05.16.099648

Mordechai, S., Gradstein, L., Pasanen, A., Ofir, R., El Amour, K., Levy, J., et al. (2011). High myopia caused by a mutation in LEPREL1, encoding prolyl 3-hydroxylase 2. *Am. J. Hum. Genet.* 89, 438–445. doi: 10.1016/j.ajhg.2011.08.003

Morgan, I. G., Ohno-Matsui, K., and Saw, S.-M. (2012). Myopia. *Lancet* 379, 1739–1748.

Pan, C.-W., Dirani, M., Cheng, C.-Y., Wong, T.-Y., and Saw, S.-M. (2015). The age-specific prevalence of myopia in Asia: a meta-analysis. *Optom. Vis. Sci.* 92, 258–266. doi: 10.1097/opx.0000000000000516

Pedersen, L., Hjortdal, J., and Ehlers, N. (2005). Central corneal thickness in high myopia. *Acta Ophthalmol. Scand.* 83, 539–5425. doi: 10.1111/j.1600-0420.2005.00498.x

Percival, S. (1987). Redefinition of high myopia: the relationship of axial length measurement to myopic pathology and its relevance to cataract surgery. *Dev. Ophthalmol.* 14:42. doi: 10.1159/000414364

Rong, S. S., Ma, S. T. U., Yu, X., Ma, L., Chu, W. K., Chan, T. C. Y., et al. (2017). Genetic associations for keratoconus: a systematic review and meta-analysis. *Sci. Rep.* 7:4620.

Schwarz, J. M., Rödelsperger, C., Schuelke, M., and Seelow, D. (2010). MutationTaster evaluates disease-causing potential of sequence alterations. *Nat. Methods* 7, 575–576. doi: 10.1038/nmeth0810-575

Shi, Y., Li, Y., Zhang, D., Zhang, H., Li, Y., Lu, F., et al. (2011a). Exome sequencing identifies ZNF644 mutations in high myopia. *PLoS Genet.* 7:e1002084. doi: 10.1371/journal.pgen.1002084

Shi, Y., Qu, J., Zhang, D., Zhao, P., Zhang, Q., Tam, P. O. S., et al. (2011b). Genetic variants at 13q12. 12 are associated with high myopia in the Han Chinese population. *Am. J. Hum. Genet.* 88, 805–813.

Tham, Y.-C., Lim, S. H., Shi, Y., Chee, M. L., Zheng, Y. F., Chua, J., et al. (2018). Trends of visual impairment and blindness in the Singapore Chinese population over a decade. *Sci. Rep.* 8:12224.

Tran-Viet, K.-N., Powell, C., Barathi, V. A., Klemm, T., Maurer-Stroh, S., Limviphuvadh, V., et al. (2013). Mutations in SCO2 are associated with autosomal-dominant high-grade myopia. *Am. J. Hum. Genet.* 92, 820–826. doi: 10.1016/j.ajhg.2013.04.005

Ughade, S. N., Zodpey, S. P., and Khanolkar, V. A. (1998). Risk factors for cataract: a case control study. *Indian J. Ophthalmol.* 46, 221–227.

Vyas, S., Chesarone-Cataldo, M., Todorova, T., Huang, Y. H., and Chang, P. (2013). A systematic analysis of the PARPprotein family identifies new functions critical for cell physiology. *Nat. Commun.* 4:2240.

Wakazono, T., Miyake, M., Yamashiro, K., Yoshikawa, M., and Yoshimura, N. (2016). Association between SCO2 mutation and extreme myopia in Japanese patients. *Jpn. J. Ophthalmol.* 60, 319–325. doi: 10.1007/s10384-016-0442-4

Wan, L., Deng, B., Wu, Z., and Chen, X. (2018). Exome sequencing study of 20 patients with high myopia. *PeerJ* 6:e5552. doi: 10.7717/peerj.5552

Wu, H., Jiang, L., Zheng, R., Luo, D., Liu, X., Hao, F., et al. (2018). Genetic association study between the COL11A1 and COL18A1 genes and high myopia in a Han Chinese population. *Genet. Test. Mol. Biomark.* 22, 359–365. doi: 10.1089/gtmb.2017.0235

Xia, Z., Bi, X., Lian, J., Dai, W., He, X., Zhao, L., et al. (2020). Slc39a5-mediated zinc homeostasis plays an essential role in venous angiogenesis in zebrafish. *Open Biol.* 10:200281. doi: 10.1098/rsob.200281

Xiao, X., Li, S., Jia, X., Guo, X., and Zhang, Q. (2016). X-linked heterozygous mutations in ARR3 cause female-limited early onset high myopia. *Mol. Vis.* 22, 1257–1266.

Xing, D. J., Zhang, H. X., Huang, N., Wu, K. C., Huang, X. F., Huang, F., et al. (2014). Comprehensive molecular diagnosis of Bardet-Biedl syndrome by high-throughput targeted exome sequencing. *PLoS One* 9:e90599. doi: 10.1371/journal.pone.0090599

Young, T. L., Metlapally, R., and Shay, A. E. (2007). Complex trait genetics of refractive error. *Arch. Ophthalmol.* 125, 38–48. doi: 10.1001/archopht.125.1.38

Zhang, Q. (2015). Genetics of refraction and myopia. *Prog. Mol. Biol. Transl. Sci.* 134, 269–279. doi: 10.1016/bs.pmbts.2015.05.007

Zhao, F., Wu, J., Xue, A., Su, Y., Wang, X., Lu, X., et al. (2013). Exome sequencing reveals CCDC111 mutation associated with high myopia. *Hum. Genet.* 132, 913–921. doi: 10.1007/s00439-013-1303-6

Zhou, G. H., Ma, Y., Li, M. L., Zhou, X. Y., Mou, H., and Jin, Z. B. (2020). ATP1A3 mutation as a candidate cause of autosomal dominant cone rod dystrophy. *Hum. Genet.* 139, 1391–1401. doi: 10.1007/s00439-020-02182-y

18

Absence of Cytochrome P450-1b1 Increases Susceptibility of Pressure-Induced Axonopathy in the Murine Retinal Projection

*Naseem Amirmokhtari[1,2], Brian D. Foresi[1], Shiv S. Dewan[1], Rachida A. Bouhenni[3] and Matthew A. Smith[1,3]**

[1] Department of Pharmaceutical Sciences, Northeast Ohio Medical University, Rootstown, OH, United States, [2] Integrated Pharmaceutical Medicine Graduate Program, Northeast Ohio Medical University, Rootstown, OH, United States, [3] Rebecca D. Considine Research Institute, Vision Center, Akron Children's Hospital, Akron, OH, United States

***Correspondence:**
Matthew A. Smith
msmith13@neomed.edu

Mutations in the cytochrome P450-1B1 (Cyp1b1) gene is a common genetic predisposition associated with various human glaucomas, most prominently in primary congenital glaucoma (PCG). The role of Cyp1b1 in the eye is largely unknown, however, its absence appears to drive the maldevelopment of anterior eye structures responsible for aqueous fluid drainage in murine models. Nevertheless, vision loss in glaucoma ultimately results from the structural and functional loss of retinal ganglion cells (RGCs). Cyp1b1's influence in the development and support of retinal ganglion cell structure and function under normal conditions or during stress, such as elevated ocular pressure; the most common risk factor in glaucoma, remains grossly unknown. Thus, to determine the role of Cyp1b1 in normal retinal projection development we first assessed the strucutrual integrity of RGCs in the retina, optic nerve, and superior colliculus in un-manipulated (naïve) Cyp1b1-knockout (Cyp1b1$^{-/-}$) mice. In addition, in a separate cohort of Cyp1b1$^{-/-}$ and wildtype mice, we elevated and maintained intraocular pressure (IOP) at glaucomatous levels for 5-weeks, after which we compared RGC density, node of Ranvier morphology, and axonal transport between the genotypes. Our results demonstrate that naïve Cyp1b1$^{-/-}$ mice develop an anatomically intact retinal projection absent of overt glaucomatous pathology. Following pressure elevation, Cyp1b1$^{-/-}$ accelerated degradation of axonal transport from the retina to the superior colliculus and altered morphology of the nodes of Ranvier and adjacent paranodes in the optic nerves. Together this data suggests the absence Cyp1b1 expression alone is insufficient to drive murine glaucomatous pathology, however, may increase the vulnerability of retinal axons to disease relevant elevations in IOP.

Keywords: glaucoma, retinal ganglion cell, microbead occlusion model, nodes of Ranvier, axonal transport disruption

INTRODUCTION

Glaucoma is a group of heterogeneous neuro-ophthalmologic conditions that impair vision through the functional disruption and eventual degeneration of retinal ganglion cells (RGCs), the neuronal substrates responsible for eye-brain communication (Davis et al., 2016; Quigley and Broman, 2006). Glaucoma is most often attributed to the aging adult (Davis et al., 2016; Tham et al., 2014), however, befalls pediatric and adolescent populations (Kaur et al., 2011), thereby placing it in a unique group of neurodegenerative conditions that afflict populations on both ends of the lifespan.

Primary congenital glaucoma (PCG) is the most prevalent form of pediatric glaucoma manifesting at birth or within 3 years of age (Aponte et al., 2010). PCG is characterized most often by elevated intraocular pressure (IOP), buphthalmos (enlarged globe), and significant maldeveloped ocular drainage structures (i.e., trabecular meshwork and iridocorneal angle) (Hoskins et al., 1984; Libby et al., 2003). Much like other forms of glaucoma, the etiology of PCG remains unknown but likely arises from an orchestration of genetic and post-translational factors. PCG can be difficult to diagnose and if not managed effectively will result in progressive vision loss which can have critical ramifications on a child's overall development and long-term quality of life (Mandal et al., 2004; Khitri et al., 2012).

Genetic mapping of PCG populations over the last decade has identified recessive inheritance of several mutations in the cytochrome P450-1B1 (Cyp1b1) gene on the GLC3A locus (Sarfarazi et al., 1995; Akarsu et al., 1996) as a common predisposition. This has led many to assert Cyp1b1 as a causative gene for PCG. Interestingly, additional evidence suggests the involvement of Cyp1b1 mutations in several other forms of glaucoma including juvenile and adult primary open angle glaucoma (POAG) (Vincent et al., 2002; Su et al., 2012). Cyp1b1 is a membrane bound protein located in the endoplasmic reticulum or the inner mitochondrial membrane of cells found in most parts of the body (Stoilov et al., 2001; Bansal et al., 2014). Its general somatic involvement is in both endogenous and exogenous metabolism of xenobiotics and steroid synthesis (Murray et al., 2001). The role of Cyp1b1 in the eye is not well understood, however, its mRNA and protein expression in various ocular tissues including the cornea, ciliary body, trabecular meshwork, and the retina is evident (Muskhelishvili et al., 2001; Bejjani et al., 2002; Doshi et al., 2006).

The majority of studies seeking to understand the role of Cyp1b1 in the eye and its influence on the onset of PCG have focused primarily on signaling pathways integral in anterior eye structure development necessary for aqueous humor drainage. Cyp1b1 is involved in the metabolism of vitamin A (retinol) to the bioactive retinoic acid (RA). RA serves as a signaling molecule during a number of developmental and physiological processes, playing multiple roles during embryonic ocular and retinal development (Molotkov et al., 2006; Matt et al., 2008; Vasiliou and Gonzalez, 2008). Of the few murine studies conducted, deletion of Cyp1b1 *in vivo* yielded modest dysgenic anterior ocular drainage structures (trabecular meshwork and ciliary body) resembling defects seen in human PCG patients (Libby et al., 2003; Teixeira et al., 2015). While understanding the role of Cyp1b1 in anterior eye structure maldevelopment and causative signaling mechanisms holds significant value in understanding the onset and development of PCG; an avenue that remains overlooked is the contribution of Cyp1b1 in the retina and retinal projection dysfunction and degeneration underlying glaucomatous pathophysiology.

Glaucoma including PCG, involves an increased sensitivity of RGCs to changes in IOP. This increased sensitivity to elevations in IOP alters the axons of the RGCs (axonopathy) which encompass but are not limited to cytoskeletal alterations (Wilson et al., 2016), synaptic hypertrophy (Smith et al., 2016), aberrant morphology of axonal nodes of Ranvier (Smith et al., 2018) and defects in axonal transport (Dengler-Crish et al., 2014). The latter two appearing as the earliest pathological manifestations preceding overt degeneration of RGC axons in the optic nerve and somal loss in the retina (Smith et al., 2016). These pre-degenerative axonopathies represent key factors in the pathophysiological sequalae of glaucoma, which likely drive or follow changes in RGC physiology that is equally necessary for maintaining proper eye-brain communication (Baltan et al., 2010; Risner et al., 2018; Smith et al., 2018). To our knowledge no prior examination has been completed to determine the integrity of the retinal projections in the absence of Cyp1b1 under normal and stressed conditions (i.e., pathological elevation in IOP).

To address this gap in understanding of the role of Cyp1b1 in glaucoma, we compared the progression of RGC axonopathy in Cyp1b1$^{-/-}$ and wildtype mice following pathological elevation in IOP using the magnetic microbead occlusion model. We found more pronounced RGC axonal transport deficits and abnormal node of Ranvier morphometry in Cyp1b1$^{-/-}$ compared to wildtypes subjects following 5-weeks IOP elevation. We propose that the absence of Cyp1b1 expression alone is insufficient to drive murine glaucomatous pathology, however, the lack of its expression may increase the vulnerability of retinal neurons to disease relevant mechanisms following pathological elevations in IOP.

MATERIALS AND METHODS

Subjects

Adult mixed sex Cyp1b1$^{-/-}$ [129S6.129 × 1(B6)-Cyp1b1^{TM1Gonz}/Mmnc] mice were obtained from the Mutant Mouse Resource and Research Center (MMRRC) at JAX (Jackson Laboratories) and genotyped before experimentation to confirm the transgene. These mice have a targeted mutation caused by a disrupted coding sequence associated with exon three of the Cyp1b1 gene. Age-matched 129S6.129 × 1(B6) mice were used as wildtype controls (Buters et al., 1999; Libby et al., 2003). Mice were maintained in the Comparative Medicine Unit at Northeast Ohio Medical University on a 12-hour light/dark cycle with standard rodent chow available *ad libitum*. All experimental procedures were approved by the Northeast Ohio Medical University Institutional Animal Care and Use

Committee and conducted in accordance with the Guide for Care and Use of Laboratory Animals published by the National Institutes of Health.

Groups, Sample Size, and Ages

Thirty-six mice were used for this study to create equivalent groups of mice based on genotype, and experimental conditions. For initial studies assessing Cyp1b1$^{-/-}$ optic projection development a total combined cohort of twelve Cyp1b1$^{-/-}$ (n = 6) and wildtype (n = 6) subjects were used. Each retina, optic nerve, and corresponding contralateral superior colliculus (SC) were analyzed as independent measures within each animal, as glaucomatous pathophysiology is known to differentially affect each eye and projection (Schlamp et al., 2006; Crish et al., 2010). Therefore, from the total cohort of twelve subjects, a total of 24 (n = 12 per group) optic projections were collected and analyzed. All tissues were collected in 4–6-month old subjects across both genotypes.

For subsequent studies aimed at determining the impact of Cyp1b1$^{-/-}$ in the optic projection under conditions of ocular stress (i.e., induced ocular hypertension), an additional cohort of twenty-four 8–10 month old Cyp1b1$^{-/-}$ (n = 12) and wildtype (n = 12) subjects were utilized. Each retina, optic nerve, and corresponding contralateral superior colliculus were analyzed as separate, independent measures within each animal. The left eye/projections across both genotype groups underwent microbeads occlusion to induced ocular pressure elevation constituting the "hypertensive" subgroup while the right eye/projection remained un-elevated, "normotensive" to serve as internal sham control.

Intraocular Pressure Elevation Induction in Subjects

Intraocular pressure was raised to glaucomatous levels in our Cyp1b1$^{-/-}$ and wildtype subjects using the microbead occlusion method as described in Lambert et al. (2019) and Smith et al. (2018) (**Figure 2**). Briefly, twelve Cyp1b1$^{-/-}$ mice and twelve wildtype subjects were anesthetized using inhaled isoflurane (3% to induce and 1.5% to maintain sedation) and secured in a custom-made mount to reduce head and body movement during procedure. Baseline IOP readings were taken using a tonometer (TonoLab, Icare). Topical tropicamide (1%) was applied to both eyes for pupillary dilation, and a glass pipette (borosilicate glass capillaries 1.0/0.75 mm OD/ID pulled to 150-μm diameter; World Precision Instruments) attached to a Micro4 MicroSyringe Pump Injection system (World Precision Instruments) was used to deliver 1 μl (2.4 × 106 beads/ml) of COMPEL magnetic microspheres (mean diameter 7.90 μm; Bangs Laboratories Inc.) into the anterior chamber of the left eye for each animal. After completion of injections, a small neodymium magnet (Amazing Magnets) was used to pull beads to the margin of the eye. Each animal received a sham injection in the right eye with sterile saline used in place of microspheres as a procedural control. Animals were allowed to recover and IOP readings were recorded at 24- and 72-h and each week post injection for a 5-week survival time. After 5-weeks of IOP elevation, subjects underwent anterograde transport labeling procedures as detailed in section "Anterograde Axonal Transport Labeling" before being sacrificed following procedures detailed in section "Tissue Collection and Preparation."

Anterograde Axonal Transport Labeling

In order to assess the integrity of RGC anterograde axonal transport mechanisms in our subjects, we used axonal transport labeling techniques as we previously described (Dengler-Crish et al., 2014; Smith et al., 2016). Anterograde transport labeling was performed in all subjects across genotype and conditions. Subjects were placed prone in a stereotaxic device (Stoelting, Wood Dale, IL, United States) equipped with a nose cone that delivered 2.5% isoflurane at 0.8 ml/min. Injections (1.5 μl) of 0.1% cholera toxin subunit B (CTB) conjugated to Alexa Fluor-488 (Molecular Probes, C-34775) in sterile phosphate buffered saline (PBS) were administered into the vitreal chamber of each eye using a 33-ga needle attached to a 25 μl Hamilton syringe.

Tissue Collection and Preparation

All subjects were sacrificed via an overdose of Beuthanasia-D (300 mg/kg, i.p.) and transcardially perfused with PBS followed by 4% paraformaldehyde (PFA). Retinas, optic nerves, and brains were dissected and submerged into 4% PFA for an additional post-fixation step. Post-fixation time was dependent on the tissue type. Retinas underwent 30-min post-fixation, whereas optic nerves and brains were post-fixed overnight. After post-fixation, tissues were cryoprotected in 20% sucrose/PBS overnight. Using a freezing sliding microtome, 50 μm-thick coronal serial sections through the rostral-caudal extent of the superior colliculus, and 15 μm-thick longitudinal optic nerve sections were collected. Retina were dissected from the eye and prepared as flattened whole-mounts.

Examining the Structural Integrity of the Retinal Projections

In order to assess whether any anatomical differences exist regarding RGCs in the retinal-brain projections of the Cyp1b1$^{-/-}$ mouse, we used immunohistochemistry to label all components of the RGCs including somas in the retina, nodes of Ranvier in the optic nerve, and the distal projection axons and terminals in the superior colliculus. Retina, optic nerve, and brain tissues were incubated at 37°C for 1 h in a blocking solution containing 5% normal donkey serum and 0.1% Triton-X 100 in PBS, followed by overnight incubation at room temperature in a primary antibody solution containing 3% serum, 0.1% Triton. Primary antibodies used were: Brn3a (mouse 1:500; Santa Cruz Biotenchonology) to label the retinal ganglion cell nuclei, Caspr (mouse 1:500; Millipore) for axon paranode junctions, Nav1.6 (rabbit 1:500; Alamone) for axonal sodium channels at the nodes of Ranvier, ERRβ (rabbit 1:500; Sigma-Aldrich) for terminating retinal ganglion cell axons, Vglut2 (guinea pig 1:500; Synaptic Systems) for the synaptic terminals in the superior colliculus. After primary antibody incubations, tissues were washed, and then incubated at room temperature for 2 h in CF-Dye conjugated (488, 594, and 647 dyes) secondary antibody solution (Biotium) at a dilution of 1:200 in 1% serum/0.1% Triton/PBS. Following the final washes, tissues were mounted onto slides and coverslipped with ProLong Glass mounting media (Thermo Fisher).

Microscopy

All images were collected on a Zeiss Axio Imager M2 equipped with a digital high-resolution camera (Hamamatsu Flash4.0 V3 Digital CMOS; Japan), motorized Z and X-Y stage and an Apotome. Two structured illumination systems using 20×/0.8, 63×/1.4, and 150×/1.35 NA Plan-Apochromat objectives (Zeiss, Jena, Germany); all ran from the Zen operating software equipped with deconvolution and extended-depth-of-field modules. For retina imagining, multi-frame z-stacked acquisition was used to create a montage image composite of the entire retinal surface (Simons et al., 2021). For the optic nerve, optical sections (0.3 μm) through longitudinal sections were collected using the Apotome 2. Images were collected at two distinct regions at the center length of each nerve (Smith et al., 2018). For the superior colliculus, every third section of the serial right superior colliculus section was imaged.

Image Analysis

All analysis detailed in the section was conducted by multiple participants that were blinded to the genotype and condition from which the tissue was derived as slides were de-identified and assignment of an arbitrary numerical sequence was used to allow for minimal identification across subjects and study groups.

To determine the density of the RGC somas in the retina of Cyp1b1$^{-/-}$ compared to wildtype controls we used ImagePro (Media Cybernetics; Rockville, MD, United States) software to count and calculate Brn3a-labeled RGCs in the retina. Densities (cells/mm^2) were derived by dividing the total number of Brn3a-positive RGCs counted in each retina by the total area of that retina.

To assess the integrity of axonal transport, and intactness of distal RGC axons in naïve, normotensive and hypertensive Cyp1b1$^{-/-}$ mice, we quantified CTB, ERRβ, and Vglut2 signal density in multiple slices of the superior colliculus using a custom-written macro for NIH ImageJ. We set background intensity for each superior colliculus section by selecting a region of non-retinorecipient (i.e., periaqueductal gray) for comparison with the retinorecipient superior colliculus. We selected only the retinorecipient layers of the superior colliculus and binned pixels running from medial to lateral superior colliculus. The number of pixels within bins with CTB, ERRβ, or Vglut2 signal brighter than background was divided by the total number of pixels in the bin to provide a signal density for each serial section. The signal density from each serial superior colliculus section was averaged for each animal and compared across all genotypes and manipulation.

Node and paranode lengths, were derived from raw image z-stacks analyzed with the Zen 2 software analysis module as previously described (Smith et al., 2018). Node of Ranvier length was defined as the minimum distance separating adjacent Caspr terminal ends with the paranode length defined as the distance across a single unilateral Caspr signal determined from z-stacks of nodes that were linearly oriented to the imaging plane.

Statistical Analysis

Statistical data analysis was performed using IBM SPSS 26 Software. Raw data were screened for outliers, normalcy, and homogeneity of variance. We used two-way factorial analyses of variance (ANOVA) to determine differences in the magnitude of transport and structural label in the superior colliculus and retina between genotypes. Only CTB label was analyzed across subjects between genotypes in microbead occlusion experiments. Average node and paranode lengths were compared between genotype/microbead occlusions groups using factorial ANOVA models with Bonferroni's corrected pairwise comparisons to elucidate subgroup differences. Microbead occlusions IOP data were analyzed using an omnibus mixed model within subjects (ANOVA) to determine whether IOP changed in each eye after model induction as a function of bead implantation (hypertensive) or control saline injection (normotensive).

RESULTS

CYP1B1$^{-/-}$ Develop Structurally Intact Visual Projections

As summarized in **Figure 1**, we did not find any major differences in the structural integrity of RGC at the level of the retina, optic nerve, or superior colliculus in naïve Cyp1b1$^{-/-}$ mice compared to wildtype subjects. Using tonometry to record IOPs in both left and right eyes in Cyp1b1$^{-/-}$ mice aging from postnatal day 16 (P16) to 12-months there was no significant difference in IOP between the left and right eyes across all ages (**Figure 1A**; $F_{1,28}$ = 0.18, $p > 0.1$). Qualitatively, recorded IOPs from Cyp1b1$^{-/-}$ mice at all examined ages did not extend outside of physiological ranges of 10–15 mmHg as reported in mice of similar genetic background with normal ocular phenotypes (Savinova et al., 2001).

In comparing RGC densities across flat-mount naïve Cyp1b1$^{-/-}$ and wildtype retina, no statistical difference was observed in retinal Brn3a cell density (**Figure 1B**, upper panel) between the two genotypes (**Figure 1B**; $F_{1,22}$ = 0.23, $p > 0.1$). Using the optic nerves to compare node of Ranvier and paranode lengths (**Figure 1C**, upper image) across naïve wildtype and Cyp1b1$^{-/-}$ subjects yielded no significant differences in node (**Figure 1C**, lower left; $F_{1,388}$ = 0.36, $p > 0.1$) or paranode length (**Figure 1C**, lower right; $F_{1,388}$ = 0.46, $p > 0.1$). Cyp1b1$^{-/-}$ node and paranode lengths adhered to expected ranges for mice of equivalent age (Stahon et al., 2016). Although not quantified, sodium channels (**Figure 1C**, upper image; red) appeared present and normally distributed within the nodes. Lastly, to determine anterograde transport integrity and distal RGC axon/synaptic connectivity to/in the superior colliculus within Cyp1b1$^{-/-}$ subjects; CTB, Vglut2, and Errβ label were independently compared across subjects. No differences were observed in the percent area fraction of CTB, Vglut2, and Errβ label in the superior colliculus of naïve Cyp1b1$^{-/-}$ subjects

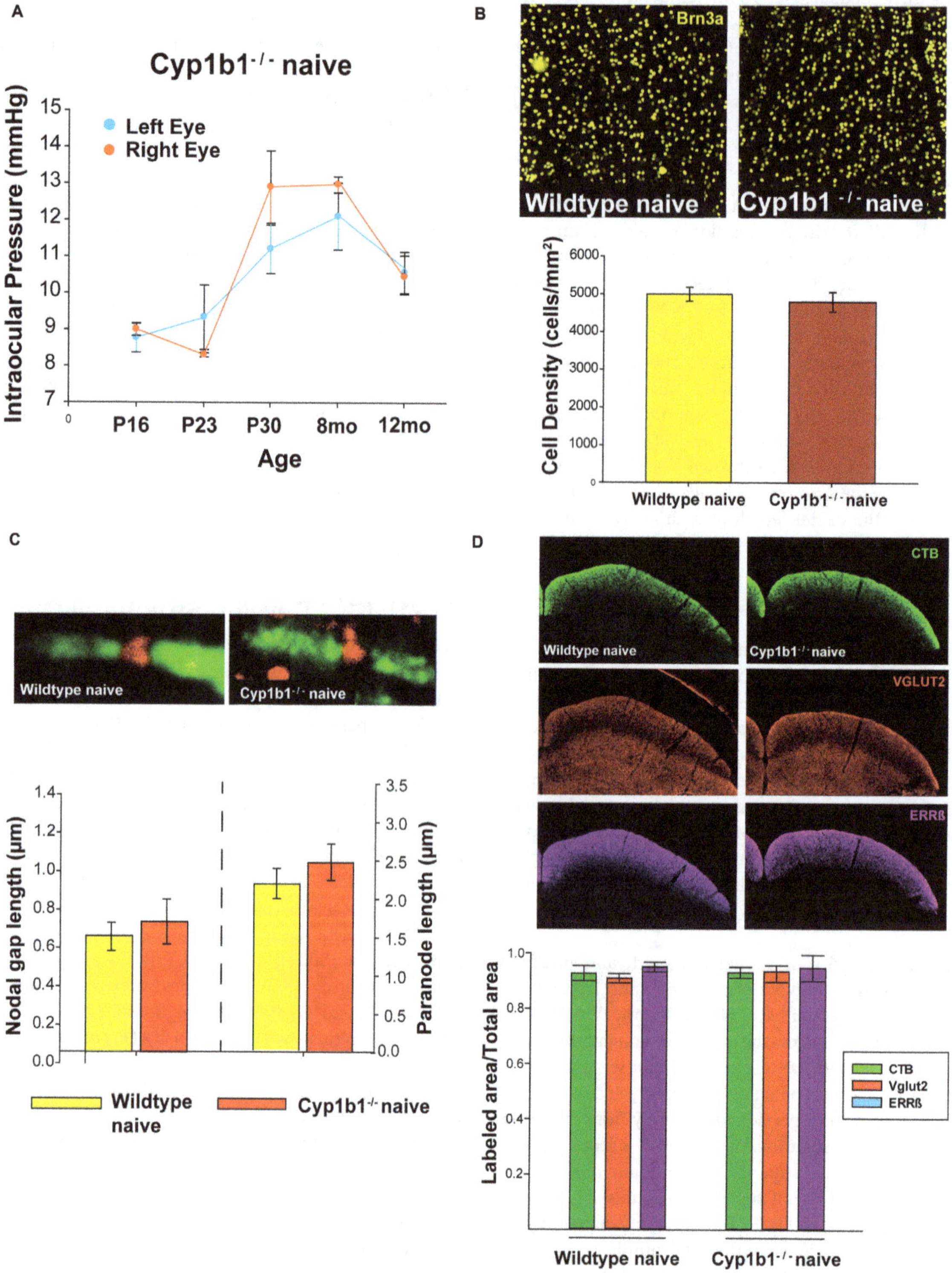

FIGURE 1 | Cyp1b1$^{-/-}$ develop structurally intact visual projections. **(A)** Cyp1b1$^{-/-}$ ocular pressure readings across the lifespan (P16 to 12-mo, *n* = 6) maintained within normal physiological range in both eyes. **(B)** Retinal ganglion cell density in naïve wildtype vs. Cyp1b1$^{-/-}$ mice. High magnification retinal whole-mount images immunostained for Brn3a, a marker for RGC nuclei. Naïve Cyp1b1$^{-/-}$ (red; *n* = 12) RGC densities do not differ from naïve wildtype retina (yellow; *n* = 12). **(C)** Cyp1b1$^{-/-}$ nodes of Ranvier appear absent of major morphometric changes in the node (Nav1.6, red; *n* = 200) and paranode (Caspr, green; *n* = 200). **(D)** A 50 μm coronal cross section through the superior colliculus of a Cyp1b1$^{-/-}$ mouse that received an intravitreal injection of cholera toxin-B conjugated –alexafluor 488 (CTB488, green) and immunostained for VGlut2 (red, RGC synapses) and estrogen related receptor-β (magenta, RGC axon + axon terminals). Graph depicts superior colliculus label density (labeled area/total area) for each marker. No differences in label density were present between Cyp1b1$^{-/-}$ and wildtype (*n* = 24).

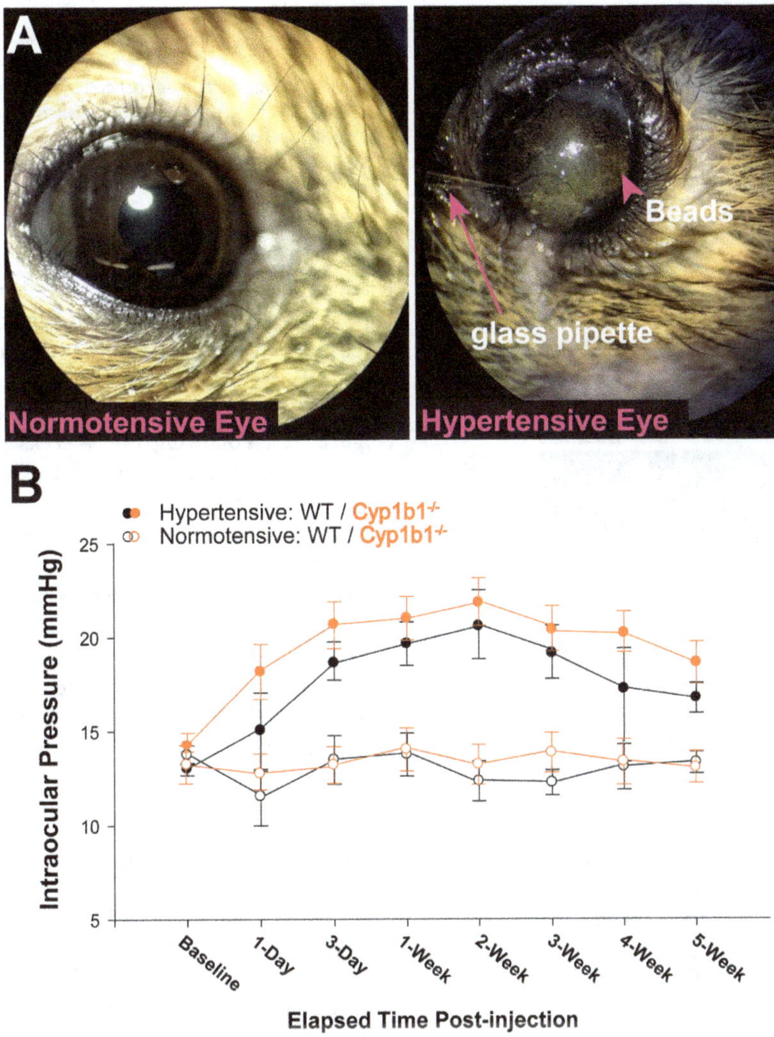

FIGURE 2 | Microbead occlusion model. **(A)** Example image of procedure being performed. Left shows saline injected eye, right shows glass pipette insertion into anterior chamber of subject delivering a solution containing 8 μm magnetic microbeads. **(B)** Intraocular pressure (IOP) readings from Cyp1b1$^{-/-}$ subjects (orange lines) and wildtype (black lines) following injection of microbeads (hypertensive and solid circles) or saline (normotensive and open circles) over 5 weeks (n = 24).

compared to wildtypes (**Figure 1D**; CTB; $F_{1,22} = 1.23, p > 0.1$), Vglut2; $F_{1,22} = 1.34, p > 0.1$), and ERRβ, $F_{1,22} = 1.23, p > 0.1$).

CYP1B1$^{-/-}$ Accelerates Axonopathy in the Rretinal Projection Following Ocular Pressure Elevation

A single unilateral injection of magnetic microbeads (**Figure 2A**) significantly elevated IOP in both Cyp1b1$^{-/-}$ and wildtype eyes by 38% for 5-weeks compared to the corresponding saline injected (normotensive) eyes (**Figure 2B**, $F_{3,26} = 1.70$, $p > 0.1$). Cyp1b1$^{-/-}$ IOPs in the injected eye (hypertensive) (**Figure 2B**, solid circle- orange) was not significantly different from hypertensive wildtype eyes (**Figure 2B**, solid circle-black; $F_{1,26} = 1.70, p > 0.1$).

As summarized in **Figure 3**, we observed significant differences in the structural integrity of RGCs at the level of the retina, optic nerve, and superior colliculus following ocular hypertension in Cyp1b1$^{-/-}$ and wildtype subjects. In the retina, following ocular hypertension, hypertensive Cyp1b1$^{-/-}$ and hypertensive wildtype subjects exhibited substantial reductions (75 and 60%, respectively) in Brn3a density compared to saline injected controls (**Figures 3A,B**; $F_{3,44} = 101.1$, $p < 0.01$). However, hypertensive Cyp1b1$^{-/-}$ retina did not exhibit any difference in Brn3a destiny compared to hypertensive wildtype retina (**Figures 3A,B**; $F_{3,44} = 3.08, p = 0.09$).

In the optic nerve, significant alterations in node and paranode lengths were observed (**Figure 3C**). Hypertensive Cyp1b1$^{-/-}$ optic nerve nodes of Ranvier were 27% longer compared to nodes within the hypertensive wildtype optic nerve (**Figure 3D** left; $F_{1,446} = 226.76$, $p < 0.05$) and the contralateral normotensive Cyp1b1$^{-/-}$ optic nerve ($F_{1,446} = 203.23, p < 0.05$). Hypertensive Cyp1b1$^{-/-}$ paranode lengths were 21% shorter in comparison to hypertensive wildtype (**Figure 3D** right; $F_{1,446} = 207.94, p < 0.05$) and normotensive Cyp1b1$^{-/-}$ optic nerves ($F_{1,446} = 220.65$, $p < 0.05$). Although not directly quantified, qualitatively, sodium

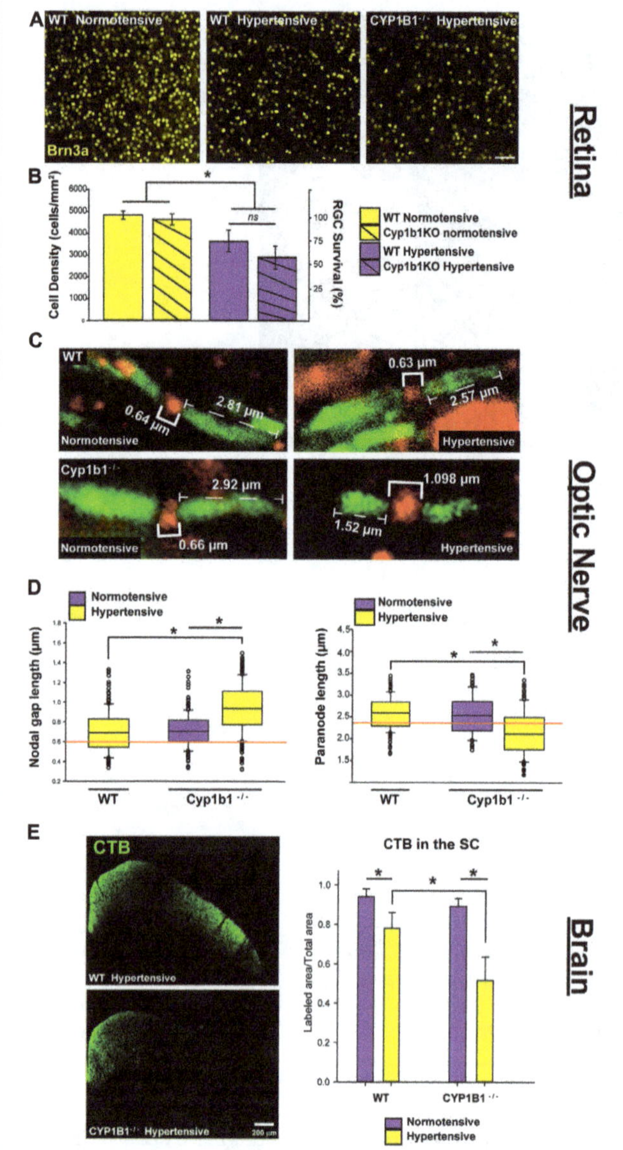

FIGURE 3 | Cyp1b1$^{-/-}$ accelerates axonopathy in the retinal projections following ocular pressure elevation. **(A)** Brn3a immunofluorescence in normotensive and hypertensive flat mount retina from wildtype and Cyp1b1$^{-/-}$ subjects (scale bar = 50 μm). **(B)** Hypertensive Cyp1b1$^{-/-}$ (solid magenta) and wildtype (dashed magenta) retina demonstrate a significant reduction in Brn3a density compared to normotensive wildtype (solid yellow) and Cyp1b1$^{-/-}$ (dashed yellow) retina. Hypertensive Cyp1b1$^{-/-}$ demonstrate no greater loss in Brn3a density compared to hypertensive wildtype retina. **(C)** Longitudinal optic nerve sections immunolabeled for Nav1.6 (red) and Caspr (green) to visualize nodes of Ranvier and adjacent paranode in normotensive and hypertensive Cyp1b1$^{-/-}$ and wildtype optic nerves. Brackets indicate node and paranode length in microns. **(D)** Node lengths increased (left) while paranode lengths decreased (right) in hypertensive (yellow) Cyp1b1$^{-/-}$ optic nerves following 5-week elevation in IOP compared to normotensive (magenta) nerves corresponding to the saline injected eye in the same animal. Nodes and paranode lengths associated with the hypertensive wildtype optic nerves were comparable to wildtype naïve (orange line; indicates average) and normotensive Cyp1b1$^{-/-}$ (magenta) lengths. **(E)** Epifluorescent images contrasting CTB label in unilateral coronal sections through the superior colliculus of hypertensive Cyp1b1$^{-/-}$ and *(Continued)*

FIGURE 3 | Continued
wildtype subjects. Superior colliculi corresponding to hypertensive eyes (yellow) in both Cyp1b1$^{-/-}$ and wildtype subjects demonstrate significant deficits in axonal transport evidenced by reduced CTB labels compared to colliculi corresponding to the saline injected normotensive eye (magenta). Collicular CTB drop-out was more pronounced in Cyp1b1$^{-/-}$ subjects compared to wildtypes following equivalent period of IOP elevation. Asterisk denotes statistical significance ($p < 0.01$).

channel density across axons and distribution within the node appeared consistent across groups and conditions.

Lastly, we compared the progression of anterograde transport deficits in the superior colliculus of Cyp1b1$^{-/-}$ and wildtype mice following induced ocular hypertension (**Figure 3E**). Following the 5-weeks period of IOP elevation, the superior colliculus of both Cyp1b1$^{-/-}$ and wildtype subjects demonstrated 45% ($F_{1,22} = 299.57$, $p < 0.01$) and 20% ($F_{1,22} = 104.54$, $p < 0.01$) depletion of CTB coverage, respectively. However, most interestingly, Cyp1b1$^{-/-}$ demonstrated a 33% greater depletion in CTB transport in the superior colliculus compared to hypertensive wildtype subjects ($F_{1,22} = 106.47$, $p < 0.01$). Colliculi corresponding to the saline injected normotensive eyes in both subjects revealed >95% CTB coverage with statistical difference reflected across genotypes.

DISCUSSION

Axonopathy is one of the earliest hallmarks of neurodegeneration in glaucoma which encompasses degradation of active transport from the retina to the colliculus, and alterations in node of Ranvier morphology, both of which occur before outright axon degeneration in the optic nerve and soma loss in the retina (Dengler-Crish et al., 2014; Smith et al., 2016; Smith et al., 2018). In the current study, we showed evidence that absence of Cyp1b1 alone is insufficient to drive glaucomatous-like axonopathy and RGC neurodegeneration in the mouse visual system. This finding was not surprising given that these animals do not develop abnormal elevations in IOP over their lifespan. This seems to align with previous studies that also did not report abnormal IOPs in these mice, and provide evidence suggesting that the abnormal development in anterior eye structures is restricted to only modest focal points across these drainage structures and therefore are not substantial enough to alter the aqueous fluid drainage (Libby et al., 2003).

Our most interesting finding is that after a 5-weeks period of an equivalent pathological elevation in IOP, deficits in anterograde transport to the colliculus were more severe in Cyp1b1$^{-/-}$ mice than in age-matched wildtype mice. Additionally, IOP elevation altered node of Ranvier morphology, where node gap lengths were longer and paranode lengths were shorter in Cyp1b1$^{-/-}$ hypertensive optic nerves compared to equivalently stressed wildtype subjects. This observation is further intriguing given that alterations in node of Ranvier morphology are not typically reported following IOP elevation induced by microbead occlusion, but rather in naturally occurring animal models such as the DBA2/J mouse (Smith et al., 2018). It is important to note that despite the nuanced alterations in node/paranode morphology and the exacerbated transport loss, Cyp1b1$^{-/-}$ subjects did not demonstrate any greater difference in RGC somal loss in the retina compared to wildtypes following ocular hypertension. Given that RGC degeneration in glaucoma occurs in a retrograde fashion occurring first in the distal axon and dying back toward cell bodies at varied rates, timing is critical. Our data represent a single time point following elevation whereby the percent change in RGC densities would have to be analyzed across multiple earlier and later time points to elucidate effects on RGC apoptosis in the retina. In any case, clinical manifestation and treatment strategies are not wholly left to preventing RGC loss and these exacerbated deficits in axonal transport and node of Ranvier alterations stand to have immense impact on RGC function.

In terms of possible mechanisms, our findings lack the support of additional literature therefore, much is left to speculation until further studies are conducted. Nevertheless, we assert that interesting linkages can be made across our findings by focusing on the bioactive metabolites produced by Cyp1b1. As mentioned, Cyp1b1 participates in the conversion of retinol to retinoic acid (RA) and metabolism of unbound arachidonic acid (AA) (Choudhary et al., 2004). Several studies have proposed various beneficial effects of RA in central nervous system injury noting RAs ability to downregulate pro-inflammatory cytokines such as IL-1β and TNFα in order to alter macrophage and microglial activation and reactive oxygen species production (Choi et al., 2005; Dheen et al., 2005; Xu and Drew, 2006; De La Rosa-Reyes et al., 2019) and in mediating RGC survival following optic nerve injury (Duprey-Díaz et al., 2016). RA has been shown to be released from NG2 cells in the central nervous system (Mey et al., 2005). NG2 cells play an intimate supporting role at the node of Ranvier where their processes are shown to insert (Serwanski et al., 2017) in order to serve as sensors to communicate changes in neuron environment in times of stress/injury (Wu et al., 2008). While it is not understood, we can speculate that RA release from NG2 cells at the node may provide additional support to mediate anti-inflammatory processes following injury or stress (Palenski et al., 2013). In the absence of Cyp1b1, diminished RA levels may lead to increased neuroinflammation (Falero-Perez et al., 2019) at the node altering their morphology in response to stress placed on axons following IOP elevation.

In addition, arachidonic acid (AA), a fatty acid that is released from cell membrane phospholipids following mechanical stimulation or hypoxia is partly metabolized by Cyp1B1. AA concentrations have been described in the retina, optic nerve, and brain and may play a role in other axonopathies/neurodegenerative disorders such as Alzheimer's disease which share several similarities to glaucoma (Conquet et al., 1975; Corcoran et al., 2004). AA has been shown to influence synaptic functions by acting as a retrograde messenger stimulating opening Kv channels (Angelova and Müller, 2009). Given that Cyp1b1 appears localized within the inner plexiform layer of the retina, it would in theory allow for maintained high concentration of AA levels at the bipolar-RGC synapse. This may alter RGC activity in Cyp1b1$^{-/-}$ projections whereby increased levels of AA could alter RGC excitability through retrograde synaptic signaling through inhibited sodium/potassium currents and synaptic transmission (Fraser et al., 1993). Additionally, AA has been described to be involved in tau hyperphosphorylation (King et al., 2000). AA activates several kinases, including protein kinase α, which directly contribute to increased tau phosphorylation levels (Kochs et al., 1993). Tau hyperphosphorylation is evident in the glaucomatous optic nerve and can disrupt axonal transport mechanisms (Wilson et al., 2016). It is possible that absence of Cyp1b1 exacerbates axonal transport deficits through increasing intra-axonal RGC tau hyperphosphorylation.

CONCLUSION

Absence of Cyp1b1 alone is not sufficient to alter visual function but does increase RGC susceptibility to axonopathy following pressure elevation. Thus, Cyp1b1 may contribute to the ability of RGCs to respond to stress or injury through internal or external signaling mechanisms mediated through bioactive metabolites.

ETHICS STATEMENT

The animal study was reviewed and approved by the Northeast Ohio Medical University Institutional Animal Care and Use Committee.

AUTHOR CONTRIBUTIONS

NA contributed extensively to experimental design, the data collection, reporting of initial results, and writing of the manuscript. BF and SD assisted with immunofluorescence assays and the data analysis. RB assisted in the data collection, interpretation of the results, and manuscript review. MS designed the study, performed and assisted in the data collection and analysis, interpreted results, and prepared the manuscript. All authors contributed to the article and approved the submitted version.

REFERENCES

Akarsu, A. N., Turacli, M. E., Aktan, S. G., Barsoum-Homsy, M., Chevrette, L., Sayli, B. S., et al. (1996). A second locus (GLC3B) for primary congenital glaucoma (Buphthalmos) maps to the 1p36 region. *Hum. Mol. Genet.* 5, 1199–1203.

Angelova, P. R., and Müller, W. S. (2009). Arachidonic acid potently inhibits both postsynaptic-type Kv4.2 and presynaptic-type Kv1.4 I_A potassium channels. *Eur. J. Neurosci.* 29, 1943–1950. doi: 10.1111/j.1460-9568.2009.06737.x

Aponte, E. P., Diehl, N., and Mohney, B. G. (2010). Incidence and clinical characteristics of childhood glaucoma: a population-based study. *Arch. Ophthalmol.* 128, 478–482. doi: 10.1001/archophthalmol.2010.41.Incidence

Baltan, S., Inman, D. M., Danilov, C. A., Morrison, R. S., Calkins, D. J., and Horner, P. J. (2010). Metabolic vulnerability disposes retinal ganglion cell axons to dysfunction in a model of glaucomatous degeneration. *J. Neurosci.* 30, 5644–5652. doi: 10.1523/JNEUROSCI.5956-09.2010

Bansal, S., Leu, A. N., Gonzalez, F. J., Guengerich, F. P., Chowdhury, A. R., Anandatheerthavarada, H. K., et al. (2014). Mitochondrial targeting of cytochrome P450 (CYP) 1B1 and its role in polycyclic aromatic hydrocarbon-induced mitochondrial dysfunction. *J. Biol. Chem.* 289, 9936–9951. doi: 10.1074/jbc.M113.525659

Bejjani, B. A., Xu, L., Armstrong, D., Lupski, J. R., and Reneker, L. W. (2002). Expression patterns of cytochrome P4501B1 (Cyp1b1) in FVB/N mouse eyes. *Exp. Eye Res.* 75, 249–257.

Buters, J. T., Sakai, S., Richter, T., Pineau, T., Alexander, D. L., Savas, U., et al. (1999). Cytochrome P450 CYP1B1 determines susceptibility to 7, 12-dimethylbenz[*a*]anthracene-induced lymphomas. *Proc. Natl. Acad. Sci. U. S. A.* 96, 1977–1982. doi: 10.1073/pnas.96.5.1977

Choi, W.-H., Ji, K.-A., Jeon, S.-B., Yang, M.-S., Kim, H., Min, K.-J., et al. (2005). Anti-inflammatory roles of retinoic acid in rat brain astrocytes: suppression of interferon-γ-induced JAK/STAT phosphorylation. *Biochem. Biophys. Res. Commun.* 329, 125–131.

Choudhary, D., Jansson, I., Stoilov, I., Sarfarazi, M., and Schenkman, J. B. (2004). Metabolism of retinoids and arachidonic acid by human and mouse cytochrome P450 1b1. *Drug Metabol. Disposit.* 32, 840–847. doi: 10.1124/dmd.32.8.840

Conquet, P., Plazonnet, B., and Le Douarec, J. C. (1975). Arachidonic acid-induced elevation of intraocular pressure and anti-inflammatory agents. *Invest. Ophthalmol.* 14, 772–775.

Corcoran, J. P. T., So, P. L., and Maden, M. (2004). Disruption of the retinoid signalling pathway causes a deposition of amyloid beta in the adult rat brain. *Eur. J. Neurosci.* 20, 896–902.

Crish, S. D., Sappington, R. M., Inman, D. M., Horner, P. J., and Calkins, D. J. (2010). Distal axonopathy with structural persistence in glaucomatous neurodegeneration. *Proc. Natl. Acad. Sci. U. S. A.* 107, 5196–5201. doi: 10.1073/pnas.0913141107

Davis, B. M., Crawley, L., Pahlitzsch, M., Javaid, F., and Cordeiro, M. F. (2016). Glaucoma: the retina and beyond. *Acta Neuropathol.* 132, 807–826. doi: 10.1007/s00401-016-1609-2

De La Rosa-Reyes, V., Duprey, M. V., Blagburn, J. M., and Blanco, R. E. (2019). Retinoic acid application affects optic nerve microglia and macrophages after optic nerve injury in frog Rana pipiens. *FASEB J.* 33, 450.6–450.6. doi: 10.1096/fasebj.2019.33.1_supplement.450.6 ***450.6-450.6,

Dengler-Crish, C. M., Smith, M. A., Inman, D. M., Wilson, G. N., Young, J. W., and Crish, S. D. (2014). Anterograde transport blockade precedes deficits in retrograde transport in the visual projection of the DBA/2J mouse model of glaucoma. *Front. Neurosci.* 8:290. doi: 10.3389/fnins.2014.00290

Dheen, S. T., Jun, Y., Yan, Z., Tay, S. S. W., and Ling, E. A. (2005). Retinoic acid inhibits expression of TNF-α and iNOS in activated rat microglia. *GLIA* 50, 21–31.

Doshi, M., Marcus, C., Bejjani, B. A., and Edward, D. P. (2006). Immunolocalization of CYP1B1 in normal, human, fetal and adult eyes. *Exp. Eye Res.* 82, 24–32. doi: 10.1016/j.exer.2005.04.016

Duprey-Díaz, M. V., Blagburn, J. M., and Blanco, R. E. (2016). Exogenous modulation of retinoic acid signaling affects adult RGC survival in the frog visual system after optic nerve injury. *PLoS One* 11:e0162626. doi: 10.1371/journal.pone.0162626

Falero-Perez, J., Sorenson, C. M., and Sheibani, N. (2019). Cyp1b1-deficient retinal astrocytes are more proliferative and migratory and are protected from oxidative stress and inflammation. *Am. J. Physiol. Cell Physiol.* 316, C767–C781. doi: 10.1152/ajpcell.00021.2019

Fraser, D. D., Hoehn, K., Weiss, S., and MacVicar, B. A. (1993). Arachidonic acid inhibits sodium currents and synaptic transmission in cultured striatal neurons. *Neuron* 11, 633–644. doi: 10.1016/0896-6273(93)90075-3

Hoskins, H. D., Shaffer, R. N., and Hetherington, J. (1984). Anatomical classification of the developmental glaucomas. *Arch. Ophthalmol.* 102, 1331–1336. doi: 10.1001/archopht.1984.01040031081030

Kaur, K., Mandal, A. K., and Chakrabarti, S. (2011). Primary congenital glaucoma and the involvement of CYP1B1. *Middle East Afr. J. Ophthalmol.* 18, 7–16. doi: 10.4103/0974-9233.75878

Khitri, M. R., Mills, M. D., Ying, G.-S., Davidson, S. L., and Quinn, G. E. (2012). Visual acuity outcomes in pediatric glaucomas. *J. Am. Assoc. Pediatr. Ophthalmol. Strabismus.* 16, 376–381. doi: 10.1016/j.jaapos.2012.05.007

King, M. E., Gamblin, T. C., Kuret, J., and Binder, L. I. (2000). Differential assembly of human tau isoforms in the presence of arachidonic acid. *J. Neurochem.* 74, 1749–1757. doi: 10.1046/j.1471-4159.2000.0741749.x

Kochs, G., Hummel, R., Meyer, D., Hug, H., Marmé, D., and Sarre, T. F. (1993). Activation and substrate specificity of the human protein kinase C α and ζ isoenzymes. *Eur. J. Biochem.* 216, 597–606. doi: 10.1111/j.1432-1033.1993.tb18179.x

Lambert, W. S., Carlson, B. J., Ghose, P., Vest, V. D., Yao, V., and Calkins, D. J. (2019). Towards a microbead occlusion model of glaucoma for a non-human primate. *Sci. Rep.* 9:11572. doi: 10.1038/s41598-019-48054-y

Libby, R. T., Smith, R. S., Savinova, O. V., Zabaleta, A., Martin, J. E., Gonzalez, F. J., et al. (2003). Modification of ocular defects in mouse developmental glaucoma models by tyrosinase. *Science* 299, 1578–1581.

Mandal, A. K., Bhatia, P. G., Bhaskar, A., and Nutheti, R. (2004). Long-term surgical and visual outcomes in Indian children with developmental glaucoma operated on within 6 months of birth. *Ophthalmology* 111, 283–290. doi: 10.1016/j.ophtha.2003.05.027

Matt, N., Ghyselinck, N. B., Pellerin, I., and Dupé, V. (2008). Impairing retinoic acid signalling in the neural crest cells is sufficient to alter entire eye morphogenesis. *Devel. Biol.* 320, 140–148. doi: 10.1016/j.ydbio.2008.04.039

Mey, J., Morassutti, D. J., Brook, G., Liu, R.-H., Zhang, Y.-P., Koopmans, G., et al. (2005). Retinoic acid synthesis by a population of NG2-positive cells in the injured spinal cord. *Eur. J. Neurosci.* 21, 1555–1568. doi: 10.1111/j.1460-9568.2005.03928.x

Molotkov, A., Molotkova, N., and Duester, G. (2006). Retinoic acid guides eye morphogenetic movements via paracrine signaling but is unnecessary for retinal dorsoventral patterning. *Development* 133, 1901–1910. doi: 10.1242/dev.02328

Murray, G. I., Melvin, W. T., Greenlee, W. F., and Burke, M. D. (2001). Regulation, function, and tissue-specific expression of cytochrome P450 CYP1B1. *Annu. Rev. Pharmacol. Toxicol.* 41, 297–316. doi: 10.1146/annurev.pharmtox.41.1.297

Muskhelishvili, L., Thompson, P. A., Kusewitt, D. F., Wang, C., and Kadlubar, F. F. (2001). In situ hybridization and immunohistochemical analysis of cytochrome P450 1B1 expression in human normal tissues. *J. Histochem. Cytochem.* 49, 229–236. doi: 10.1177/002215540104900210

Palenski, T. L., Sorenson, C. M., Jefcoate, C. R., and Sheibani, N. (2013). Lack of Cyp1b1 promotes the proliferative and migratory phenotype of perivascular supporting cells. *Lab. Invest.* 93, 646–662. doi: 10.1038/labinvest.2013.55

Quigley, H. A., and Broman, A. T. (2006). The number of people with glaucoma worldwide in 2010 and 2020. *Br. J. Ophthalmol.* 90, 262–267.

Risner, M. L., Pasini, S., Cooper, M. L., Lambert, W. S., and Calkins, D. J. (2018). Enhanced ganglion cell excitability in glaucoma. *Proc. Natl. Acad. Sci.U.S.A.* 115, E2393–E2402. doi: 10.1073/pnas.1714888115

Sarfarazi, M., Akarsu, A. N., Hossain, A., Turacli, M. E., Aktan, S. G., Barsoum-Homsy, M., et al. (1995). Assignment of a locus (GLC3A) for primary congenital glaucoma (Buphthalmos) to 2p21 and evidence for genetic heterogeneity. *Genomics* 30, 171–177.

Savinova, O. V., Sugiyama, F., Martin, J. E., Tomarev, S. I., Paigen, B. J., Smith, R. S., et al. (2001). Intraocular pressure in genetically distinct mice: an update and strain survey. *BMC Genet.* 2:12. doi: 10.1186/1471-2156-2-12

Schlamp, C. L., Li, Y., Dietz, J. A., Janssen, K. T., and Nickells, R. W. (2006). Progressive ganglion cell loss and optic nerve degeneration in DBA/2J mice is variable and asymmetric. *BMC Neurosci.* 7:66. doi: 10.1186/1471-2202-7-66

Serwanski, D. R., Jukkola, P., and Nishiyama, A. (2017). Heterogeneity of astrocyte and NG2 cell insertion at the node of ranvier. *J. Comp. Neurol.* 525, 535–552. doi: 10.1002/cne.24083

Simons, E. S., Smith, M. A., Dengler-Crish, C. M., and Crish, S. D. (2021). Retinal ganglion cell loss and gliosis in the retinofugal projection following intravitreal exposure to amyloid-beta. *Neurobiol. Dis.* 147:105146. doi: 10.1016/j.nbd.2020.105146

Smith, M. A., Plyer, E. S., Dengler-Crish, C. M., Meier, J., and Crish, S. D. (2018). Nodes of Ranvier in Glaucoma. *Neuroscience* 390, 104–118. doi: 10.1016/j.neuroscience.2018.08.016

Smith, M. A., Xia, C. Z., Dengler-Crish, C. M., Fening, K. M., Inman, D. M., Schofield, B. R., et al. (2016). Persistence of intact retinal ganglion cell terminals after axonal transport loss in the DBA/2J mouse model of glaucoma. *J. Comp. Neurol.* 524, 3503–3517. doi: 10.1002/cne.24012

Stahon, K. E., Bastian, C., Griffith, S., Kidd, G. J., Brunet, S., and Baltan, S. (2016). Age-related changes in axonal and mitochondrial ultrastructure and function in white matter. *J. Neurosci.* 36, 9990–10001. doi: 10.1523/JNEUROSCI.1316-16.2016

Stoilov, I., Jansson, I., Sarfarazi, M., and Schenkman, J. B. (2001). Roles of cytochrome p450 in development. *Drug Metabol. Drug Interact.* 18, 33–55.

Su, C. C., Liu, Y. F., Li, S. Y., Yanget, J. J., and Yen, Y. C. (2012). Mutations in the CYP1B1 gene may contribute to juvenile-onset open-angle glaucoma. *Eye* 26, 1369–1377. doi: 10.1038/eye.2012.159

Teixeira, L. B., Zhao, Y., Dubielzig, R. R., Sorenson, C. M., and Sheibani, N. (2015). Ultrastructural abnormalities of the trabecular meshwork extracellular matrix in Cyp1b1-deficient mice. *Vet. Pathol.* 52, 397–403.

Tham, Y. C., Li, X., Wong, T. Y., Quigley, H. A., Aung, T., and Cheng, C. Y. (2014). Global prevalence of glaucoma and projections of glaucoma burden through 2040: a systematic review and meta-analysis. *Ophthalmology* 121, 2081–2090. doi: 10.1016/j.ophtha.2014.05.013

Vasiliou, V., and Gonzalez, F. J. (2008). Role of CYP1B1 in glaucoma. *Annu. Rev. Pharmacol. Toxicol.* 48, 333–358. doi: 10.1146/annurev.pharmtox.48.061807.154729

Vincent, A. L., Billingsley, G., Buys, Y., Levin, A. V., Priston, M., Trope, G., et al. (2002). Digenic inheritance of early-onset glaucoma: CYP1B1, a potential modifier gene. *Am. J. Hum. Genet.* 70, 448–460. doi: 10.1086/338709

Wilson, G. N., Smith, M. A., Inman, D. M., Dengler-Crish, C. M., and Crish, S. D. (2016). Early cytoskeletal protein modifications precede overt structural degeneration in the DBA/2J mouse model of glaucoma. *Front. Neurosci.* 10:494. doi: 10.3389/fnins.2016.00494

Wu, Y. J., Tang, Y. F., Xiao, Z. C., Bao, Z. M., and He, B. P. (2008). NG2 cells response to axonal alteration in the spinal cord white matter in mice with genetic disruption of neurofilament light subunit expression. *Mol. Neurodegener.* 3:18. doi: 10.1186/1750-1326-3-18

Xu, J., and Drew, P. D. (2006). 9-cis-retinoic acid suppresses inflammatory responses of microglia and astrocytes. *J. Neuroimmunol.* 171, 135–144.

19

Mitochondrial Mutations in Ethambutol-Induced Optic Neuropathy

Xiao-Hui Zhang[1,2], Yue Xie[2], Quan-Gang Xu[1], Kai Cao[2], Ke Xu[2], Zi-Bing Jin[2], Yang Li[2*] and Shi-Hui Wei[1*]*

[1] Department of Ophthalmology, The Chinese People's Liberation Army General Hospital, The Chinese People's Liberation Army Medical School, Beijing, China, [2] Beijing Ophthalmology and Visual Sciences Key Laboratory, Beijing Institute of Ophthalmology, Beijing Tongren Eye Center, Beijing Tongren Hospital, Capital Medical University, Beijing, China

***Correspondence:**
Zi-Bing Jin
jinzb@mail.eye.ac.cn
Yang Li
yilbio@163.com
Shi-Hui Wei
weishihui706@hotmail.com

Background: Ethambutol-induced optic neuropathy (EON) is a well-recognized ocular complication in patients who take ethambutol as a tuberculosis treatment. The aim of the current study was to investigate the presence of mitochondrial mutations, including *OPA1* and Leber's hereditary optic neuropathy (LHON)-mitochondrial DNA (mtDNA), in patients with EON and to determine their effect on clinical features of these patients.

Methods: All 47 patients underwent clinical evaluations, including best-corrected visual acuity, fundus examination, and color fundus photography; 37 patients were then followed up over time. Molecular screening methods, including PCR-based sequencing of the *OPA1* gene and LHON-mtDNA mutations, together with targeted exome sequencing, were used to detect mutations.

Results: We detected 15 *OPA1* mutations in 18 patients and two LHON-mtDNA mutations in four patients, for an overall mutation detection rate of 46.8%. The mean presentation age was significantly younger in the patients with the mitochondrial mutations (27.5 years) than in those without mutations (48 years). Fundus examination revealed a greater prevalence of optic disc hyperemia in the patients with mutations (70.5%) than without mutations (48%). Half of the patients with mutations and 91% of the patients without mutations had improved vision. After adjusting for confounders, the logistic regression revealed that the patients with optic disc pallor on the first visit ($p = 0.004$) or the patients with the mitochondrial mutations ($p < 0.001$) had a poorer vision prognosis.

Conclusion: Our results indicated that carriers with *OPA1* mutations might be more vulnerable for the toxicity of EMB to develop EON.

Keywords: ethambutol, optic neuropathy, *OPA1*, mitochondrial DNA, mutation

INTRODUCTION

Ethambutol (EMB), one of the first-line drugs used to treat tuberculosis, works by inhibiting the arabinosyl transferase of mycobacteria (Belanger et al., 1996). However, its use is associated with a well-recognized ocular complication, ethambutol-induced optic neuropathy (EON), which is characterized by blurring of the vision, dyschromatopsia, and central or cecocentral scotoma

(Carr and Henkind, 1962). The ocular symptoms usually appear after 7 to 8 months of treatment with EMB, and the development of EON is both time- and dose-dependent (Fraunfelder et al., 2006; Lee et al., 2008). The incidence of EON is about 1% in patients prescribed an EMB dose at 15 mg/kg/d (Santaella and Fraunfelder, 2007; Yang et al., 2016). The risk factors for the occurrence of EON include older age, low body weight, and renal dysfunction (Chen et al., 2012). About 30 to 54% of the patients have varying degrees of vision recovery at 3 to 7 months after EMB discontinuation (Lee et al., 2008; Ezer et al., 2013); however, some patients have severe and permanent visual loss, even without the known risk factors. Therefore, other predisposing factors might exist for EON.

At present, the pathophysiology of EON still remains unclear. Several previous studies have indicated that EMB disrupts energy metabolism and the network structure of mitochondria by inducing severe vacuole formation and by decreasing membrane potential (Chung et al., 2009; Guillet et al., 2010). Dotti et al. (1998) first described the m.G11778A mitochondrial DNA (mtDNA) mutation in an EON patient, pointing to a relationship between mitochondrial mutation and the development of EON. Leber's hereditary optic neuropathy (LHON) is caused by mtDNA mutations that disrupt complex I activity of the mitochondrial respiratory chain and ATP synthesis (Zhang et al., 2018). Autosomal dominant optic atrophy (ADOA) is another form of mitochondrial optic neuropathy that is caused by mutations of the *OPA1* gene (Delettre et al., 2000). The *OPA1* gene encodes a dynamin-related GTPase, which is localized at the inner membrane of mitochondria and plays a role in mitochondrial fusion (Kao et al., 2015).

Both LHON and ADOA have a common pathophysiological outcome, which is mitochondrial energy deficiency and retinal ganglion cell apoptosis (Kao et al., 2015; Zhang et al., 2018). The current literature reports 8 patients carrying LHON mtDNA mutations and 2 patients harboring *OPA1* mutations who developed optic neuropathy during the use of EMB (Dotti et al., 1998; De Marinis, 2001; Hwang et al., 2003; Chowdhury et al., 2006; Ikeda et al., 2006; Guillet et al., 2010; Pradhan et al., 2010; Seo et al., 2010). Most of these studies are case reports, and the final clinical diagnosis is controversial for those patients. The relationship between the mitochondrial mutations and the clinical features of EON has not been fully studied.

In the present study, we investigated the presence of mitochondrial mutations (*OPA1* and LHON-mtDNA) in a cohort of 47 patients with EON. We also studied the effects of these mutations on the clinical features of the patients by performing genetic analysis and identified disease-causing gene mutations in 22 patients.

MATERIALS AND METHODS

Patients

This study was approved by the Medical Ethics Committee of Beijing Tongren Hospital. All investigations followed the tenets of the Declaration of Helsinki. Clinical data were retrospectively collected from outpatient and hospitalized patients diagnosed with EON from 2011 to 2018 at the Department of Ophthalmology in Chinese People's Liberation Army General Hospital and at the Genetics Laboratory of the Beijing Institute of Ophthalmology at Beijing Tongren Hospital. Blood was taken at initial presentation for genetic analysis with the patients' or their parents'/guardians' consent. We recruited a total of 47 unrelated patients, and 37 patients were followed up either by revisit evaluation (two patients) or by telephone surveys (35 patients). All patients underwent ophthalmological evaluations, including the best corrected visual acuity (BCVA), slit-lamp biomicroscopy, fundus examination, and color fundus photography. Some patients had color perception tests (Lanthony 15-Hue, Farnsworth D-15, or Ishihara color plates), Octopus or Humphry visual field tests, and spectral domain OCT examinations. We extracted genomic DNA from peripheral blood leukocytes from all patients and from available family members, following the manufacturer's instructions (Vigorous, Beijing, China).

The inclusion criteria for EON were based on previous guidelines (Fraunfelder et al., 2006; Lee et al., 2008). The diagnosis had to satisfy the major criterion and at least two of the minor criteria. The major criterion is vision loss appearing only after taking EMB and within 2 months after discontinuation of the drug. The minor criteria are: (1) abnormal results on color perception tests, and (2) central, paracentral, or cecocentral scotoma or temporal hemianopia on visual field examinations, and (3) optic disc hyperemia or pallor on color fundus photography. Exclusion criteria include optic neuritis, glaucoma, and other retinal diseases.

PCR-Based Sequencing of the *OPA1* Gene and Leber's Hereditary Optic Neuropathy-mtDNA

All coding regions of the *OPA1* gene and 19 primary LHON-mtDNA mutations were amplified by PCR in 36 patients. The primer sequences and the product lengths for amplification were described previously (Chen et al., 2014). The 19 primary LHON-mtDNA mutations included m.11778G > A, m.3460G > A, m.14484T > C, m.3376G > A, m.3635G > A, m.3697G > A, m.3700G > A, m.3733G > A, m.4171C > A, m.10197G > A, m.10663T > C, m.13051G > A, m.13094T > C, m.14459G > A, m.14482C > A, m.14482C > G, m.14495A > G, m.14502T > C, and m.14568C > T [1]. Purified PCR products were sequenced with an ABI PRISM 3730 DNA sequencer (Applied Biosystems, Foster City, CA, United States). Sequencing data were compared with the GenBank sequence for the *OPA1* gene (NM_015560) and mtDNA sequence (AC_000021.2).

Targeted Exome Sequencing

Eleven patients were investigated by TES with a capture panel including 194 known neuro-ophthalmological genes (**Supplementary Table 1**). The Illumina library preparation and capture experiments were performed as previously reported (Sun et al., 2018). Briefly, genomic DNA was fragmented

[1] https://www.mitomap.org

by endonuclease digestion and used to capture the targeted genomic sequences. The amplicon-based enrichment library was sequenced on an Illumina NextSeq 500 (Illumina, Inc., San Diego, CA, United States). After removing the sequencing adapters, low quality reads, and duplicated reads, the high quality reads were aligned with the reference human genome (hg19) using the Burrows-Wheeler Aligner. Single nucleotide polymorphisms and insertions or deletions were called using the Genomic Analysis Toolkit Haplotype Caller.

Bioinformatics Analysis

The potential functional impacts of missense mutations were evaluated with Polyphen-2 [2], Mutation Taster [3], and SIFT[4]. The effect of splicing mutations was analyzed with NetGene2[5] and BDGP [6]. The allele frequency of the variants was confirmed in the 1,000 Genome Project[7] and ExAC[8]. Co-segregation analysis was performed in available family members to verify the suspected mutations. We classified the variants into pathogenic, likely pathogenic, uncertain of significant, likely benign, and benign according to the guidelines published by the American Academy of Medical Genetics and Genomics (ACMG) (Richards et al., 2015).

Statistical Analysis

We converted the Snellen ratios into logarithm of the minimum angle of resolution (logMAR) values for statistical purpose. LogMAR values of 0, 1.0, and 2.0 are equal to a Snellen vision of 1.0, 0.1, and counting fingers, respectively (Holladay, 1997). The Wilcoxon rank sum test and Pearson Chi-square or Fisher's exact test were used to analyze the quantitative and categorical data, respectively. The Kruskal–Wallis test or multivariate logistic regression was used to analyze correlations. We performed all statistical analysis using SPSS version 22 software (IBM Corporation, New York, United States). The statistical significance level was 5%.

RESULTS

Mitochondrial Mutation Detection Rate and Related Mutations

We detected *OPA1* and LHON-mtDNA mutations in 22 of the 47 patients with EON, for an overall mutation detection rate of 46.8%. Mutations in 15 patients were detected by Sanger sequencing and mutations in 7 patients were detected by TES (**Supplementary Table 2**). The average coverage of the TES was 99.8%. The average sequencing depth was 288X. About 99% of the data had a depth of 10X or more.

We identified 15 distinct mutations of the *OPA1* gene in 18 patients (**Supplementary Figure 1**), for a detection rate of 38.3%. According to the ACMG guidelines, 13 mutations were defined as pathogenic and two mutations were defined as likely pathogenic (**Table 1**). Of these mutations, 8 were newly detected in the current study. These mutations included five (33.3%) nonsense, four (26.5%) frameshift indels, three (20%) splicing defects, two (13.3%) missense, and one (7%) large deletion mutation (**Table 1**). The most common mutation was c.2708_2711delTTAG (p.V903Gfs*3), with an allele frequency of 22.2% (4/18); the remaining 14 mutations were detected only once. The eight novel mutations included three frameshift indels, two missense, one splicing effect, one nonsense, and one large deletion. None of these novel mutations were observed in the public databases. The two missense mutations were predicted as disease-causing by three *in silico* analysis programs (**Table 1**).

We detected the m.11778G > A mutation in two patients and the m.14484T > C mutation in two patients. The detection rate of LHON-mtDNA mutations was 8.5%.

Demographics and Clinical Characteristics of All Patients

The 47 patients in the current study included 31 males and 16 females, for a male-to-female ratio of 1.9:1 (**Supplementary Table 2**). Of these patients, seven had a family history of optic neuropathy, two carrying an *OPA1* mutation and four harboring an mtDNA mutation. The mean age of presentation was 39 years (range 16–74 years). The mean daily dose of EMB was 12.9 mg/kg (range 3.8–29.2 mg/kg) and the mean medication duration was 4 months (range 1–24 months). All patients had a major complaint of blurred vision, and 41 (87.2%) of them experienced the visual impairment simultaneously in both eyes. The mean course of the disease, defined as the time interval from the vision loss to the first visit, was 2 months (range 0.5–24 months). Eight patients had a complaint of ocular pain, numbness of a lower extremity, or hearing loss. Their mean BCVA was 1.0 (logMAR; range 0.5–1.3), which was not correlated with their daily EMB dose ($p = 0.646$), their medication duration ($p = 0.099$), or the course of their disease ($p = 0.939$).

Fundus examination revealed a symmetrical fundus appearance in 43 patients (91.5%). Of the 94 eyes, 46 (48.9%) showed optic disc hyperemia and retinal nerve fiber layer (RNFL) swelling, 15 (16.0%) had temporal disc pallor, nine (9.6%) presented with nasal disc hyperemia and temporal disc pallor, four (4.2%) showed total disc pallor, and 20 (21.3%) presented a normal optic disc appearance (**Figure 1**). Unilateral retinal hemorrhage was observed in four patients (**Figure 2**). The result of logistic regression showed that the patients with optic disc pallor had a longer course of disease compared with patients with optic disc hyperemia or with normal optic disc appearance ($p < 0.001$).

Of the 33 patients (61 eyes) who had a color perception test, 23 eyes (37.7%) presented with red/green color vision impairment, 22 eyes (36.1%) showed total color blindness, eight eyes (13.1%) presented with yellow/blue color vision impairment, and eight eyes (13.1%) showed normal color perception. Of the

[2] http://genetics.bwh.harvard.edu/pph2/
[3] http://www.mutationtaster.org/
[4] http://provean.jcvi.org/index.php
[5] http://www.cbs.dtu.dk/services/NetGene2/
[6] http://www.fruitfly.org/seq_tools/splice.html
[7] http://browser.1000genomes.org/index.html
[8] http://exac.broadinstitute.org/

TABLE 1 | Fifteen mutations of the *OPA1* gene identified in this study.

cDNA change	Protein change	Protein domain	Allele number	Polyphen-2	Mutation Taster	SIFT	PROVEAN	NetGene2	BDGP	1000G	ExAC	gnomAD	References	ACMG
c.32 + 1G > C	-	basic	1		DC			donor loss	donor loss	N	N	N	This study	P
c.154C > T	p.R52X	basic	1		DC					N	N	4.02E-06	Ban et al., 2007	P
c.544_545 insT	p.T184Yfs*11	-	1		DC					N	N	N	This study	P
c.934C > T	p.R312X	GTPase	1		DC					N	N	N	Cardaioli et al., 2006	P
exon12-17 deletion	-	GTPase, dynamin	1		-					N	N	N	This study	P
c.1516 + 1G > A	-	GTPase	1		DC			donor loss	donor loss	N	N	N	Santarelli et al., 2015	P
c.1631T > A	p.L544X	dynamin	1		DC					N	N	N	This study	P
c.1847 + 1_+ 4del	-	dynamin	1		DC			donor loss	donor loss	N	N	N	Ferré et al., 2009	P
c.1808A > C	p.D603A	dynamin	1	PD	DC	D	Deleterious	no splice sites change	no splice sites change	N	N	N	This study	LP
c.2111T > A	p.V704D	dynamin	1	PD	DC	D	Deleterious	no splice sites change	no splice sites change	N	N	N	This study	LP
c.2121_2124del	p.S708Lfs*14	dynamin	1		DC					N	N	N	This study	P
c.2131C > T	p.R711X	dynamin	1		DC					N	N	N	Delettre et al., 2001	P
c.2197C > T	p.R733X	dynamin	1		DC					N	N	N	Li et al., 2008	P
c.2246_2247insTTA	p.E749Dfs*2	dynamin	1		DC					N	N	N	This study	P
c.2708_2711delTTAG	p.V903Gfs*3	GTPase effector	4		DC					N	N	N	Delettre et al., 2000	P

PD, probably damaging; DC, disease causing; D, damaging; N, none; P, pathogenic; LP, likely pathogenic.

33 patients (66 eyes) who had a visual field examination, 31 eyes (47%) presented with central scotoma, 23 eyes (34.8%) showed cecocentral scotoma, six eyes (9.1%) presented with paracentral scotoma, and six eyes (9.1%) showed temporal hemianopia.

The 37 patients were followed up over time (range 1–87 months), with a mean follow-up time of 15 months. Patient E005, carrying *OPA1* mutation p.R52X, and patient A3124, without mutations, underwent revisit examinations. After 4 years of follow-up, the BCVA of patient E005 improved from 0.02 in the right eye and 0.04 in the left eye to 0.1 in both eyes. The RNFL thickness at the temporal side of binocular optic discs was below the limits (**Figure 3**). After 11 months of follow-up, the BCVA of patient A3124 improved from 0.05 in the right eye and 0.03 in the left eye to 0.5 and 0.3, respectively. Fundus photography showed the optic disc hyperemia resolved at follow-up in both eyes (**Figure 3**). Of the remaining patients, 26 patients stated their VA had improved, eight patients reported their VA was unchanged, and one patient said his VA had worsened. None of patients with VA improved underwent cataract surgery or other intervention that would affect the assessment of visual outcome. The mean recovery time of the VA was 4 months (range 1–12 months). After adjusting for any confounders, the logistic regression revealed that the patients with optic disc pallor on the first visit ($p = 0.004$) or the patients with the mitochondrial mutations ($p < 0.001$) had a poorer vision prognosis (**Supplementary Table 3**).

Comparison of Patients With Mitochondrial Mutations and Without Mutations

To simplify the description and statistical analysis, we divided the 47 patients into two groups: group 1 consisted of the patients carrying mitochondrial mutations and group 2 included the patients without mitochondrial mutations. We compared the difference in the demographics, EMB medications (**Table 2**), and clinical characteristics (**Table 3**) between the patients in the two groups. The mean visiting age was significantly younger in group 1 (27.5 years) than in group 2 (48 years). The percentage of patients with a family history was statistically higher in group 1 (27%) than in group 2 (4%). The percentage of eyes with optic disc hyperemia was higher in group 1 than in group 2. The visual outcome was better for group 2 than for group 1. Among the nine patients whose VA did not improve, six patients (66.7%) carried *OPA1* mutations and one patient (11.1%) carried the m.G11778A mutation.

DISCUSSION

The current study investigated the mitochondrial mutations in 47 unrelated patients with EON and described the clinical characteristics of the patients. We identified *OPA1* mutations in 18 (38.3%) patients and LHON-mtDNA mutations in four (8.5%) patients. EON is a dose-dependent form of toxic neuropathy related to several other risk factors, such as renal dysfunction and older age (Santaella and Fraunfelder, 2007; Chen et al., 2012; Yang et al., 2016). In the current cohort, 91.5% of the patients with EON had taken low-dose EMB (≤ 15mg/kg/day),

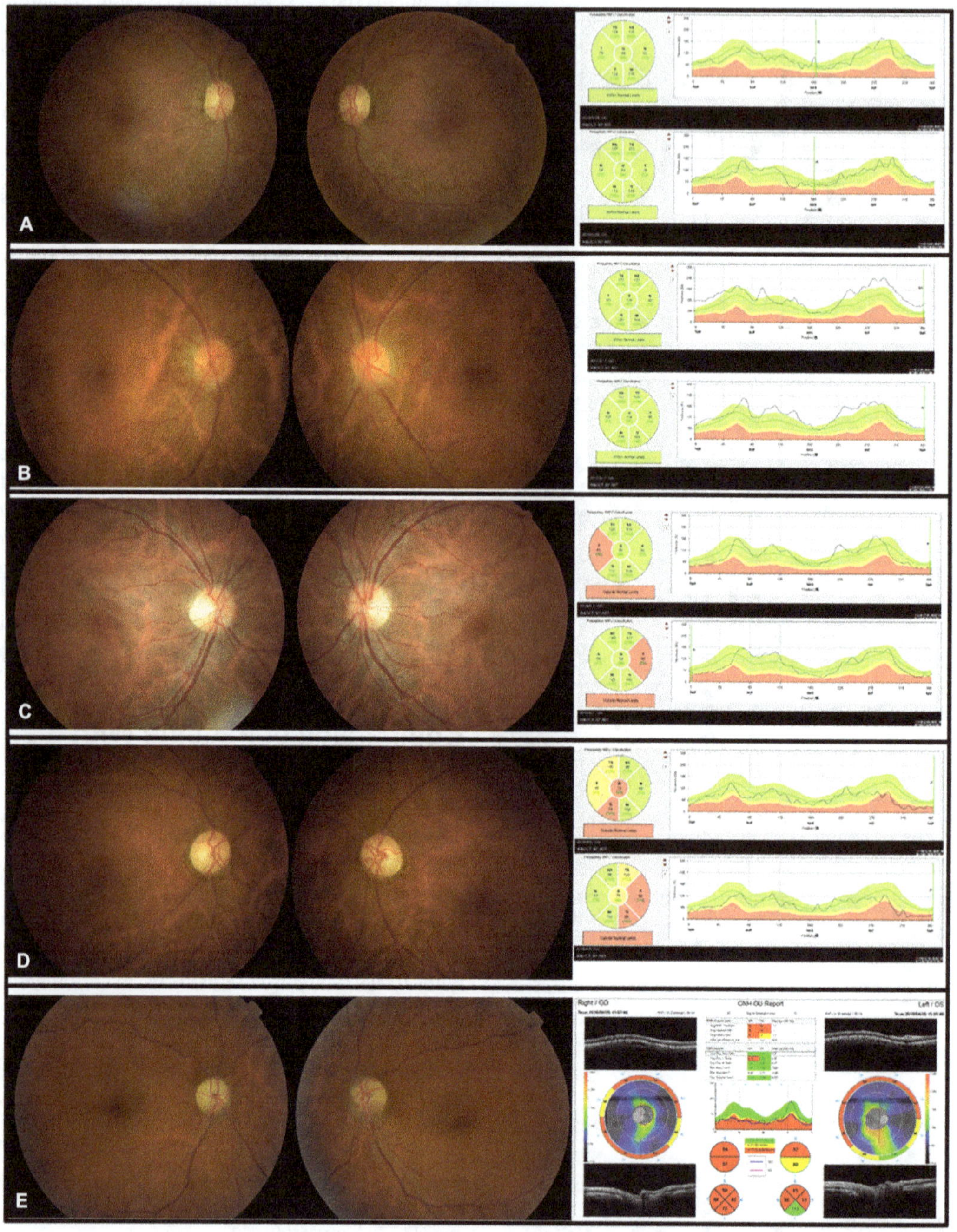

FIGURE 1 | Five kinds of disc appearances and OCT images in five patients with EON. **(A)** The disc appearance and the RNFL thickness were normal. **(B)** The optic discs were hyperemic. The superior, temporal, and inferior RNFL was thickened. **(C)** The border of the nasal discs was blurred and the temporal discs were pale. The temporal RNFL thickness was thinner than normal. **(D)** The temporal discs were pale and the temporal RNFL became thin. **(E)** The optic discs were pale, with the inferior border of the disc blurred in the left eye.

95.7% of the patients had a normal renal function, and 89.4% of the patients were younger than 60 years; therefore, the risk of developing ocular toxicity was relatively low in our cohort. Our results suggested that mitochondrial genetic variations, and especially *OPA1* mutations, are major predisposing factors for the occurrence of toxic optic neuropathy.

Mutations of the *OPA1* gene are responsible for 50–70% of ADOA, (Cohn et al., 2007; Yu-Wai-Man et al., 2010) which is the most common form of inherited optic neuropathy. *OPA1*-related ADOA is usually a mild and slowly progressive disorder (Cohn et al., 2007). Typically, patients suffer an insidious, symmetrical, and progressive visual defect in their childhood; however, the

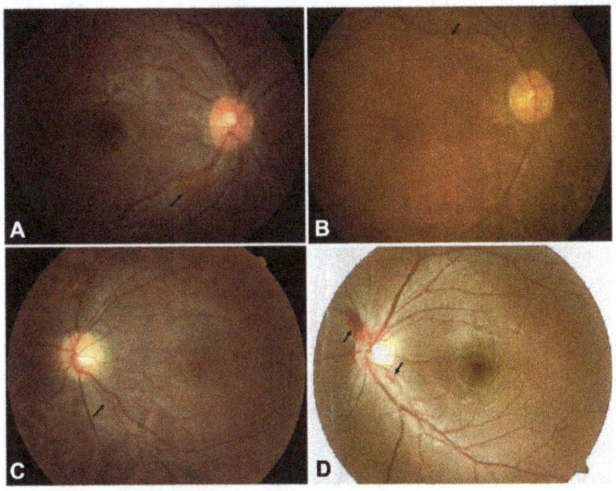

FIGURE 2 | Fundus appearance of 4 patients with retinal hemorrhage (black arrows). **(A)** Retinal hemorrhage located at the inferior temporal side of the optic disc in the right eye of the patient A781. **(B)** Retinal hemorrhage located at the superior temporal side of the optic disc in the right eye of the patient A2579. **(C)** Retinal hemorrhage located at the inferior temporal side of the optic disc in the left eye of the patient A3198. **(D)** Retinal hemorrhages located at the border of the optic disc in the left eye of the patient E004.

severity of visual impairment is highly variable (Cohn et al., 2007). About 10–20% of mutation carriers are "asymptomatic," as they have a normal visual acuity or only a subtle visual disturbance (Cohn et al., 2007; Yu-Wai-Man et al., 2010). In the current cohort, we identified different kinds of mutations of the *OPA1* gene, but the type and location of these mutations were similar to those reported in typical patients with ADOA, (Cohn et al., 2007; Ferré et al., 2009; Yu-Wai-Man et al., 2010; Chen et al., 2014) except for the low frequency (13%, 2/15) of missense mutations. This frequency was only the half rate observed previously in patients with ADOA (approximately 27%) (Chen et al., 2014). Another previous study indicated that vision loss was usually more severe in patients with missense mutations than with null mutations (Yu-Wai-Man et al., 2010). Unlike the typical patients with ADOA, the *OPA1* mutation carriers in the current study all experienced a subacute visual loss while taking EMB therapy, and none of them noticed a visual abnormality before the treatment; therefore, they might be "asymptomatic" cases. In addition, 71% of the *OPA1* mutation carriers presented optic disc hyperemia, which has never been observed in typical patients with ADOA. By contrast, only 20% of those carriers showed temporal disc pallor, which is a prominent optic appearance in patients with ADOA (41–86%) (Cohn et al., 2007; Yu-Wai-Man et al., 2010; Chen et al., 2014). Four patients harboring the most common mutation c.2708_2711delTTAG had different fundus appearance. We speculate that the difference in the fundus performance may be due to the different course of vision loss of patients. In a previous study, Pradhan et al. described a 36-year old man who suffered a bilateral, painless visual loss during his anti-tuberculosis treatment that included EMB

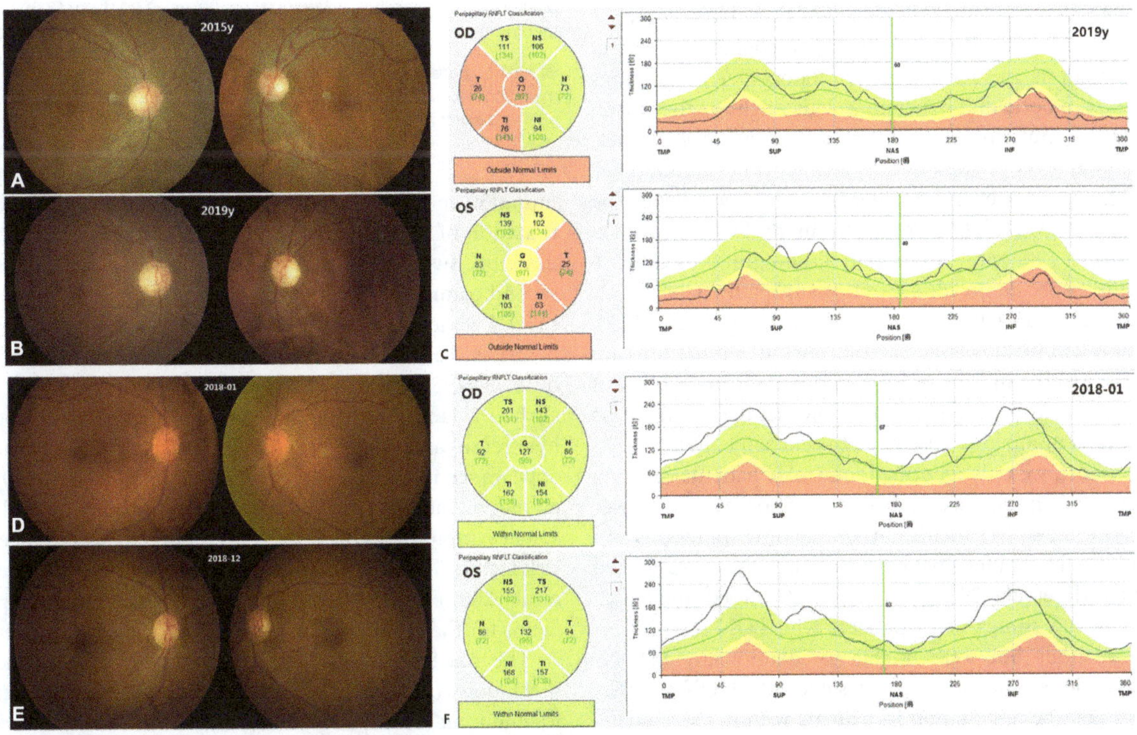

FIGURE 3 | Fundus appearance and OCT images on the first visit and at follow-up for patient E005 **(A–C)** and patient A3124 **(D–F)**. In the patient E005, the fundus appearance did not change. The temporal RNFL in both eyes was below the normal limits at follow-up **(C)**. In the patient A3124, the color and border of the optic discs turned normal. The RNFL was thickened in both eyes on the first visit **(F)**.

TABLE 2 | Comparison of the demographic and the EMB medication of the two groups of patients.

	Group 1	Group 2	*P* value
No. of patients	22	25	–
OPA1 mutant allele, *N* (%)	18 (81.8)	0	–
MtDNA mutant allele, *N* (%)	4 (18.2)	0	–
Male, N (%)	17 (77.27)	14 (56.00)	0.125‡
Mean age at presentation, years (range)	27.50 (16.00–73.00)	48.00 (17.00–74.00)	0.006†
Family history, *N* (%)	6 (27.27)	1 (4.00)	0.025‡
Smoking, *N* (%)	3 (15.00)	2 (8.00)	0.458‡
Renal dysfunction, *N* (%)	0 (0.00)	2 (9.52)	0.179§
Mean daily dose, mg/kg/d (range)	12.90 (3.80–16.90)	12.90 (8.80–29.20)	0.943†
Mean medication time, months (range)	3.75 (1.40–22.00)	5.00 (1.00–24.00)	0.864†

Group 1, patients with mitochondrial mutations; Group 2, patients without mitochondrial mutations; ‡Pearson χ2 test; † Wilcoxon rank sum test; § Fisher's exact test.

TABLE 3 | Comparison of the clinical characteristic of the two groups of patients.

	Group 1	Group 2	*P* value
Mean LogMAR BCVA (range)	1.22 (0.10–1.70)	1.00 (0.10–2.00)	0.453†
Mean course of the vision loss, months (range)	2.00 (0.50–10.00)	2.00 (0.50–24.00)	0.497†
Disc appearance, eyes (%)	44 (100.00)	50 (100.00)	0.020‡
Normal	4 (9.09)	16 (32.00)	
Hyperemia	31 (70.45)	24 (48.00)	
Pallor	9 (20.46)	10 (20.00)	
Color vision, eyes (%)	24 (100.00)	37 (100.00)	0.607‡
Normal	3 (12.50)	5 (13.51)	
Red/green color vision impairment	7 (29.17)	16 (43.24)	
Yellow/blue color vision impairment	3 (12.50)	5 (13.51)	
Total color blindness	11 (45.83)	11 (29.74)	
Visual field, eyes (%)	34 (100.00)	32 (100.00)	0.059§
Central scotoma	18 (52.94)	13 (40.63)	
Paracentral scotoma	4 (11.76)	2 (6.25)	
Cecocentral scotoma	12 (35.30)	11 (34.38)	
Temporal hemianopia	0 (0.00)	6 (18.74)	
Vision outcomes, patients (%)	14 (100.00)	23 (100.00)	0.016‡
Improved	7 (50.00)	21 (91.30)	
Unchanged	6 (42.86)	2 (8.70)	
Decreased	1 (7.14)	0 (0.00)	
Mean recovery time, months (range)	6.00 (2.00–12.00)	3.00 (1.00–12.00)	0.107†

Group 1, patients with mitochondrial mutations; Group 2, patients without mitochondrial mutations; †Wilcoxon rank sum test; ‡Pearson χ2 test; §Fisher's exact test.

(Pradhan et al., 2010). This patient also had optic disc hyperemia and peripapillary hemorrhage. After a series of differential diagnoses, the researchers finally identified a nonsense p.R38X *OPA1* mutation in this patient and inferred that the visual loss in that patient had been exacerbated following EMB therapy. We speculate that optic disc hyperemia is an acute response to the toxic effect of EMB; consequently, a concomitant effect of *OPA1* mutations and EMB toxicity renders *OPA1* mutations carriers prone to optic disc hyperemia. This might be the reason why the *OPA1* mutations carriers presented more optic disc hyperemia than was observed in the patients without mutations, even though both groups had a similar disease time course. The mutation rate (38.3%) of *OPA1* mutations in this EON cohort was higher than that (9.6 and 7.6%) reported in a group of Chinese patients with suspected hereditary optic neuropathy (Chen et al., 2014) and other Han Chinese population (Zhang et al., 2017). One reason might be the patients harboring *OPA1* mutations are more sensitive to the toxicity of EMB and present more obvious visual defects as our mentioned above. Another reason might be due to the small number of patients in the current cohort.

In this cohort, we only identified four male patients carrying a LHON-mtDNA mutation, and this rate (8.5%) was much lower than the rate (38.3%) in patients harboring *OPA1* mutations and the rate (33%) in Chinese patients with LHON or suspected with LHON (Ji et al., 2008; Yu et al., 2010). Hwang et al. (2003) screened a cohort of 24 patients with EON for LHON-mtDNA mutations but were unable to identify any LHON-mtDNA mutations. Therefore, the existence of LHON-mtDNA mutations might be uncommon in patients with EON. To date, twelve patients (including our four patients) have been reported to develop optic neuropathy while taking EMB (**Table 4**; Dotti et al., 1998; De Marinis, 2001; Chowdhury et al., 2006; Ikeda et al., 2006; Seo et al., 2010). Ten of these patients carried mutation m.11778G > A, which is the most common primary mutation of LHON (Chen et al., 2014). In the present study, we described two patients carrying the m.14484T > C mutation (the second commonest primary mutation of LHON) who developed LHON while taking EMB (**Table 4**). Unlike the eight previously described cases, the four patients in our cohort had a younger onset age (48 years vs. 21.5 years). In addition, these four patients all had a family history, and three of them showed optic disc hyperemia and RNFL pseudoedema, which is a typical fundus appearance in the acute stage of LHON (Chen et al., 2014). Not all individuals who carry LHON-mtDNA mutations will develop visual symptoms, as the occurrence of LHON usually needs other risk factors, like heavy smoking and alcohol consumption (Sadun et al., 2003). EMB might have been a trigger or an epigenetic factor for the manifestation of LHON in these four patients.

The toxicity of EMB is related to its zinc-chelating effect and its metabolites (Chung et al., 2009). At present, the exact mechanism for the toxic neuropathy induced by EMB remains unclear, but increasing evidence indicates a relationship with mitochondrial dysfunction. In an early study, Heng et al. found that EMB was specifically toxic to retinal ganglion cells and that it caused ganglion cell degeneration by a glutamate excitotoxic pathway

TABLE 4 | Clinical features of reported patients with EMB-induced LHON.

ID	Onset age (years)	Gender	Medication time (months)	BCVA (OD/OS)	Follow-up time (months)	Follow-up BCVA (OD/OS)	Optic disc finding (OD/OS)	Mutation	References
1	50–55	M	8	0.5/0.04	24	0.5/0.04	TEP/TEP	m.G11778A	Dotti et al., 1998
2	50–55	M	11	0.5/0.04	21	1.0/0.7	normal/normal	m.G11778A#	De Marinis, 2001
3	65–70	F	12	0.2/0.05	6	0.3/0.09	–	m.G11778A	Ikeda et al., 2006
4	65–70	F	3	0.03/0.03	12	0.01/0.01	normal/normal	m.G11778A	Ikeda et al., 2006
5	30–35	M	4	0.3/0.15	1	0.06/HM	H/H	m.G11778A	Chowdhury et al., 2006
6	40–45	M	4	0.1/0.1	5	FC/FC	normal/H	m.G11778A	Seo et al., 2010
7	20- 25	M	12	0.6/1.0	15	FC/FC	H/H	m.G11778A	Seo et al., 2010
8	30–35	F	4	FC/FC	-	-	TOP/TOP	m.G11778A	Seo et al., 2010
A2061	15–20	M	12	0.06/0.06	-	-	H/H	m.G11778A	This study
A2290	20–25	M	18	FC/FC	24	FC/FC	TEP/TEP	m.G11778A	This study
A781	15–20	M	12	0.8/0.02	–	–	H*/H	m.T14484C	This study
A1780	25–30	M	7	0.1/0.3	–	–	H/H	m.T14484C	This study

*F, female; M, male; FC, finger counting; HM, hand move; TEP, temporal pallor; H, hyperemia; TOP, total pallor; *hemorrhage; #heteroplasmic.*

(Heng et al., 1999). LHON-mtDNA and *OPA1* mutations also cause damage to the small-caliber papillomacular bundle axons (Barboni et al., 2010) therefore, the clinical features of EON, LHON, and ADOA partially overlap. All three conditions show color vision abnormality and visual field defects. In the current cohort, most patients presented central or cecocentral scotoma, which could be observed in both EON and LHON or ADOA, whereas only three patients in group 2 showed temporal hemianopia, which is a typical visual field defect of EMB-related optic chiasmopathy (Jayanetti et al., 2017). In this cohort, the majority of patients presented with red/green color vision impairment or total color blindness, while only two patients carrying *OPA1* mutations displayed yellow/blue color vision impairment, which is a typical color defect of ADOA (Cohn et al., 2007). Fundus hemorrhage is not common in LHON or ADOA, and three of the four patients with fundus hemorrhage were in group 2, indicating it to be one of the EON clinical features. Our results showed that the mean age was significantly younger in the patients with mitochondrial mutations (27.5 years; group 1) than in the patients without mutations (48 years; group 2), further demonstrating that mitochondrial mutation was an important risk factor for the occurrence of EON, especially in young tuberculosis patients. Patients carrying mitochondrial mutations (*OPA1* or mtDNA) may be more vulnerable to the toxicity of EMB. Of the seven patients with a family history, six patients were mutation carriers; therefore, physicians should carefully question patients with tuberculosis or their family members about ophthalmic problems before EMB is prescribed.

Consistent with the observation by Lee et al. (2008) we found that the visual prognosis was related to the initial fundus appearance of the patients with EON. Up to 79.8% of the patients in our cohort showed normal optic disc appearance or optic disc hyperemia, which suggested they were in the early stage of EON. This might be a reason why our patients had a higher visual recovery rate (75.7%) than the rates described in other EON studies (23.1–47%) (Lee et al., 2008; Ezer et al., 2013). Another reason for this high rate might be due to that the 94.6% VA improvement was reported by patients subjectively; this is one limitation of the current study. Nevertheless, we still observed that the visual outcome was better in the patients in group 2 than in group 1, suggesting that the mitochondrial mutations were a critical factor affecting visual prognosis of patients with EON. Of the eight patients carrying mutation m.11778G > A, only one patient who harbored a heteroplasmic mutation showed VA improvement, (De Marinis, 2001) whereas the other patients all experienced VA decreases or no change during their follow-up (**Table 4**). Another limitation of the current study is that we did not take into account the ocular toxicity of other anti-tuberculosis drugs, such as isoniazid. The third limitation is that since the study was retrospective in nature, the examinations were not standardized.

In conclusion, our results indicated that carriers with *OPA1* mutations might be more vulnerable for the toxicity of EMB to develop EON, whereas the exact effect of these *OPA1* mutations has not been confirmed in future functional assays. Although mitochondrial mutation screening is not possible in all patients prior to anti-tuberculosis medication, genetic analysis should be strongly recommended for patients with a family history of optic neuropathy.

ETHICS STATEMENT

The studies involving human participants were reviewed and approved by Medical Ethics Committee of Beijing Tongren Hospital. The patients/participants provided their written informed consent to participate in this study.

AUTHOR CONTRIBUTIONS

X-HZ participated in the data collection, data analysis, and manuscript preparation. YX, KX, and KC participated in the data collection and analysis. Q-GX contributed in the study design and data collection. Z-BJ, YL, and S-HW participated in the study design and the manuscript revision. All authors contributed to the article and approved the submitted version.

REFERENCES

Ban, Y., Yoshida, Y., Kawasaki, S., and Mochida, C. (2007). A novel mutation of the OPA1 gene in a Japanese patient with autosomal dominant optic atrophy. *Graefes Arch. Clin. Exp. Ophthalmol.* 245, 1581–1583. doi: 10.1007/s00417-007-0598-1

Barboni, P., Carbonelli, M., Savini, G., Ramos Cdo, V., Carta, A., Berezovsky, A., et al. (2010). Natural history of Leber's hereditary optic neuropathy: longitudinal analysis of the retinal nerve fiber layer by optical coherence tomography. *Ophthalmology* 117, 623–627. doi: 10.1016/j.ophtha.2009.07.026

Belanger, A. E., Besra, G. S., Ford, M. E., Mikusová, K., Belisle, J. T., Brennan, P. J., et al. (1996). The embAB genes of Mycobacterium avium encode an arabinosyl transferase involved in cell wall arabinan biosynthesis that is the target for the antimycobacterial drug ethambutol. *Proc. Natl. Acad. Sci. U. S. A.* 93, 11919–11924. doi: 10.1073/pnas.93.21.11919

Cardaioli, E., Gallus, G. N., Da Pozzo, P., Rufa, A., Franceschini, R., Motolese, E., et al. (2006). A novel mutation producing premature termination codon at the OPA1 gene causes autosomal dominant optic atrophy. *J. Neurol.* 253, 672–673. doi: 10.1007/s00415-005-0057-z

Carr, R. E., and Henkind, P. (1962). Ocular manifestations of ethambutol, Toxic amblyopia after administration of an experimental antituberculous drug. *Arch. Ophthalmol.* 67, 566–571. doi: 10.1001/archopht.1962.00960020566009

Chen, H. Y., Lai, S. W., Muo, C. H., Chen, P. C., and Wang, I. J. (2012). Ethambutol-induced optic neuropathy: a nationwide population-based study from Taiwan. *Br. J. Ophthalmol.* 96, 1368–1371. doi: 10.1136/bjophthalmol-2012-301870

Chen, J., Xu, K., Zhang, X., Jiang, F., Liu, L., Dong, B., et al. (2014). Mutation screening of mitochondrial DNA as well as OPA1 and OPA3 in a Chinese cohort with suspected hereditary optic atrophy. *Invest. Ophthalmol. Vis. Sci.* 55, 6987–6995. doi: 10.1167/iovs.14-14953

Chowdhury, B., Nagpaul, A. K., and Chowdhury, D. (2006). Leber's hereditary optic neuropathy masquerading as ethambutol-induced optic neuropathy in a young male. *Indian J. Ophthalmol.* 54, 218–219. doi: 10.4103/0301-4738.27091

Chung, H., Yoon, Y. H., Hwang, J. J., Cho, K. S., Koh, J. Y., and Kim, J. G. (2009). Ethambutol-induced toxicity is mediated by zinc and lysosomal membrane permeabilization in cultured retinal cells. *Toxicol. Appl. Pharmacol.* 235, 163–170. doi: 10.1016/j.taap.2008.11.006

Cohn, A. C., Toomes, C., Potter, C., Towns, K. V., Hewitt, A. W., Inglehearn, C. F., et al. (2007). Autosomal dominant optic atrophy: penetrance and expressivity in patients with OPA1 mutations. *Am. J. Ophthalmol.* 143, 656–662. doi: 10.1016/j.ajo.2006.12.038

De Marinis, M. (2001). Optic neuropathy after treatment with anti-tuberculous drugs in a subject with Leber's hereditary optic neuropathy mutation. *J. Neurol.* 248, 818–819. doi: 10.1007/s004150170103

Delettre, C., Griffoin, J. M., Kaplan, J., Dollfus, H., Lorenz, B., Faivre, L., et al. (2001). Mutation spectrum and splicing variants in the OPA1 gene. *Hum. Genet.* 109, 584–591. doi: 10.1007/s00439-001-0633-y

Delettre, C., Lenaers, G., Griffoin, J. M., Gigarel, N., Lorenzo, C., Belenguer, P., et al. (2000). Nuclear gene OPA1, encoding a mitochondrial dynamin-related protein, is mutated in dominant optic atrophy. *Nat. Genet.* 26, 207–210. doi: 10.1038/79936

Dotti, M. T., Plewnia, K., Cardaioli, E., Manneschi, L., Rufa, A., Alemà, G., et al. (1998). A case of ethambutol-induced optic neuropathy harbouring the primary mitochondrial LHON mutation at nt 11778. *J. Neurol.* 245, 302–303. doi: 10.1007/s004150050223

Ezer, N., Benedetti, A., Darvish-Zargar, M., and Menzies, D. (2013). Incidence of ethambutol-related visual impairment during treatment of active tuberculosis. *Int. J. Tuberc. Lung Dis.* 17, 447–455. doi: 10.5588/ijtld.11.0766

Ferré, M., Bonneau, D., Milea, D., Chevrollier, A., Verny, C., Dollfus, H., et al. (2009). Molecular screening of 980 cases of suspected hereditary optic neuropathy with a report on 77 novel OPA1 mutations. *Hum. Mutat.* 30, E692–E705.

Fraunfelder, F. W., Sadun, A. A., and Wood, T. (2006). Update on ethambutol optic neuropathy. *Expert Opin. Drug Saf.* 5, 615–618.

Guillet, V., Chevrollier, A., Cassereau, J., Letournel, F., Gueguen, N., Richard, L., et al. (2010). Ethambutol-induced optic neuropathy linked to OPA1 mutation and mitochondrial toxicity. *Mitochondrion* 10, 115–124. doi: 10.1016/j.mito.2009.11.004

Heng, J. E., Vorwerk, C. K., Lessell, E., Zurakowski, D., Levin, L. A., and Dreyer, E. B. (1999). Ethambutol is toxic to retinal ganglion cells via an excitotoxic pathway. *Invest. Ophthalmol. Vis. Sci.* 40, 190–196.

Holladay, J. T. (1997). Proper method for calculating average visual acuity. *J. Refract. Surg.* 13, 388–391. doi: 10.3928/1081-597x-19970701-16

Hwang, J. M., Kim, J., and Park, S. S. (2003). Leber's hereditary optic neuropathy mutations in ethambutol-induced optic neuropathy. *J. Neurol.* 250, 87–89. doi: 10.1007/s00415-003-0960-0

Ikeda, A., Ikeda, T., Ikeda, N., Kawakami, Y., and Mimura, O. (2006). Leber's hereditary optic neuropathy precipitated by ethambutol. *Jpn. J. Ophthalmol.* 50, 280–283. doi: 10.1007/s10384-005-0308-7

Jayanetti, V., Rossiter-Thornton, M., Azar, D., and Fraser, C. L. (2017). Sibling Ethambutol optic chiasmopathy. *Neuroophthalmology* 42, 40–43. doi: 10.1080/01658107.2017.1322616

Ji, Y., Zhang, A. M., Jia, X., Zhang, Y. P., Xiao, X., Li, S., et al. (2008). Mitochondrial DNA haplogroups M7b1'2 and M8a affect clinical expression of leber hereditary optic neuropathy in Chinese families with the m.11778G->a mutation. *Am. J. Hum. Genet.* 83, 760–768. doi: 10.1016/j.ajhg.2008.11.002

Kao, S. H., Yen, M. Y., Wang, A. G., Yeh, Y. L., and Lin, A. L. (2015). Changes in mitochondrial morphology and bioenergetics in human lymphoblastoid cells with four novel OPA1 mutations. *Invest. Ophthalmol. Vis. Sci.* 56, 2269–2278. doi: 10.1167/iovs.14-16288

Lee, E. J., Kim, S. J., Choung, H. K., Kim, J. H., and Yu, Y. S. (2008). Incidence and clinical features of ethambutol-induced optic neuropathy in Korea. *J. Neuroophthalmol.* 28, 269–277. doi: 10.1097/wno.0b013e31818e3c6b

Li, Y., Deng, T., Tong, Y., Peng, S., Dong, B., He, D., et al. (2008). Identification of two novel OPA1 mutations in Chinese families with autosomal dominant optic atrophy. *Mol. Vis.* 14, 2451–2457.

Pradhan, M., Sharp, D., Best, S., Vincent, A., and Vaphiades, M. (2010). Drug-induced optic neuropathy-TB or not TB. *Surv. Ophthalmol.* 55, 378–385. doi: 10.1016/j.survophthal.2009.10.005

Richards, S., Aziz, N., Bale, S., Bick, D., Das, S., Gastier-Foster, J., et al. (2015). Standards and guidelines for the interpretation of sequence variants: a joint consensus recommendation of the American College of Medical Genetics and Genomics and the Association for Molecular Pathology. *Genet. Med.* 17, 405–424. doi: 10.1038/gim.2015.30

Sadun, A. A., Carelli, V., Salomao, S. R., Berezovsky, A., Quiros, P. A., Sadun, F., et al. (2003). Extensive investigation of a large Brazilian pedigree of 11778/haplogroup J Leber hereditary optic neuropathy. *Am. J. Ophthalmol.* 136, 231–238. doi: 10.1016/s0002-9394(03)00099-0

Santaella, R. M., and Fraunfelder, F. W. (2007). Ocular adverse effects associated with systemic medications: recognition and management. *Drugs* 67, 75–93. doi: 10.2165/00003495-200767010-00006

Santarelli, R., Rossi, R., Scimemi, P., Cama, E., Valentino, M. L., La Morgia, C., et al. (2015). OPA1-related auditory neuropathy: site of lesion and outcome of cochlear implantation. *Brain* 138, 563–576. doi: 10.1093/brain/awu378

Seo, J. H., Hwang, J. M., and Park, S. S. (2010). Antituberculosis medication as a possible epigenetic factor of Leber's hereditary optic neuropathy. *Clin. Exp. Ophthalmol.* 38, 363–366. doi: 10.1111/j.1442-9071.2010.02240.x

Sun, T., Xu, K., Ren, Y., Xie, Y., Zhang, X., Tian, L., et al. (2018). Comprehensive molecular screening in Chinese Usher syndrome patients. *Invest. Ophthalmol. Vis. Sci.* 59, 1229–1237. doi: 10.1167/iovs.17-23312

Yang, H. K., Park, M. J., Lee, J. H., Lee, C. T., Park, J. S., and Hwang, J. M. (2016). Incidence of toxic optic neuropathy with low dose ethambuol. *Int. J. Tuberc. Lung Dis.* 20, 261–264. doi: 10.5588/ijtld.15.0275

Yu, D., Jia, X., Zhang, A. M., Li, S., Zou, Y., Zhang, Q., et al. (2010). Mitochondrial DNA sequence variation and haplogroup distribution in Chinese patients with LHON and m.14484T>C. *PLoS One* 5:e13426. doi: 10.1371/journal.pone.0013426

Yu-Wai-Man, P., Griffiths, P. G., Burke, A., Sellar, P. W., Clarke, M. P., Gnanaraj, L., et al. (2010). The prevalence and natural history of dominant optic atrophy due to OPA1 mutations. *Ophthalmology* 117, 1538–1546. doi: 10.1016/j.ophtha.2009.12.038

Zhang, A. M., Bi, R., Hu, Q. X., Fan, Y., Zhang, Q., and Yao, Y. G. (2017). The OPA1 gene mutations are frequent in Han Chinese patients with suspected optic neuropathy. *Mol. Neurobiol.* 54, 1622–1630. doi: 10.1007/s12035-016-9771-z

Zhang, J., Ji, Y., Lu, Y., Fu, R., Xu, M., Liu, X., et al. (2018). Leber's hereditary optic neuropathy (LHON)-associated ND5 12338T > C mutation altered the assembly and function of complex I, apoptosis and mitophagy. *Hum. Mol. Genet.* 27, 1999–2011. doi: 10.1093/hmg/ddy107

20

Screening and Functional Analysis of TEK Mutations in Chinese Children With Primary Congenital Glaucoma

Yunsheng Qiao[1], *Yuhong Chen*[1,2,3], *Chen Tan*[1], *Xinghuai Sun*[1,2,3], *Xueli Chen*[1,2,3]* *and Junyi Chen*[1,2,3]*

[1]*Department of Ophthalmology and Visual Science, Eye and ENT Hospital, Shanghai Medical College, Fudan University, Shanghai, China,* [2]*NHC Key Laboratory of Myopia, Chinese Academy of Medical Sciences, Shanghai Key Laboratory of Visual Impairment and Restoration (Fudan University), Shanghai, China,* [3]*State Key Laboratory of Medical Neurobiology and MOE Frontiers Center for Brain Science, Institutes of Brain Science, Fudan University, Shanghai, China*

Correspondence:
Junyi Chen
chenjy@fudan.edu.cn
Xueli Chen
xueli_chen@fudan.edu.cn

Purposes: Recent studies have suggested that loss-of-function mutations of the tunica intima endothelial receptor tyrosine kinase (TEK) are responsible for approximately 5% of primary congenital glaucoma (PCG) cases in diverse populations. However, the causative role of TEK mutations has not been studied in Chinese PCG patients. Here, we report the mutation spectrum of TEK after screening a large cohort of PCG patients of Chinese Han origin and analyze the identified variants in functional assays.

Methods: TEK-targeted next-generation sequencing (NGS) was performed in 200 PCG patients. Candidate variants were prioritized by mutation type and allele frequency in public datasets. Plasmids containing wild type and identified variants of TEK were constructed and used to assess protein expression, solubility, receptor auto-phosphorylation, and response to ligand stimulation in cell-based assays.

Results: Ten missense and one nonsense heterozygous variants were detected by NGS in 11 families. The clinical features of TEK variants carriers were comparable to that of TEK-mutated patients identified in other populations and CYP1B1-mutated individuals from in-house database. Functional analysis confirmed four variants involving evolutionarily conserved residues to be loss-of-function, while one variant (p.R1003H) located in tyrosine kinase domain seemed to be an activating mutation. However, our results did not support the pathogenicity of the other five variants (p.H52R, p.M131I, p.M228V, p.H494Y, and p.L888P).

Conclusion: We provide evidence for TEK variants to be causative in Chinese PCG patients for the first time. Attention needs to be paid to TEK mutations in future genetic testing.

Keywords: TEK receptor tyrosine kinase, primary congenital glaucoma, next generation sequencing, mutations, functional analysis

INTRODUCTION

In healthy eyes, the intraocular pressure (IOP) is maintained by dynamic balance between aqueous humor production *via* ciliary body and drainage through trabecular and uveoscleral pathway (Johnson et al., 2017). Developmental defects of aqueous outflow structures can give rise to elevated IOP and early-onset glaucoma, causing buphthalmos, cornea stretching, optic disc cupping, and irreversible blindness (Lewis et al., 2017). Affecting children in the first 3 years of life, primary congenital glaucoma (PCG) is the most common form of infantile glaucoma with isolated angle anomalies (Young et al., 2020).

Genetic factors serve a critical role in the pathogenesis of PCG. To date, mutations of CYP1B1, LTBP2, MYOC, FOXC1, TEK, and ANGPT1 have been implicated in PCG patients from diverse populations (Stoilov et al., 1997; Kaur et al., 2005; Ali et al., 2009; Chakrabarti et al., 2009; Souma et al., 2016; Thomson et al., 2017). However, the molecular basis of PCG remains largely unrevealed, especially for patients of Chinese Han origin with CYP1B1 heterozygous and homozygous mutations accounting for only 17.2% of cases and no mutations of LTBP2 being identified (Chen et al., 2008; Chen et al., 2016).

Haploinsufficiency of TEK (Tunica intima endothelial receptor tyrosine kinase, Gene ID: 7010) caused by heterozygous loss-of-function mutations was reported to be causative for 5% of multiethnic PCG patients characterized by autosomal dominant inheritance with decreased penetrance and variable expressivity (Souma et al., 2016). This gene encodes a transmembrane receptor tyrosine kinase (Tie2) involved in cardiovascular development and homeostasis (Saharinen et al., 2017). Activating mutations of TEK have been identified as the genetic causes for most inherited and sporadic cases of venous malformation (VM) (Vikkula et al., 1996; Limaye et al., 2009). Notably, TEK is also expressed in the endothelia of Schlemm's canal (SC) and collector channels, vital components of conventional aqueous outflow pathway (van Zyl et al., 2020). Conditional knockout of TEK from embryonic day 17.5 caused completely absent SC and significantly increased IOP, while heterozygous TEK deletion led to a severely hypomorphic SC and elevated IOP in mice (Souma et al., 2016). This dose–effect relationship clearly demonstrated that the normal function of Tie2 is indispensable during angle development.

For the first time, we performed TEK-targeted next generation sequencing in a large cohort of Chinese PCG patients aiming to verify the causative role and depict the mutation spectrum of TEK in this population.

MATERIALS AND METHODS

Study Participants

Two hundred patients along with their parents were enrolled *via* the Eye and ENT Hospital Biobank from 2004 to 2018. The diagnosis of PCG must agree with the following criteria: (1) expansion of corneal diameter, corneal clouding, or Haab's striae; (2) IOP >21 mm Hg; (3) optic nerve cupping or asymmetric cup-to-disc ratio; and (4) disease onset before age 3. Other developmental glaucoma or secondary glaucoma, such as Peter's anomaly, Axenfeld–Rieger syndrome, and aniridia were excluded.

All PCG cases were confirmed by glaucoma specialists before surgery under general anesthesia. Anterior segment examination and corneal diameter measurement were performed with the aid of surgical microscopes. IOP was measured using a Tono-PEN tonometry (Mentor, Norwell, MA, United States). The structures of anterior chamber angle and the optic disc were observed under gonioscopy whenever possible. Five milliliters of venous blood was collected from each PCG patient and his/her parents and preserved in the biobank for genomic DNA extraction.

Next Generation Sequencing and Variants Prioritization

In this study, a customized panel with 58 pairs of primers was designed to cover the coding regions and 50-bp sequences flanking the splice sites of TEK gene (**Supplementary Table S1**). DNA samples were amplified by multiplex PCR and sequenced by a Hiseq4000 platform (Illumina, San Diego, CA). Sequencing reads were aligned to the human reference genome assembly (hg19). Variants were called by Genome Analysis Toolkit (version 3.70) and annotated by ANNOVAR (Wang et al., 2010). Exonic and splice site (±5 bp) variants with an allele frequency <0.1% in the Genome Aggregation database (gnomAD_all and gnomAD_eas) were validated by Sanger sequencing and selected for further analysis. Additionally, four probands were exome sequenced using a SureSelect Human All Exon Kit (Aglient, Santa Clara, CA, United States) and the aforementioned Hiseq4000 platform. When available, parental DNA samples were also subjected to Sanger sequencing for co-segregation analysis.

In Silico Functional Study

Twelve *in silico* tools were integrated to predict the pathogenicity of non-synonymous variations, including SIFT (Sim et al., 2012), Polyphen-2 (Adzhubei et al., 2010), LRT (Chun and Fay, 2009), MutationTaster (Schwarz et al., 2014), MutationAssessor (Reva et al., 2011), FATHMM (Shisha et al., 2013), PROVEN (Choi and Chan, 2015), VEST (Carter et al., 2013), Meats (Kim et al., 2017), M-CAP (Jagadeesh et al., 2016), CADD (Kircher et al., 2014), and DANN (Quang et al., 2015). Multiple Tie2 protein sequences from different species were retrieved to evaluate the evolutionary conservation of affected residues. To assess the effect of residue substitution on protein structure and stability, the FoldX plugin for YASARA (Van Durme et al., 2011) was used to calculate the free energy change induced by specific mutations with three repetitions each, and the resulting structures were visualized with YASARA View (Krieger and Vriend, 2014). For variants located within immunoglobulin (Ig)-like domains and the epidermal growth factor (EGF)-like domain, the Tie2 ligand-binding domain crystal structure (PDB ID: 2GY5, 23-445 aa) was utilized as the template (Barton et al., 2006). Additionally, crystal structure of the membrane proximal three fibronectin type III (FNIII) domains of Tie2 (PDB ID: 5UTK, 438-741 aa) and Tie2 kinase domain (PDB: 1FVR, 798-1124 aa) were used as templates for respective missense variants (Moore et al., 2017) (Shewchuk et al., 2000).

Cloning of TEK-Expressing Plasmids

The full-length human TEK cDNA (reference sequence: NM_000459.5, 4,683 bp) with 3x Flag (DYKDDDDK) tag was cloned into the pCDNA3.1-ZsGreen vector (**Supplementary Figure S1A**). Site-directed mutagenesis was performed to introduce mutations into TEK-expressing vectors. Specifically, two plasmids (Y1024X-Flag and TEK1023-Flag, **Supplementary Figures S1B, C**) were generated to verify the nonsense mutation p.Y1024*. All plasmids were validated by Sanger sequencing.

Western Blot Analysis

Wild-type (WT) or mutant TEK-Flag plasmids (1 μg) were transfected into subconfluent 293T cells in six-well dishes using Lipofectamine 2000 (Life Technologies, Carlsbad, CA). Twenty-four hours later, cells were lysed by 1% Triton X-100, centrifuged, and separated into supernatant and insoluble pellets. Radioimmunoprecipitation assay (RIPA) buffer was added to the pellets before sonication. Same amount of proteins (15 μg) was separated by electrophoresis and transferred to polyvinylidene fluoride (PVDF) membranes. After blocking with 5% non-fat milk, antibodies against phosphotyrosine (1:3,000; ab179530, Abcam, Cambridge, United Kingdom) and Flag (1:5,000; 20543-1-AP, Proteintech, Rosemont, IL, United States) were used to detect the phosphorylation and expression of Flag-tagged Tie2, respectively. β-Actin (1:5,000; 66009-1-Ig, Proteintech, Rosemont, IL, United States) was used as a loading control. For proteasomal inhibition assay, transfected 293T cells were treated with 5 μM MG132 (MedChemExpress, Shanghai, China) for 24 h before harvest.

Quantitative Real-Time PCR

Total RNA was extracted from 293T cells using EZ-press RNA Purification Kit (EZBioscience, Roseville, MN, United States) 24 h after transfection. One thousand nanograms of RNA was used for reverse transcription and subsequent quantitative PCR in CFX96TM real-time system (Bio-Rad, Hercules, CA, United States). The housekeeping gene ACTB was used as the internal control. All mRNA variants were normalized to WT-TEK using the δ-delta Ct method. The primers are listed below: forward primer, 5′-TCCAGGCAACTTGACTTCGG-3; reverse primer, 5′-CCTTGAACCTTGTAACGGATAG-3.

TEK Localization Assay

Human umbilical vein endothelial cells (HUVECs) were obtained from ScienCell and cultured using endothelial cell medium (ScienCell, Carlsbad, CA, United States). Cells were transfected with either WT or mutant TEK-Flag plasmids by electroporation with Neon transfection system (Thermo Fisher, MA, United States) following the manufacturer's instructions. The transfected cells were seeded on glass coverslips in 24-well dishes. After 48 h, cells were either directly fixed with 4% paraformaldehyde for 15 min at room temperature or stimulated with 600 ng/ml recombinant human Angiopoietin 1 (R&D systems, Minneapolis, MN, United States) for another 30 min at 37°C before fixation. Cells were then permeabilized and blocked by 5% goat serum and 0.3% TritonX-100 in phosphate-buffered saline (PBS) for an hour at room temperature and incubated overnight at 4°C with anti-Flag antibody (1:200; 66008-3-Ig, Proteintech, Rosemont, IL, United States) and anti-ZO1 antibody (1:500; 21773-1-AP, Proteintech, Rosemont, IL, United States). Cyanine3- and Cyanine5-conjugated secondary antibodies (Thermo Fisher, MA, United States) were used to detect Flag and ZO-1 signals, respectively. Cell nuclei were stained by 4,6-diamidino-2-phenylindole (DAPI) (1 μg/ml; Sigma-Aldrich, St. Louis, MO, United States) for 5 min. Images were taken with a fluorescence microscope (DM4000 B, Leica, Wetzlar, Germany).

Statistical Analysis

Statistical analysis was performed with Stata software (15.1, StataCorp). Continuous variables were compared using Student's *t*-test or paired *t*-test, while Pearson chi-square test was applied to comparing categorical variables. A p value <0.05 was considered statistically significant.

RESULTS

Identification of Rare/Novel TEK Variants

An average read depth of 1,938.3 was achieved in this study, while 99.3% of the targeted regions had 100x coverage per base. In total, 44 TEK variants were detected in 199 samples. Among these, 11 rare or novel heterozygous nonsynonymous variants were identified in 11 unrelated patients (**Table 1** and **Supplementary Figure S2**). Four variants (p.R1003H, p.H52R, p.H494Y, and p.Y1024*) co-segregated with the glaucoma phenotype. Other six variants were inherited from unaffected parents, consistent with the autosomal dominant pattern with decreased penetrance and variable expressivity suggested by Souma and others (Souma et al., 2016).

One mutation (p.A841V) was previously identified in a large American pedigree by Young et al. (2020). In addition, a different amino acid change in proline residue 244 (p.P244R) was also reported in the same study. The nonsense mutation (p.Y1024*) was confirmed by Western blotting (**Supplementary Figure S1D**). The truncated protein lacks tyrosine residues for phosphorylation in C-terminus (e.g., 1,102 and 1,108), which are indispensable in mediating cellular signals. Therefore, it was reasonable to speculate that these variants were detrimental to protein function.

The remaining eight missense variants differed in pathogenicity prediction. Half of them (p.C264F, p.L504P, p.L888P, and p.R1003H) involved evolutionarily conserved residues (**Supplementary Figure S3**) and evaluated as destabilizing by FoldX (**Table 1**), whereas the other four variants (p.H52R, p.M131I, p.M228V, and p.H494Y) were predicted to be benign by most *in silico* tools.

Since family 01-07 were previously confirmed negative for CYP1B1 and LTBP2 mutations, probands from family 08-11 were exome sequenced to explore mutations in other known disease-causing genes. C-354 was found to inherit the nonsense mutation of TEK (p.Y1024*) and a missense variant of CYP1B1 (p.L107V) from his affected father. C-350 carried an additional missense

TABLE 1 | TEK variants identified in 11 families.

Family ID	Patient ID	Chromosomal position	Exons	DNA change	Amino acid change	gnomAD_all	gnomAD_eas	In silico predictions	Average ddG
01	C-9	27217702	exon19	c.3008G > A	p.R1003H	0.000012	0.000054	11|12	2.55
02	C-56	27168521	exon3	c.393G > A	p.M131I			2|12	0.81
03	C-39	27192508	exon11	c.1511T > C	p.L504P			8|12	4.16
04	C-64	27172667	exon5	c.682A > G	p.M228V	0.000032	0.000272	0|12	0.36
05	C-99	27209206	exon16	c.2663T > C	p.L888P			10|12	2.33
06	C-151	27157931	exon2	c.155A > G	p.H52R	0.000028	0	0|12	−0.55
07	C-165	27172715	exon5	c.730C > T	p.P244S			8|12	4.00
08	C-270	27206737	exon15	c.2522C > T	p.A841V	0.000004	0	11|12	1.40
09	C-290	27190679	exon10	c.1480C > T	p.H494Y			0|12	−0.55
10	C-350	27173250	exon6	c.791G > T	p.C264F			10|12	8.48
11	C-354	27218784	exon20	c.3072T > A	p.Y1024X			3|3	NA

Chromosomal positions correspond to GRCh37/hg19 assembly. Reference TEK mRNA, sequence, NM_000459.4. Reference TEK, protein sequence, NP_000450.2. gnomAD_all, allele frequency in all populations from gnomAD, dataset. gnomAD_eas, allele frequency in East Asian populations from gnomAD, dataset. In silico *predicitons were made combining 12 programs listed in* Methods, *and presented as "Number of deleterious predictions | Number of total predictions". Changes in Gibbs free energy were calculated via FoldX plugin for YASARA (average of three repetitions).*

TABLE 2 | Comparison of clinical characteristics of TEK-mutated PCG cohorts.

	Souma et al. (2016)	Young et al. (2020)	This study	*p*-value
Mutation rate (%)	10/189 (5.3)	NA	11/200 (5.5)	0.931[a]
Penetrance (%)	14/22 (63.6)	13/21 (61.9)	13/19 (68.4)	0.979[a]
Sex (male: female)	9:5	6:11	8:3	0.103[a]
Bilaterally: unilaterally involvement	6:6	10:4	7:4	0.470[a]
Age at onset (month, mean ± SD)	3.73 ± 7.1	7.27 ± 7.2	9.55 ± 10.2	0.162[b]

[a]*Pearson's chi squared test.*
[b]*Kruskal–Wallis test.*

variant of LTBP2 (p.T886K) from her mother compared to her unaffected father. No rare or novel variants of MYOC, FOXC1, and ANGPT1 were detected (**Supplementary Table S2**).

Clinical Characteristics of TEK-Mutated PCG Patients

In this study, 5.5% of PCG patients carried rare or novel variants of TEK (**Table 2**). Of the carriers, 13 out of 19 (68.4%) exhibited clinically identifiable glaucoma phenotypes starting from 9.5 months after birth on average. There appeared to be a gender predilection, as most cases were male. In addition, more patients were bilaterally affected. Eight patients were followed up for disease prognosis (**Table 3**). Most of them (5/8) remained stable after initial trabeculotomy. Two patients underwent secondary angle surgeries, and one was enucleated for ocular components.

There were no statistically significant difference between TEK-mutated PCG groups with regard to clinical features listed in **Table 2**. Similarly, the clinical presentations were comparable between Chinese patients with TEK mutations and those with CYP1B1 mutations or unidentified causes (**Table 4**).

Functional Impact of TEK Variants

All PCG-related TEK missense variants but p.A841V were tested in cell-based assays to evaluate their impact on protein expression, solubility, auto-phosphorylation, and response to ligand stimulation. First, WT and mutant TEK plasmids were overexpressed in 293T cells. The transcription levels of missense variants were all comparable to WT (**Supplementary Figure S4**). Three variants (p.P244S, p.C264F, and p.L504P) located in the ectodomain of Tie2 led to a dramatic reduction in protein expression in both soluble and insoluble fractions (**Figure 1**). After inhibition of proteosomal activity by MG132, the insoluble fraction of p.P244S and p.C264F mutant was remarkably increased, suggesting significant protein degradation, whereas p.L504P was insensitive to MG132 treatment. P244 together with P243 is critical in the structure of a β-turn (**Figure 2**). Substitution of proline (non-polar) to a serine (polar) is likely to change protein conformation. As C264 forms a disulfide bond with C255, we inferred that the p.C264F variant might lead to the disruption of the disulfide bridge and misfolding of translation product. L504 locates in the E β-strand of fibronectin type IIIa (FNIIIa) domain, which contributes to a classical antiparallel β-sheet motif (Moore et al., 2017). The replacement of leucine by proline disrupted intra-strand hydrogen bond resulting in an energetically unstable structure.

Both protein expression and auto-phosphorylation levels of the other four variants in the ectodomain (p.H52R, p.M131I, p.M228V, and p.H494Y) were comparable to that of WT (**Supplementary Figure S5**), consistent with the *in silico* prediction of pathogenicity and structural analysis

TABLE 3 | Clinical information for TEK-mutated patients.

Family ID	Patient ID	Amino acid change	Sex	Age at onset	Eyes	Preoperative IOP (mmHg)	Cornea clouding	Corneal diameter (mm)	Cup–disc ratio	Treatment
01	C-9	p.R1003H	M	Birth	OD	20.6	No	12	0.5	Loss to follow-up
					OS	20.6	Haab's striae	13	0.7	
02	C-56	p.M131I	M	2y	OD	20.6	Macula	13	0.4	1 trabeculotomy
03	C-39	p.L504P	M	2y	OD	31	Clear	14.5	0.4	1 trabecolotomy in both eyes
					OS	48.5	Yes	16.5	0.9	
04	C-64	p.M228V	F	3 m	OD	34	Yes	14.5	0.9	Initial trabeculotomy and loss to follow-up
					OS	25	Yes	14.5	0.8	
05	C-99	p.L888P	M	2y	OD	50.62	Haab's striae	14	0.8	2 trabeculotomies in both eyes
					OS	54.66	Haab's striae	13	0.8	
06	C-151	p.H52R	F	Birth	OD	–	–	–	–	1 trabeculotomy and 1 trabecolectomy in both eyes
					OS	–	–	–	–	With subsequent tube shunt and enucleation of the left eye
07	C-165	p.P244S	M	Birth	OS	28	–	13.5	1.0	1 trabeculotomy
08	C-270	p.A841V	M	2 m	OS	42	Yes	13	1.0	1 trabeculotomy
09	C-290	p.H494Y	M	1y	OS	45	Yes	13	1.0	2 trabeculotomies
10	C-350	p.C264F	F	1y	OD	28	Haab's striae	13.5	1.0	1 trabeculotomy in both eyes
					OS	30.4	Haab's striae	13.5	1.0	
11	C-354	p.Y1024X	M	4 m	OD	31.8	–	13	–	Initial trabeculotomy in both eyes and loss to follow-up
					OS	29	–	12.5	–	

Sex: M, male; F, female. Age at onset: m, month; y, year. Eyes: OD, right eye; OS, left eye.

TABLE 4 | Comparison of clinical characteristics of PCG subgroups.

	CYP1B1	TEK	Unknown causes	*p*-value
Mutation rate (%)	20/124 (16.1)	11/200 (5.5)	NA	0.004[a]
Sex (Male: Female)	14:6	8:3	68:29	0.983[a]
Bilaterally: unilaterally involvement	12:8	7:4	46:51	0.398[a]
Age at onset (month, mean ± SD)	11.18 ± 13.04	9.55 ± 10.2	11.84 ± 12.49	0.647[b]
Preoperative IOP (mmHg)	40.94 ± 11.03	35.34 ± 5.89	35.45 ± 11.73	0.143[b]
Corneal diameter (mm)	13.26 ± 1.30	13.78 ± 1.15	13.35 ± 1.00	0.587[b]
Age at operation (day)	972.21 ± 1008.5	665.3 ± 564.5	718.51 ± 703.3	0.876[b]

[a]*Pearson's chi squared test.*
[b]*Kruskal–Wallis test.*

(**Supplementary Figure S6**). Notably, p.R1003H mutant was overexpressed in the insoluble component with increased auto-phosphorylation in the soluble fraction, matching the features of activating mutations (**Figure 3**). Structural analysis indicated that the *de novo* variant p.R1003H was likely to cause the disruption a hydrogen bond connecting R1003 with M1024 (**Figure 2**). However, variant p.L888P could not be distinguished from WT in our cell-based assay (**Figure 3**).

The ectodomain of Tie-2 consists of three Ig-like domains and an EGF-like domain, which are responsible for ligand binding (Yu et al., 2013), and a FNIII domain that is involved in ligand-induced receptor multimerization (Moore et al., 2017). Variants in these regions have the potential to weaken or disrupt ligand-mediated signaling. Thus, we transiently expressed all variants in HUVECs and explored their response to stimulation by potent agonist angiopoeitin-1 (ANGPT1). As anticipated, the WT TEK was diffusely expressed on the cytomembrane of HUVECs and relocalized to cell–cell junctions when treated with ANGPT1 (**Figure 4**). Surprisingly, the expression of variants p.P244S, p.C264F, and p.L504P was greatly reduced, consistent with the results of Western blotting. However, the other seven mutants did not exhibit significant alteration in response to ligand stimulation

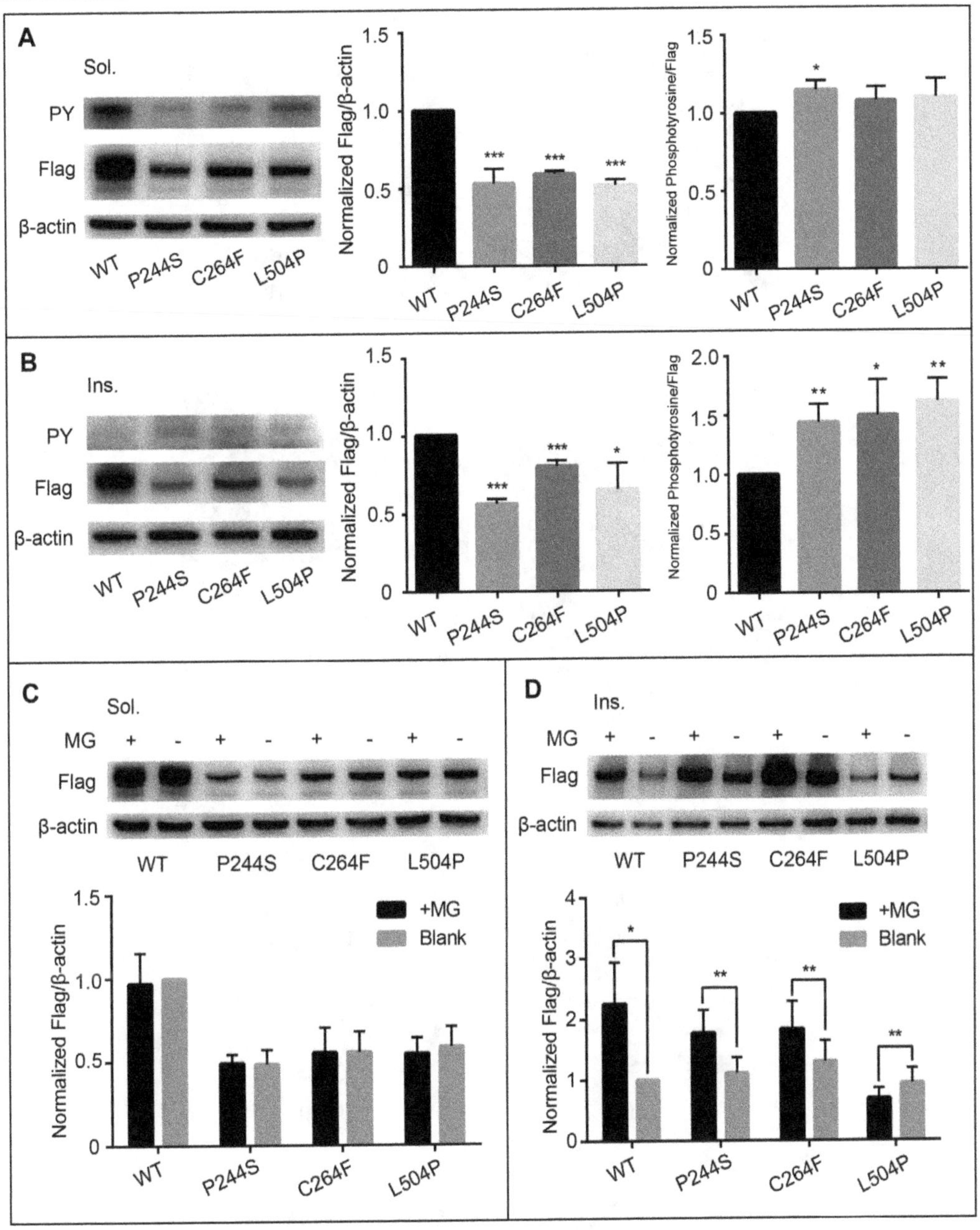

FIGURE 1 | Functional assessment of variants p.P244S, p.C264F, and p.L504P. The expression of soluble protein was significantly reduced **(A)** and remained unchanged after MG132 treatment **(C)**. No dramatic change in auto-phosphorylation was detected **(A)**. The expression of insoluble protein was also significantly reduced with increased phosphorylation level **(B)**. In addition, protein degradation was reversed in p.P244S and p.C264F, while p.L504P was unresponsive to proteasomal inhibition **(D)**. Sol, soluble; Ins, insoluble; PY, phosphotyrosine; WT, wild type; MG, MG132.

(**Figure 4**). A summary of functional analysis results is provided in **Supplementary Table S3**.

DISCUSSION

In this study, we screened for TEK mutations in a large cohort of Chinese PCG patients for the first time. Deep-targeted NGS yielded 10 rare/novel potentially pathogenic variants and one previously confirmed mutation. Subsequent cell-based functional study was able to classify four variants (p.P244S, p.C264F, p.L504P, and p.Y1024*) as loss-of-function, one (p.R1003H) as gain-of-function, while the remaining 5 (p.H52R, p.M131I, p.M228V, p.H494Y, and p.L888P) appeared to be benign.

The development of the vascular and lymphatic system relies upon the orderly expression of TEK (Dumont et al., 1994; Thomson et al., 2014). As an essential part of aqueous humor drainage pathway, SC shares striking similarities with lymphatic

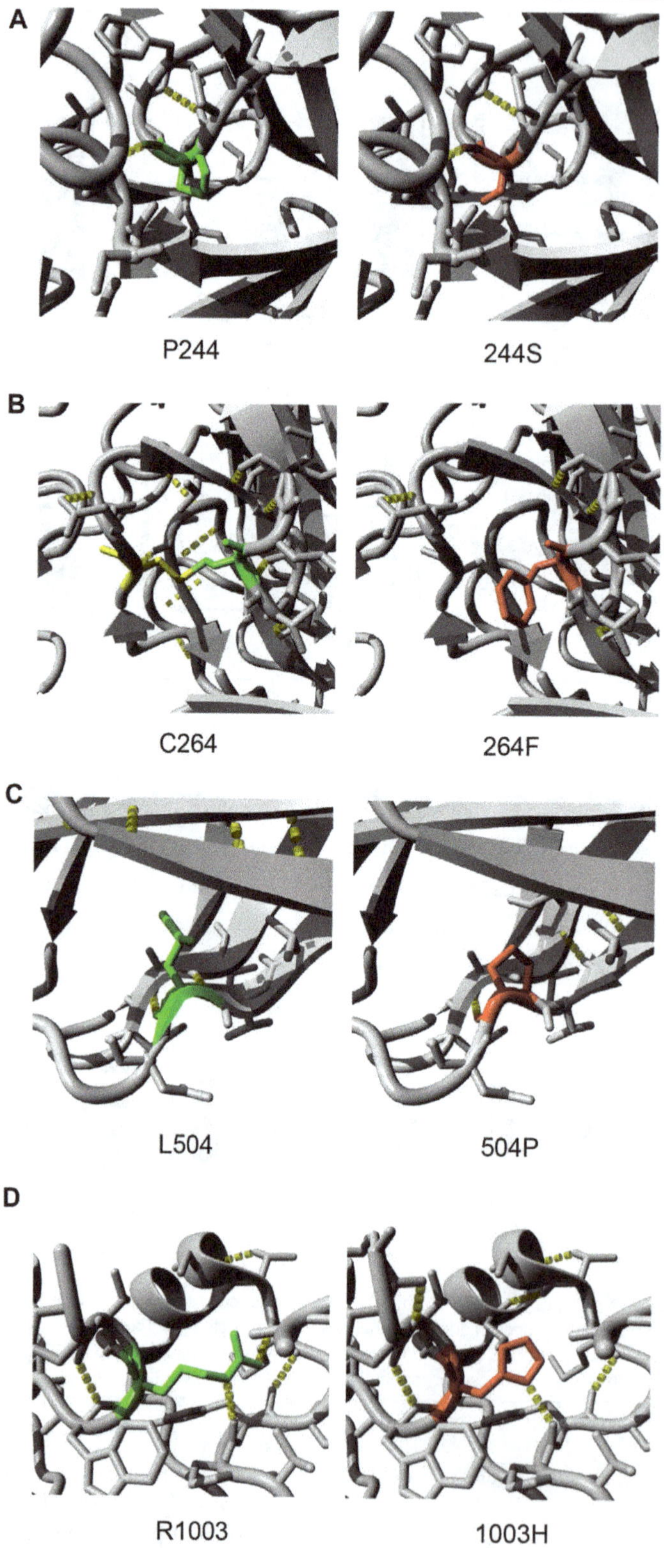

FIGURE 2 | Crystal structures of four pathogenic TEK mutants **(A)**. p.P244S substitutes a nonpolar proline to polar serine, which may influence the structure of a β-turn **(B)**. Cysteine-264 forms a disulfide bond with Cysteine-255. Thus, substitution of C264 was predicted to be destabilizing due to the disruption of a disulfide bond **(C)**. p.L504P is within a β-sheet of the FNIII domain; the substitution is likely to cause loss of hydrogen bonds, as is the case in p.R1003H **(D)**. Green, wild-type residue; red, mutated residue; yellow, cysteine-255; yellow dots, hydrogen bonds.

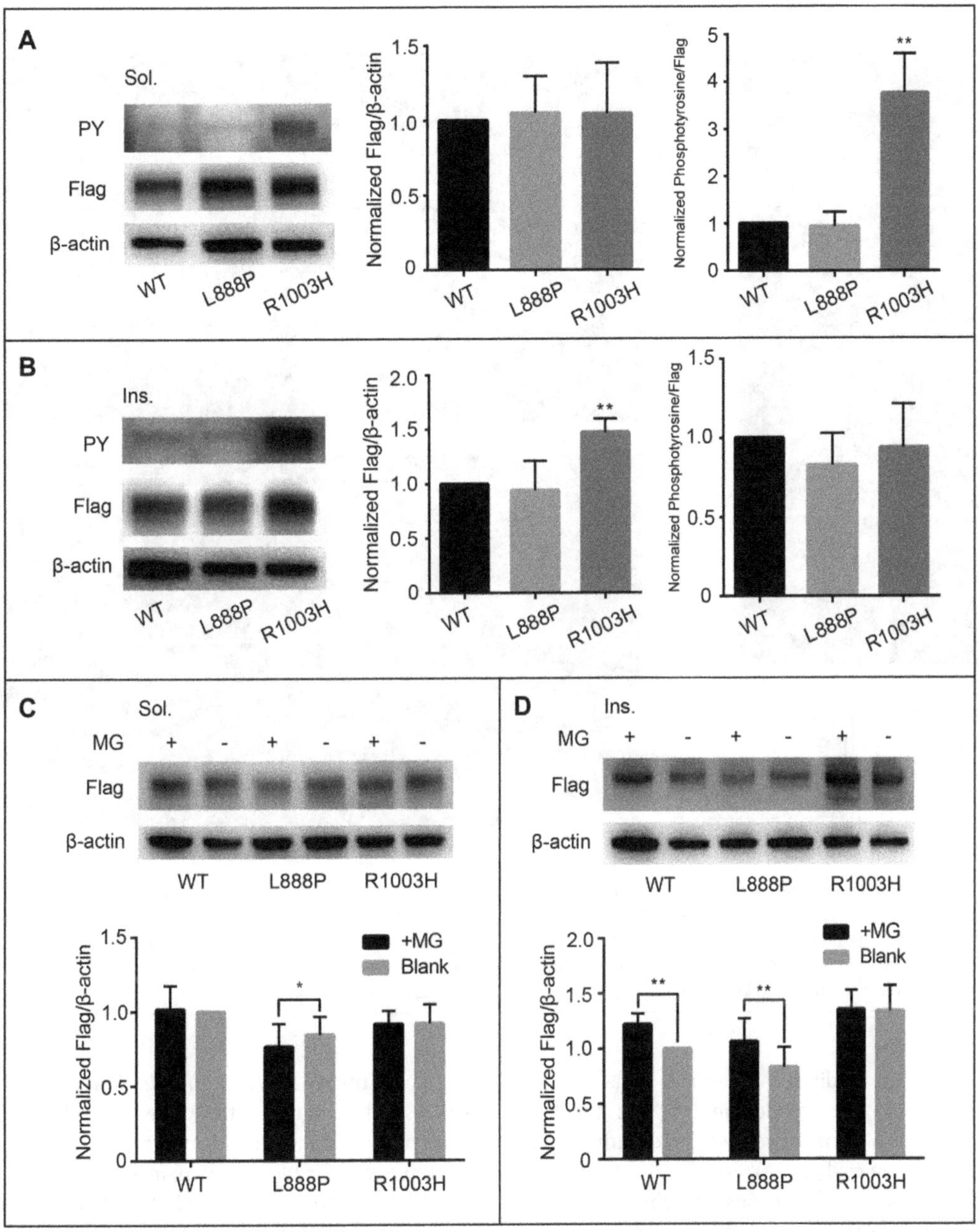

FIGURE 3 | Functional assessment of cytodomain variants p.L888P and p.R1003H. The protein expression and auto-phosphorylation levels of p.L888P are comparable to that of wild type **(A, B)**. However, p.R1003H is significantly phosphorylated in soluble portion **(A)** and enriched in insoluble fraction **(B)**, which does not respond to MG132 treatment **(C, D)**. Sol, soluble; Ins, insoluble; PY, phosphotyrosine; WT, wild type; MG, MG132.

vascular system (Aspelund et al., 2014). Indeed, some studies suggested SC as a specialized hybrid vessel with both lymphatic and vascular features (Ramos et al., 2007; Kizhatil et al., 2014). However, it was not until 2014 that an unintentional discovery linked the unique properties of SC and the pathogenesis of PCG (Thomson et al., 2014). Further studies delineated a clear dose effect between TEK function and SC morphology (Souma et al., 2016). Since then, more loss-of-function TEK mutations were reported in PCG patients with different ethnic backgrounds (Kabra et al., 2017; Young et al., 2020).

Despite being exhaustively investigated, the genetic cause of PCG remained largely unknown for most outbred populations (Mashima et al., 2001; Lim et al., 2013; Mohanty et al., 2013). In China, mutations in confirmed pathogenic genes only accounts for approximately 20% of PCG patients (Chen et al., 2008; Chen et al., 2016). Our results depicted the mutation spectrum of the recently reported causative gene and suggested the necessity of incorporating TEK in targeted panel for genetic diagnosis of PCG.

The incidence of TEK mutations in this study was similar to that of earlier reports (Souma et al., 2016; Kabra et al., 2017;

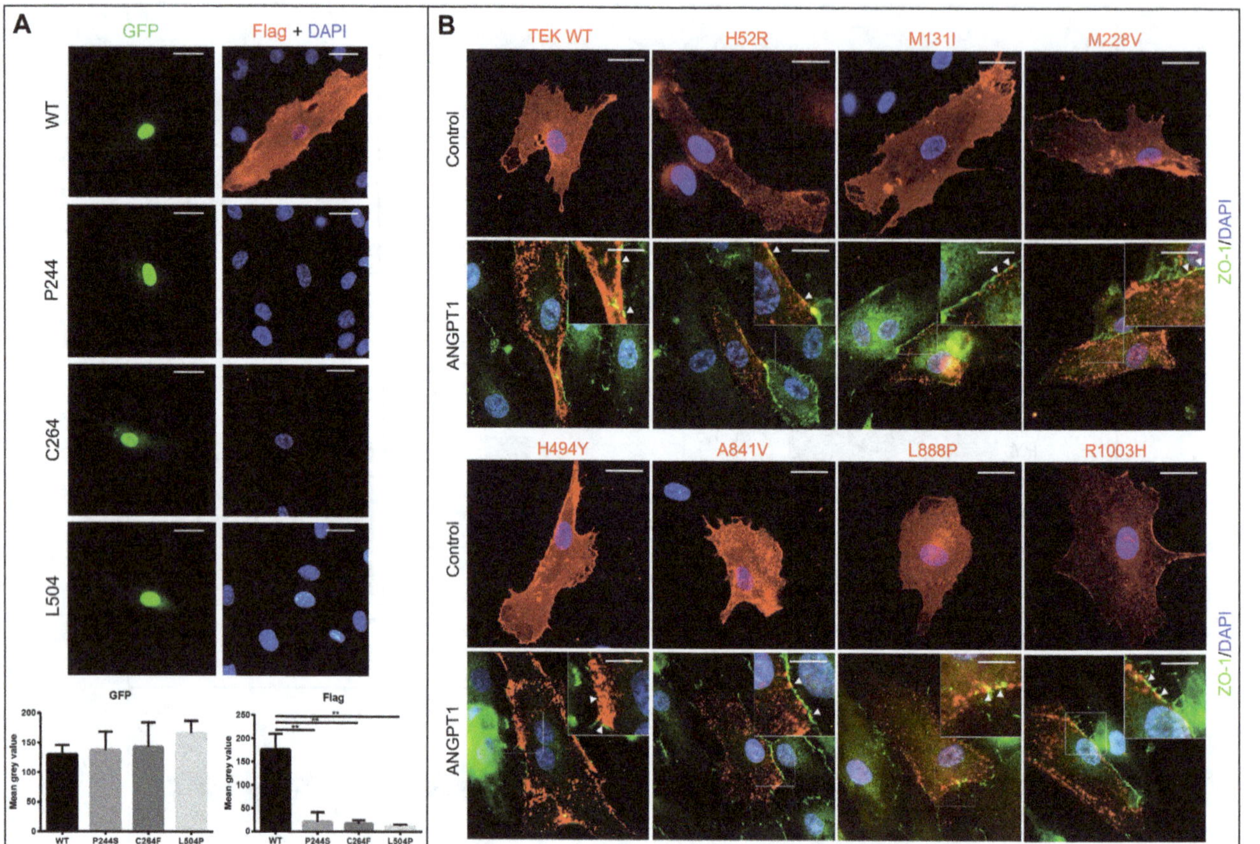

FIGURE 4 | Expression and ligand responsiveness of TEK variants **(A)**. Expression of p.P244S, p.C264F, and p.L504P were greatly decreased in HUVECs. GFP (green) signals indicated cells were successfully transfected. Wild-type Tie2 (anti-Flag, red) was diffusely distributed in cellular membrane of quiescent HUVECs (first row). However, Flag signals for three loss-of-function variants were notably reduced. Scale bars indicate 25 μm. **(B)** After stimulation by Angiopoietin-1 for 30 min **(lower panel)**, TEK proteins were relocated to cell–cell junctions as indicated by anti-ZO-1 (green). Nuclei were stained by DAPI (blue). Scale bars indicate 25 μm in upper panel and 12.5 μm in lower panel for magnified images. Pictures presented were representative of four biological replicates.

Young et al., 2020). In addition, identified variants were predominantly located in the ectodomain of Tie2 (7/11), a distinctive feature varying from those associated with familial or sporadic VM (Saharinen et al., 2017). Possibly due to the wide coverage of coding sequence (23 exons, 4683bp for longest transcript), disease-associated variants rarely recur. Nevertheless, one of our patients shared a missense mutation (p.A841V) with a multigeneration pedigree reported by Young et al. (2020). This family was unique in terms of high disease penetrance, complex phenotypes, and refractoriness to treatment. A modifier gene, SVEP1, was proposed to explain the remarkable clinical features. Carrying the same TEK mutation, proband from family 8 presented relatively mild symptoms, such as unilateral involvement, limited penetrance, and favorable prognosis. Subsequent WES failed to detect any variants in SVEP1, which possibly explained the phenotypic disparities.

Based on the conservation analysis, missense variants identified in this study can be categorized into two groups. Variants p.H52R, p.M131I, p.M228V, and p.H494Y involve revolutionarily un-conservative residues, while the rest locates in conserved positions. p.H52R and p.H494Y both co-segregated with phenotype; however, *in silico* predictions and functional studies did not support their causative roles. Previous structural analysis revealed that the ligand–receptor interface is confined to the top of the Tie2 Ig2 domain, including the loops B-C (147-150 aa), C, (158–161 aa), and F-G (195–200 aa), strand C (151–157 aa), and strand C(162–167 aa) (Yu et al., 2013). Thus, amino acid changes in position 52, 131, and 228 are theoretically function sparing. Of note, we identified a rare *de novo* activating mutation (p.R1003H) in one patient. Unfortunately, we could not confirm whether this patient presented with VM or not since she was lost to follow-up. However, based on previous reports, this variant should not be considered as the cause of PCG. Similarly, there was not enough evidence to classify variant p.L888P to be pathogenic judging from structural and functional analysis. There might be other mechanisms through which those variants could lead to PCG. For instance, variants in other genes involved in ANG-Tie2 pathway could contribute jointly to the phenotype. It is necessary to screen relevant genes in future studies. Another possibility is that those variants could interfere the expression of TEK gene *in vivo*, which might be revealed using gene-edited animals. Additionally, TEK variants are likely to influence the phosphorylation level of particular amino acid sites (Souma et al., 2016). To this end, technologies of proteomics are required (e.g., mass spectrometry).

Mutant TEK proteins were previously shown to exhibit diminished or reduced interaction with CYP1B1, suggesting a potential digenic inheritance (Kabra et al., 2017). Interestingly, coexistence of variants in different pathogenic genes for PCG was noticed in our patients. The CYP1B1 variants that co-occurred with TEK mutations in this study were also found in healthy controls from Asian populations (Kim et al., 2011; Gong et al., 2015; Do et al., 2016). Nevertheless, how the cytoplasmic receptor Tie2 comes into direct contact with endoplasmic reticulum-targeted enzyme and what is the biological implication of this protein complex require further investigation.

There are some shortcomings to our study. First, limited by sequencing methods, it is outside the scope of this study to illustrate the mutation profile of other known disease-causing genes or uncover new potentially causal genes in this cohort. Considering the critical role of ANG-Tie2 signaling in SC development, it is tempting to screen genes encoding other component involved in this pathway (e.g., ANGPT1, ANGPT2, ANGPT4, and TIE1). In addition, the number of patients identified with TEK mutations was small, which limited the statistic power of comparison between patient groups and precluded any meaningful genotype–phenotype association analysis.

In summary, we confirmed the causative role of TEK mutation in Chinese PCG patients for the first time. The majority of disease-associated mutations are heterozygous missense variants involving evolutionarily conserved amino acid residues. Although TEK mutations account for <5% of total cases, due attention should be given in future genetic testing.

ETHICS STATEMENT

The studies involving human participants were reviewed and approved by the Institutional Review Board of Eye and ENT Hospital, Fudan University. Written informed consent to participate in this study was provided by the participants' legal guardian/next of kin.

AUTHOR CONTRIBUTIONS

JC, XC, and XS contributed in the conception and design of the study and revised the manuscript. YC and CT recruited the patients. YQ acquired and analyzed the data and drafted the article. All authors approved the manuscript.

ACKNOWLEDGMENTS

The samples used for the analyses described in this manuscript were obtained from the EENT Biobank. We would like to thank all the participants and the staffs for their valuable contribution to this research.

REFERENCES

Adzhubei, I. A., Schmidt, S., Peshkin, L., Ramensky, V. E., Gerasimova, A., Bork, P., et al. (2010). A Method and Server for Predicting Damaging Missense Mutations. *Nat. Methods* 7, 248–249. doi:10.1038/nmeth0410-248

Ali, M., Mckibbin, M., Booth, A., Parry, D. A., Jain, P., Riazuddin, S. A., et al. (2009). Null Mutations in LTBP2 Cause Primary Congenital Glaucoma. *Am. J. Hum. Genet.* 84, 664–671. doi:10.1016/j.ajhg.2009.03.017

Aspelund, A., Tammela, T., Antila, S., Nurmi, H., Leppänen, V.-M., Zarkada, G., et al. (2014). The Schlemm's Canal Is a VEGF-C/VEGFR-3-responsive Lymphatic-like Vessel. *J. Clin. Invest.* 124, 3975–3986. doi:10.1172/jci75395

Barton, W. A., Tzvetkova-Robev, D., Miranda, E. P., Kolev, M. V., Rajashankar, K. R., Himanen, J. P., et al. (2006). Crystal Structures of the Tie2 Receptor Ectodomain and the Angiopoietin-2-Tie2 Complex. *Nat. Struct. Mol. Biol.* 13, 524–532. doi:10.1038/nsmb1101

Carter, H., Douville, C., Stenson, P. D., Cooper, D. N., and Karchin, R. (2013). Identifying Mendelian Disease Genes with the Variant Effect Scoring Tool. *BMC Genomics* 14 (Suppl. 3), S3. doi:10.1186/1471-2164-14-S3-S3

Chakrabarti, S., Kaur, K., Rao, K. N., Mandal, A. K., Kaur, I., Parikh, R. S., et al. (2009). The Transcription Factor GeneFOXC1Exhibits a Limited Role in Primary Congenital Glaucoma. *Invest. Ophthalmol. Vis. Sci.* 50, 75–83. doi:10.1167/iovs.08-2253

Chen, X., Chen, Y., Fan, B. J., Xia, M., Wang, L., and Sun, X. (2016). Screening of the LTBP2 Gene in 214 Chinese Sporadic CYP1B1-Negative Patients with Primary Congenital Glaucoma. *Mol. Vis.* 22, 528–535.

Chen, Y., Jiang, D., Yu, L., Katz, B., Zhang, K., Wan, B., et al. (2008). CYP1B1 and MYOC Mutations in 116 Chinese Patients with Primary Congenital Glaucoma. *Arch. Ophthalmol.* 126, 1443 1447. doi:10.1001/archopht.126.10.1443

Choi, Y., and Chan, A. P. (2015). PROVEAN Web Server: a Tool to Predict the Functional Effect of Amino Acid Substitutions and Indels. *Bioinformatics* 31, 2745–2747. doi:10.1093/bioinformatics/btv195

Chun, S., and Fay, J. C. (2009). Identification of Deleterious Mutations within Three Human Genomes. *Genome Res.* 19, 1553–1561. doi:10.1101/gr.092619.109

Do, T., Shei, W., Chau, P. T. M., Trang, D. L., Yong, V. H. K., Ng, X. Y., et al. (2016). CYP1B1 and MYOC Mutations in Vietnamese Primary Congenital Glaucoma Patients. *J. Glaucoma* 25, e491–e498. doi:10.1097/ijg.0000000000000331

Dumont, D. J., Gradwohl, G., Fong, G. H., Puri, M. C., Gertsenstein, M., Auerbach, A., et al. (1994). Dominant-negative and Targeted Null Mutations in the Endothelial Receptor Tyrosine Kinase, Tek, Reveal a Critical Role in Vasculogenesis of the Embryo. *Genes Develop.* 8, 1897–1909. doi:10.1101/gad.8.16.1897

Gong, B., Qu, C., Li, X., Shi, Y., Lin, Y., Zhou, Y., et al. (2015). Mutation Spectrum ofCYP1B1in Chinese Patients with Primary Open-Angle Glaucoma. *Br. J. Ophthalmol.* 99, 425–430. doi:10.1136/bjophthalmol-2014-306054

Jagadeesh, K. A., Wenger, A. M., Berger, M. J., Guturu, H., Stenson, P. D., Cooper, D. N., et al. (2016). M-CAP Eliminates a Majority of Variants of Uncertain Significance in Clinical Exomes at High Sensitivity. *Nat. Genet.* 48, 1581–1586. doi:10.1038/ng.3703

Johnson, M., Mclaren, J. W., and Overby, D. R. (2017). Unconventional Aqueous Humor Outflow: A Review. *Exp. Eye Res.* 158, 94–111. doi:10.1016/j.exer.2016.01.017

Kabra, M., Zhang, W., Rathi, S., Mandal, A. K., Senthil, S., Pyatla, G., et al. (2017). Angiopoietin Receptor TEK Interacts with CYP1B1 in Primary Congenital Glaucoma. *Hum. Genet.* 136, 941–949. doi:10.1007/s00439-017-1823-6

Kaur, K., Reddy, A., Mukhopadhyay, A., Mandal, A., Hasnain, S., Ray, K., et al. (2005). Myocilin Gene Implicated in Primary Congenital Glaucoma. *Clin. Genet.* 67, 335–340. doi:10.1111/j.1399-0004.2005.00411.x

Kim, H. J., Suh, W., Park, S. C., Kim, C. Y., Park, K. H., Kook, M. S., et al. (2011). Mutation Spectrum of CYP1B1 and MYOC Genes in Korean Patients with Primary Congenital Glaucoma. *Mol. Vis.* 17, 2093–2101.

Kim, S., Jhong, J.-H., Lee, J., and Koo, J.-Y. (2017). Meta-analytic Support Vector Machine for Integrating Multiple Omics Data. *BioData Mining* 10, 2. doi:10.1186/s13040-017-0126-8

Kircher, M., Witten, D. M., Jain, P., O'roak, B. J., Cooper, G. M., and Shendure, J. (2014). A General Framework for Estimating the Relative Pathogenicity of Human Genetic Variants. *Nat. Genet.* 46, 310–315. doi:10.1038/ng.2892

Kizhatil, K., Ryan, M., Marchant, J. K., Henrich, S., and John, S. W. M. (2014). Schlemm's Canal Is a Unique Vessel with a Combination of Blood Vascular and Lymphatic Phenotypes that Forms by a Novel Developmental Process. *Plos Biol.* 12. e1001912 doi:10.1371/journal.pbio.1001912

Krieger, E., and Vriend, G. (2014). YASARA View-Molecular Graphics for All Devices-From Smartphones to Workstations. *Bioinformatics* 30, 2981–2982. doi:10.1093/bioinformatics/btu426

Lewis, C. J., Hedberg-Buenz, A., Deluca, A. P., Stone, E. M., Alward, W. L. M., and Fingert, J. H. (2017). Primary Congenital and Developmental Glaucomas. *Hum. Mol. Genet.* 26, R28–r36. doi:10.1093/hmg/ddx205

Lim, S.-H., Tran-Viet, K.-N., Yanovitch, T. L., Freedman, S. F., Klemm, T., Call, W., et al. (2013). CYP1B1, MYOC, and LTBP2 Mutations in Primary Congenital Glaucoma Patients in the United States. *Am. J. Ophthalmol.* 155, 508–517. doi:10.1016/j.ajo.2012.09.012

Limaye, N., Wouters, V., Uebelhoer, M., Tuominen, M., Wirkkala, R., Mulliken, J. B., et al. (2009). Somatic Mutations in Angiopoietin Receptor Gene TEK Cause Solitary and Multiple Sporadic Venous Malformations. *Nat. Genet.* 41, 118–124. doi:10.1038/ng.272

Mashima, Y., Suzuki, Y., Sergeev, Y., Ohtake, Y., Tanino, T., Kimura, I., et al. (2001). Novel Cytochrome P4501B1 (CYP1B1) Gene Mutations in Japanese Patients with Primary Congenital Glaucoma. *Invest. Ophthalmol. Vis. Sci.* 42, 2211–2216.

Mohanty, K., Tanwar, M., Dada, R., and Dada, T. (2013). Screening of the LTBP2 Gene in a north Indian Population with Primary Congenital Glaucoma. *Mol. Vis.* 19, 78–84.

Moore, J. O., Lemmon, M. A., and Ferguson, K. M. (2017). Dimerization of Tie2 Mediated by its Membrane-Proximal FNIII Domains. *Proc. Natl. Acad. Sci. USA* 114, 4382–4387. doi:10.1073/pnas.1617800114

Quang, D., Chen, Y., and Xie, X. (2015). DANN: a Deep Learning Approach for Annotating the Pathogenicity of Genetic Variants. *Bioinformatics* 31, 761–763. doi:10.1093/bioinformatics/btu703

Ramos, R. F., Hoying, J. B., Witte, M. H., and Daniel Stamer, W. (2007). Schlemm's Canal Endothelia, Lymphatic, or Blood Vasculature? *J. Glaucoma* 16, 391–405. doi:10.1097/ijg.0b013e3180654ac6

Reva, B., Antipin, Y., and Sander, C. (2011). Predicting the Functional Impact of Protein Mutations: Application to Cancer Genomics. *Nucleic Acids Res.* 39, e118. doi:10.1093/nar/gkr407

Saharinen, P., Eklund, L., and Alitalo, K. (2017). Therapeutic Targeting of the Angiopoietin-TIE Pathway. *Nat. Rev. Drug Discov.* 16, 635–661. doi:10.1038/nrd.2016.278

Schwarz, J. M., Cooper, D. N., Schuelke, M., and Seelow, D. (2014). MutationTaster2: Mutation Prediction for the Deep-Sequencing Age. *Nat. Methods* 11, 361–362. doi:10.1038/nmeth.2890

Shewchuk, L. M., Hassell, A. M., Ellis, B., Holmes, W. D., Davis, R., Horne, E. L., et al. (2000). Structure of the Tie2 RTK Domain. *Structure* 8, 1105–1113. doi:10.1016/s0969-2126(00)00516-5

Shihab, H. A., Gough, J., Cooper, D. N., Stenson, P. D., Barker, G. L. A., Edwards, K. J., et al. (2013). Predicting the Functional, Molecular, and Phenotypic Consequences of Amino Acid Substitutions Using Hidden Markov Models. *Hum. Mutat.* 34, 57–65. doi:10.1002/humu.22225

Sim, N.-L., Kumar, P., Hu, J., Henikoff, S., Schneider, G., and Ng, P. C. (2012). SIFT Web Server: Predicting Effects of Amino Acid Substitutions on Proteins. *Nucleic Acids Res.* 40, W452–W457. doi:10.1093/nar/gks539

Souma, T., Tompson, S. W., Thomson, B. R., Siggs, O. M., Kizhatil, K., Yamaguchi, S., et al. (2016). Angiopoietin Receptor TEK Mutations Underlie Primary Congenital Glaucoma with Variable Expressivity. *J. Clin. Invest.* 126, 2575–2587. doi:10.1172/jci85830

Stoilov, I., Akarsu, A. N., and Sarfarazi, M. (1997). Identification of Three Different Truncating Mutations in Cytochrome P4501B1 (CYP1B1) as the Principal Cause of Primary Congenital Glaucoma (Buphthalmos) in Families Linked to the GLC3A Locus on Chromosome 2p21. *Hum. Mol. Genet.* 6, 641–647. doi:10.1093/hmg/6.4.641

Thomson, B. R., Heinen, S., Jeansson, M., Ghosh, A. K., Fatima, A., Sung, H.-K., et al. (2014). A Lymphatic Defect Causes Ocular Hypertension and Glaucoma in Mice. *J. Clin. Invest.* 124, 4320–4324. doi:10.1172/jci77162

Thomson, B. R., Souma, T., Tompson, S. W., Onay, T., Kizhatil, K., Siggs, O. M., et al. (2017). Angiopoietin-1 Is Required for Schlemm's Canal Development in Mice and Humans. *J. Clin. Invest.* 127, 4421–4436. doi:10.1172/jci95545

Van Durme, J., Delgado, J., Stricher, F., Serrano, L., Schymkowitz, J., and Rousseau, F. (2011). A Graphical Interface for the FoldX Forcefield. *Bioinformatics* 27, 1711–1712. doi:10.1093/bioinformatics/btr254

Van Zyl, T., Yan, W., Mcadams, A., Peng, Y.-R., Shekhar, K., Regev, A., et al. (2020). Cell Atlas of Aqueous Humor Outflow Pathways in Eyes of Humans and Four Model Species Provides Insight into Glaucoma Pathogenesis. *Proc. Natl. Acad. Sci. USA* 117, 10339–10349. doi:10.1073/pnas.2001250117

Vikkula, M., Boon, L. M., Iii, K. L. C., 3rd, Calvert, J. T., Calvert, A. J., Goumnerov, B., et al. (1996). Vascular Dysmorphogenesis Caused by an Activating Mutation in the Receptor Tyrosine Kinase TIE2. *Cell* 87, 1181–1190. doi:10.1016/s0092-8674(00)81814-0

Wang, K., Li, M., and Hakonarson, H. (2010). ANNOVAR: Functional Annotation of Genetic Variants from High-Throughput Sequencing Data. *Nucleic Acids Res.* 38, e164. doi:10.1093/nar/gkq603

Young, T. L., Whisenhunt, K. N., Jin, J., Lamartina, S. M., Martin, S. M., Souma, T., et al. (2020). SVEP1 as a Genetic Modifier of TEK-Related Primary Congenital Glaucoma. *Invest. Ophthalmol. Vis. Sci.* 61, 6. doi:10.1167/iovs.61.12.6

Yu, X., Seegar, T. C. M., Dalton, A. C., Tzvetkova-Robev, D., Goldgur, Y., Rajashankar, K. R., et al. (2013). Structural Basis for Angiopoietin-1-Mediated Signaling Initiation. *Proc. Natl. Acad. Sci.* 110, 7205–7210. doi:10.1073/pnas.1216890110

Permissions

All chapters in this book were first published by Frontiers; hereby published with permission under the Creative Commons Attribution License or equivalent. Every chapter published in this book has been scrutinized by our experts. Their significance has been extensively debated. The topics covered herein carry significant findings which will fuel the growth of the discipline. They may even be implemented as practical applications or may be referred to as a beginning point for another development.

The contributors of this book come from diverse backgrounds, making this book a truly international effort. This book will bring forth new frontiers with its revolutionizing research information and detailed analysis of the nascent developments around the world.

We would like to thank all the contributing authors for lending their expertise to make the book truly unique. They have played a crucial role in the development of this book. Without their invaluable contributions this book wouldn't have been possible. They have made vital efforts to compile up to date information on the varied aspects of this subject to make this book a valuable addition to the collection of many professionals and students.

This book was conceptualized with the vision of imparting up-to-date information and advanced data in this field. To ensure the same, a matchless editorial board was set up. Every individual on the board went through rigorous rounds of assessment to prove their worth. After which they invested a large part of their time researching and compiling the most relevant data for our readers.

The editorial board has been involved in producing this book since its inception. They have spent rigorous hours researching and exploring the diverse topics which have resulted in the successful publishing of this book. They have passed on their knowledge of decades through this book. To expedite this challenging task, the publisher supported the team at every step. A small team of assistant editors was also appointed to further simplify the editing procedure and attain best results for the readers.

Apart from the editorial board, the designing team has also invested a significant amount of their time in understanding the subject and creating the most relevant covers. They scrutinized every image to scout for the most suitable representation of the subject and create an appropriate cover for the book.

The publishing team has been an ardent support to the editorial, designing and production team. Their endless efforts to recruit the best for this project, has resulted in the accomplishment of this book. They are a veteran in the field of academics and their pool of knowledge is as vast as their experience in printing. Their expertise and guidance has proved useful at every step. Their uncompromising quality standards have made this book an exceptional effort. Their encouragement from time to time has been an inspiration for everyone.

The publisher and the editorial board hope that this book will prove to be a valuable piece of knowledge for researchers, students, practitioners and scholars across the globe.

List of Contributors

Xiao-Fang Wang, Hui Chen, Peng-Juan Huang, Zhuo-Kun Feng, Zi-Qi Hua, Xiang Feng, Xiao-Tao Xu and Huan-Yun Yu
School of Ophthalmology and Optometry, The Eye Hospital, Wenzhou Medical University, Wenzhou, China

Fang Han
Beijing Ophthalmology and Visual Sciences Key Laboratory, Beijing Institute of Ophthalmology, Beijing Tongren Eye Center, Beijing Tongren Hospital, Capital Medical University, Beijing, China

Ren-Juan Shen
Division of Ophthalmic Genetics, The Eye Hospital, Wenzhou Medical University, National Center for International Research in Regenerative Medicine and Neurogenetics, Wenzhou, China
Beijing Institute of Ophthalmology, Beijing Tongren Eye Center, Beijing Tongren Hospital, Capital Medical University, Beijing Ophthalmology and Visual Sciences Key Laboratory, Beijing, China

Zi-Bing Jin
Division of Ophthalmic Genetics, The Eye Hospital, Wenzhou Medical University, National Center for International Research in Regenerative Medicine and Neurogenetics, Wenzhou, China
Beijing Institute of Ophthalmology, Beijing Tongren Eye Center, Beijing Tongren Hospital, Capital Medical University, Beijing Ophthalmology and Visual Sciences Key Laboratory, Beijing, China
Beijing Advanced Innovation Center for Big Data-Based Precision Medicine, Beihang University and Capital Medical University, Beijing Tongren Hospital, Beijing, China

Xiaohong Meng, Yanling Long, Jiayun Ren, Gang Wang, Xin Yin and Shiying Li
Department of Ophthalmology, Southwest Hospital, Army Medical University (Third Military Medical University), Chongqing, China
Key Laboratory of Visual Damage and Regeneration and Restoration of Chongqing, Chongqing, China

Qing Zhu
Zhengzhou University People's Hospital, Henan Provincial People's Hospital, Zhengzhou, China

Xue Rui and Xun-Lun Sheng
Ningxia Clinical Research Center of Blinding Eye Disease, Ningxia Eye Hospital, People's Hospital of Ningxia Hui Autonomous Region, First Affiliated Hospital of Northwest University for Nationalities, Yinchuan, China

Ya Li, Ya You and Bo Lei
Zhengzhou University People's Hospital, Henan Provincial People's Hospital, Zhengzhou, China
Henan Branch of National Clinical Research Center for Ocular Diseases, Henan Eye Institute and Henan Eye Hospital, Henan Provincial People's Hospital, Zhengzhou, China

Ting Xiao, Xin Zhang, Ke Xu and Yang Li
Beijing Ophthalmology & Visual Sciences Key Lab, Beijing Tongren Eye Center, Beijing Institute of Ophthalmology, Beijing Tongren Hospital, Capital Medical University, Beijing, China

De-Fu Chen and Hua Gao
School of Ophthalmology and Optometry, The Eye Hospital, Wenzhou Medical University, Wenzhou, China

Haoyu Chang, Xiaohui Zhang and Yue Xie
Beijing Ophthalmology and Visual Science Key Laboratory, Beijing Tongren Eye Center, Beijing Tongren Hospital, Beijing Institute of Ophthalmology, Capital Medical University, Beijing, China

Belén García Bohórquez, Ana Rodríguez Muñoz, Gema García García and José M. Millán
Molecular, Cellular and Genomics Biomedicine, Health Research Institute La Fe, Valencia, Spain
CIBER of Rare Diseases, Madrid, Spain

Elena Aller and Teresa Jaijo
Molecular, Cellular and Genomics Biomedicine, Health Research Institute La Fe, Valencia, Spain
CIBER of Rare Diseases, Madrid, Spain
Unit of Genetics, University Hospital La Fe, Valencia, Spain

Wei Li
BGI Education Center, University of Chinese Academy of Sciences, Shenzhen, China
College of Life Sciences, University of Chinese Academy of Sciences, Beijing, China
Shenyang Industrial Technology Institute of Ophthalmology, Shenyang, China

Ning Qu and Wei-Ping Qian
Department of Reproductive Medicine, Peking University Shenzhen Hospital, Shenzhen, China

Jian-Kang Li, Kang Shao, Wen Yang and Lu-Sheng Wang
City University of Hong Kong Shenzhen Research Institute, Shenzhen, China

Chen Liang
School of Basic Medicine, Qingdao University, Qingdao, China

Yu-Xin Li and Le Tian
BGI Education Center, University of Chinese Academy of Sciences, Shenzhen, China
College of Life Sciences, University of Chinese Academy of Sciences, Beijing, China
School of Basic Medicine, Qingdao University, Qingdao, China

Yi-Xi Chen
School of Biology and Biological Engineering, South China University of Technology, Guangzhou, China

Zhuo-Shi Wang and Wei He
Shenyang Industrial Technology Institute of Ophthalmology, Shenyang, China
He Eye Specialists Hospital, He University, Shenyang, China

Xuan Chen
College of Plant Protection, Hunan Agricultural University, Changsha, China

Xiao-Ying Jin
College of Informatics, HuaZhong Agricultural University, Wuhan, China

Dong-Ming Han and Zi-Wei Wang
BGI Education Center, University of Chinese Academy of Sciences, Shenzhen, China
College of Life Sciences, University of Chinese Academy of Sciences, Beijing, China

Jinfeng Kong and Lei Feng
Eye Center, The Second Affiliated Hospital of Zhejiang University School of Medicine, Hangzhou, China

Si Chen
Eye Center, The Second Affiliated Hospital of Zhejiang University School of Medicine, Hangzhou, China
Department of Ophthalmology, Jinshan Branch of Shanghai Sixth People's Hospital, Shanghai, China

Huatuo Dai and Yunqing Ren
Department of Dermatology, The Children's Hospital, Zhejiang University School of Medicine, National Clinical Research Center for Child Health, Hangzhou, China
Department of Dermatology, The Second Affiliated Hospital of Zhejiang University School of Medicine, Hangzhou, China

Rajkumar Dorajoo
Genome Institute of Singapore, Agency for Science, Technology and Research, Singapore, Singapore

Jianjun Liu
Genome Institute of Singapore, Agency for Science, Technology and Research, Singapore, Singapore
Department of Medicine, Yong Loo Lin School of Medicine, National University of Singapore, Singapore, Singapore

Xianyong Yin
Department of Biostatistics and Center for Statistical Genetics, University of Michigan School of Public Health, Ann Arbor, MI, United States

Imen Habibi
IRO-Institute for Research in Ophthalmology, Sion, Switzerland

Yosra Falfoul, Khaled El Matri, Ahmed Chebil and Leila El Matri
Oculogenetic Laboratory LR14SP01, Faculty of Medicine of Tunis, Hedi Rais Institute of Ophthalmology (Department B), Tunis El Manar University, Tunis, Tunisia

Hoai Viet Tran
Hôpital Ophtalmique Jules-Gonin, Unité d'oculogénétique, Lausanne, Switzerland

Daniel F. Schorderet
IRO-Institute for Research in Ophthalmology, Sion, Switzerland
Faculty of Biology and Medicine, University of Lausanne, Lausanne, Switzerland
Faculty of Life Sciences, Ecole Polytechnique Fédérale de Lausanne, Lausanne, Switzerland

Shihao Chen
Center for Refractive Surgery, The Eye Hospital, Wenzhou Medical University, Wenzhou, China

Xing-Yong Li
Center for Refractive Surgery, The Eye Hospital, Wenzhou Medical University, Wenzhou, China
Division of Ophthalmic Genetics, The Eye Hospital, Wenzhou Medical University, National Center for International Research in Regenerative Medicine and Neurogenetics, Wenzhou, China

Jia-Jia Jin, Jian-Yang Mao, Fei-Fei Cheng and Zhen-Ji Chen
Division of Ophthalmic Genetics, The Eye Hospital, Wenzhou Medical University, National Center for International Research in Regenerative Medicine and Neurogenetics, Wenzhou, China

Emmanouela Linardaki
DNA Analysis, Molecular Biology and Genetics Center, Heraklion, Greece

Stavroula Voulgaraki
Emmetropia Mediterranean Eye Institute, Heraklion, Greece

Ioannis M. Aslanides
Center for Refractive Surgery, The Eye Hospital, Wenzhou Medical University, Wenzhou, China
Emmetropia Mediterranean Eye Institute, Heraklion, Greece

Panfeng Wang, Xiaoyun Jia, Xueshan Xiao, Shiqiang Li, Yuxi Long, Mengchu Liu, Yongyu Li, Jun Li and Qingjiong Zhang
State Key Laboratory of Ophthalmology, Zhongshan Ophthalmic Center, Sun Yat-sen University, Guangzhou, China

Yan Xu
State Key Laboratory of Ophthalmology, Zhongshan Ophthalmic Center, Sun Yat-sen University, Guangzhou, China
Guangdong Provincial Key Laboratory of Reproductive Medicine, Reproductive Medicine Center, The First Affiliated Hospital, Sun Yat-sen University, Guangzhou, China

Leming Fu
Henan University People's Hospital, Henan Provincial People's Hospital, Zhengzhou, China

Bo Lei
Henan University People's Hospital, Henan Provincial People's Hospital, Zhengzhou, China
Henan Branch of National Clinical Research Center for Ocular Diseases, Henan Eye Institute/Henan Eye Hospital, People's Hospital of Zhengzhou University, Henan Provincial People's Hospital, Zhengzhou, China

Ya Li, Shun Yao and Qingge Guo
Henan Branch of National Clinical Research Center for Ocular Diseases, Henan Eye Institute/Henan Eye Hospital, People's Hospital of Zhengzhou University, Henan Provincial People's Hospital, Zhengzhou, China

Xianjun Zhu
Department of Laboratory Medicine, Sichuan Provincial People's Hospital, School of Medicine, University of Electronic Science and Technology of China, Chengdu, China

Milton A. English and Anand Swaroop
Neurobiology-Neurodegeneration and Repair Laboratory, National Eye Institute, National Institutes of Health, Bethesda, MD, United States

Rinki Ratnapriya
Neurobiology-Neurodegeneration and Repair Laboratory, National Eye Institute, National Institutes of Health, Bethesda, MD, United States
Department of Ophthalmology, Baylor College of Medicine, Houston, TX, United States

Samuel G. Jacobson, Artur V. Cideciyan, Alejandro J. Roman, Alexander Sumaroka and Rebecca Sheplock
Department of Ophthalmology, Perelman School of Medicine, Scheie Eye Institute, University of Pennsylvania, Philadelphia, PA, United States

Giulia Ascari, Marieke De Bruyne, Miriam Bauwens, Mattias Van Heetvelde, Elfride De Baere, Thalia Van Laethem, Toon Rosseel, Björn Menten and Alfredo Dueñas Rey
Center for Medical Genetics Ghent, Ghent University Hospital, Ghent, Belgium
Department of Biomolecular Medicine, Ghent University, Ghent, Belgium

Nanna D. Rendtorff
The Kennedy Center, Department of Clinical Genetics, Rigshospitalet, Copenhagen University Hospital, Copenhagen, Denmark

Julie De Zaeytijd
Department of Ophthalmology, Ghent University Hospital, Ghent, Belgium

Michel Van Lint
Department of Ophthalmology, Antwerp University Hospital, Antwerp, Belgium

Gavin Arno
Great Ormond Street Hospital, London, United Kingdom
Moorfields Eye Hospital, London, United Kingdom
UCL Institute of Ophthalmology, London, United Kingdom

Julie Jacob
Department of Ophthalmology, University Hospitals Leuven, Leuven, Belgium

David Creytens, Jo Van Dorpe
Department of Pathology, Ghent University Hospital, Ghent, Belgium
Department of Diagnostic Sciences, Ghent University, Ghent, Belgium

Tim De Pooter, Peter De Rijk and Mojca Strazisar
Neuromics Support Facility, VIB Center for Molecular Neurology, VIB, Antwerp, Belgium
Neuromics Support Facility, Department of Biomedical Sciences, University of Antwerp, Antwerp, Belgium

Wouter De Coster
Applied and Translational Neurogenomics Group, VIB Center for Molecular Neurology, VIB, Antwerp, Belgium
Applied and Translational Neurogenomics Group, Department of Biomedical Sciences, University of Antwerp, Antwerp, Belgium

Mette Bertelsen
The Kennedy Center, Department of Clinical Genetics, Rigshospitalet, Copenhagen University Hospital, Copenhagen, Denmark
Departmentof Ophthalmology, Rigshospitalet-Glostrup, University of Copenhagen, Glostrup, Denmark

Lisbeth Tranebjaerg
The Kennedy Center, Department of Clinical Genetics, Rigshospitalet, Copenhagen University Hospital, Copenhagen, Denmark
Institute of Clinical Medicine, University of Copenhagen, Copenhagen, Denmark

Junwen Wang, Xueshan Xiao and Wenmin Sun
State Key Laboratory of Ophthalmology, Zhongshan Ophthalmic Center, Sun Yat-sen University, Guangzhou, China

Chengshou Zhang and Yibo Yu
Eye Center of the Second Affiliated Hospital, School of Medicine, Zhejiang University, Hangzhou, China

Jianghua Hu
Eye Center of the Second Affiliated Hospital, School of Medicine, Zhejiang University, Hangzhou, China
Department of Ophthalmology, Jiande Branch, The Second Affiliated Hospital, School of Medicine, Zhejiang University, Hangzhou, China

Yang Liu and Juan Liu
School of Basic Medical Sciences, Third Clinical Medical College of Ningxia Medical University (People's Hospital of Ningxia Hui Autonomous Region), Yinchuan, China

Jin-Jin Zhang
Clinical Medical College, Ningxia Medical University, Yinchuan, China

Shun-Yu Piao, Wen-Juan Zhuang and Wen Zhang
Ningxia Eye Hospital, People's Hospital of Ningxia Hui Autonomous Region, Third Clinical Medical College of Ningxia Medical University, Yinchuan, China

Ya Ma
Beijing Institute of Ophthalmology, Beijing Tongren Eye Center, Beijing Tongren Hospital, Capital Medical University, Beijing Ophthalmology and Visual Science Key Laboratory, Beijing, China

Zhong-Qi Xue
Department of Ophthalmology, Affiliated Hospital of Qingdao Binhai University, Qingdao, China

Naseem Amirmokhtari
Department of Pharmaceutical Sciences, Northeast Ohio Medical University, Rootstown, OH, United States
Integrated Pharmaceutical Medicine Graduate Program, Northeast Ohio Medical University, Rootstown, OH, United States

Brian D. Foresi and Shiv S. Dewan
Department of Pharmaceutical Sciences, Northeast Ohio Medical University, Rootstown, OH, United States

Rachida A. Bouhenni
Rebecca D. Considine Research Institute, Vision Center, Akron Children's Hospital, Akron, OH, United States

Matthew A. Smith
Department of Pharmaceutical Sciences, Northeast Ohio Medical University, Rootstown, OH, United States
Rebecca D. Considine Research Institute, Vision Center, Akron Children's Hospital, Akron, OH, United States

Quan-Gang Xu and Shi-Hui Wei
Department of Ophthalmology, The Chinese People's Liberation Army General Hospital, The Chinese People's Liberation Army Medical School, Beijing, China

Xiao-Hui Zhang
Department of Ophthalmology, The Chinese People's Liberation Army General Hospital, The Chinese People's Liberation Army Medical School, Beijing, China
Beijing Ophthalmology and Visual Sciences Key Laboratory, Beijing Institute of Ophthalmology, Beijing Tongren Eye Center, Beijing Tongren Hospital, Capital Medical University, Beijing, China

Kai Cao
Beijing Ophthalmology and Visual Sciences Key Laboratory, Beijing Institute of Ophthalmology, Beijing Tongren Eye Center, Beijing Tongren Hospital, Capital Medical University, Beijing, China

Yunsheng Qiao and Chen Tan
Department of Ophthalmology and Visual Science, Eye and ENT Hospital, Shanghai Medical College, Fudan University, Shanghai, China

Yuhong Chen, Xinghuai Sun, Xueli Chen and Junyi Chen
Department of Ophthalmology and Visual Science, Eye and ENT Hospital, Shanghai Medical College, Fudan University, Shanghai, China
NHC Key Laboratory of Myopia, Chinese Academy of Medical Sciences, Shanghai Key Laboratory of Visual Impairment and Restoration (Fudan University), Shanghai, China
State Key Laboratory of Medical Neurobiology and MOE Frontiers Center for Brain Science, Institutes of Brain Science, Fudan University, Shanghai, China

Index

P

R

S

T

W

www.ingramcontent.com/pod-product-compliance
Lightning Source LLC
LaVergne TN
LVHW082159200926
848484LV00008B/2185
9798887403489